Horizons in
Medicine No. 7

Horizons in

Medicine

No. 7

EDITED BY
STAFFORD LIGHTMAN
PhD, MB, BChir, FRCP

Department of Medicine
University of Bristol
Bristol Royal Infirmary
Bristol

Royal College of Physicians of London

Blackwell Science

© 1996 by
Blackwell Science Ltd
Editorial Offices:
Osney Mead, Oxford OX2 0EL
25 John Street, London WC1N 2BL
23 Ainslie Place, Edinburgh EH3 6AJ
238 Main Street, Cambridge
  Massachusetts 02142, USA
54 University Street, Carlton
  Victoria 3053, Australia

Other Editorial Offices:
Arnette Blackwell SA
  224, Boulevard Saint Germain
  75007 Paris, France

Blackwell Wissenschafts-Verlag GmbH
  Kurfürstendamm 57
  10707 Berlin, Germany

  Zehetnergasse 6
  A-1140 Wien
  Austria

First published 1996

Set by Setrite Typesetters, Hong Kong
Printed and bound in Great Britain
at the University Press, Cambridge

The Blackwell Science logo is a
trade mark of Blackwell Science Ltd,
registered at the United Kingdom
Trade Marks Registry

DISTRIBUTORS

Marston Book Services Ltd
PO Box 269
Abingdon
Oxon OX14 4YN
(*Orders*: Tel: 01235 465500
          Fax: 01235 465555)

USA
Blackwell Science, Inc.
238 Main Street
Cambridge, MA 02142
(*Orders*: Tel: 800 215-1000
              617 876-7000
          Fax: 617 492-5263)

Canada
Copp Clark, Ltd
2775 Matheson Blvd East
Mississauga, Ontario
Canada, L4W 4P7
(*Orders*: Tel: 800 263-4374
              905 238-6074)

Australia
Blackwell Science Pty Ltd
54 University Street
Carlton, Victoria 3053
(*Orders*: Tel: 3 9347 0300
          Fax: 3 9347 5001)

A catalogue record for this title
is available from the British Library
and the Library of Congress

ISBN 0-86542-756-9
ISSN 0957-5804

Contents

v

Colour plates fall between pp. 304 and 305

List of contributors

DAVID J. P. BARKER MD PhD FRCP *Professor & Director, MRC Environmental Epidemiology Unit, University of Southampton, Southampton General Hospital, Southampton SO16 6YD*

JAN C. BIRKENHÄGER *Professor of Medicine, Department of Internal Medicine III, Erasmus University Medical School, PO Box 1738, 3000 DR Rotterdam, The Netherlands*

DAVID P. DE BONO MD FRCP FESC *British Heart Foundation Professor, Division of Cardiology, Department of Medicine, University of Leicester, Clinical Sciences Wing, Glenfield General Hospital, Leicester LE3 9QP*

FIONULA M. BRENNAN PhD *Kennedy Institute of Rheumatology, Sunley Building, 1 Lurgan Avenue, Hammersmith, London W6 8LW*

MORRIS J. BROWN MA MD MSc FRCP *Professor of Clinical Pharmacology, Clinical Pharmacology Unit, F & G Block, Level 2, Addenbrooke's Hospital, Hills Road, Cambridge CB2 2QQ*

KEITH D. BUCHANAN MD PhD FRCP FRCP(Ed) FRCP(Glas) FRCP(I) *Professor of Metabolic Medicine, Department of Medicine, The Queen's University of Belfast, Royal Victoria Hospital, Belfast BT12 6BJ*

J. STEWART CAMERON MD FRCP *Emeritus Professor of Renal Medicine, Clinical Science Laboratories, 17th Floor, Guy's Tower, Guy's Hospital, St Thomas's Street, London SE1 9RT*

V. KRISHNA K. CHATTERJEE MA FRCP *Wellcome Senior Clinical Research Fellow & Honorary Consultant Physician, Department of Medicine, University of Cambridge, Level 5, Addenbrooke's Hospital, Hills Road, Cambridge CB2 2QQ*

SHARA B. A. COHEN PhD *Kennedy Institute of Rheumatology, Sunley Building, 1 Lurgan Avenue, Hammersmith, London W6 8LW*

HELEN CONNOR BPharm PhD MRPharmS *Research Associate, Glaxo Research and Development Ltd, Park Road, Ware SG12 0DP*

NICHOLAS P. CURZEN BM MRCP(UK) *MRC Training Fellow & Honorary Registrar in Critical Care & Cardiology, Unit of Critical Care, National Heart & Lung Institute, Royal Brompton Hospital, Sydney Street, London SW3 6NP*

DAVID B. DUNGER MD FRCP *Consultant Paediatric Endocrinologist, Department of Paediatrics, University of Oxford, Level 4, John Radcliffe Hospital, Headington, Oxford OX3 9DU*

ALUN E. EVANS MD FRCP FFPHM(I) *Professor & Head of the Department of Epidemiology & Public Health, The Queen's University of Belfast, Mulhouse Building, Institute of Clinical Science, Grosvenor Road, Belfast BT12 6BJ*

TIMOTHY W. EVANS MD PhD FRCP *Reader in Critical Care Medicine, National Heart & Lung Institute & Consultant Physician in Thoracic & Intensive Care Medicine, Department of Anaesthesia & Intensive Care, Royal Brompton Hospital, Sydney Street, London SW3 6NP*

TERRY G. FEEST MD FRCP *Consultant Nephrologist, The Richard Bright Renal Unit, Southmead General Hospital, Westbury on Trym, Bristol BS10 5NB*

MARC FELDMANN MB PhD FRCPath MRCP *Professor of Cellular Immunology, Kennedy Institute of Rheumatology, Sunley Building, 1 Lurgan Avenue, Hammersmith, London W6 8LW*

R. J. GIBBONS DPhil MRCP *Wellcome Fellow, MRC Molecular Haematology Unit, Institute of Molecular Medicine, John Radcliffe Hospital, Headington, Oxford OX3 9DU*

GUY M. GOODWIN DPhil FRCP(Ed) FRCPsych *MRC Professor of Psychiatry, University of Edinburgh & MRC Brain Metabolism Unit, Royal Edinburgh Hospital, Morningside Park, Edinburgh EH10 5HF*

GEORGE E. GRIFFIN PhD FRCP FRCP(Ed) *Professor of Infectious Diseases & Medicine, Head of Division of Infectious Diseases, Departments of Medicine & Cellular & Molecular Sciences, St George's Hospital Medical School, Cranmer Terrace, London SW17 0RE*

ABRAHAM GUZ MD FRCP *Professor Emeritus, Department of Medicine, Charing Cross & Westminster Medical School, London W6 8RF*

DAVID R. HADDEN MD FRCP *Consultant Physician, Sir George E Clark Metabolic Unit, Royal Victoria Hospital, Belfast BT12 6BA & Honorary Professor of Endocrinology, The Queen's University of Belfast*

PETER S. HARPER CBE DM FRCP *Professor & Head of Department, Institute of Medical Genetics, University of Wales College of Medicine, Heath Park, Cardiff CF4 4XN*

PETER C. HARRIS PhD *MRC Senior Scientist, MRC Molecular Haematology Unit, Institute of Molecular Medicine, John Radcliffe Hospital, Headington, Oxford OX3 9DU*

ANDREW T. HATTERSLEY BM BCh MRCP *Senior Lecturer & Consultant Physician, Department of Diabetes Research & Vascular Medicine, Postgraduate Medical School, Royal Devon and Exeter Hospital, Barrack Road, Exeter EX2 5AX*

ROGELIO HERNANDEZ-PANDO *Department of Pathology, Instituto Nacional de la Nutricion, Salvador Zubiran, Calle Vasco de Quiroga 15, Delegacion Tlalpan, 14000 Mexico DF*

TIM W. HIGENBOTTAM MD BSc FRCP *Professor of Respiratory Medicine, Department of Medicine & Pharmacology, Section of Respiratory Medicine, University of Sheffield Medical School, Beech Hill Road, Sheffield, S10 2RX*

DOUGLAS R. HIGGS DSc(Med) FRCP FRCPath *MRC Senior Scientist & Honorary Consultant Haematologist, MRC Molecular Haematology Unit, Institute of Molecular Medicine, John Radcliffe Hospital, Headington, Oxford OX3 9DU*

STEPHEN T. HOLGATE MD DSc FRCP *MRC Clinical Professor of Immunopharmacology, University Department of Medicine, Level D, Centre Block, Southampton General Hospital, Southampton SO9 4XY*

JEFF M. P. HOLLY BSc PhD *Senior Lecturer, University Department of Medicine, Dorothy Crowfoot Hodgkin Laboratories, Jenner Yard, Bristol Royal Infirmary, Bristol BS2 8HW*

IEUAN A. HUGHES MD FRCP FRCP(C) *Professor of Paediatrics, University of Cambridge, Addenbrooke's Hospital, Hills Road, Cambridge CB2 2QQ*

PATRICK P. A. HUMPHREY DSc BPharm PhD FRPharmS
Professor & Director, Glaxo Institute of Applied Pharmacology, Department of Pharmacology, University of Cambridge, Tennis Court Road, Cambridge CB2 1QJ

HOWARD S. JACOBS MD FRCP FRCOG *Professor of Reproductive Endocrinology, Division of Endocrinology, Department of Medicine, University College London Medical School, The Middlesex Hospital, Mortimer Street, London W1N 8AA*

PETER KATSIKIS *Kennedy Institute of Rheumatology, Sunley Building, 1 Lurgan Avenue, Hammersmith, London W6 8LW*

PETER G. E. KENNEDY MD DSc FRCP FRCP(Glas) FRSE *Professor of Neurology, University of Glasgow Department of Neurology, Institute of Neurological Sciences, Southern General Hospital NHS Trust, Glasgow G51 4TF*

KAY-TEE KHAW MB BChir MSc FRCP *Professor of Clinical Gerontology, University of Cambridge School of Medicine, F & G Block, Level 2, Addenbrooke's Hospital, Cambridge CB2 2QQ*

RICHARD A. KNIGHT MB BS PhD *Senior Lecturer, Department of Cystic Fibrosis, National Heart & Lung Institute, Emmanuel Kaye Building, Manresa Road, London SW3 6LR*

ROBERT I. LECHLER MB PhD FRCP FRCPath *Professor of Molecular Immunology & Honorary Consultant in Medicine & Head of Department of Immunology, Royal Postgraduate Medical School, Hammersmith Hospital, Du Cane Road, London W12 0NN*

ANDREW LEVY PhD MRCP *Consultant Senior Lecturer in Medicine, Endocrinology & Diabetes, Department of Medicine, Bristol Royal Infirmary, Marlborough Street, Bristol BS2 8HW*

CLAIRE E. LEWIS MA DPhil *Senior Lecturer in Molecular & Cellular Pathology, Department of Pathology, University of Sheffield Medical School, Beech Hill Road, Sheffield S10 2RX*

W. IAN McDONALD MB PhD FRCP FRACP FRCOphth *Professor of Clinical Neurology, Institute of Neurology, The National Hospital, Queen Square, London WC1N 3BG*

JAMES O'D. McGEE MD FRCP FRCPath *Professor & Head of Nuffield Department of Pathology & Bacteriology, University of Oxford, Level 4, Academic Centre, John Radcliffe Hospital, Headington, Oxford OX3 9DU*

R. N. MAINI MB BChir FRCP FRCP(Ed) *Director, The Mathilda and Terence Kennedy Institute of Rheumatology, Kennedy Building, 6 Bute Gardens, Hammersmith, London W6 7DW*

THOMAS W. MEADE CBE DM FRCP FRS *Director, MRC Epidemiology & Medical Care Unit, Wolfson Institute of Preventive Medicine, St Bartholomew's & the Royal London School of Medicine & Dentistry, Charterhouse Square, London EC1M 6BQ*

ROBERTO MONTESANO MD *Professor of Histology & Cell Biology, Department of Morphology, University Medical Center, 1 Rue Michel-Servet, 1211 Geneva 4, Switzerland*

ROBYN E. O'HEHIR PhD FRACP FRCP *Professor, Department of Allergy & Clinical Immunology, The Alfred Healthcare Group, PO Box 315, Prahan, Victoria 3181, Australia*

MARK F. OLIVER CBE MD FRCP FRCP(Ed) *Professor Emeritus, National Heart & Lung Institute, Dovehouse Street, London SW3 6LY*

MARK B. PEPYS MD PhD FRCP FRCPath *Professor of Immunological Medicine/Honorary Consultant Physician, Immunological Medicine Unit, Royal Postgraduate Medical School, Hammersmith Hospital, Du Cane Road, London W12 0NN*

D. J. PICKETTS PhD *MRC Scientist, MRC Molecular Haematology Unit, Institute of Molecular Medicine, John Radcliffe Hospital, Headington, Oxford OX3 9DU*

HUIBERT A. P. POLS *Senior Endocrinologist, Department of Internal Medicine III, Erasmus University Medical School, PO Box 1738, 3000 DR Rotterdam, The Netherlands*

GEORGE K. RADDA CBE DPhil FRS *British Heart Foundation Professor of Molecular Cardiology, MRC Biochemical & Clinical Magnetic Resonance Unit, John Radcliffe Hospital, Headington, Oxford OX3 9DU*

GRAHAM A. W. ROOK MD *Professor of Medical Microbiology, University College London Medical School, 67–73 Riding House Street, London W1P 7LD*

NILESH J. SAMANI MD FRCP *Senior Lecturer & Honorary Consultant Cardiologist, Department of Cardiology, Clinical Sciences Wing, Glenfield General Hospital, Groby Road, Leicester LE3 9QP*

JONATHAN R. SECKL PhD FRCP(Ed) *Wellcome Senior Clinical Fellow & Senior Lecturer in Medicine/Honorary Consultant Physician, Molecular Endocrinology Laboratory, Department of Medicine, University of Edinburgh, Western General Hospital, Edinburgh EH4 2XU*

I. STEINER *The Laboratory of Neurovirology, Department of Neurology, Hadassah University Hospital, Hebrew University-Hadassah Medical School, Jerusalem, Israel 91120*

JOHANNES P. T. M. VAN LEEUWEN *Senior Investigator, Department of Internal Medicine III, Erasmus University Medical School, PO Box 1738, 3000 DR Rotterdam, The Netherlands*

TRUDY VINK-VAN WIJNGAARDEN PhD *Department of Internal Medicine III, Erasmus University Medical School, PO Box 1738, 3000 DR Rotterdam, The Netherlands*

MARITA WALMSLEY BsC *Kennedy Institute of Rheumatology, Sunley Building, 1 Lurgan Avenue, Hammersmith, London W6 8LW*

MARK J. WALPORT MB PhD FRCP MRCPath *Professor of Medicine & Head of the Rheumatology Unit, Royal Postgraduate Medical School, Hammersmith Hospital, Du Cane Road, London W12 0NN*

DAVID A. WARRELL DM DSc FRCP *Professor of Tropical Medicine & Infectious Diseases & Director, Centre for Tropical Medicine & Infectious Diseases, University of Oxford, Nuffield Department of Clinical Medicine, John Radcliffe Hospital, Headington, Oxford OX3 9DU*

Preface

Organizing meetings and editing the subsequent publication is normally a chore which I try to avoid like the plague. In the case of the 15th Advanced Medicine Conference of the Royal College of Physicians and Volume 7 of *Horizons in Medicine*, it was more a privilege. The opportunity to invite a broad range of the most exciting medical researchers to a conference in which they could enthuse over their research has been unique — and it certainly provided the opportunity to hear speakers whose work I have admired from the distance of their publications.

Medical science is moving forward at an unprecedented rate on all fronts. Contrary to the perception of many, it is not only the molecular sciences which are leading the way. Molecular biology certainly has played a major role in our understanding of disease as evidenced in many of the chapters of this book, but epidemiology, new imaging techniques, biochemistry of tissue regulatory factors and new techniques in immunology, microbiology and neuroscience have given us the opportunity to ask basic questions about disease processes which would have been thought impossible to address just a few years ago. Examples of the powers of all of these techniques are clearly provided within the contributions to this book.

It would be quite inappropriate to pick out specific lectures from amongst the superb talks which were given at this meeting. Suffice it to say that the audience was treated to a unique and exciting view of the growing points or 'horizons' of medicine and were clearly stimulated by what they heard. I hope this book conveys the excitement both of the contributors and the audience which was palpable at the conference.

I should like to thank Philada Dann and her colleagues in the College for all their great help both in running the conference and in helping, together with Blackwell Science, to produce this volume. Finally — and most importantly — I must thank all the contributors for their time and effort in creating such a successful conference and for supplying the manuscripts which form the basis of this book.

STAFFORD LIGHTMAN

PART 1
LECTURES

A new appraisal of reducing cholesterol in the prevention of coronary heart disease

MICHAEL F. OLIVER

When the facts change, I change my mind. What do you do?
(Maynard Keynes.)

The evidence relating raised plasma cholesterol concentrations to a high incidence of atherosclerosis and increased risk of coronary heart disease (CHD) no longer stirs argument within medical circles. But the view that not only this risk but also the mortality from CHD and from all causes can be reduced by lowering raised plasma cholesterol concentrations has, until very recently, remained controversial. Polarization of views has led over the last 20 years to the emergence of enthusiasts for whom cholesterol lowering and the prevention of CHD are almost synonymous, and sceptics who attribute to lipid reduction more harm than good. This debate, which is frequently exploited by the media, has led many in the medical profession and the general public to believe that the case for treatment of raised cholesterol is flawed and can be disregarded. The publication recently of several definitive trials [1–5] indicates that this attitude is no longer tenable for patients who have already developed CHD and is also unacceptable for men with hypercholesterolaemia at high risk for CHD [6].

BACKGROUND

The data incriminating raised concentrations of plasma low-density lipoproteins (LDL) as an important pathogenic factor in the development of atherosclerosis, and hence CHD, are overwhelming. They are derived from extensive evidence that induction of atherosclerosis occurs in experimental animals as a result of raising plasma LDL; the powerful relationship in humans between raised LDL in familial hypercholesterolaemia, both homozygote and heterozygote varieties, with coronary atherosclerosis and premature CHD; the moderately strong epidemiological relationship between raised LDL in communities with a high incidence of CHD in contrast to those with a low incidence; and the fact that in individuals raised LDL increases the relative risk of CHD.

There are, however, several important unanswered questions regarding atheroma formation. These include the role of oxidized LDL uptake by monocyte-macrophages [7]; why and how oxidation occurs; to what extent unstable long chain polyunsaturated fatty acids, liable to undergo peroxidation, are involved; whether or not local antioxidant forces are relevant; knowledge of exactly how the LDL and macrophage endothelial interactions are initiated and modulated; and the role of cytokines in these interactions.

Similarly, how are high concentrations of high-density lipoproteins (HDL) protective against CHD [8]? We do not yet understand the factors influencing 'reverse cholesterol transport' [9] and the mechanisms through which cholesterol leaves the arterial wall; is it reasonable to expect extracellular crystals of cholesterol to be mobilized and removed from the endothelial space; what is the role of apoprotein A_1 and of the cholesterol transferase proteins in promoting this efflux; and how might HDL be raised pharmacologically?

Also, what determines that an atheromatous plaque becomes unstable [10]? Why does it fissure, often precipitating acute myocardial ischaemia or infarction, when it does? What is the role of platelet-fibrin formation in normal flowing blood and when there is endothelial damage? To what extent does nitric oxide-endothelium-dependent modulation [11] influence the formation of atheromatous lesions?

REGRESSION STUDIES

A few years ago, there was genuine doubt as to whether it is possible either to prevent progression of atheromatous lesions in humans or to induce partial regression, even though both had been demonstrated in animals in which atheroma had been induced after relatively short periods of feeding with high-fat/cholesterol diets. This doubt resulted from consideration of the pathology, particularly of coronary atherosclerosis. Atheromatous lesions include extracellular deposition of cholesterol (often with crystal formation), extensive collagen responses and fibrosis, plain muscle disruption and even calcification, and incorporation of fibrin degradation products. They take many years to develop and are often very extensive in the coronary arterial tree, as well as causing focal obstructions. The chances of this process being stopped or even reversed in middle-aged people and with clinical benefit seemed unlikely. Even if the process could be arrested, does it follow that the recipient organ (myocardium, brain or legs) would receive improved perfusion and therefore better viability [12]?

Several small and short-term trials of various cholesterol-lowering regimes have produced encouraging results. Now, with the long follow-up of the Program on the Surgical Control of the Hyperlipidemias

(POSCH) study [13] using regional ileal bypass surgery as a means of reducing hypercholesterolaemia and the results of several statin trials [1–4], there can no longer be any doubt that marked reduction of raised plasma LDL cholesterol does indeed slow progression and induces regression of coronary atheroma in some patients, albeit a minority. The extent of the changes is small, however. Improvements of 0.1–0.2 mm or less occur in minimal and mean arterial diameters; this needs to be judged in the context that a 50% arterial occlusion equals about 2 mm intrusion into the lumen (Fig. 1). They also take several years to become evident (Figs 2 and 3). The POSCH study has also indicated that structural improvements to the diseased arteries take many years.

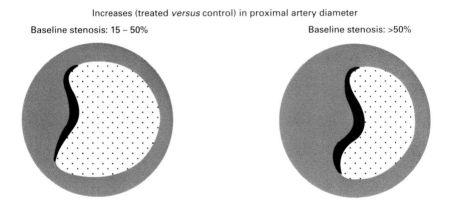

Increases (treated *versus* control) in proximal artery diameter

Baseline stenosis: 15 – 50%   Baseline stenosis: >50%

Fig. 1 The approximate extent of regression (black area) which has been recorded in quantitative angiographic trials of cholesterol lowering by statins. (The spotted area represents the lumen.)

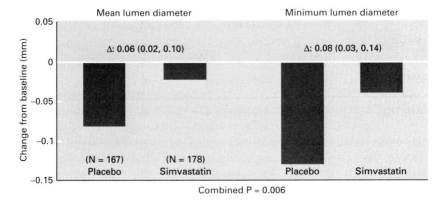

Fig. 2 The differences in mean and minimum lumen diameter in the Multicentre Anti-Atheroma Study (MAAS) trial [2] after 4 years of simvastatin treatment.

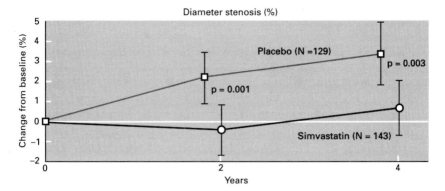

Fig. 3 The differences in diameter stenosis in the MAAS trial [2] after 4 years of simvastatin treatment.

Not all the regression trials have demonstrated a concurrent clinical benefit. In general, the smaller the trial and the less well it was blinded, the quicker the apparent improvement [14]. The large POSCH trial of 860 patients took over 12 years to show a significant difference in CHD mortality between the surgically treated and control groups [15]. Some of the reasons for the apparent discrepancy between atheroma regression and clinical events are that trials using nicotinic acid or a resin were, by definition, not blinded and soft endpoints, such as referral to coronary artery bypass grafting (CABG) or percutaneous transluminal coronary angioplasty (PTCA) were used to score clinical events. Also most trials have been too small and were not designed with the statistical power to demonstrate a result in clinical events. Endothelial-dependent vasoconstriction in response to acetylcholine is increased in human coronary arteries in the presence of hypercholesterolaemia [16] and it is lessened by lowering LDL [17]. This suggests that improvement in arterial tone (remodelling) may occur in some responsive individuals at an early stage. But it seems intrinsically unlikely that functional improvement in myocardial perfusion (which is the ultimate aim), resulting from material changes in arteries with advanced atherosclerosis, will occur within months.

In my view, there is no need for further invasive coronary artery regression trials in order to study the effects of reducing raised LDL. We now know that atheroma can regress in those who are initially hypercholesterolaemic. Various meta-analyses have been performed and, although like has not always been compared with like since the patients, duration of treatment and the treatment itself differ from trial to trial, a beneficial trend is evident [18]. But it appears that, for patients with initially normal concentrations of cholesterol and LDL, regression of coronary atheroma does not occur even with very marked reduction of these plasma moieties over $2^1/2$ years [19]. Improvements of non-invasive methods of assessment are needed. Already, precision carotid ultra-sonography has indicated that reduction of LDL by a statin leads to less atheroma in these arteries [20].

SECONDARY PREVENTION

The largest and longest secondary prevention trial — the 4S — led to significant reductions in all-cause mortality and in CHD mortality [5]. The trial was conducted over 5 years in 4444 patients, mostly men, and on admission to the trial the serum cholesterol 'window' was 5.5–8.0 mmol/l. The extent of reduction of LDL cholesterol (– 35%) achieved was greater than in any previous trial and simvastatin produced a 30% reduction (P < 0.0003) in the relative risk of deaths from all causes, a 42% reduction in deaths from CHD and a 34% reduction in CHD morbidity (P < 0.0001). These benefits applied equally to all baseline quartiles of LDL and at all ages up to 65 years. There were also significantly fewer CABG in the treated group but no difference in the subsequent requirement for PTCA between the groups. Interestingly, in view of the discussion in the previous paragraph, it took between 18 and 24 months before a significant trend emerged in favour of the simvastatin group.

This successful trial has revolutionized thinking about the need for reduction of raised LDL concentrations in patients with established CHD. Now there is no excuse not to treat most patients with CHD, when plasma cholesterol or LDL concentrations are also raised; these are the patients we must identify. There may be two exceptions: one is PTCA, since there is no evidence that the statins reduce the restenosis rate and or that restenosis is related to plasma cholesterol concentrations; and the other is cardiac failure where the prognosis is determined by the degree of ventricular impairment rather than the extent of coronary atherosclerosis. But it is not yet appropriate to give a statin to all CHD patients, since we do not yet know whether the clinical benefits will apply also to those with lower lipid levels where, for example, the thrombotic component of the disease may be dominant.

We have procrastinated for long enough, even though it was justified earlier to do so. Now that the facts are in, the message must be passed on. There is evidence that in the UK the majority of patients with CHD, particularly those in their 60s and 70s, never even have their plasma lipids measured [21], let alone receive treatment. This conservatism must be overcome.

PRIMARY PREVENTION

A similar change in policy is now needed for the management of raised cholesterol in people without overt CHD. The recently completed West of Scotland trial [6] of pravastatin in 6595 hypercholesterolaemic 45–65-

year-old men over a period of nearly 5 years is a seminal report. Most men were otherwise healthy; none had previous myocardial infarction and only 5% had self-reported stable angina on admission to the trial. The criteria for entry to the trial comprised LDL cholesterol concentrations > 4.0 mmol/l (~ 155 mg/dl) at both key screening visits, or > 4.5 mmol/l (~ 175 mg/dl) at one of these screening visits, but < 6.0 mmol/l (~ 230 mg/dl). Pravastatin reduced total cholesterol by 20%, LDL cholesterol by 26%, triglycerides by 12% and HDL cholesterol was raised by 5%. There were no side-effects or adverse reactions. In the pravastatin-treated group the risk of CHD death or non-fatal myocardial infarction, and non-fatal infarction alone, was reduced by 31% (P < 0.001); deaths definitely due to CHD were reduced by 28% ($P = 0.13$) and from all causes by 22% ($P = 0.051$); and the need for coronary angiography was reduced by 31% and PTCA or CABG by 37% ($P < 0.001$). The clinical benefits of pravastatin treatment were equivalent in the 84% without and the 16% with prior vascular risk; and also in those below and above the median of cholesterol concentrations at baseline.

The West of Scotland primary prevention trial is the fifth long-term randomized study to show benefit from reducing hypercholesterolaemia in healthy men at high risk for CHD and the first to use a statin. The results of the Los Angeles Veterans diet trial [22], the World Health Organization (WHO) clofibrate trial [23], the Lipid Research Clinics cholestyramine trial [24] and the Helsinki Heart trial using gemfibrozil [25] all pointed in the same direction but used measures which reduced LDL cholesterol by less than half that of the statins.

The West of Scotland trial showed clinical benefit within 2 years of starting treatment with pravastatin. This contrasts with the experiences of the earlier primary prevention trials using diet, fibrates or cholestyramine, where benefit was not established until after 3 or 4 years of treatment. This early benefit may be a consequence of the greater extent of reduction of LDL cholesterol achieved by statins, or a manifestation of rapid improvement in endothelial-dependent vasorelaxation with LDL reduction [26], or of less platelet aggregation, rather than stabilization of atheromatous plaques, which is probably slower.

The earlier trials also showed an increase in non-cardiovascular mortality. Various meta-analyses have been carried out on these and other smaller primary prevention trials and this adverse finding is significant ($2P < 0.02$) [27]. It is particularly evident for those not initially at high risk for CHD [28]. Neither the 4S nor the West of Scotland trials showed an excess of non-cardiovascular deaths; indeed, both had a minor but non-significant reduction. While the issue will not be finally resolved until the results of an ongoing mega trial [29] are available, we can now approach cholesterol lowering in those at high risk without the caution of recent years.

It may be concluded, now, that men *with* risk factors and a raised plasma cholesterol or LDL level should be treated with a statin. But the question of whether or not all men who have plasma cholesterol concentrations of > 5.5 mmol/l (or LDL cholesterol > 4.0 mmol/l or a total cholesterol/HDL ratio > 5) *without* additional CHD risk factors should be treated with statins will be debated intensively by physicians, health economists and pharmaceutical companies. The usual recommendation for these men at lower risk is to decrease dietary saturated fat intake and increase the polyunsaturated/saturated fat ratio, but this is often ineffective outside clinic conditions (see later), and therefore an effective and safe drug assumes more importance.

Some additional perspective about the extent of benefit may help with these decisions [30]. Of 1000, 55-year-old men living in the UK at all categories of CHD risk, 87% will be alive 10 years later. CHD is the cause of 36% of the deaths occurring over this period and, since the West of Scotland trial indicates that one-third of these CHD deaths might be prevented, the 10-year overall survival might be improved by about 1.5% and the 5-year survival rate by rather less than 1%. Alternatively, it can be estimated that for middle-aged men there will be nine fewer deaths and about 20 fewer non-fatal myocardial infarcts per 1000, when treated with a statin over 5 years. Since statins must be taken for life and a year's treatment costs between £400 and £600, exclusive of physician or laboratory charges, the cost–benefit ratio is equivocal in such men. My preference, therefore, is to focus on those most at risk — with plasma cholesterol levels above about 6 mmol/l.

LOW CHOLESTEROL AND NON-CARDIAC DISEASES

At present, the relation between low plasma cholesterol concentrations and non-cardiac diseases should be regarded as a separate issue from that of the safety of lowering cholesterol from previously high levels. A J-relation exists between plasma cholesterol and disease. This is best illustrated through the Multiple Risk Factor Intervention Trial (MRFIT) data [31] (Fig. 4). The left limb of the J is due to a miscellany of diseases, including cancer, but also comprising a higher than expected prevalence of haemorrhagic stroke and suicides. The important National Heart, Lung and Blood Institute (NHLBI) report [32] on the relations between low blood cholesterol and mortality provides detail. Occult cancer appears to be the main explanation [33], but the consistently higher than expected incidence of haemorraghic stroke is unexplained.

WHAT CAN BE ACHIEVED THROUGH DIET?

The short answer to this question, so far as CHD is concerned, is very

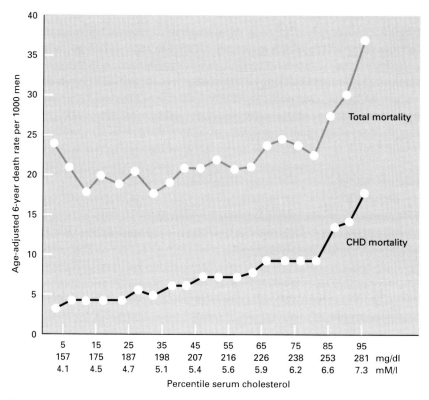

Fig. 4 Age-adjusted 6-year coronary heart disease and total death rates per 1000 men screened for the MRFIT study [31] according to serum cholesterol percentiles.

little [34]. There are two reasons for this. One is that the degree of reduction in LDL concentrations with a low-fat, low-cholesterol diet is small (usually < 5%) [35], and the other is that compliance is poor outside strict clinic conditions [36]. Several long-term trials indicate that such a diet alone has not had any beneficial effect on CHD or all-cause mortality [37]. The Oslo Heart Study [38] does, on the other hand, indicate that reduction of cigarette smoking in conjunction with dietary reduction of raised cholesterol concentrations may be beneficial.

Successive government reports, recommendations from the American Heart Association, for example, and even the recently published guidelines from the European Society of Cardiology [39], have been insufficiently critical regarding the failure of the standard low-fat, low-cholesterol diet to reduce CHD. There is an air of wishful thinking and unreality about the subject. Many dieticians are employed expensively by the National Health Service without evidence that their dietary advice has had or is having any impact on CHD [36]. Meanwhile, obesity is increasing in middle-aged men and women in the UK!

But diets with an increase in polyunsaturated fats do appear to reduce CHD incidence. The first large long-term trial using a polyunsaturated/saturated (P/S) ratio of 1.5 led to fewer CHD deaths and all-cause deaths [22]. Two recent trials [40,41] of n-3 fatty acid-enriched diets also suggest that there is benefit. Interestingly, the latter two trials were not associated with reduction in plasma cholesterol or LDL concentrations. The evidence that fish oil diets reduce a thrombotic tendency is strong [42]. More attention should be paid to the quality of the fat in the diet rather than the total fat calories consumed.

CONCLUSIONS

Many questions remain regarding the mechanisms through which high concentrations of LDLs lead to coronary atheroma and high concentrations of HDLs protect against it. But there should no longer be any argument or controversy regarding the need and benefits of lowering raised plasma cholesterol and LDL concentrations in patients with manifest CHD. The preferred treatment is a statin. Inaction is no longer acceptable. Undertreatment of those at continuing high risk is one problem.

Reduction of hypercholesterolaemia in otherwise healthy men leads to less CHD. The priority should be to treat those with additional risk factors. Since the cost–benefit ratio of action is inversely related to cholesterol concentrations, treatment of healthy people without additional risk factors needs individual consideration.

REFERENCES

1 Waters D, Higginson L, Gladstone P et al. Effects of monotherapy with an HMGCoA reductase inhibitor on the progression of coronary atherosclerosis as assessed by serial quantitative arteriography: the Canadian Coronary Atherosclerosis Intervention Trial. *Circulation* 1994;**89**:959–968.

2 MAAS Investigators. Effect of simvastatin on coronary atheroma: a multicentre antiatheroma study. *Lancet* 1994;**344**:633–638.

3 Jukema JW, Bruschke AVG, van Boven AJ et al. Effects of lipid lowering by pravastatin on progression and regression of coronary artery disease in symptomatic men with normal to moderately elevated serum cholesterol levels. The regression growth evaluation statin study (REGRESS). *Circulation* 1995;**91**:2528–2540.

4 Pitt B, Mancini GBJ, Ellis SG et al. Pravastatin limitation of atherosclerosis in the coronary arteries (PLAC I): reduction in atherosclerosis progression and clinical events. *J Am Coll Cardiol* 1995;**26**:1133–1139.

5 Scandinavian Simvastatin Survival Study Group. Randomised trial of cholesterol lowering in 4444 patients with coronary heart disease: the Scandinavian Simvastatin Survival Study (4 S). *Lancet* 1994;**344**:1383–1389.

6 Shepherd J, Cobbe SM, Ford I et al. Prevention of coronary heart disease with pravastatin in men with hypercholesterolemia. *N Engl J Med* 1995;**333**:1301–1307.

7 Steinberg D, Parthasarathy S, Carew TE et al. Beyond cholesterol: modifications of low-density lipoprotein that increase its atherogenicity. *N Engl J Med* 1989;**320**:915–924.

8 Miller NE. *High Density Lipoproteins and Atherosclerosis*, vol. II. Elsevier, Amsterdam, 1989.

9   Durrington PN. How HDL protects against atheroma. *Lancet* 1993;**342**:1315–1316.
10 Libby P. Molecular bases of the acute coronary syndromes. *Circulation* 1995;**91**:2844–2850.
11 Moncada S, Higgs A. The L-arginine–nitric oxide pathway. *N Engl J Med* 1993;**329**:2002–2012.
12 Oliver MF. Perspective of trials of regression of coronary atherosclerosis. *Cardiovasc Risk Factors* 1992;**2**:234–238.
13 Buchwald H, Varco RL, Matts JP and the POSCH group. Effect of partial ileal bypass surgery on mortality and morbidity from coronary heart disease in patients with hypercholesterolemia. *N Engl J Med* 1990;**323**:946–955.
14 Brown G, Albers JJ, Fisher LD *et al*. Regression of coronary artery disease as a result of intensive lipid-lowering therapy in men with high levels of apolipoprotein-B. *N Engl J Med* 1990;**323**:1289–1298.
15 Buchwald H, Campos CT, Boen JR *et al*. Disease-free intervals after partial ileal bypass in patients with coronary heart disease and hypercholesterolemia: report from the program on the surgical control of the hyperlipidemias (POSCH). *J Am Coll Cardiol* 1995;**26**:351–357.
16 Dexter H, Zeiher AM. Endothelial function in human coronary arteries *in vivo*. *Hypertension* 1991;**18**:90–99.
17 Treasure CB, Klein JL, Weintraub WS *et al*. Beneficial effects of cholesterol-lowering therapy on the coronary endothelium in patients with coronary artery disease. *N Engl J Med* 1995;**332**:481–487.
18 Vos JW. Retardation and arrest of progression or regression of coronary artery disease: a review. *Prog Cardiovasc Dis* 1993;**35**:435–454.
19 The Harvard Atherosclerosis Reversibility Project (HARP). *Lancet* 1994;**344**:1182–1186.
20 Furberg CD, Adams HP, Applegate WB *et al*. Effect of lovastatin on early carotid atherosclerosis and cardiovascular events. *Circulation* 1994;**90**:1679–1687.
21 Aspire Steering Group. A British Cardiac Society survey of the potential for the secondary prevention of coronary disease: ASPIRE (Action on secondary prevention through intervention to reduce events). *Heart* 1996;**75**:334–342.
22 Dayton S, Pearce ML, Hashimoto S *et al*. A controlled clinical trial of a diet high in unsaturated fat preventing complications in atherosclerosis. *Circulation* 1969;**39/40** (suppl. II):63.
23 Report from Committee of Principal Investigators. A cooperative trial in the primary prevention of ischaemic heart disease using clofibrate. *Br Heart J* 1978;**40**:1069–1118.
24 Lipid Research Clinics Coronary Prevention Trial. *JAMA* 1984;**251**:351–374.
25 Frick MH, Elo O, Haapa K *et al*. Helsinki Heart Study: primary prevention trial with gemfibrozil in middle-aged men with dyslipidaemia. *N Engl J Med* 1987;**317**:1237–1245.
26 Stroes ESG, Koomans HA, de Bruin TWA, Rabelink TJ. Vascular function in the forearm of hypercholesterolaemic patients off and on lipid-lowering medication. *Lancet* 1995;**346**:467–471.
27 Peto R, Yusuf S, Collins R. Cholesterol-lowering trial results in their epidemiologic context. *J Am Coll Cardiol* 1991;**17**:III–451.
28 Davey Smith G, Song F, Sheldon TA. Cholesterol lowering and mortality; the importance of considering initial level of risk. *Br Med J* 1993;**306**:1367–1373.
29 Collins R, Keech A, Peto R *et al*. Cholesterol and total mortality: need for larger trials. *Br Med J* 1992;**304**:1689.
30 Oliver MF. Statins prevent coronary heart disease. *Lancet* 1995;**346**:1378–1379.
31 Neaton JD, Blackburn H, Jacobs D *et al*. Serum cholesterol level and mortality: findings for men screened in the Multiple Risk Factor Intervention Trial. *Arch Intern Med* 1992;**152**:1490–1500.
32 Jacobs D, Blackburn H, Higgins M *et al*. Report of the conference on low blood cholesterol: mortality associations. *Circulation* 1992;**86**:1046–1060.
33 Wannamethee G, Shaper AG, Whincup PH, Walker M. Low serum cholesterol concentrations and mortality in middle aged British men. *Br Med J* 1995;**311**:409–413.
34 Oliver MF. Should the amount of fat in the diet be reduced? *Am J Clin Nutr* (in press).

35 Ramsay LE, Yeo WW, Jackson PR. Dietary reduction of cholesterol concentration: time to think again. *Br Med J* 1993;**303**:953–957.

36 Neil HAW, Roe L, Godlee JW *et al.* Randomised trial of lipid lowering dietary advice in general practice: the effects on serum lipids, lipoproteins, and antioxidants. *Br Med J* 1995;**310**:569–573.

37 Holme I. Relation of coronary heart disease incidence and total mortality to plasma cholesterol reduction in randomized trials: use of meta-analysis. *Br Heart J* 1993;**69**:S42–S50.

38 Hjermann I, Velve Byre K, Holme I, Leren P. Effect of diet and smoking on the incidence of coronary heart disease. *Lancet* 1981;**ii**:1303–1310.

39 Pyörälä K, De Backer G, Poole-Wilson P, Wood D. Prevention of coronary heart disease in clinical practice. Recommendations of the Task Force of the European Society of Cardiology, European Atherosclerosis Society and European Society of Hypertension. *Eur Heart J* 1994;**15**:1300–1331.

40 Burr ML, Fehily AM, Gilbert JF *et al.* Effects of changes in fat, fish, and fibre intakes on death and myocardial reinfarction: diet and reinfarction trial (DART). *Lancet* 1989;**ii**:757–761.

41 de Lorgeril M, Renaud S, Mamelle N *et al.* Mediterranean alpha-linolenic acid-rich diet in secondary prevention of coronary heart disease. *Lancet* 1994;**343**:1454–1459.

42 Dyerberg J, Bang HO, Stofferson E, Moncada S, Vane JR. Eicosapentaenoic acid and prevention of thrombosis and atherosclerosis? *Lancet* 1978;**2**:117–119.

New genes for old diseases: the molecular basis of myotonic dystrophy and Huntington's disease

PETER S. HARPER

In medicine, as in many other fields, the science of genetics has shown its power most strikingly by its ability to throw new light on old and apparently insoluble problems. In this lecture I hope to illustrate this from my own experience in research and in clinical practice, in relation to two genetic disorders, myotonic dystrophy (dystrophia myotonica) and Huntington's disease.

These two inherited disorders have formed the cornerstone of my work for a period of almost 25 years since I entered the new field of medical genetics. I have studied them from all angles, clinical and genetic, have written books on both [1,2], but only very recently, with the isolation of the genes for each disorder, and the recognition of the remarkable mutational mechanism involved, have many of the puzzling features that I have documented over the years been resolved.

The title of my lecture is intended to highlight the insights that genetic analysis has provided for these diseases. The phrase 'new genes' indicates that in both instances the genes have been newly isolated (in 1992 and 1993), while previous biochemical and other studies had given no clue as to what their nature or function might be. Even more remarkably, both are an example of a completely new type of mutation: unstable or dynamic mutations in an expanded triplet repeat of bases, now recognized as forming a distinct and growing family of disorders due to trinucleotide repeat expansions.

By contrast the term 'old diseases' reflects the fact that they have been recognized for many years, over a century in the case of George Huntington's classical description of the disease [3] in 1872 (with even earlier reports now known to be the same disorder), and a long history also in the case of myotonic dystrophy, first described by Steinert [4] in Germany and by Batten and Gibb [5] in Britain in 1909. Both disorders were also among the first to be recognized as following mendelian dominant inheritance, proposed for Huntington's disease in 1908 by Punnett [6] and for myotonic dystrophy in 1918 by Fleischer [7].

The term 'old diseases' has taken on added significance since the molecular basis has been discovered since, as will be seen, the original mutations predisposing to the disorders may indeed be very old — possibly many thousands of years.

At the time I started to work on these two disorders neither I nor anyone else had reason to suspect that they might be in any way related to each other; as can be seen from Table 1 the clinical features are very different, Huntington's disease being a disorder of the central nervous system, while myotonic dystrophy, in addition to the muscular wasting and characteristic myotonia, shows a remarkable degree of multisystem involvement. When looked at from the viewpoint of the clinical geneticist, however, (Table 2) a number of common features start to emerge, not simply the dominant pattern of inheritance but the variability in age at onset, the apparent rarity of new mutations and, most notably, the existence of unusual childhood forms of the two disorders and the occurrence of 'anticipation', a phenomenon to be discussed in detail shortly.

Both myotonic dystrophy and Huntington's disease have traditionally been considered as disorders of adult life, and it was many years before it was recognized that they might occur in early childhood. Juvenile Huntington's disease was first fully recognized in the 1920s [8], though a likely case in a family had been noted as long ago as 1888 [9]; the distinctive congenital form of myotonic dystrophy was not documented until 1960

Table 1 Clinical features.

Myotonic dystrophy	Huntington's disease
Progressive muscle weakness and wasting; myotonia	Progressive CNS degeneration
Multisystem disorder	No other systems primarily involved
Smooth and cardiac muscle involvement	Particular involvement of caudate nucleus and cerebral cortex
Endocrine disturbance, cataract and CNS involvement all frequent	Premature neuronal cell death the main feature

CNS, Central nervous system.

Table 2 Classical genetic studies.

Myotonic dystrophy	Huntington's disease
Autosomal dominant	Autosomal dominant
Exceptionally variable in clinical picture and age at onset	Very variable age at onset
New mutations apparently very rare	New mutations apparently very rare
Atypical congenital form	Atypical juvenile form
Anticipation (marked)	Anticipation (moderate)

[10]. These childhood forms played a major role in shaping my own research in this field, notably congenital myotonic dystrophy, whose clinical and genetic features I studied extensively both in the USA [11] and in the UK [12,13] in the 1970s. Not only do the clinical features of this condition differ markedly from the classical adult form, but it is almost invariably transmitted by an affected mother, in contrast to what would be expected from autosomal dominant inheritance. During the course of my early research on myotonic dystrophy, I recognized the parallel with Huntington's disease (Table 3) where the rare childhood form also showed marked clinical differences from most adult-onset cases, and where a striking parent-of-origin effect is also seen, but in this case with most cases paternally transmitted [14], the opposite to the maternal transmission of myotonic dystrophy. Thus in both disorders genetic studies were producing unusual, puzzling and remarkably comparable findings, despite the apparent dissimilarity of the conditions. This situation was heightened by the recognition that both disorders appeared to demonstrate anticipation, a finding central to the later molecular explanation of the genetic features, which merits some discussion at this point.

The term 'anticipation' can be defined as the occurrence of a disorder with earlier age at onset (and usually greater severity) in successive generations [15]. Arising out of the rather confused concept of degeneration, especially in relation to mental illness, it was first documented in a precise and accurate form by Fleischer [7] in 1918, who observed that apparently unrelated patients with myotonic dystrophy could be linked in previous generations through individuals who had cataracts in later life but no muscle disease. Since cataract was already a known clinical feature of myotonic dystrophy, Fleischer suggested perceptively (and, we now know, correctly) that cataract in these patients was a precursor for the full disorder in subsequent generations and that the disorder worsened and occurred with earlier onset with each transmission.

These observations were widely accepted (though not explained) for several decades, until the analysis of Penrose [16] in 1948 suggested

Table 3 Childhood forms of myotonic dystrophy and Huntington's disease.

Congenital myotonic dystrophy	Juvenile Huntington's disease
Severe — often fatal around birth	Not from birth, but can occur as early as 5 years
Clinical picture different from adult form — hypotonia, mental retardation, little myotonia	Clinical picture differs from adult form — rigidity, general neurodegeneration
Occurs in same families as classical cases	Occurs in same families as classical cases
Almost always transmitted by affected mother	Usually paternally transmitted

that anticipation in myotonic dystrophy did not represent a biological phenomenon but could be explained by the natural variability of the disorder, by biases of observation and by effects of the opposite allele. Penrose was strongly influenced by the difficulty in imagining any mechanism by which a gene could change in successive generations, as well as by the unscientific way in which anticipation had originally been proposed for mental illness and mental handicap.

Following Penrose's paper, the concept of anticipation virtually vanished from the literature for 30 years, but the underlying facts relating to myotonic dystrophy were more obstinate and eventually demanded reassessment. My own observations on the congenital form, with a possible maternal effect [11–13], showed that myotonic dystrophy could indeed worsen if transmitted by a female, while thorough studies by Höweler and colleagues [17] in the Netherlands, of families that had been observed continually for decades, showed that progressively earlier onset was a fact even when the biases had been eliminated. Finally, an interesting parallel could be seen for anticipation in another disorder, fragile X mental retardation, where the possibility of a two-step mechanism of mutation had already been raised [18]; in 1989 I suggested that something comparable might be occurring in myotonic dystrophy [19]. On a wider front it was becoming clear that anticipation was also seen in Huntington's disease [20], although only in the male line of transmission, and that this was likely to underlie the puzzling paternal transmission of the juvenile form, already mentioned. Thus by 1990 it was clear that anticipation was real (Table 4); the only problem was that no obvious biological mechanism was known, either from humans or from other species, which could explain it. This explanation had to await the development of the techniques of molecular genetics and the isolation of the genes involved, and it is to this aspect of the story that we must now turn.

For the first decade of my research on myotonic dystrophy and Huntington's disease, the genes involved were abstract concepts, not tangible entities that could be studied directly. Patterns of transmission and variation within families and populations could tell us much about

Table 4 Anticipation in myotonic dystrophy and Huntington's disease.

Myotonic dystrophy	Huntington's disease
1918 First proposed (Fleischer)	Not suspected in early genetic studies
1948 Explained by 'bias' (Penrose)	1969 Paternal transmission of juvenile Huntington's disease
1989 Again suspected as 'real' from pedigree studies (Höweler)	1988 Anticipation shown in male line only
1991 Unstable DNA in fragile X suggested a biological mechanism	

the nature of the inheritance, as I have indicated, but we were totally ignorant as to what were the characteristics of these genes, or what was the nature of the proteins they produced. There were not even any substantial clues from biochemical research as to what type of protein might be expected. Thus the possibility of positional cloning, the isolation of a gene through molecular techniques based solely on its position on the chromosome, proved to be of special importance for both myotonic dystrophy and Huntington's disease.

The full story of the isolation of these two genes has been told elsewhere [21,22], but I consider myself exceptionally fortunate to have been part of the Cardiff team that was, along with international collaborators, responsible for the successful achievement of this goal for both genes and to have been involved from beginning to end. It seems unjust to summarize 10 years of intensive — and at times frustrating — work in a single table (Table 5), but now that the genes themselves are isolated, the path along the way is of less direct relevance to clinicians. It is worth noting, however, that the extensive gene mapping around these two chromosome regions, chromosome 19 in myotonic dystrophy and chromosome 4 in Huntington's disease, has resulted in a major general contribution to the human genome project, with a series of genes discovered that have proved to be completely different to those being looked for, even though physically near by. For example, one gene originally analysed in relation to Huntington's disease proved to be that for an important growth factor and to be responsible for the bone disorder achondroplasia [23].

Table 5 Positional cloning of the myotonic dystrophy and Huntington's disease genes.

Myotonic dystrophy	Huntington's disease
No clues from biochemistry	No clues from biochemistry
9-year search from first chromosomal location	10-year search from first chromosomal location
Single locus on chromosome 19	Single locus on chromosome 4
All candidate genes misleading	Confusion over exact location from recombinants
Gene and mutation identified in 1992	Gene and mutation identified in 1993

The process of moving from gene mapping based on family studies to actually identifying and isolating the genes proved extremely difficult for both diseases, but one valuable clue, a particular contribution of our Cardiff group [24,25], was the recognition of the precise location by finding strong allelic association or linkage disequilibrium between specific marker alleles and the disease. In both disorders this helped greatly to narrow the region

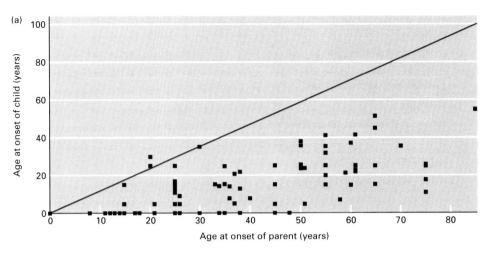

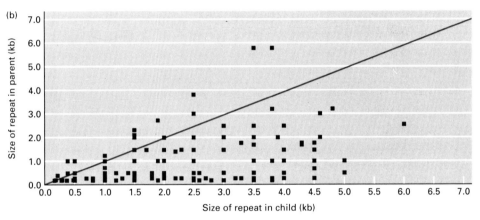

Fig. 2 Anticipation at the clinical and molecular levels. Comparison of parental and childhood generations in myotonic dystrophy showing close correspondence of anticipation in the same series of families for: (a) age at onset, with onset predominantly at earlier age in offspring; (b) increased size of mutational expansion in offspring. (Courtesy of Dr Helen Harley.)

Table 6 Genetic instability in myotonic dystrophy and Huntington's disease.

Myotonic dystrophy	Huntington's disease
Normal range less than 30 repeats	Normal range less than 35 repeats
Disease range extreme (50–2000 + repeats)	Disease range moderate — mostly 40–60 repeats
Somatic variation marked	Little somatic variation seen
Germ-line and somatic expansions may differ considerably	Expansion in spermatogenesis (possibly little in oogenesis)

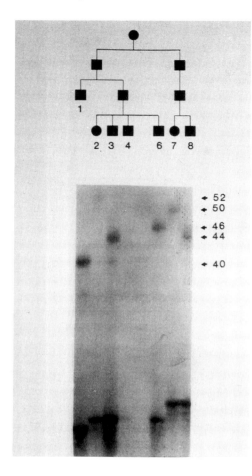

Fig. 3 Unstable DNA sequence
in Huntington's disease.
Molecular analysis for the
Huntington's disease mutation in
a single kindred, showing the
variable degree of expansion in
different family members.
(Expanded abnormal alleles
arrowed.) Reproduced with
permission from [46]. (Courtesy
of Dr Russell Snell.)

molecular distribution show any degree of constancy in relation to age of
onset or severity. It is clear that other factors have an important influence
on clinical expression of the genes.

Can we explain why in myotonic dystrophy the severe congenital cases
are almost all maternally transmitted, while in Huntington's disease the
opposite occurs (Table 7)? In fact, this paradox can be readily explained
if we take into consideration the size of the expansions. In congenital
myotonic dystrophy these are very large indeed — up to several thousand
repeats; pooled data between centres show that in paternal transmission
there seems to be a size limit and that beyond this the repeat number
is more likely to decrease than increase [34]; possibly sperm carrying
very large expansions are less viable. No such limit exists for female
transmissions, thus explaining the maternal transmission of the most severe
cases.

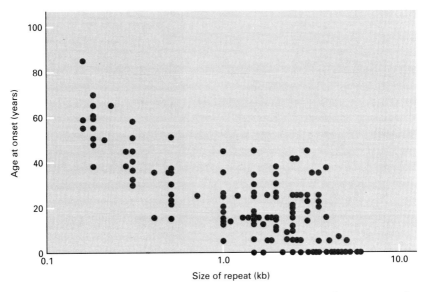

Fig. 4 Correlation of phenotype and genotype in myotonic dystrophy. Age at onset and mutation expansion. (Courtesy of Dr Helen Harley.)

When we look at the situation for Huntington's disease we find that even the most severe juvenile cases have quite small expansions (rarely over 100 repeats). Analysis of sperm samples from male Huntington's disease patients shows a more variable and generally larger repeat number than found in blood from the same individual [35], suggesting that in this range spermatogenesis is more likely to produce large expansions, and thus juvenile disease, than is transmission from an affected mother. For myotonic dystrophy, patients with around 100 repeats will mostly be mildly affected, and it is of interest that such mild cases are also most often of paternal origin — thus there is no real difference between the disorders provided one is comparing similar size ranges of the mutation.

At the beginning of this lecture, I mentioned that for these two 'old diseases' the original mutations might themselves be very ancient. Our

Table 7 Childhood forms of disease: the molecular basis.

Congenital myotonic dystrophy	Juvenile Huntington's disease
Largest expansions, may exceed 2000 repeats (but overlap non-congenital range)	Largest expansions (but rarely over 100 repeats)
Parental expansions also larger than average	Usually occur when parent already has substantial expansion
Size limit of expansion through male meiosis, so female transmission of congenital cases	Male transmission explained by increased mean repeat size in sperm compared with other tissues

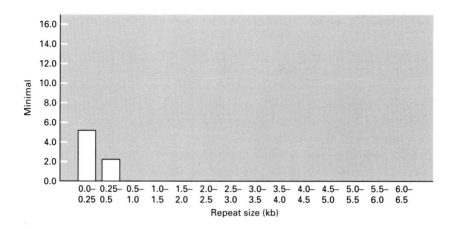

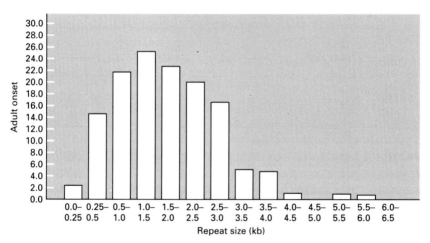

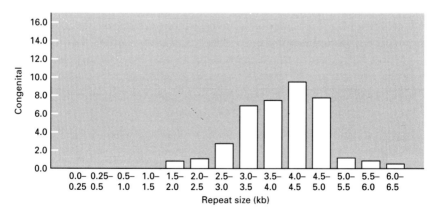

Fig. 5 Correlation of phenotype and genotype in myotonic dystrophy. Main clinical groups and mutation expansion.

new molecular understanding is raising some remarkable possibilities in this respect, although the situation is far from being fully resolved. It has long been recognized for both Huntington's disease and myotonic dystrophy that truly isolated cases likely to represent new mutations are very unusual. If care is taken, almost all cases can be shown to be derived from an affected parent (often minimally affected) or can be linked through ancestors to other branches of the family who have the disorder.

Our new concept of unstable or dynamic mutation, with the associated anticipation, now explains why these linking ancestors are so mildly affected or even entirely healthy. Where available for testing they commonly show a molecular repeat number that is at the borderline between normal and abnormal ranges [36,37]; some of these individuals may develop symptoms if they live long enough, while others will remain unaffected, only being recognized if they have passed on an expanded sequence to their descendants. Such individuals may provide links between families extending back many generations; thus the many families in Northern Quebec with myotonic dystrophy [38], where the frequency of the disease approaches 1 in 400, can almost all be traced back to a single individual born in France in the 16th century.

The origin of the mutations may go back much further than this. Almost all patients with myotonic dystrophy studied around the world have shown the same unstable type of mutation, but it could be argued that this had arisen separately on many occasions. However, if one analyses DNA markers around the gene to give a composite pattern or haplotype, one finds that this also seems to be unique for myotonic dystrophy over most of Europe and beyond [24], suggesting that most cases may have a common origin. Study of the normal range of repeats at the myotonic dystrophy locus shows considerable variation between ethnic groups, with the polymorphism clearly present in non-human primates [39]. Thus the original change eventually leading to myotonic dystrophy may have occurred many thousands of years ago, with a gradual increase over many generations until the number of repeats reached a point where it became significantly unstable and started to produce clinical problems.

One allied observation that may prove to be related to the origin of the myotonic dystrophy mutation is that the disorder is exceptionally rare in Africa south of the Sahara [40], whereas over most European and Asiatic populations, including Japan, it is relatively common. It is thus possible that the original mutation occurred after African races had diverged from others, but before any separation of Asiatic and Caucasian races. An alternative suggestion is that there could be a predisposing haplotype, absent or rare in Africans, from which the myotonic dystrophy mutation might have arisen more than once. Whatever the outcome, it can be seen how important the study of these disease mutations is becoming as part of the analysis of our general evolutionary history.

So far I have mentioned nothing about the nature of the genes themselves, but have concentrated on the properties of the mutations; it is indeed remarkable how many clinical and genetic aspects can be explained purely on the basis of the instability and patterns of transmission of the trinucleotide repeat. What do we know about the genes for these two diseases (Table 8), their function, and the proteins that they produce? This is an area of work where progress is inevitably much slower, and I can only touch on it in this lecture.

Table 8 Properties of the normal gene.

Myotonic dystrophy	Huntington's disease
Moderate size — 15 exons	Large gene — 67 exons
Sequence predicts protein to be a serine-threonine protein kinase	No clues from sequence as to function of protein
Specific localization in muscle	Expressed in all cell types
Probably important in controlling activity of ion channels	Protein localized in cytoplasm, not nucleus
Expanded trinucleotide repeat (CTG) in 3′ untranslated region of gene	Expanded trinucleotide repeat (CAG) in 5′ translated region of gene

One of the striking developments of molecular biology has been the increasing feasibility of sequencing large stretches of DNA. Once the myotonic dystrophy and Huntington's disease genes and mutations had been identified, sequence data could be generated and predictions made from computer-stored sequence databases, regarding the structural and functional properties to be expected from the amino acid sequence of the proteins. In the case of myotonic dystrophy, this prediction strongly suggested that the protein would be a member of the serine-threonine protein kinase family [41–43], something now receiving confirmation by identification of the protein biochemically and by functional studies. This actually fits well with what we know about the physiological basis of myotonia; a series of non-progressive myotonic disorders have been shown to result from defects of the sodium and chloride ion channels in muscle, and it can be speculated that the myotonic dystrophy protein kinase may modify the activity of these ion channels, as well as being important for the integrity of the muscle membrane.

For Huntington's disease, by contrast, the sequence prediction showed no suggestions of possible function [30], nor was there any homology with sequences previously described (this at least was of some relief to the teams involved, since it would have been an anticlimax to 10 years of search if it had turned out that the gene was already known in some other species!). Research in progress shows that the protein produced is widely distributed in brain and elsewhere, but it will be some time before we are clear as to what it actually does.

In this lecture, I hope that I have already shown the importances of combining clinical and molecular approaches in understanding inherited disorders, and also the value of looking across between apparently unrelated diseases. The insights gained from identifying the genes and unstable mutations for myotonic dystrophy, Huntington's disease and also fragile X syndrome have led to the recognition that we are dealing with a general mechanism of mutation and with a growing family of genetic disorders showing a number of common properties, as well as significant differences.

Table 9 shows the chronological sequence of this growth; other members may well have joined the group by the time this is read in print (Friedreich's ataxia is a recent and unexpected addition). Perhaps of greater relevance, however, is the recognition that the conditions can also be grouped functionally in a way that can allow us to understand important similarities and differences. In the right-hand part of Table 9 myotonic dystrophy and fragile X syndrome are grouped together, but separately from Huntington's disease and other disorders now known to show trinucleotide repeat expansions. These first two conditions show the most striking anticipation and range of clinical variation, reflecting the extent of the expansions seen and the consequent genetic instability, which is

Table 9 Trinucleotide repeat expansions: the wider grouping.

Chronological sequence	Functional grouping
1991 Spinobulbar muscular atrophy (SBMA)	*Group 1* (sequence untranslated)
1992 Fragile X syndrome (type A) Myotonic dystrophy	Fragile X syndrome (types A and E) Myotonic dystrophy Friedreich's ataxia
1993 Huntington's disease Spinocerebellar ataxia (SCA1) Fragile X syndrome (type E)	*Group 2* (sequence translated) SBMA Huntington's disease
1994 Dentatorubropallido-Luysian atrophy (DRPLA) Machado–Joseph disease (SCA3)	SCA1 DRPLA Machado–Joseph disease (SCA3)
1996 Friedreich's ataxia	

itself strongly size-dependent. They also show the greatest somatic variation between tissues. Huntington's disease and the others, by contrast, show a much more modest range of expansion, little somatic variation and, as already mentioned, a lesser degree of anticipation mainly in the male line. It is also striking that all the members of this second group are central nervous system degenerations, with differences in cell types affected, but with molecular defects so similar in their ranges of expansion that figure legends reporting these could be transposed between the disorders without it being noticed. How can we explain the real differences between the two groups?

The most logical answer, and the simplest (Table 10), seems to be that in the first group (myotonic dystrophy and fragile X) the trinucleotide repeat showing expansion is not located in the coding sequence of the gene and thus does not actually appear in the protein product. Precisely how the expansion produces disease pathology is still uncertain, but in simple terms some interference with the normal gene function can be envisaged, the degree of which is directly related to the size of the expanded repeat. Small expansions cause little or no clinical pathology, and the repeat has to expand to a massive degree before the most severe consequences are seen.

Table 10 Trinucleotide repeat expansions: untranslated and translated groups.

Untranslated	Translated
Myotonic dystrophy and fragile X	Huntington's disease and other CNS degenerations
Nature of repeat varies	All are CAG repeats
Phenotype varies	All are CNS degenerations
Expansion and instability often extreme; much somatic variation	Expansion and instability moderate; little somatic variation
Anticipation marked	Anticipation modest

CNS, Central nervous system.

In the second group, by contrast, the repeat sequence in all cases is placed in the coding region near the 5′ end of the gene; it can thus be expected to appear in the protein product and has been proved to do so in Huntington's disease and also in Kennedy's disease (spinobulbar muscular atrophy), the first disease in which a trinucleotide repeat mutation was identified, but whose significance was only recognized later. A further point of considerable significance is that in all members of this second group the repeat trinucleotide is CAG, coding for glutamine, unlike the first group, which is CTG in the case of myotonic dystrophy and CGG in fragile X.

The classification of unstable trinucleotide repeat disorders into these two categories, untranslated and translated, has considerable clinical consequences and greatly influences how one thinks about the ways in which mutation and disease are related. In the translated group it seems likely that only a modest expansion can be produced without lethal effect, since the structure and function of the protein will be affected directly by its altered sequence; thus only a moderate degree of instability will be seen, with relatively little somatic variation and only modest anticipation. In the untranslated group, by contrast, expansion of the repeat sequence can reach a massive degree, at which point marked anticipation and somatic variability due to the extreme instability will be seen.

If we ask how many more trinucleotide repeat disorders could still await discovery, my personal view would be that myotonic dystrophy may well be the only dominantly inherited disorder in the untranslated group, since it would be surprising if clinicians and geneticists were to have overlooked in other disorders the spectacular degree of anticipation seen and recognized so long ago in myotonic dystrophy. The group of translated CAG repeats, however, with Huntington's disease as the prototype, has already been joined by several other central nervous system degenerations where a slight degree of anticipation had been documented, while others, such as familial spastic paraplegia, seem likely candidates. A personal speculation, justified a little later, would be that any new diseases in this group will also be central nervous system degenerations, not disorders of other systems, while if there are any further to be found in the first group, they might affect any organs.

Following through on this speculation (Table 11) has led me to suggest that grouping of these conditions as untranslated (myotonic dystrophy) and translated (Huntington's disease) is fundamental to research strategies for understanding the conditions and their pathogenesis. If an expanded repeat sequence does not appear in the protein, then it can only produce pathology by interfering with the normal function of the gene. Thus, for myotonic dystrophy, the nature and normal role of the protein kinase are critical, and will relate directly to our understanding of the disease once we understand its function in different tissues. Thinking ahead to future therapy, this may well be related to factors which can restore or alter the normal gene function. Pharmacological agents could well be imagined as effective, at least in arresting progression of adult-onset cases.

For Huntington's disease and others in the untranslated group, future directions might be quite different. It seems likely that the presence of an expanded glutamine repeat in the protein molecule may have direct effects on gene function [44], and that the effect might be to some extent comparable regardless of the specific function of the gene concerned. Until we know more about the exact nature of these genes, this is perhaps a rash speculation, but we already have some evidence from one member

Table 11 Trinucleotide repeat expansions and pathogenesis of disease — some speculations.

Untranslated group	Translated group
Pathology through interference with normal gene function	Pathology may directly involve repeat sequence — gene function may be little affected
Phenotype will reflect function of specific gene involved — widely different according to nature of gene	Phenotype related to neuronal effects of glutamine repeat in protein — similar despite differences in gene function
Understanding and future therapy for disease likely to be related to understanding of specific gene function	Understanding and therapy could prove more related to mechanism of effects of repeat on neurons than to specific genes involved

of the group, Kennedy's disease, where the mutation is in the androgen receptor [45]; other mutations that destroy the function of this gene have no neurological effects, while in Kennedy's disease itself the endocrine features are minimal. It might seem heretical to suggest that the pathogenesis of Huntington's disease will have nothing to do with the function of the Huntington's gene! Nor would I advocate this view, but it may well prove that the direct effects of the mutation are as relevant as the specific properties and function of the gene in which it is placed. Again this could be relevant to therapeutic approaches, which might turn out to be fruitfully related to those factors influencing the neuronal effects of glutamine repeats.

It can be seen that the new understanding being made possible by the molecular advances that I have described is truly revolutionizing the way we look at these 'old diseases' and at the old problems which classical genetic and clinical studies had identified but could not solve without the new molecular techniques. It is salutary, though, to appreciate to what a large extent these new advances have rested upon the old foundations; without the recognition of anticipation, of the unexpected parent-of-origin effects, the clinical variability and the apparent lack of mutations, the new discoveries would have been considerably delayed — indeed, we might not yet have the 'new genes' to describe!

Standing at the interface of clinical medicine and molecular genetics perhaps enables me to see more clearly the value of the different types of observation and experiment, and how important it is for those with clinical and scientific trainings to communicate and collaborate with each other. I have been especially privileged to see this happen for the two disorders — myotonic dystrophy and Huntington's disease — that have been my main interest for almost 25 years, and to be able to look ahead to a time when we can consider using our new understanding in devising treatment for the many patients who remain afflicted by these serious, relatively frequent, and challenging genetic disorders.

ACKNOWLEDGEMENTS

I am deeply grateful to many colleagues in Cardiff who over a period of many years have undertaken much of the work described here, to the collaborating groups around the world with whom we have worked closely, to the numerous funding bodies for their generous and continuing support, and to the many patients and families whose cooperation has been essential for all of the work.

REFERENCES

1   Harper PS. *Myotonic Dystrophy*, 2nd edn. W.B. Saunders, London. 1989.
2   Harper PS. (ed.) *Huntington's Disease.* W.B. Saunders, London. 1991.
3   Huntington G. On chorea. *Med Surg Reporter* 1872;**26**:320–321.
4   Steinert H. Myopathologische Beitrage 1. Uber das klinische und anatomische bild des Muskelschwunds der Myotoniker. *Dtsch Z Nervenheilkd* 1909;**37**:58–104.
5   Batten FE, Gibb HP. Myotonia atrophica. *Brain* 1909;**32**:187–205.
6   Punnett RC. Mendelian inheritance in man. *Proc R Soc Med* 1908;**1**:135–168.
7   Fleischer B. Uber myotonische dystrophie mit katarakt. Albrecht von Graefes. *Arch Klin Ophthalmol* 1918;**96**:91–133.
8   Entres JL. Uber Huntington'sche chorea. *Z Gesamte Neurol Psychiatrie* 1921;**73**:541–551.
9   Hoffmann J. Uber chorea chronica progressiva (Huntingtonsche chorea hereditaria). *Virchows Arch* Pathol Anat 1888;**111**:513–548.
10 Vanier TM. Dystrophia myotonica in childhood. *Br Med J* 1960;**2**:1284–1288.
11 Harper PS, Dyken PR. Early onset dystrophia myotonica — evidence supporting a maternal environmental factor. *Lancet* 1972;**2**:53–55.
12 Harper PS. Congenital myotonic dystrophy in Britain 1. Clinical aspects. *Arch Dis Child* 1975;**50**:505–513.
13 Harper PS. Congenital myotonic dystrophy in Britain 2. Genetic basis. *Arch Dis Child* 1975;**50**:514–521.
14 Merrit AD, Conneally PM, Rahman NF, Drew AL. Juvenile Huntington's chorea. In: *Progress in Neurogenetics 1*, edited by Barbeau A, Brunnette JR. Excerpta Medica, Amsterdam. 1969.
15 Harper PS, Harley HG, Reardon W *et al.* Anticipation in myotonic dystrophy: new light on an old problem. *Am J Hum Genet* 1992;**51**:10.
16 Penrose LS. The problem of anticipation in pedigrees of dystrophia myotonica. *Ann Eugen (Lond)* 1948;**14**:125–232.
17 Höweler CJ, Busch HFM, Geraedts JPM, Niermeijer MR, Staal A. Anticipation in myotonic dystrophy: fact or fiction. *Brain* 1989;**112**:779–797.
18 Sherman S, Jacobs PA, Morton N *et al.* Further segregation analysis of the fragile X syndrome with special reference to transmitting males. *Hum Genet* 1985;**69**:289–299.
19 Harper PS. *Myotonic Dystrophy.* W.B. Saunders, 1989, pp. 309–312.
20 Ridley RM, Frith CD, Crow TJ, Conneally PM. Anticipation in Huntington's disease is inherited through the male line but may originate in the female. *J Med Genet* 1988;**25**:589–595.
21 Nowak R. Geneticists prove clinicians' hunches right about myotonic dystrophy. *J NIH Res* 1992;**4**:49.
22 Harper PS. The gene for Huntington's disease — a personal view. *MRC News* 1993; Autumn 38–40.

23 Shiang R, Thompson IM, Zhu YZ, Church DM. Mutations in the transmembrane domain of FGFR3 cause the most common genetic form of dwarfism, achondroplasia. *Cell* 1994;**78**:335–342.

24 Harley HG, Brook JD, Floyd J *et al.* Detection of linkage disequilibrium between the myotonic dystrophy locus and a new polymorphic DNA marker. *Am J Hum Genet* 1991;**49**:68.

25 Snell RG, Lazarou LP, Youngman S *et al.* Linkage disequilibrium in Huntington's disease: an improved localisation for the gene. *J Med Genet* 1989;**26**:673–675.

26 Harley HG, Brook JD, Rundle SA *et al.* Expansion of an unstable DNA region and phenotypic variation in myotonic dystrophy. *Nature* 1992;**355**:545.

27 Oberle I, Rousseau F, Helz D *et al.* Instability of a 550 base-pair DNA segment and abnormal methylation in fragile X syndrome. *Science* 1991;**262**:1097–1102.

28 Buxton J, Shelbourne P, Davies J *et al.* Detection of an unstable fragment of DNA specific to individuals with myotonic dystrophy. *Nature* 1992;**355**:547.

29 Aslanidis C, Jensen G, Amemiya C *et al.* Cloning of the essential myotonic dystrophy region and mapping of the putative defect. *Nature* 1992;**255**:548.

30 The Huntington's Disease Collaborative Research Group. A novel gene containing a trinucleotide repeat that is expanded and unstable on Huntington's disease chromosomes. *Cell* 1993;**72**:971–983.

31 Harley HG, Rundle SA, MacMillan J *et al.* Size of the unstable CTG repeat sequence in relation to phenotype and parental transmission in myotonic dystrophy. *Am J Hum Genet* 1993;**52**:1164.

32 Snell RG, MacMillan JC, Cheadle JP *et al.* Relationship between trinucleotide repeat expansion and phenotypic variation in Huntington's disease. *Nature Genetics* 1993;**4**:393–397.

33 Harley HG, Rundle SA, Reardon W *et al.* Unstable DNA sequence in myotonic dystrophy. *Lancet* 1992;**339**:1125.

34 Ashizawa T, Anvret M, Baiget M *et al.* Characteristics of intergenerational contractions of the CTG repeat in myotonic dystrophy. *Am J Hum Genet* 1994;**54**:414–423.

35 MacDonald ME, Barnes G, Srinidhi J *et al.* Gametic but not somatic instability of CAG repeat length in Huntington's disease. *J Med Genet* 1993;**30**:982–986.

36 Reardon W, Harley HG, Brook JD *et al.* Minimal expression of myotonic dystrophy: a clinical and molecular analysis. *J Med Genet* 1992;**29**:770.

37 Goldberg YP, Andrew SW, Theilmann J *et al.* Familial predisposition to recurrent mutations causing Huntington's disease: genetic risk to sibs of sporadic cases. *J Med Genet* 1993;**30**:987–990.

38 Mathieu J, De Braekeleer M, Prevost C. Genealogical reconstruction of myotonic dystrophy in the Saguenay-Lac-Saint-Jean area. *Neurology* 1990;**40**:839.

39 Imbert G, Kretz C, Johnson K, Mandel J-L. Origin of the expansion mutation in myotonic dystrophy. *Nature Genet* 1993;**4**:72.

40 Goldman A, Ramsay M, Jenkins T. Absence of myotonic dystrophy in Southern African negroids is associated with a significantly lower number of CTG trinucleotide repeats. *J Med Genet* 1994;**31**:41–44.

41 Brook JD, McCurrach ME, Harley HG *et al.* Molecular basis of myotonic dystrophy: expansion of a trinucleotide (CTG) repeat at the 3′ end of a transcript encoding a protein kinase family member. *Cell* 1992;**68**:799.

42 Fu Y-H, Pizzuti A, Fenwick RG *et al.* An unusual triplet repeat in a gene related to myotonic dystrophy. *Science* 1992;**255**:1256.

43 Mahadevan M, Tsilfidis C, Sabourin L *et al.* Myotonic dystrophy mutation: an unstable CTG repeat in the 3′ untranslated region of a candidate gene. *Science* 1992;255:1253–1255.

44 Perutz MF, Johnson T, Suzuki M *et al.* Glutamine repeats as polar zippers: their possible role in inherited neurodegenerative disease. *Proc Natl Acad Sci* 1994;**91**:5355–5358.

45 LaSpada AR, Wilson EM, Lubahn DB *et al.* Androgen receptor gene mutations in X-linked spinal and bulbar muscular atrophy. *Nature* 1991;**352**:77–79.

46 MacMillan JC, Davies P, Harper PS. Molecular diagnostic analysis for Huntington's disease: a prospective evaluation. *J Neurol Neurosurg Psychiatry* 1993;**58**:496–498.

The molecular control of angiogenesis and epithelial tubulogenesis

ROBERTO MONTESANO

A central issue in developmental biology concerns the control of morphogenesis, i.e. the process by which groups of interacting cells give rise to precisely organized three-dimensional structures. Within this vast field, we have focused on the mechanisms of two clinically relevant morphogenetic processes: the formation of new capillary blood vessels (angiogenesis), and the generation of branching epithelial tubules (tubulogenesis), which is a crucial event in the development of most parenchymal organs. In this review, we will describe the elaboration of *in vitro* models of angiogenesis and epithelial tubulogenesis, and discuss the role of paracrine-acting growth factors and cell–extracellular matrix interactions in these processes.

THE MOLECULAR CONTROL OF ANGIOGENESIS

The establishment of a vascular supply is an absolute requirement for inflow of nutrients, outflow of waste products, and gas exchange in most tissues and organs. Not surprisingly, the cardiovascular system is the first organ system to develop and reach a functional state in the embryo. Two processes have been implicated in blood vessel formation: vasculogenesis, the *in situ* differentiation of mesodermal precursors into endothelial cells, and angiogenesis, the formation of new capillary blood vessels by a process of sprouting from pre-existing vessels. While vasculogenesis appears to be limited to the early embryonic period, angiogenesis can occur throughout life. Under normal conditions, capillary proliferation is tightly controlled in adult tissues and only occurs during the female reproductive cycle (e.g. in the corpus luteum and regenerating endometrium), in the placenta during pregnancy, and as a result of tissue injury such as wound healing or ischaemia. Angiogenesis may however be detrimental to the organism. This occurs in pathological conditions such as proliferative retinopathy and childhood haemangioma. Angiogenesis is also necessary for the continued growth of solid tumours, and allows the haematogenous dissemination of tumour cells and the formation of metastases (reviewed in [1]).

The series of morphogenetic events which result in the formation of new capillary blood vessels has been well-described [1]. Angiogenesis begins with localized breakdown of the basement membrane of the parent vessel. Endothelial cells then migrate into the surrounding matrix within which they form a capillary sprout. As the sprouts elongate by migration and proliferation of endothelial cells, a lumen is gradually formed proximal to the migrating front. Contiguous tubular sprouts subsequently anastomose to form functional capillary loops, and vessel maturation is completed by reconstitution of the basement membrane [2]. Alterations in at least three endothelial cell functions thus occur during this series of events:

1 modulation of interactions with the extracellular matrix, which requires alterations of cell–matrix contacts and the production of matrix-degrading proteolytic enzymes;

2 an initial increase and subsequent decrease in locomotion (migration), which allows the cells to translocate towards the angiogenic stimulus and to stop once they reach their destination;

3 an increase in proliferation, which provides new cells for the growing and elongating vessel, and a subsequent return to the quiescent state once the vessel is formed.

In view of the physiological and pathological importance of angiogenesis, much work has been dedicated over the last decade to the identification of factors capable of regulating this process. A number of polypeptide growth factors produced by both normal and tumour cells have been shown to stimulate formation of new capillary blood vessels *in vivo*. The most thoroughly characterized of these angiogenic cytokines are acidic and basic fibroblast growth factors (aFGF, bFGF), vascular endothelial growth factor (VEGF; also known as vascular permeability factor), transforming growth factor β_1 (TGF-β_1) and tumour necrosis factor α (TNF-α), (reviewed in [3]). However, while bFGF and VEGF are mitogenic for endothelial cells, TGF-β and TNF-α inhibit their growth. The angiogenic effect of the latter two cytokines is therefore believed to be mediated in part by direct-acting angiogenesis factors released from chemoattracted inflammatory cells.

Despite our detailed knowledge of the sequential steps of the neovascularization process from descriptive *in vivo* studies and the identification of a host of angiogenesis-modulating cytokines, the molecular mechanisms of angiogenesis remain poorly understood. Two of the most widely used methods for studying angiogenesis *in vivo* are the chick chorioallantoic membrane assay and the rabbit corneal micropocket assay [1]. These assays have been used for many years to describe the morphological events of angiogenesis, to identify stimulators and inhibitors of angiogenesis, and to quantitate the neovascular response to test compounds. Although these *in vivo* assays are essential to establish whether a given molecule stimulates blood vessel formation *in vivo*, their interpretation is complicated by the fact that an angiogenic response can be elicited indirectly through the recruitment of inflammatory cells. To circumvent this drawback and to facilitate the study of the target cells, *in vitro* assays have now been developed for several of the cellular mechanisms of the angiogenic process. These include assays for endothelial cell proliferation, migration and production of proteolytic enzymes, as well as assays for formation of capillary-like cords or tubes. In an attempt to understand better the mechanisms that regulate angiogenesis, we have developed a number of additional experimental models in which important components of this process can be accurately recapitulated, modulated and analysed under well-defined *in vitro* conditions. In particular, in order to approximate the *in vivo* situation as closely as possible, we have designed three-dimensional culture systems which allow the re-establishment of interactions between microvascular endothelial cells and the surrounding extracellular matrix.

Collagen matrix promotes the organization of endothelial cells into capillary-like tubules

In vivo, microvascular endothelial cells experience a different extracellular matrix environment, depending on whether they are in a resting state or are undergoing sprouting and migration during angiogenesis. In the normal quiescent state, endothelial cells rest on a specialized extracellular matrix, the basement membrane, which contains predominantly type IV collagen and laminin. During angiogenesis, however, these cells focally degrade their investing basement membrane, and subsequently migrate into the interstitial matrix of the surrounding connective tissue, which consists mainly of type I collagen [2]. In an attempt to understand the role of the extracellular matrix in the process of angiogenesis, we have studied the interactions of endothelial cells with three-dimensional gels of reconstituted type I collagen fibrils. When a monolayer of microvascular endothelial cells on the surface of a collagen gel is covered with a second layer of collagen, it reorganizes within a few days into a network of branching and anastomosing tubules (Fig. 1). These experiments demonstrated that a three-dimensional interaction with collagen fibrils plays an important role in the organization of endothelial cells into capillary-like tubes [4].

The induction of the invasive phenotype

In the studies described above [4], formation of capillary-like tubules was experimentally induced by embedding endothelial cells within a three-dimensional collagen matrix. During angiogenesis *in vivo*, however, the morphogenetic events that culminate in the formation of new blood capillaries are intimately associated with the activation of an invasive

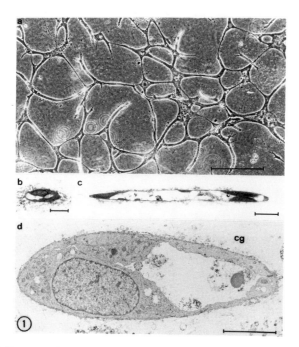

Fig. 1 (a) Collagen matrix promotes the organization of endothelial cells into capillary-like tubules. Phase-contrast microscopy of a culture of microvascular endothelial cells grown initially on top of a collagen gel and subsequently covered with a second layer of collagen. Four days after being overlaid, the existing monolayer has reorganized into a network of branching and anastomosing cords of endothelial cells. (b–d) Sections for light (b,c) and electron (d) microscopy perpendicular to a culture of capillary endothelial cells sandwiched between two collagen layers as in (a). The endothelial cells surround a central lumen so as to form capillary-like tubular structures. cg, Collagen gel.
(a) Bar = 200 μm; (b) bar = 10 μm; (c) bar = 20 μm; (d) bar = 5 μm. Reproduced with permission from [40].

process, i.e. the local breakdown of the microvascular basement membrane and the penetration of endothelial sprouts into the interstitial extracellular matrix. Central to the understanding of the mechanisms of angiogenesis is therefore the question of how normally quiescent endothelial cells acquire invasive properties that endow them with the ability to migrate through the extracellular matrix.

Our earlier studies [4] had shown that endothelial cells grown on a collagen gel form a monolayer on the surface of the gel and do not invade the underlying matrix. We asked whether it might be possible to induce the endothelial cells to penetrate into the collagen matrix, as they do during angiogenesis *in vivo*. Cell invasiveness in angiogenesis and in other biological processes is believed to require the elaboration of matrix-degrading proteolytic enzymes, which include metalloproteases such as collagenases, and serine proteases such as plasminogen activators (PAs) [5]. To investigate the possible role of proteases in endothelial cell invasiveness *in vitro*, confluent monolayers of either microvascular or large-vessel endothelial cells on collagen gels were treated with phorbol myristate acetate (PMA), a tumour promoter that markedly stimulates their production of collagenase and PAs [5]. Whereas control endothelial cells were confined to the surface of the gels, PMA-treated endothelial cells invaded the underlying collagen matrix, within which they formed capillary-like tubular structures. This phenomenon was associated with the degradation of collagen fibrils and was prevented by 1,10-phenanthroline, an inhibitor of metalloproteases, which suggested the involvement of a collagenase in the invasive process [6,7].

bFGF induces angiogenesis *in vitro*

The experiments described above [6,7] indicated that endothelial cells, even after repeated passage in culture, retain the potential to express a latent angiogenic programme, that may be switched on by appropriate signals. To establish whether physiological messengers could elicit an angiogenic response similar to that induced by PMA, microvascular endothelial cells grown on collagen gels were treated with bFGF, one of the best characterized angiogenic polypeptides (for review, see [1,3]). bFGF induced the endothelial cells to invade the underlying collagen matrix and to form capillary-like tubules (Fig. 2), as previously observed in response to PMA. Concomitantly, bFGF stimulated the endothelial cells to produce PAs [8]. These results showed that, *in vitro*, bFGF can induce two essential components of angiogenesis, namely invasion of a three-dimensional extracellular matrix and morphogenesis of endothelial tubules. In addition, since bFGF is unable to induce tubule formation in conventional culture systems, these studies highlighted the importance of cell–matrix interactions in the response of endothelial cells to angiogenic factors.

Synergism between VEGF and bFGF in the induction of angiogenesis *in vitro*

VEGF, also known as vascular permeability factor, is an endothelial cell-specific mitogen which is angiogenic *in vivo* (for a review, see [9]). We found that, like bFGF [8], VEGF induces microvascular endothelial cells grown on collagen gels to invade the underlying matrix, within which they form capillary-like tubules [10]. The most striking effect of VEGF, however, was observed in combination with bFGF: when added simultaneously, VEGF and bFGF induced an *in vitro* angiogenic response which was far greater than additive [10]. These results demonstrate that, by acting in concert, these two cytokines have a potent synergistic effect on the induction of angiogenesis *in vitro*. The synergism between these two cytokines has recently been confirmed in a rabbit model of hind-limb

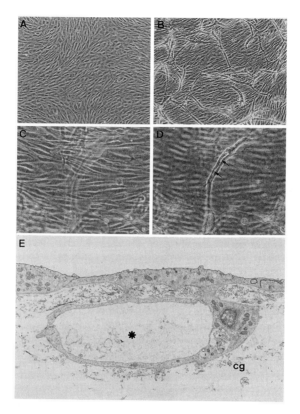

Fig. 2 Basic fibroblast growth factor (bFGF) induces *in vitro* angiogenesis in the collagen gel invasion assay. (A) Microvascular endothelial cells grown on a collagen gel form a monolayer of closely apposed cells. (B) Three days after addition of bFGF, the cells have formed a network of branching cords. (C,D) Higher magnification of a bFGF-treated culture. The same field is shown at two different planes of focus. In (C), the focus is on the gel surface. By focusing beneath the surface monolayer (D), an endothelial cell cord containing a lumen-like translucent space (arrows) can be seen. The cord appears blurred in (C). When viewed in cross-section by electron microscopy (E), a cell cord invading the collagen gel (cg) is seen to contain a lumen (asterisk), and is structurally similar to capillaries *in vivo*. (A,B) = 70×; (C,D) = 175×; (E) = 5400×. (E), is reproduced with permission from [8].

ischaemia, in which coadministration of bFGF and VEGF resulted in a marked stimulation of collateral blood vessel formation [11]. The finding of a synergism between bFGF and VEGF may therefore have important therapeutic applications.

Proteolytic balance and capillary morphogenesis

The coordinate modulation of invasive behaviour and PAs production by PMA [5,6,12], bFGF [8,12] and VEGF [10,13], together with our demonstration of an increase in urokinase-type PA (u-PA) and u-PA receptor expression [14,15] in endothelial cells migrating from the edge of an experimental wound *in vitro*, supported the proposed role for the PA-plasmin system [5] in angiogenesis. The expression of proteolytic activity by endothelial cells must, however, be tightly controlled in order to prevent inappropriate matrix degradation. That the balance between proteases and protease inhibitors might be essential for capillary morphogenesis was first demonstrated in experiments in which fibrin gels were substituted for collagen gels, the reasoning being that angiogenesis often occurs in a fibrin-rich matrix, for example during wound healing. When grown on the surface of a three-dimensional fibrin gel and treated with PMA [16] or bFGF [12], endothelial cells progressively lysed their underlying substrate. The absence of a three-dimensional substrate therefore precluded invasion and formation of capillary-like tubules. However, inhibition of fibrinolysis by addition of serine protease inhibitors allowed the preservation of a three-dimensional matrix scaffold into which endothelial cells could be induced to migrate to form tube-like structures. These results suggested that neutralization of excess proteolytic activity by protease inhibitors plays an important permissive role in angiogenesis by preventing inappropriate or premature degradation of the extracellular matrix [12,16].

Additional indirect support for this hypothesis came from the finding that agents which induce invasion and tube formation *in vitro*, namely PMA [6], bFGF [8] and VEGF [10], increase not only u-PA [5,8,12,13], but also the physiological inhibitor of u-PA, PA inhibitor type 1 (PAI-1) [12,13,17] in microvascular endothelial cells, as well as by the finding of a concomitant increase in u-PA and PAI-1 in endothelial cells migrating in two dimensions from the edge of a wounded monolayer [14,18]. A detailed analysis of the role of u-PA and PAI-1 in capillary-like tube formation *in vitro* was performed using two cytokines, namely bFGF and TGF-β_1, which have opposite effects on endothelial cell proteolytic activity [17]. bFGF, which increases proteolysis (as reflected by the ratio of u-PA to PAI-1 messenger RNA), induced endothelial cells to form tube-like structures with large ectatic lumina in fibrin gels, whereas coaddition of TGF-β_1, which decreases the u-PA/PAI-1 ratio, reduced lumen size [12,19].

What happens then when there is excessive and uncontrolled proteolysis? The answer to this question was provided by the study of endothelial cells expressing the polyomavirus middle T (mT) oncogene, which have been shown to induce formation of cyst-like endothelial tumours (endotheliomas) when injected into mice [20]. We have developed an *in vitro* correlate of endothelioma formation by embedding mT-expressing endothelial cells into three-dimensional fibrin gels. In contrast to normal endothelial cells, which formed a network of capillary-like tubules, mT-expressing endothelial cells formed large cysts which bear a striking resemblance to the endotheliomas which were seen *in vivo* (Fig. 3). In

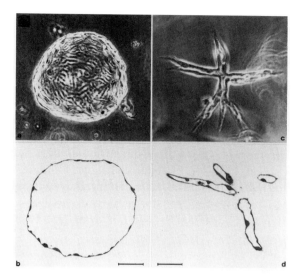

Fig. 3 Morphogenetic behaviour of middle T (mT)-expressing endothelial cells grown within fibrin gels under control conditions or in the presence of exogenously added serine protease inhibitors. (a) Spherical cyst formed by mT-expressing endothelial cells grown within a fibrin gel (phase-contrast microscopy). In this picture, the focus is approximately on the equatorial plane of the cyst. The endothelial cells lining the floor and the roof of the cavity appear blurred in the centre of the cyst. (b) Semithin section of an endothelial cyst. The large cavity is lined by a continuous monolayer of flattened endothelial cells. (c,d) Branching capillary-like tubules formed by mT-expressing endothelial cells grown within a fibrin gel in the presence of the serine protease inhibitors ε-aminocaproic acid (c) or Trasylol (d). (a,b) Bar = 100 μm; (c,d) bar = 50 μm. Reproduced with permission from [41].

addition, mT-expressing endothelial cells produced greater PA activity but very little PAI-1 when compared to endothelial cells not expressing mT. Neutralization of the unbalanced proteolytic activity of mT-expressing endothelial cells by addition of exogenous serine protease inhibitors to the culture system corrected their aberrant morphogenetic behaviour and resulted in the formation of capillary-like branching tubules [21]. Taken together, the results described above suggest that a precisely regulated balance between proteases and protease inhibitors is necessary for normal capillary morphogenesis (for a more detailed discussion of the notion of endothelial proteolytic balance, see [22,23]).

Potential clinical implications of *in vitro* studies of angiogenesis

Angiogenesis plays an important role in a wide range of physiological and pathological processes. Modulation of the angiogenic process has therefore been proposed as an alternative or adjunct to current therapeutic modalities in several diseases characterized by local hyper- or hypovascularity. *Inhibition of angiogenesis* has long been recognized as a potential strategy for cancer treatment [24]. Although angiogenesis is required for the growth of solid tumours beyond $1-2 \text{ mm}^3$, under physiological conditions it is only required for wound healing and reproductive functions. Complete inhibition of angiogenesis should therefore be well-tolerated by most adults. Inhibition of angiogenesis is also of potential benefit in the treatment of ocular neovascularization (e.g. diabetic proliferative retinopathy) and of life-threatening childhood haemangiomas. The redundancy of angiogenesis-stimulating cytokines may however hinder therapeutic strategies based on neutralization of angiogenic factors. Since sprouting endothelial cells must invade and translocate across the extracellular matrix regardless of the nature of the angiogenic stimulus, targeting cellular processes such as extracellular proteolysis or integrin-mediated cell–matrix interactions may overcome the problems of growth factor redundancy. We therefore believe that a better understanding of the molecular mechanisms of angiogenesis may allow the design of angiostatic agents capable of inhibiting inappropriate blood vessel growth in a variety of clinical settings. Identification of additional inhibitors of angiogenesis is potentially of great importance, because different anti-angiogenic agents may act through diverse mechanisms and may therefore achieve maximum therapeutic effect when administered in appropriate combinations.

Stimulation of angiogenesis, on the other hand, can accelerate the healing of wounds and peptic ulcers, and promotes growth of collateral vessels in ischaemic diseases. Coronary atherosclerosis, peripheral arterial occlusion and cerebral vascular insufficiency are amongst the commonest causes of morbidity and mortality in western societies. Under normal conditions, the ischaemia caused by obstruction of an artery stimulates the development of collateral vessels, which however are often insufficient to maintain normal tissue perfusion. This situation may result in myocardial infarction, stroke or gangrene of the extremities. Recent work has demonstrated that administration of angiogenic factors can enhance the growth of collateral vessels in animal models of myocardial, peripheral and cerebral arterial insufficiency (reviewed in [25,26]). Considering that no effective drug therapy currently exists for many patients with critical leg ischaemia or disabling claudication, these results suggest that 'therapeutic angiogenesis may have an immense clinical potential' [26]. We are confident that the use of *in vitro* systems may contribute to the development of therapeutic angiogenesis by allowing the identification of additional physiological stimulators of angiogenesis and of other examples of synergistic interactions, as we have shown previously for the combination of bFGF and VEGF [10]. Evidence from recent *in vivo* studies [11] suggests that in situations where stimulation of angiogenesis is desired, the benefit derived from coaddition of two cytokines whose interaction is synergistic would be greater than that derived from the addition of one of these cytokines alone.

THE MOLECULAR CONTROL OF EPITHELIAL TUBULOGENESIS

The formation of epithelial organs during embryonic development involves an ordered sequence of morphogenetic processes that ultimately result in the construction of precisely organized multicellular structures. Remarkably, different epithelia acquire diverse forms that are appropriate for their specific functions, such as the thyroid follicles, the kidney tubules and the complex branching ducts found in the lung and exocrine glands. Although a great deal has been learned about the general principles underlying the biogenesis of polarized epithelial monolayers, the mechanisms responsible for the generation of tissue-specific patterns of epithelial architecture are less well-understood [27].

During embryogenesis, definitive epithelial organs frequently arise from pre-existing epithelial tissues. Commonly, these developing epithelia are surrounded by mesenchyme, and it has long been recognized that epithelial–mesenchymal interactions are required to bring about proper epithelial morphogenesis. Thus, using tissue dissociation techniques, it has been demonstrated that the embryonic epithelia of the kidney, lung, salivary glands and pancreas fail to undergo branching morphogenesis if separated from the adjacent mesenchyme, and that morphogenesis resumes when the components are recombined *in vitro*. However, the molecular mechanisms involved in these inductive interactions have only recently begun to be elucidated [27,28]. Postulated mesenchymal factors include:
(a) components of the extracellular matrix;
(b) cell surface-associated molecules acting by direct contact; and
(c) diffusible factors.
The notion that extracellular matrix components mediate, at least in part, the inducing effect of mesenchyme on epithelial morphogenesis is now supported by a large body of experimental evidence. For example, numerous *in vitro* studies have shown that reconstituted matrices such as collagen or basement membrane gels promote the organization of epithelial cells into three-dimensional, tissue-like structures. Thus, when embedded in collagen gels, thyroid follicular cells form follicles [29], whereas pancreatic endocrine cells form islet-like organoids [30]. It is noteworthy, however, that the epithelial structures formed under these experimental conditions do not always accurately reproduce the *in vivo* architecture of the tissue of origin, which suggests that additional cues are required for histotypic morphogenesis.

At the beginning of this decade, despite the increasing recognition of the involvement of polypeptide growth factors in early embryonic development, virtually nothing was known about the role of soluble mediators in the morphogenesis of epithelial structures. This paucity of knowledge was due in part to the lack of suitable model systems in which simple morphogenetic processes could be recapitulated, modulated and analysed under well-defined *in vitro* conditions. Considering that adult epithelia remain responsive to inductive influences from connective tissue [31], our approach to this problem has been to assess the effect of diffusible stromal factors on the morphogenetic properties of well-differentiated epithelial cells grown in a three-dimensional collagen matrix.

Fibroblast-derived soluble factors induce morphogenesis of branching tubules by kidney epithelial cells

The Madin-Darby canine kidney (MDCK) cell line represents a parti- cularly attractive model system for studying the factors that govern the ordered assembly of epithelial cells into spatially organized multicellular units. MDCK cells have been shown to retain several anatomical and functional properties of kidney distal tubule or collecting duct epithelium and to generate tubule-like structures *in vivo*. However, when grown within three-dimensional collagen gels, MDCK cells form spherical cysts [32]. These observations raised an interesting question: have MDCK cells irreversibly lost the capacity to organize into epithelial tubules *in vitro*, or have they retained a latent tubulogenic potential that can be unmasked by specific signals which are missing in the collagen matrix? To address this issue, we set out to investigate whether the morphogenetic properties of MDCK cells might be influenced by diffusible factors released by neighbouring mesenchymal or stromal cells. Our strategy has been to design an *in vitro* system in which MDCK cells are cocultured in collagen gels with embryonic or adult fibroblasts under conditions precluding heterocellular contact.

By using this experimental approach, we have obtained evidence that fibroblast-derived soluble factors play a crucial role in the control of epithelial morphogenesis. This evidence is based on the following obser- vations: first, MDCK cells suspended within a collagen gel contiguous to a fibroblast-populated gel layer formed branching tubules, instead of the spherical cysts that developed under control conditions, i.e. in the absence of fibroblasts (Fig. 4). Second, MDCK cells grown as a monolayer on a cell-free collagen gel cast on top of a fibroblast-containing gel layer invaded the underlying collagen matrix, within which they formed a network of branching tubules. Third, fibroblast-conditioned medium mimicked the effect of coculture by eliciting tubule formation by MDCK cells [33].

To assess whether well-characterized growth and differentiation factors could mediate the tubulogenic effect of fibroblast-conditioned media, MDCK cells grown in collagen gels were incubated with epidermal

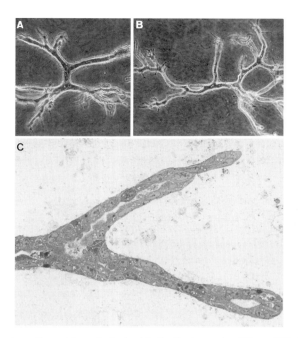

Fig. 4 Formation of branching tubules by Madin-Darby canine kidney (MDCK) cells cocultured with 3T3 fibroblasts. MDCK cells were suspended within a collagen gel layered on to a preformed collagen gel containing 3T3 fibroblasts. (A,B) Phase-contrast microscopy (125×); (C) semithin section (650×). Reproduced with permission from [33].

growth factor (EGF), bFGF, aFGF, TGF-β_1, insulin-like growth factor I (IGF-I), insulin-like growth factor II (IGF-II), platelet-derived growth factor (PDGF), or keratinocyte growth factor (KGF). None of these treatments modified the morphogenetic behaviour of MDCK cells, which formed spherical cysts as observed under control conditions. These results therefore suggested that the tubulogenic activity in fibroblast-conditioned media was distinct from a number of well-characterized cytokines, and that it could represent either a novel molecule(s) or a hitherto unsuspected function of a known molecule(s) [33].

Hepatocyte growth factor is a paracrine mediator of morphogenetic epithelial–mesenchymal interactions

While we were attempting to identify the fibroblast-derived factors responsible for the induction of tubule formation by MDCK cells (see above), it was reported that hepatocyte growth factor (HGF), a polypeptide considered to be a humoral mediator of liver regeneration [34], is produced by cultured fibroblasts and stimulates the proliferation of a broad spectrum of epithelial cells [35]. These new data prompted us to explore the effect of HGF in our system.

We found that MDCK cells grown in collagen gels in the presence of HGF formed linear or branching tubular structures. In addition, MDCK cells grown in the presence of fibroblast-conditioned medium that had been preincubated with specific anti-HGF antibodies exclusively formed spherical cysts similar to those observed in control cultures, i.e. in the absence of conditioned medium. Anti-HGF antibodies also suppressed tubulogenesis in cocultures of MDCK cells and fibroblasts (Fig. 5). These data demonstrated that the fibroblast-derived factor that induces tubule formation by MDCK cells is HGF [36].

HGF was originally identified in rat serum as a potent mitogen for cultured hepatocytes, and was therefore considered to have a narrow target cell specificity and to act primarily as a humoral mediator of liver regeneration after partial hepatectomy or hepatic injury [34]. However, it has subsequently been shown that HGF is the same molecule as scatter factor (SF), a fibroblast-derived polypeptide which was identified by its ability

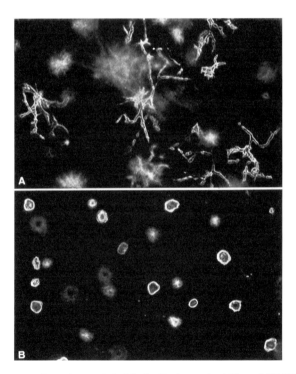

Fig. 5 Suppression of tubulogenesis in Madin-Darby canine kidney (MDCK) cells/ fibroblast cocultures by antibodies to hepatocyte growth factor (HGF). MDCK cells were suspended in a collagen gel layered on to a collagen gel containing MRC-5 fibroblasts and grown for 6 days either (A) in the absence or (B) in the presence of anti-HGF immunoglobulin Gs (IgGs) (dark-field illumination). (A) MDCK cells incubated under control conditions (i.e. in the absence of anti-HGF antibody) have formed branching tubules. (B) MDCK cells incubated with anti-HGF IgGs (2 µg/ml) have formed spherical cysts. (A,B) 80×. Reproduced with permission from [36].

to dissociate epithelial cell colonies in monolayer culture [37]. The identity of HGF and SF raises the important question as to why the same molecule induces formation of well-organized tubules by MDCK cells grown in collagen gels, while causing dissociation of MDCK cell colonies grown in conventional tissue culture dishes [37]. Since we have observed that HGF induces scattering of MDCK colonies grown either in plastic dishes or *on top* of collagen gels, the critical factor that dictates whether these cells will dissociate or organize into tubules in response to HGF/SF is likely to be the geometry of cell–substrate interactions (i.e. two-dimensional versus three-dimensional interactions). It is well-known that epithelial cells grown *on the surface* of collagen gels spread extensively and form a monolayer, whereas they organize into three-dimensional tissue-like structures when embedded *within* a collagen gel (see, for example, [29,30]). It is therefore conceivable that the stimulating effect of HGF/SF on cell motility and migration may elicit different biological responses depending upon the geometrical relationships between the target cells and their substratum. Thus, stimulation of cell motility in monolayer cultures may result solely in dissociation and scattering of preformed epithelial colonies. In contrast, the complex topographical and mechanical cues conveyed by a three-dimensional extracellular matrix scaffolding may precisely guide and orient cell movement, in such a way that ordered cell repositioning and establishment of new organizational patterns are achieved without disruption of intercellular contacts. An alternative possibility is that substrate-dependent alterations of cell shape and cytoskeletal organization transduce intracellular signals that modify cell responsiveness to HGF/SF.

Based on the considerations outlined above, we propose that cell scattering as observed on a planar substratum represents a frustrated form of morphogenetic cell movement resulting from the lack of an appropriate permissive environment. The finding that HGF can induce either dissociation or morphogenetic rearrangement of MDCK epithelial cells depending on their topological relationships with the substratum provides a vivid illustration of the concept that the biological effects of cytokines are profoundly influenced by the interaction of target cells with the surrounding extracellular matrix [38].

The finding that stroma-derived factors induce the formation of branching tubules in cultures of kidney-derived MDCK cells raised the question of whether paracrine epithelial–mesenchymal interactions might induce tubulogenesis in other types of epithelial cells. To address this issue, we investigated whether diffusible factors released by fibroblasts could promote formation of duct-like structures by mammary gland epithelial cells embedded in collagen gels. Using a clone (TAC-2) derived in our laboratory from the normal murine mammary gland (NMuMG) epithelial cell line, we found that addition of fibroblast-conditioned

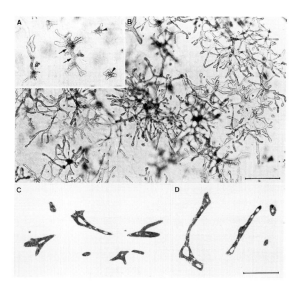

Fig. 6 Fibroblast-conditioned medium stimulates formation of branching tubules by TAC-2 mammary gland epithelial cells grown in collagen gels. (A) TAC-2 cells grown in collagen gels for 7 days under control conditions have formed small colonies with a variety of morphologies ranging from irregularly shaped cell aggregates (arrowheads) to poorly branched structures (arrows). (B) TAC-2 cells grown in collagen gels for 7 days in the presence of fibroblast-conditioned medium have formed an extensive network of highly arborized branching cords. (C,D) Semithin sections of collagen gel cultures of TAC-2 cells incubated with fibroblast-conditioned medium reveal the formation of duct-like tubular structures. (A,B) Bar = 50 µm; (C,D) bar = 100 µm. Reproduced with permission from [39].

medium to cultures of TAC-2 cells stimulated the development of an extensive system of highly arborized duct-like structures, which in appropriate sections were seen to contain a central lumen (Fig. 6). The effect of fibroblast-conditioned medium was completely abrogated by antibodies to HGF, whereas addition of exogenous HGF to the cultures mimicked the tubulogenic activity of conditioned medium (Fig. 7). The effect of HGF was markedly potentiated by the simultaneous addition of hydrocortisone, which also enhanced lumen formation [39]. These results indicate that the morphogenetic activity of HGF is not restricted to a single epithelial cell type. They also suggest that HGF is an important stroma-derived paracrine mediator of mammary gland tubulogenesis.

CONCLUDING REMARKS

Taken together, the results presented in the two parts of this review support the notion that morphogenesis of capillary blood vessels and epithelial tissues is governed by the interplay of two different classes of signalling molecules — paracrine-acting growth factors and insoluble extracellular

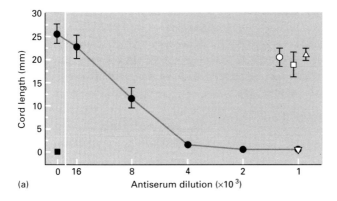

(a)

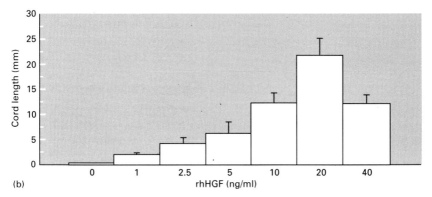

(b)

Fig. 7 Demonstration that the tubulogenic activity of fibroblast-conditioned medium (CM) on TAC-2 cells is due to hepatocyte growth factor (HGF). (a) Antiserum to HGF inhibits the tubulogenic activity of CM from MRC-5 fibroblasts. MRC-5 CM was preincubated with the indicated dilutions of rabbit anti-HGF antiserum (filled circles), anti-proalbumin antiserum (open square), anti-secretin antiserum (open circle) or non-immune serum (open triangle) prior to addition to cultures of TAC-2 cells. Values are mean cord length per colony ± s.e.m. Inverted open triangle: complete culture medium (without MRC-5 CM) preincubated with anti-HGF antiserum; filled square: complete culture medium alone. n = at least three experiments. (b) Dose-dependent induction of epithelial cord formation by recombinant human HGF (rhHGF). TAC-2 cells were suspended in collagen gels and incubated with the indicated concentrations of rhHGF for 9 days. Values are mean cord length per colony ± s.e.m. Values for all concentrations of rhHGF are significantly different from control ($P < 0.001$); n = at least three experiments for all conditions. Reproduced with permission from [39].

matrix components. Interactions of cells with the surrounding extracellular matrix, in addition to directly promoting morphogenetic events, are crucial determinants of cell responses to growth factors.

ACKNOWLEDGEMENTS

I would like to thank Drs Michael Pepper, Jean-Dominique Vassalli and

Jesus Soriano for their important contribution to the work presented in this review, and my mentor Dr Lelio Orci for enthusiastic support, encouragement, inspiration and constructive criticism. We apologize for not having been able to cite many important papers because of editorial policy limiting the length of the reference list. This work was supported by grants from the Swiss National Science Foundation.

REFERENCES

1 Folkman J, Klagsbrun M. Angiogenic factors. *Science* 1987;**235**:442–447.
2 Ausprunk DH, Folkman J. Migration and proliferation of endothelial cells in preformed and newly formed blood vessels during angiogenesis. *Microvasc Res* 1977;**14**:53–65.
3 Folkman J, Shing Y. Angiogenesis. *J Biol Chem* 1992;**267**:10931–10934.
4 Montesano R, Orci L, Vassalli P. *In vitro* rapid organization of endothelial cells into capillary-like networks is promoted by collagen matrices. *J Cell Biol* 1983;**97**:1648–1652.
5 Gross JL, Moscatelli D, Jaffe EA, Rifkin DB. Plasminogen activator and collagenase production by cultured capillary endothelial cells. *J Cell Biol* 1982;**95**:974–981.
6 Montesano R, Orci L. Tumor-promoting phorbol esters induce angiogenesis *in vitro*. *Cell* 1985;**42**:469–477.
7 Montesano R, Orci L. Phorbol esters induce angiogenesis *in vitro* from large vessel endothelial cells. *J Cell Physiol* 1987;**130**:284–291.
8 Montesano R, Vassalli J-D, Baird A, Guillemin R, Orci L. Basic fibroblast growth factor induces angiogenesis *in vitro*. *Proc Natl Acad Sci USA* 1986;**83**:7297–7301.
9 Ferrara N, Jackeman LB, Houck KA, Leung DW. Molecular and biological properties of the vascular endothelial growth factor family of proteins. *Endocr Rev* 1992;**13**:1–15.
10 Pepper MS, Ferrara N, Orci L, Montesano R. Potent synergism between vascular endothelial growth factor (VEGF) and basic fibroblast growth factor (bFGF) in the induction of angiogenesis *in vitro*. *Biochem Biophys Res Commun* 1992;**189**:824–831.
11 Asahara T, Bauters C, Zheng LP *et al*. *In vivo* synergistic effects of vascular endothelial growth factor and basic fibroblast growth factor on angiogenesis in a rabbit ischemic hind limb. *Circulation* 1994;**90**:I-585 (abstract).
12 Pepper MS, Belin D, Montesano R, Orci L, Vassalli J-D. Transforming growth factor-beta 1 modulates basic fibroblast growth factor-induced proteolytic and angiogenic properties of endothelial cells *in vitro*. *J Cell Biol* 1990;**111**:743–755.
13 Pepper MS, Ferrara N, Orci L, Montesano R. Vascular endothelial growth factor (VEGF) induces plasminogen activators and plasminogen activator inhibitor-1 in microvascular endothelial cells. *Biochem Biophys Res Commun* 1991;**181**:902–906.
14 Pepper MS, Vassalli J-D, Montesano R, Orci L. Urokinase-type plasminogen activator is induced in migrating capillary endothelial cells. *J Cell Biol* 1987;**105**:2535–2541.
15 Pepper MS, Sappino A-P, Stocklin R, Montesano R, Orci L, Vassalli J-D. Upregulation of urokinase receptor expression on migrating endothelial cells. *J Cell Biol* 1993;**122**:673–684.
16 Montesano R, Pepper MS, Vassalli J-D, Orci L. Phorbol ester induces cultured endothelial cells to invade a fibrin matrix in the presence of fibrinolytic inhibitors. *J Cell Physiol* 1987;**132**:509–516.
17 Saksela O, Moscatelli D, Rifkin DB. The opposing effects of basic fibroblast growth factor and transforming growth factor beta on the regulation of plasminogen activator activity in capillary endothelial cells. *J Cell Biol* 1987;**105**:957–963.
18 Pepper MS, Sappino A-P, Montesano R, Orci L, Vassalli J-D. Plasminogen activator inhibitor-1 is induced in migrating endothelial cells. *J Cell Physiol* 1992;**153**:129–139.
19 Pepper MS, Vassalli J-D, Orci L, Montesano R. Biphasic effect of transforming growth factor-beta-1 on *in vitro* angiogenesis. *Exp Cell Res* 1993;**204**:356–363.

20 Williams RL, Risau W, Zerwes HG, Drexler H, Aguzzi A, Wagner EF. Endothelioma cells expressing the polyoma middle T oncogene induce hemangiomas by host cell recruitment. *Cell* 1989;**57**:1053–1063.

21 Montesano R, Pepper MS, Möhle-Steinlein U, Risau W, Wagner EF, Orci L. Increased proteolytic activity is responsible for the aberrant morphogenetic behavior of endothelial cells expressing the middle T oncogene. *Cell* 1990;**62**:435–445.

22 Pepper MS, Montesano R. Proteolytic balance and capillary morphogenesis. *Cell Differ Dev* 1990;**32**:319–328.

23 Pepper MS, Vassalli J-D, Orci L, Montesano R. Angiogenesis *in vitro*: cytokine interactions and balanced extracellular proteolysis. In: *Angiogenesis. Molecular Biology, Clinical Aspects*, edited by Maragoudakis ME, Gullino PM, Lelkes PI. Plenum Press, New-York, 1994;149–170.

24 Folkman J. Tumor angiogenesis: therapeutic implications. *N Engl J Med* 1971;**285**:1182–1186.

25 Höckel M, Schlenger K, Doctrow S, Kissel T, Vaupel P. Therapeutic angiogenesis. *Arch Surg* 1993;**128**:423–429.

26 Symes JF, Sniderman AD. Angiogenesis: potential therapy for ischaemic disease. *Curr Opin Lipidol* 1994;**5**:305–312.

27 Gumbiner BM. Epithelial morphogenesis. *Cell* 1992;**69**:385–387.

28 Birchmeier C, Birchmeier W. Molecular aspects of mesenchymal–epithelial interactions. *Annu Rev Cell Biol* 1993;**9**:511–540.

29 Chambard M, Gabrion J, Mauchamp J. Influence of collagen gel on the orientation of epithelial cell polarity: follicle formation from preformed monolayers. *J Cell Biol* 1981;**91**:157–166.

30 Montesano R, Mouron P, Amherdt M, Orci L. Collagen matrix promotes reorganization of pancreatic endocrine cell monolayers into islet-like organoids. *J Cell Biol* 1983;**97**:935–939.

31 Cunha GR, Bigsby RM, Cooke PS, Sugimura Y. Stroma–epithelial interactions in adult organs. *Cell Differ* 1985;**17**:137–148.

32 McAteer JA, Evan AP, Gardner KD. Morphogenetic clonal growth of kidney epithelial cell line MDCK. *Anat Rec* 1987;**217**:229–239.

33 Montesano R, Schaller G, Orci L. Induction of epithelial tubular morphogenesis *in vitro* by fibroblast-derived soluble factors. *Cell* 1991;**66**:697–711.

34 Nakamura T, Nishizawa T, Hagiya M *et al.* Molecular cloning and expression of human hepatocyte growth factor. *Nature* 1989;**342**:440–443.

35 Rubin JS, Chan AM-L, Bottaro DP *et al.* A broad spectrum human lung fibroblast-derived mitogen is a variant of hepatocyte growth factor. *Proc Natl Acad Sci USA* 1991;**88**:415–419.

36 Montesano R, Matsumoto K, Nakamura T, Orci L. Identification of a fibroblast-derived epithelial morphogen as hepatocyte growth factor. *Cell* 1991;**67**:901–908.

37 Gherardi E, Stoker M. Hepatocytes and scatter factor. *Nature* 1990;**346**:228.

38 Nathan C, Sporn M. Cytokines in context. *J Cell Biol* 1991;**113**:981–986.

39 Soriano JV, Pepper MS, Nakamura T, Orci L, Montesano R. Hepatocyte growth factor stimulates extensive development of branching duct-like structures by cloned mammary gland epithelial cells. *J Cell Sci* 1995;**108**:413–430.

40 Montesano R, Pepper M, Orci L. Angiogenesis *in vitro*: morphogenetic and invasive properties of endothelial cells. *News Physiol Sci* 1990;**5**:75–79.

41 Montesano R, Pepper MS, Vassalli J-D, Orci L. The control of angiogenesis: endothelial cell-matrix interactions and extracellular proteolysis. In: *Endothelial and Mucus-Secreting Cells*, edited by Pozzi E. Masson, Milan, 1991:1–17.

MULTIPLE CHOICE QUESTIONS

1 The term angiogenesis applies to the process of
  a differentiation of endothelial cells from mesodermal precursors
  b formation of arteries and veins from existing microvessels
  c formation of anastomoses between arteries and veins

    d formation of new capillary blood vessels by a process of sprouting from large vessels

    e formation of new capillary blood vessels by a process of sprouting from existing microvessels

2 The addition of basic fibroblast growth factor to a confluent endothelial monolayer on a collagen gel induces the endothelial cells to

    a form tubular structures on the surface of the gel

    b migrate mostly as isolated cells into the underlying gel

    c invade the underlying gel mostly as solid cords of cells

    d invade the underlying gel mostly as tubular structures

    e degrade the collagen gel completely

3 The aberrant morphogenetic behaviour of endothelial cells expressing the polyoma middle T oncogene (i.e. cyst formation in fibrin gels) can be corrected by the addition of

    a plasmin

    b serine protease inhibitors

    c collagen type I

    d basic fibroblast growth factor

    e vascular endothelial growth factor

4 Tubule formation by Madin-Darby canine kidney (MDCK) epithelial cells grown in collagen gels is induced by

    a direct contact with stromal cells

    b production of extracellular matrix by stromal cells

    c production of diffusible factors by stromal cells

    d production of proteolytic enzymes by stromal cells

    e production of protease inhibitors by stromal cells

5 Addition of hepatocyte growth factor to colonies of MDCK cells grown *on the surface* of collagen gels induces

    a cell scattering

    b cyst formation

    c inhibition of growth

    d increased cell aggregation

    e tubule formation

Answers

1			2			3		
	a	False		**a**	False		**a**	False
	b	False		**b**	False		**b**	True
	c	False		**c**	False		**c**	False
	d	False		**d**	True		**d**	False
	e	True		**e**	False		**e**	False

4 a False
   b False
   c True
   d False
   e False

5 a True
   b False
   c False
   d False
   e False

The role of cytokines in rheumatoid arthritis

R. N. MAINI

GENES, IMMUNITY AND CYTOKINES IN THE PATHOGENESIS OF RHEUMATOID ARTHRITIS

When William Croone, the distinguished scientist and physician in whose memory this lecture is delivered, practised medicine in London in the years between 1660 and 1684, rheumatoid arthritis (RA) was not a recognized entity. It was Garrod, two centuries later, who first described this destructive disorder of joints with its predilection for women [1]. The relatively recent description of RA has prompted speculation that it is a disease of the modern age [2], perhaps reflecting an encounter with a recently introduced environmental agent of modern civilization. The pros and cons for this proposition continue to be debated, but there can be little doubt that epidemiological data support the case for genetic factors and an environmental agent in the causation of RA. Thus, a concordance rate of only 33% in identical twins, presumably with the same copies of DNA, against a background prevalence of around 1% in the general population, is a forceful argument for both an environmentally triggered disease and a genetic susceptibility [3,4].

In the past decade, exciting developments have revealed a link between genes in the human leukocyte antigen (HLA) system and the occurrence of RA. The genetic link is with the hypervariable region of the β chain of HLA-DR molecules encoding a pentapeptide sequence in positions 69–74 and expressed by the allelic variants of subtypes of HLA-DR4 (e.g. DW4, DW14 and DW15) and other types, e.g. DR1, DW16 and DR10 [5,6]. This region of similarity has given rise to the concept of a *shared epitope*, which equates with the genetic element of susceptibility to RA. The location of the susceptibility sequence within the antigen-binding groove of HLA molecules is consistent with the hypothesis that it might encode a functional epitope which is recognized by T-cells (Fig. 1). Thus, HLA-restricted antigen presentation to a T-cell could provide a rational explanation for the previously recognized features of RA such as activated T and B lymphocytes in the rheumatoid synovium and, via T- and B-cell cooperation, the occurrence of disease-specific autoantibodies, which include

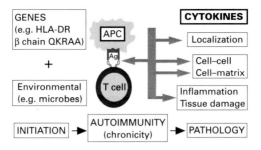

Fig. 1 The pathogenesis of rheumatoid arthritis can be viewed as a multistep process. Environmental factors (e.g. antigens of microorganisms) may initiate an immune response by antigen binding to human leukocyte antigen (HLA)-DR molecules and this bimolecular complex interacting with a T-cell receptor. The genetic susceptibility to RA has been mapped to a shared epitope expressed by some DR4 subtypes and DR1 on the β chain of HLA-DR alleles. Subsequently the immune response could be perpetuated by autoantigens (for example, by molecular mimicry or epitope spreading). Localization of the disease process to joints and other tissues involves adhesion of cytokine-activated endothelial cells to counterligands on circulating leukocytes. These leukocytes then traverse the vascular barrier under the influence of chemokines. In tissues, cell–cell and cell–matrix interactions in synovium and at the cartilage–pannus junction further perpetuate inflammation and joint damage.

rheumatoid factors of all isotypes, as well as immunoglobulin G (IgG) antiperinuclear, antikeratin and anti-RA33 (antinuclear) antibodies [7].

While disease initiation may be explained by an immune response to an environmental antigen and perpetuation (or chronicity) of disease by autoimmunity, increasing knowledge of the role of cytokines in RA provides a framework for understanding the pathophysiology of localization of the disease to joints. It illuminates our understanding of the locally destructive potential of the immunoinflammatory response and the systemic features of the disease [8]. Indeed, it can be argued that, in established chronic RA, cytokines become the dominant biological force, with the trimolecular immunological interaction between HLA molecules, peptide antigens, and T-cell receptors, which was critical at the initiation of disease, playing a low-key, but obligatory, role in its perpetuation (Fig. 2).

- Initiation
- Perpetuation
- Localization
- Inflammation
- Organ damage

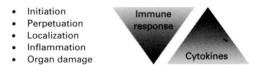

Fig. 2 The triangles show the hypothetical inverse relationship of the importance of an immune response and cytokine-mediated pathophysiology in the steps involved in the pathogenesis of rheumatoid arthritis. The immune response is more important in initiating and perpetuating chronicity and could play a part in localization to tissues, whilst cytokines are more implicated in regulation of cellular traffic, inflammation and joint damage.

Cytokines are intercellular messenger molecules which principally exert their effects on other cells in the local milieu in which they are produced by binding to their cognate receptors. In reality, many cytokines are produced in the course of a biological response to a stimulus. The interconnections, resulting in agonistic and antagonistic effects, have been referred to as a *cytokine network*. When produced in sufficient quantities to circulate in blood, they can exert effects on distant tissues. At the Kennedy Institute of Rheumatology we have found that an impressive range of cytokines and natural inhibitors is produced in rheumatoid joints. The results of these investigations have been previously reported by my colleague Professor Feldmann at the College in the Watson-Smith lecture and at an advanced medicine conference (see Feldmann *et al.*, p. 343). Here I will summarize the conclusions of these experimental observations and other preclinical work which identified cytokines as being of special significance and demonstrated the importance of tumour necrosis factor α (TNF-α) as the controlling element of the cytokine network.

An important starting point of our investigations was the demonstration of interleukin-1 (IL1), TNF-α, TNF receptors and interleukin-6 (IL-6) by immunohistology in the synovial membrane of RA joints [9–13]. Here the cytokines produced by inflammatory cells, immune cells, vascular endothelium and fibroblasts were candidate agents for orchestrating the immunoinflammatory response. More importantly, TNF-α and IL-1 were also found to be present at the cartilage-pannus junction, where they could exert their destructive potential. The predominant, but not exclusive, cell type producing IL-1, TNF-α and IL-6 appeared to be derived from the macrophage lineage.

When preparations of mononuclear synovial cells (consisting of macrophages, lymphocytes, fibroblasts and other cell types), obtained by enzymatic dissociation of surgically excised synovial membranes, were analysed, IL-1, TNF-α, IL-6, IL-8, granulocyte-macrophage colony-stimulating factor (GM-CSF) and other cytokines were detectable at messenger RNA level in increased quantities over basal levels [14–18]. Upon *in vitro* culture of these mononuclear cells, without any added stimulants, all the cytokines continued to be synthesized for several days. Most significantly from the point of view of conceptual developments, their production was suppressed by the addition of neutralizing antibodies to TNF-α. These *in vitro* experiments provided the first important cue supporting a pivotal role of TNF-α in regulating the production of other cytokines [19]. The experiments demonstrated that cytokine production in RA joints behaved more like a *cascade*, with TNF-α at its head, than a *network* of randomly connected molecules.

From this array of cytokines produced in RA joints, and their known biological activities, it was possible to construct a coherent scheme and hypotheses of their possible clinicopathological significance [8,20].

• IL-1 and TNF-α emerged as the most promising candidates involved in cartilage degradation. Singly, and synergistically, these cytokines can induce synthesis and release of inflammatory mediators, such as metalloproteinases, prostaglandins and nitric oxide in many cell types, e.g. synovial fibroblasts, macrophages and chondrocytes. The production of these inflammatory mediators could well explain the destructive effects of pannus on cartilage matrix and of pericellular degradation of matrix around chondrocytes. TNF-α and IL-1 can also inhibit synthesis of matrix components, thus hindering repair mechanisms. Their effects *in vitro* were consistent with the pathology of cartilage damage observed in RA.

• IL-1 and TNF-α mediate additional effects relevant to understanding the pathogenesis of RA. For example, both cytokines induce adhesion molecules such as E-selectin and intracellular adhesion molecule (ICAM)-1 on synovial vascular endothelium and simultaneous production of chemokines such as IL-8, macrophage inflammatory protein (MIP)-1α, MIP-1β, monocyte chemoattractant protein (MCP)-1 and RANTES by endothelium and surrounding cells [8]. The combination of adhesive molecules and chemokines brings about a microenvironment, in a highly vascular tissue, which promotes the adhesion and transmigration of circulating polymorphs, monocytes and lymphocytes into the extravascular space. Here the cytokine-rich milieu stimulates cellular activation and cell–cell interaction, providing an explanation for the immunological and inflammatory phenomena observed. These include the activation of T- and B-cells, fibroblasts and macrophages.

Of considerable interest, upon further investigation, was the finding that the RA joint is also a site at which cytokines such as IL-10 and TGF-β, with anti-inflammatory and/or immunosuppressive effects, are locally produced [21–23]. Also produced were natural inhibitors of IL-1 and TNF-α, such as soluble shed receptors of these cytokines, with neutralizing activity, and a protein with antagonistic effects, i.e. IL-1 receptor antagonist. However, these counterbalancing molecules are apparently not produced in sufficient quantities to tip the balance in favour of homeostasis and termination of the inflammatory reaction (see Feldmann *et al.*, p. 343). Conceivably, however, these molecules could explain the time scale of disease progression (years rather than months) and the typical fluctuating course of disease with occasional natural remissions.

Our initial *in vitro* experiments and predictions of the pathogenic role of cytokines and of TNF-α in particular received support from studies of animal models. The animal model data also provided encouraging results which set the scene for anti-TNF trials. First, collagen type II-induced arthritis (CIA) in DBA/1 mice, which has similarities with the pathological features of RA and shows parallelism in its response to therapeutic interventions with drugs, was significantly ameliorated by injections of monoclonal anti-TNF antibodies and soluble TNF-receptor immunoglobulin fusion proteins [24,25]. Second, in work by Kollias and his colleagues, a colony of transgenic mice expressing a human TNF-α gene was successfully established. These mice developed a rheumatoid-like disorder at 5–6 weeks of age, and the disease could be suppressed by monoclonal anti-TNF antibodies administered from birth [26].

CLINICAL TRIALS WITH MONOCLONAL ANTI-TNF-α ANTIBODIES: PROOF OF PRINCIPLE AND EFFICACY

By 1992 we had accumulated sufficient evidence to proceed to a preliminary, open-label trial of anti-TNF-α therapy of RA. A partially humanized (chimeric) monoclonal anti-TNF-α antibody, cA2, manufactured by Centocor Inc., Pennsylvania, USA, was used [27]. The agent cA2, derived from a mouse monoclonal antibody, is genetically engineered to retain its murine variable region and has engrafted to it constant domains of a human κ light chain and IgG1 heavy chains (Fig. 3). Based on the experience of dose-ranging studies in the murine CIA model, we administered a total of 20 mg/kg body weight to RA patients. This was given by intravenous infusion over 2 hours, in two (or four) divided doses evenly spaced over a fortnight. Twenty RA patients with active disease unresponsive to most drugs, many on maintenance therapy with corticosteroids, entered the trial.

An impressive improvement in clinical indices of inflammation (number of swollen and tender joints, duration of morning stiffness and pain score), locomotor function, and reduction in C-reactive protein (CRP) or erythrocyte sedimentation rate (ESR) was observed in virtually every patient [28]. A mean reduction of 60–70% from baseline was achieved within days, reaching its maximum in 4–6 weeks. A clinical response was sustained for 12–24 weeks, with eventual relapse of disease in all patients.

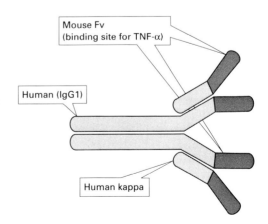

Mouse Fv
(binding site for TNF-α)

Human (IgG1)

Human kappa

Fig. 3 The cA2 anti-tumour necrosis factor-α (TNF-α) monoclonal antibody (mAb) used in clinical trials is derived from a mouse monoclonal antibody. The *variable* domain of the murine mAb is genetically engineered on to a backbone of constant domains of a human κ light chain and immunoglobulin G1 (IgG1) heavy chain. The neutralizing mAb has high affinity for TNF-α.

Although the universality, magnitude and kinetics of the antirheumatoid effect exceeded results observed with disease-modifying drugs, a multi-centre randomized placebo-controlled trial was considered to be an essential next step. Accordingly, this was undertaken in 1992–93 on a total of 73 patients with RA. As in the open-label trial, disease-modifying drugs were withdrawn for a period of at least 4 weeks prior to anti-TNF therapy and the patients stabilized on a constant dose of non-steroidal anti-inflammatory drugs (NSAIDs) and, if already on corticosteroids, on a fixed dose of prednisolone not exceeding 10 mg/day. Twenty-four patients received a single intravenous infusion of 10 mg/kg, a high dose of anti-TNF-α antibody (cA2); 25 patients received 1 mg/kg (a low dose) and 24 patients received a placebo infusion of 0.1% human serum albumin. At follow-up over the subsequent days and weeks, it was found that the patients receiving anti-TNF-α antibody showed large differences from baseline in all parameters of disease activity measured [29]. This was striking when compared to small changes in patients receiving placebo (Fig. 4).

Using a validated composite index of disease activity incorporating six clinical measurements at a 20% level of improvement [30], 79% of patients receiving the high dose of anti-TNF-α antibody, 58% of patients receiving low dose, and 8% of patients receiving placebo gave positive responses at the primary end-point of the study, i.e. at 4 weeks postinfusion [20,29] (Fig. 5).

The duration of the 20% Paulus response was used to monitor benefit and all patients were followed at weekly intervals until disease relapse. After a single dose of 10 mg/kg antibody, almost 90% of patients satisfied the response criteria in the first 4 weeks, 50% of patients maintained benefit for at least 6 weeks, and 20% of patients for over 20 weeks. Corresponding values for 1 mg/kg were 3 weeks for 50% of patients and 8 weeks for 20% of patients. In a group of patients who had previously received a placebo infusion, a 3 mg/kg dose of antibody was subsequently administered to establish a dose–response relationship. The results showed that the main difference in clinical response in the dose range used in treated groups lay in the duration of the effect, with a marginal difference in frequency of responders, and almost none in the maximum magnitude of change from baseline in individual parameters of disease activity. The higher the dose, the higher the frequency of responders and the longer the duration of benefit [31].

From this randomized clinical trial, the following was concluded:
• Anti-TNF-α antibody exerted an impressive anti-inflammatory effect within days, reaching its maximum at 3-4 weeks, and this was associated with a dramatic reduction in acute-phase proteins and ESR. These clinical and laboratory data pointed to a significant advance in the experimental therapy of RA.
• The specificity of the monoclonal antibody for TNF-α provided unequivocal evidence of the critical role played by TNF-α in regulating

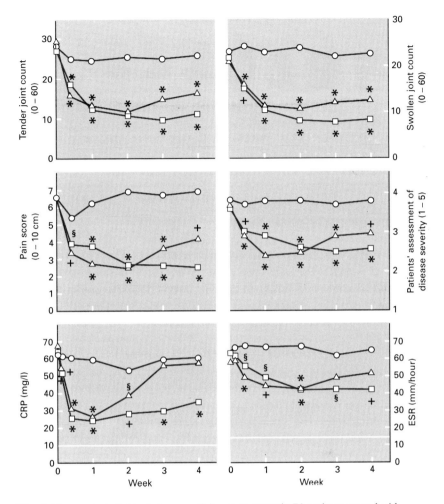

Fig. 4 Changes in individual disease activity assessments in 73 patients treated with placebo (○), 1 mg/kg (△) or 10 mg/kg (□) cA2 in a randomized, double-blind trial. Each of the clinical assessments showed marked down-modulation in both cA2 groups, compared with no significant change in the placebo group. Similar differences were observed for the two acute-phase measurements, erythrocyte sedimentation rate (ESR) and C-reactive protein (CRP). 1 mg/kg cA2 was just as effective as 10 mg/kg at week 2, but the duration of effect was shorter: see CRP graph especially. (*P* values represent significance versus placebo: +*P* < 0.05; §*P* < 0.01; **P < 0.001). Reproduced with permission from [29].

the cytokine cascade and secondary effects on inflammatory mediators involved in RA.

HOW DOES ANTI-TNF-α MONOCLONAL ANTIBODY WORK?

Treatment of RA with a monoclonal anti-TNF-α antibody provided a

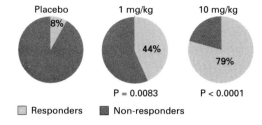

Placebo   1 mg/kg   10 mg/kg
8%   44%   79%

P = 0.0083   P < 0.0001

☐ Responders   ■ Non-responders

Fig. 5 Overall clinical responses (using the Paulus 20% response criteria) in 73 patients treated with placebo, 1 mg/kg or 10 mg/kg cA2 in a randomized, double-blind trial. Response states were assessed 4 weeks after treatment. The data show that the majority of patients treated with the higher cA2 dose responded, compared with 8% of those receiving placebo, confirming the clinical efficacy of *in vivo* tumour necrosis factor (TNF) blockade in the disease (*P* values represent significance versus placebo). Reproduced with permission from [20,29].

unique opportunity to test our fundamental hypothesis that over-production of TNF-α is at the apex of the cytokine cascade and, consequently, of cytokine-inducible secondary molecular pathways of the inflammatory response. If true, we might expect to demonstrate a down-regulation of other cytokines, such as IL-1, IL-6, IL-8 and GM-CSF, which *in vitro* analysis had shown to be regulated by TNF-α. However, since most of these cytokines were rapidly cleared from the joint and circulation, they could only be detected in picogram quantities in the local environment of the joint. Joint aspiration and synovial tissue biopsies would be required to examine the validity of the hypothesis further, but a rapid reduction of joint swelling following therapy constrained our ability to obtain joint fluids. An exception to this rule was IL-6, which was produced in sufficient quantities to give rise to stable levels which could be measured in nanograms in blood. Since IL-6 binding to hepatocytes is thought to be the main signal for CRP production, and we had observed a rapid and dramatic reduction in CRP levels following administration of anti-TNF-α antibody, it seemed likely that blood levels of IL-6 might give an indication of its regulation by TNF-α. Serial measurement of serum IL-6, allowing for diurnal variations, indeed supported our prediction, with significant reduction of IL-6 blood levels being observed within 12 hours of the administration of anti-TNF-α antibody, and preceding reduction in CRP and serum amyloid A levels by 12–24 hours [20,28,32].

Although measurement of IL-6 has provided convincing evidence that anti-TNF therapy deactivates the cytokine cascade, more direct evidence is currently being sought by examining serial synovial biopsies.

Measuring serum IL-1 levels, as expected, was unhelpful, since it was either undetectable or present in the normal range in the majority of sera. However, serum levels of IL-1 receptor antagonist (IL-1ra) showed a rapid reduction in keeping with a down-regulation of the cytokine network. At this stage it is not clear how IL-1ra production is regulated, but we suspect that TNF-α, possibly via IL-1, may be involved in its production, obeying the rules of the cytokine network in RA.

The trials with anti-TNF antibody have clearly demonstrated a dose-dependent effect lasting several weeks after a single infusion, but since all patients eventually relapse, the intervention does not permanently switch off the immunoinflammatory response. This is not inconsistent with our current views of the role of TNF-α and other proinflammatory cytokines in the pathogenesis of established chronic RA patients (see Fig. 2). It is the expected outcome of blocking the cytokine cascade downstream from the factors that induce the production of TNF-α (Fig. 6). The stimulus for TNF-α production is currently not known but probably requires T-cell–macrophage interaction involving a ligand–receptor mechanism dependent on cell–cell contact [33]. Whether anti-TNF therapy in earlier stages of RA may exert a longer-term effect, or even induce remission, will be addressed in future trials. It is conceivable that at earlier stages of disease, the disequilibrium between cytokine production and the anticytokine homeostatic response, discussed previously, is more amenable to correction. It is certainly likely that earlier intervention would exert the greatest effect in preventing cumulative effects of joint destruction on functional outcome.

An unexpected finding of the trials, however, which is not yet fully understood, is the long duration of benefit, lasting several weeks following a single infusion of a partially humanized (chimeric) antibody [27]. Such antibodies should offer an advantage over murine antibodies in being less immunogenic in humans, but are expected to show a shorter half-life following injection than human immunoglobulin. In fact, it was found that the pharmacokinetics of cA2 (anti-TNF-α antibody) is similar to a human immunoglobulin. It persists in the circulation in bioactive levels for long periods, for example, about 6 weeks following a single 10 mg/kg infusion [31]. However, there may be other reasons for the longevity of response. One explanation is suggested by the results of serial biopsies of synovium from knee joints examined before and after anti-TNF-α

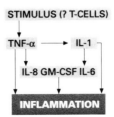

Fig. 6 This shows the dominance of tumour necrosis factor-α (TNF-α) and interleukin-1 (IL-1) in regulating the cytokine cascade in rheumatoid arthritis. There is evidence that TNF-α regulates IL-1 production in rheumatoid arthritis but the reverse may not be the case; hence TNF-α is regarded as being at the apex.

therapy. These biopsies show a reduction in the cellularity of synovium with a significant fall in the numbers of lymphocytes and macrophages per square unit of the histological section [20,34]. The reduction in synovial cellularity is associated with an increase in the circulating lymphocyte count (still within the normal range) lasting 2–4 weeks [35]. The data, therefore, suggest that anti-TNF-α therapy leads to a reduction in the flux of lymphocytes into the joints, thereby reducing the immunological signals which sustain synovitis. Other mechanisms dependent on the complement-fixing property of cA2 may play a part in reduction of macrophages, as might a down-regulation of GM-CSF and other haema-topoietic factors. However, when the neutralizing capacity of circulating anti-TNF antibody falls below the rate of TNF production, reaccumulation of cells in the synovium gradually begins again and inflammatory activity is re-established. Thus benefit of the therapy outlasts the circulating levels of neutralizing capacity of the antibody.

The concept that evolved from these observations was that a reduction of cellular traffic may significantly contribute to the mode of action of monoclonal anti-TNF-α therapy. We have recently found that this may be the case from further studies. Thus, there is a reduction in vascular adhesion molecules such as E-selectin, ICAM-1 and vascular cell adhesion molecule (VCAM)-1 expressed on the endothelium of blood vessels and detected by immunohistology of serial biopsies before and after anti-TNF therapy [20,34]. This reduction in tissues is associated with a reduction in the elevated circulating levels of soluble E-selectin and soluble ICAM-1 levels in treated patients [35]. The reduction of cell-associated and soluble circulating adhesion molecules is entirely consistent with current knowledge of the parts that TNF-α and IL-1 play in regulating their production and release from vasular endothelium [36,37].

Other, as yet uninvestigated, mechanisms could also play an important part in the therapeutic benefits of anti-TNF-α antibody. For example, we have observed a significant fall in circulating polymorphonuclear cell count in the first 2 or 3 weeks, and a small but significant rise in haemoglobin at 4 weeks postinfusion [29]. The former, we suggest, could result from antibody binding to TNF-expressing polymorphs, leading to their enhanced clearance. The latter could result from removal of the inhibitory effects of TNF-α on haemopoiesis. It is also possible that the rapid pain relief and alleviation of fatigue which treated patients report are due to blockade of the effects of TNF-α on the central nervous system. Whether anti-TNF therapy has effects on the hypothalamic–pituitary–adrenal axis is also being investigated in ongoing studies.

FUTURE PERSPECTIVES AND CONCLUSIONS

What of the future of anti-TNF-α therapy of RA? Trials with anti-TNF-α antibody (cA2) are continuing and further results are expected to define the place of this therapy of RA in the next 3–4 years. Meanwhile, other TNF-blocking agents have confirmed our experience; for example, a murine CDR-3 engrafted anti-TNF-α antibody with constant regions of human κ and IgG4 immunoglobulin [38], and two different soluble TNF receptors (p55 and p75) linked to immunoglobulin as fusion proteins produced by Immunex [39] and Roche, have all shown an anti-inflammatory effect in RA. Based on the overall experience of research and development, it is possible to make interim conclusions and look into the future.

It is clear that a single injection of anti-TNF-α antibody controls intractable flares of disease activity in RA with a marked enhancement of the quality of life for some weeks; the control of flares may therefore constitute one indication for the use of the antibody. Since anti-TNF-α antibody is not a cure and disease relapse is invariable, repeated therapy will be required. Repeated injection with benefit is possible, as judged by a trial in a small cohort of patients with up to four repeated cycles of therapy extending over a period of a year or more [40]. It is conceivable that monoclonal antibody therapy will prove to be a viable, if expensive, option for long-term control of RA in a proportion of patients. Repeated anti-TNF-α infusions at regular intervals are being tested in a current clinical trial, as is the possibility that antibody therapy may be effective used as adjunctive therapy with known disease modifying antirheumatic drugs (DMARDs) such as methotrexate.

If continued long-term therapy is possible, an important question that we will be asking is whether erosive disease of joints is halted. Protection of joints was observed following anti-TNF therapy in a murine model of arthritis [24]. In this experimental work, combination of anti-TNF antibody or a soluble TNF receptor immunoglobulin fusion protein with anti-T cell-directed therapy (anti-CD4 antibody) resulted in marked beneficial effect [25,41]. Such combination therapies could have a similar synergistic benefit in RA, but could also be associated with greater immunosuppression and associated adverse events. Immunosuppression might also occur in patients on anti-TNF-α monotherapy, since TNF-α has a protective immune function under physiological conditions. Thus it is possible that patients receiving TNF-blocking therapy will be susceptible to intracellular infections similar to those observed in murine models [42]. However, it is also possible that reversing chronic exposure to TNF-α, which is itself immunosuppressive, may on balance prove of benefit in RA. In support of this possibility is the enhancement of lymphocyte proliferative tests observed in patients receiving anti-TNF therapy [43].

Our trials with monoclonal antibodies have highlighted important principles in understanding the role of cytokines in the pathogenesis of RA and applying the emerging advance in knowledge to refining new therapies (see Feldmann *et al.*, p. 343). As regards the role of TNF-α, it is important to re-emphasize that the clinical benefit and improvement in a panoply of changes in cytokine physiology and cellular activation and kinetics consequent upon anti-TNF therapy should not be taken as evidence that only TNF-α is directly involved in mediating pathological effects. Analysis of effects of TNF via inhibition of production of other inflammatory molecules on the one hand, and its direct effects on the other, will require careful dissection in future studies. It is possible that a significant anti-inflammatory effect may be achieved by blocking the effects of other molecules (e.g. metalloproteinases) produced further downstream in the inflammatory reaction. Such selectivity could minimize the possible adverse effects of TNF-α blockade in immune defence against bacterial infections. However, the added value of TNF-α blockade by virtue of its widespread effects has been clearly demonstrated by our work and may explain why such impressive benefit was observed in clinical trials.

Since it is possible to envisage reduction of TNF-α production by interfering with intracellular pathways, e.g. signal transduction, DNA transcription, stabilization of messenger RNA and inhibition of enzymatic cleavage of TNF-α release, one may expect the development of chemical drugs which mimic the results we have seen with anti-TNF-α antibody. Reports suggest that such drugs are under development and may offer an alternative for the treatment of RA. However, these drugs are likely to lack the unique molecular specificity of a monoclonal anti-TNF-α antibody in unravelling the complexities of disease mechanisms.

Whatever the final outcome of this development, one can safely predict that TNF-directed therapy will preoccupy the agenda of research and development of drugs in the next decade and give new insights into the molecular mechanisms of rheumatoid disease.

ACKNOWLEDGEMENTS

I am grateful to the Arthritis and Rheumatism Council; to Marc Feldmann, Michael Elliott, Fionula Brennan for scientific collaboration and to Lindsay Roffe and Meg James for help with the preparation of illustrations and manuscript.

REFERENCES

1 Garrod AB. *Nature and Treatment of Gout and Rheumatic Gout.* Walton and Maberly, London, 1859.
2 Halberg P. *Rheumatoid arthritis: history.* In: *Rheumatology*, edited by Klippel JH, Dieppe PA. Mosby, London, 1994:1–4.
3 Lawrence JS. Rhematoid arthritis: nature or nurture? *Ann Rheum Dis* 1970;**29**:357–369.
4 Silman AJ, MacGregor AJ, Thomson W *et al.* Twin concordance rates for rheumatoid arthritis: results from a nationwide study. *Br J Rheumatol* 1993;**32**:903–907.
5 Gregersen PK, Silver J, Winchester RJ. The shared epitope hypothesis: an approach to

understanding the molecular genetics of susceptibility to rheumatoid arthritis. *Arthritis Rheum* 1987;**30**:1205–1213.

6 Nepom GT, Nepom BS. Prediction of susceptibility to rheumatoid arthritis based on HLA genetics. *Rheum Dis Clin North Am* 1992;**18**:785–792.

7 Maini RN, Feldmann M. *Immunopathogenesis of rheumatoid arthritis*. In: *Oxford Textbook of Rheumatology*, vol. 2, edited by Maddison PJ, Isenberg DA, Woo P, Glass DN. Oxford University Press, New York, 1993:621–638.

8 Feldmann M, Brennan FM, Maini RN. *Role of cytokines in autoimmunity*. In: *Annul Review of Immunology*, vol. 14, edited by Paul WE. Annual Reviews, Palo Alto, California, 1996;397–440.

9 Field M, Chu C, Feldmann M, Maini RN. Interleukin-6 localization in the synovial membrane in rheumatoid arthritis. *Rheumatol Int* 1991;**11**:45–50.

10 Chu CQ, Field M, Feldmann M, Maini RN. Localization of tumor necrosis factor α in synovial tissues and at the cartilage–pannus junction in patients with rheumatoid arthritis. *Arthritis Rheum* 1991;**34**:1125–1132.

11 Deleuran BW, Chu CQ, Field M *et al.* Localization of tumour necrosis factor receptors in the synovial tissue and cartilage/pannus junction in rheumatoid arthritis: implication for local actions of TNFα. *Arthritis Rheum* 1992;**35**:1170–1178.

12 Deleuran BW, Chu CQ, Field M *et al.* Localization of the interleukin-1α, type 1 interleukin-1 receptor and interleukin-1 receptor antagonist in the synovial membrane and cartilage/pannus junction in rheumatoid arthritis. *Br J Rheumatol* 1992;**31**:801–809.

13 Chu CQ, Field M, Allard S, Abney E, Feldmann M, Maini RN. Detection of cytokines at the cartilage/pannus junction in patients with rheumatoid arthritis: implications for the role of cytokines in cartilage destruction and repair. *Br J Rheumatol* 1992;**31**:653–661.

14 Buchan G, Barrett K, Turner M, Chantry D, Maini RN, Feldmann M. Interleukin-1 and tumour necrosis factor mRNA expression in rheumatoid arthritis: prolonged production of IL1α. *Clin Exp Immunol* 1988;**73**:449–455.

15 Brennan FM, Zachariae CO, Chantry D *et al.* Detection of interleukin 8 biological activity in synovial fluids from patients with rheumatoid arthritis and production of interleukin 8 mRNA by isolated synovial cells. *Eur J Immunol* 1990;**20**:2141–2144.

16 Haworth C, Brennan FM, Chantry D, Turner M, Maini RN, Feldmann M. Expression of granulocyte-macrophage colony-stimulating factor in rheumatoid arthritis: regulation by tumor necrosis factor-alpha. *Eur J Immunol* 1991;**21**:2575–2579.

17 Brennan FM, Chantry D, Jackson A, Maini RN, Feldmann M. Inhibitory effect of TNFα antibodies on synovial cell interleukin-1 production in rheumatoid arthritis. *Lancet* 1989;**2**:244–247.

18 Butler DM, Maini RN, Feldmann M, Brennan FM. Modulation of proinflammatory cytokine release in rheumatoid synovial membrane cell cultures. Comparison of monoclonal anti-TNFα antibody with the IL-1 receptor antagonist. *Eur Cyt Network* 1995;**6**:225–230.

19 Brennan FM, Maini RN, Feldmann M. TNFα: a pivotal role in rheumatoid arthritis? *Br J Rheumatol* 1992;**31**:293–298.

20 Maini RN, Elliott MJ, Brennan FM *et al.* Monoclonal anti-TNFα antibody as a probe of pathogenesis and therapy of rheumatoid arthritis. *Immunol Rev* 1995;**144**:195–223.

21 Katsikis PD, Chu CQ, Brennan FM, Maini RN, Feldmann M. Immunoregulatory role of interleukin 10 in rheumatoid arthritis. *J Exp Med* 1994;**179**:1517–1527.

22 Cohen SBA, Katsikis PD, Chu CQ *et al.* High level of interleukin-10 production by the activated T cell population within the rheumatoid synovial membrane. *Arthritis Rheum* 1995;**38**:946–952.

23 Chu CQ, Field M, Abney E *et al.* Transforming growth factor-β 1 in rheumatoid synovial membrane and cartilage/pannus junction. *Clin Exp Immunol* 1991;**86**:380–386.

24 Williams RO, Feldmann M, Maini RN. Anti-tumor necrosis factor ameliorates joint disease in murine collagen-induced arthritis. *Proc Natl Acad Sci* 1992;**89**:9784–9788.

25 Williams RO, Ghrayeb J, Feldmann M, Maini RN. Successful therapy of collagen-induced

arthritis with TNF receptor-IgG fusion protein and combination with anti-CD4. *Immunology* 1995;**84**:433–439.

26 Keffer J, Probert L, Cazlaris H *et al.* Transgenic mice expressing human tumour necrosis factor: a predictive genetic model of arthritis. *EMBO J* 1991;**10**:4025–4031.

27 Knight DM, Trinh H, Le J *et al.* Construction and initial characterisation of a mouse–human chimaeric anti-TNF antibody. *Mol Immunology* 1993;**30**:1443–1453.

28 Elliott MJ, Maini RN, Feldmann M *et al.* Treatment of rheumatoid arthritis with chimeric monoclonal antibodies to TNFα. *Arthritis Rheum* 1993;**36**:1681–1690.

29 Elliott MJ, Maini RN, Feldmann M *et al.* Randomised double-blind comparison of chimeric monoclonal antibody to tumour necrosis factor α (cA2) versus placebo in rheumatoid arthritis. *Lancet* 1994;**344**:1105–1110.

30 Paulus HE, Egger MJ, Ward JR, Williams HJ. Analysis of improvement in individual rheumatoid arthritis patients treated with disease-modifying anti-rheumatic drugs, based on the findings in patients treated with placebo. *Arthritis Rheum* 1990;**33**:477–484.

31 Maini RN, Elliott MJ, Long-Fox A *et al.* Clinical response of rheumatoid arthritis (RA) to anti-TNFα (cA2) monoclonal antibody (mab) is related to administered dose and persistence of circulating antibody. *Arthritis Rheum* 1995;**38**:S186.

32 Charles P, Elliott MJ, Davis *et al.* Regulation of cytokines and acute phase proteins following TNFα blockade in rheumatoid arthritis. 1995; (submitted for publication).

33 Isler P, Vey E, Zhang JH *et al.* Cell surface glycoproteins expressed on activated human T cells induce production of interleukin-1 beta by monocytic cells: a possible role of CD69. *Eur Cytokine Network* 1993;**4**:15–23.

34 Tak PP, Taylor PC, Breedveld FC *et al.* Reduction in cellularity and expression of adhesion molecules in rheumatoid synovial tissue after anti-TNFα monoclonal antibody treatment. *Arthritis Rheum* 1996; (in press).

35 Paleolog EM, Hunt M, Elliott MJ, Woody JN, Feldmann M, Maini RN. Monoclonal anti-tumour necrosis factor α antibody deactivates vascular endothelium in rheumatoid arthritis. *Arthritis Rheum* 1996; (in press).

36 Carlos TM, Harlan JM. Leukocyte-endothelial adhesion molecules. *Blood* 1994;**84**:2068–2101.

37 Pigott R, Dillon LP, Hemingway IH, Gearing AJ. Soluble forms of E-selectin, ICAM-1 and VCAM-1 are present in the supernatants of cytokine activated cultured endothelial cells. *Biochem Biophys Res Commun* 1992;**187**:584–589.

38 Rankin ECC, Choy EHS, Kassimos D *et al.* The therapeutic effects of an engineered human anti-tumour necrosis factor alpha antibody (CD571) in rheumatoid arthritis. *Br J Rheum* 1995;**34**:334–342.

39 Moreland LW, Margolies GR, Heck LW *et al.* Soluble tumor necrosis factor receptor (sTNFR): results of a phase I dose-escalation study in patients with rheumatoid arthritis. *Arthritis Rheum* 1994;**37**(suppl):S295.

40 Elliott MJ, Maini RN, Feldmann M *et al.* Repeated therapy with monoclonal antibody to tumour necrosis factor α (cA2) in patients with rheumatoid arthritis. *Lancet* 1994;**344**:1125–1127.

41 Williams RO, Mason LJ, Feldmann M, Maini RN. Synergy between anti-CD4 and anti-tumor necrosis factor in the amelioration of established collagen-induced arthritis. *Proc Natl Acad Sci* 1994;**91**:2762–2766.

42 Pfeffer K, Matsuyama T, Kündig TM *et al.* Mice deficient for the 55kd tumour necrosis factor receptor are resistant to endotoxic shock, yet succumb to *L. monocytogenes* infection. *Cell* 1993;**73**:457–467.

43 Cope AP, Londei M, Chu NR *et al.* Chronic exposure to tumor necrosis factor (TNF) *in vitro* impairs the activation of T cells through the T cell receptor/CD3 complex; reversal *in vivo* by anti-TNF antibodies in patients with rheumatoid arthritis. *J Clin Invest* 1994;**94**:749–760.

PART 2
CARDIOVASCULAR DISEASE

Fetal growth and coronary heart disease

DAVID J. P. BARKER

Recent research has shown that babies who are small at birth and during infancy will be at increased risk of developing coronary heart disease, stroke, diabetes or hypertension during adult life. That a person's destiny and lifespan may be determined before birth is well-known. Genetically determined diseases such as Huntington's chorea illustrate how a long period of normal development and adult life can be prematurely brought to an end by the action of inherited defects. What is new is the realization that it is not only the presence or absence of genes that controls our destiny but the way in which gene expression may be permanently changed by the nutrient environment in early life.

There are three reasons why this new field of research has developed.
1 The current explanation of coronary heart disease, a destructive model in which inappropriate adult lifestyles hasten ageing processes, fails to account for either the time trends of the disease or its geography, or why one person gets the disease and another does not.
2 The search for alternative explanations led to a strong geographical clue that the role of fetal life in the genesis of coronary heart disease might be much greater than had been thought [1].
3 Animal experiments show that changes in nutrition in early life permanently change the growth and form of the body, together with a range of its structures and functions [2]. This phenomenon is known as programming.

STUDIES IN ANIMALS

The substantial body of evidence on the plasticity of the fetus, its ability to adapt to undernutrition, and the permanent effects of these adaptations, derives from animal experiments carried out by Widdowson and others [2]. These studies allow us to make two predictions about the human fetus.
1 Lack of nutrients or oxygen will cause persisting changes, which include altered metabolism, including glucose and lipid metabolism, altered blood pressure and settings of hormonal axes, enzymes and cell receptors.

69

2 The long-term effects of undernutrition depend on the stage at which it occurs. Tissues and systems tend to be vulnerable to programming during phases of rapid cell replication, and different tissues undergo these sensitive phases of development at different times.

SMALL SIZE AT BIRTH AND IN INFANCY

It has been possible to explore the links between growth *in utero* and later coronary heart disease as a result of a search of the archives in the UK which revealed collections of birth records of men and women born 50 years and more ago in Hertfordshire, Preston and Sheffield. Figure 1 shows findings in a group of 8175 men born in the county of Hertfordshire before 1930. Their weight at 1 year of age strongly predicted their subsequent death rates from coronary heart disease [3]. Death rates fell steeply between those who were small and those who were large at 1 year. There were similar trends in coronary heart disease with birth weight in men and women. A study in Sheffield showed that the small babies with high coronary death rates in adulthood were small in relation to duration of gestation rather than because they were prematurely born.

These findings pose the question of what are the processes linking reduced early growth with adult disease. Examination of samples of men and women who were born and still live in Hertfordshire, Sheffield

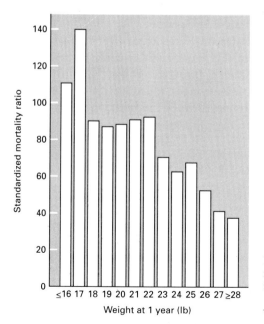

Fig. 1 Standardized mortality ratios for coronary heart disease in 8175 men born during 1911–1930 according to their weight at 1 year of age.

and Preston shows that babies who were small have, as adults, raised blood pressure, raised serum cholesterol and plasma fibrinogen concentrations, and impaired glucose tolerance — the main risk factors for coronary heart disease [4]. Table 1 shows the mean systolic pressures of men and women aged 64–71 years. Systolic pressure falls progressively between those who were small at birth and those who were large. This relation between birth weight and blood pressure has now been demonstrated in 20 studies of children and adults, and there is a secure base for saying that impaired fetal growth is strongly linked to blood pressure at all ages except during adolescence, when the tracking of blood pressure levels which begins in early childhood is perturbed by the adolescent growth spurt. Differences in blood pressure associated with birth weight are small in childhood but are magnified throughout life, suggesting that there may be amplification as well as initiation processes. It is not known what initiates high blood pressure in intrauterine life, but there are interesting clues, including the work of Edwards and colleagues in Edinburgh, which has pointed to the possible role of cortisol [5]. The fetus may be exposed to excessive cortisol either through breakdown of the enzyme barriers in the placenta which protect it from maternal cortisol, or because fetoplacental stress leads to increased cortisol production.

Table 2 shows the prevalence of non-insulin-dependent diabetes and impaired glucose tolerance according to birth weight in a group of men in Hertfordshire [6]. The prevalence falls sharply between men who were small at birth and those who were large. There are similar findings in women. This association between birth weight and diabetes has been replicated in two other studies in the UK, two studies in the USA, and one in Sweden [7].

Table 1 Mean systolic pressure (mmHg) in men and women aged 64–71 years according to birth weight.

Birth weight			
(lb)	(kg)	Men	Women
≤ 5.5	≤ 2.50	171 (18)	169 (9)
→ 6.5	→ 2.95	168 (53)	165 (33)
→ 7.5	→ 3.41	168 (144)	160 (68)
→ 8.5	→ 3.86	165 (111)	163 (48)
> 8.5	> 3.86	163 (92)	155 (26)
Total		166 (418)	161 (184)
Standard deviation		24	26

Figures in brackets are numbers of subjects.

Table 2 Prevalence of non-insulin-dependent diabetes and impaired glucose tolerance in men aged 59–70 years, according to birth weight.

Birth weight (lb)*	Number of men	% with impaired glucose tolerance or diabetes	Odds ratio adjusted for body mass index (95% confidence interval)
≤ 5.5	20	40	6.6 (1.5–28)
→ 6.5	47	34	4.8 (1.3–17)
→ 7.5	104	31	4.6 (1.4–16)
→ 8.5	117	22	2.6 (0.8–8.9)
→ 9.5†	54	13	1.4 (0.3–5.6)
> 9.5	28	14	1.0
Total	370	25	

* See Table 1 for birth weights in kg.
† 4.31 kg.

BODY PROPORTIONS AT BIRTH

Studies of men and women who were small at birth have shown that they are resistant to insulin. The occurrence of insulin resistance in adults is characterized in a syndrome, syndrome X, in which diabetes, hypertension and raised plasma triglyceride concentrations coincide. Allowing for current body mass, the relative risk of having syndrome X among people 6.5 lb (2.95 kg) or less at birth is about 10 times higher than among people who were more than 9.5 lb (4.31 kg; Table 3). This is a large difference in risk. For comparison, the risk of coronary heart disease among smokers compared with non-smokers is about 2. The insulin resistance syndrome is associated not only with low birth weight but also with thinness at birth, as measured by a low ponderal index (birth weight/length^3). Babies

Table 3 Prevalence of syndrome X (type 2 diabetes, hypertension and hyperlipidaemia) in men according to birth weight.

Birth weight (lb)*	Men		Odds ratio adjusted for body mass index (95% confidence interval)
	Total	% with syndrome X	
≤ 5.5	20	30	18.0 (2.6–118)
→ 6.5	54	19	8.4 (1.5–49)
→ 7.5	114	17	8.5 (1.5–46)
→ 8.5	123	12	4.9 (0.9–27)
→ 9.5	64	6	2.2 (0.3–14)
>9.5	32	6	1.0
Total	407	14	

* See Tables 1 and 2 for birth weights in kg.

who are thin at birth lack muscle as well as fat, and muscle in adult life is the peripheral site of insulin action. Insulin tolerance tests on men and women aged 50 confirm that those who were thin at birth are less sensitive to insulin.

Raised blood pressure in adult life is associated with both thinness at birth and with short body length in relation to head size. Short babies are thought to have encountered undernutrition in late gestation and to have sustained brain growth at the expense of the trunk, including the abdominal viscera. An analysis of mean serum cholesterol concentrations in a group of men and women aged 50 showed that total and low-density lipoprotein (LDL) cholesterol concentrations fell between people who had small and large abdominal circumferences at birth (Table 4) [8]. Abdominal circumference reflects liver size, the liver being disproportionately large in the fetus. An inference from Table 4 is that babies with impaired liver development permanently reset their cholesterol metabolism. Reduced abdominal circumference at birth is also associated with raised plasma concentrations of fibrinogen, another strong predictor of coronary heart disease. The differences in serum cholesterol and plasma fibrinogen concentrations associated with the range of abdominal circumference at birth are large, equivalent to at least a 30% difference in risk of coronary heart disease.

Other observations suggest that infant feeding may also programme adult cholesterol metabolism. Men in Hertfordshire who were breast-fed beyond 1 year were found to have raised serum LDL cholesterol concentrations and increased death rates from coronary heart disease [7]. The mechanisms by which late weaning of infants might programme lipid metabolism are a matter for speculation. One possible explanation, however, which derives from observations on baboons, is that thyroid hormones present in breast milk may down-regulate the suckling infant's thyroid function and thereby influence cholesterol metabolism.

Table 4 Mean serum lipid concentrations according to abdominal circumference at birth in men and women aged 50–53 years.

Abdominal circumference		No. of people	Total cholesterol (mmol/l)	Low-density lipoprotein cholesterol (mmol/l)
(in)	(cm)			
≤ 11.5	29.2	53	6.7	4.5
→ 12.0	30.5	43	6.9	4.6
→ 12.5	31.7	31	6.8	4.4
→ 13.0	33.0	45	6.2	4.0
> 13.0	33.0	45	6.1	4.0
Total		217	6.5	4.3

SUMMARY OF PROGRAMMING

This brief review allows a number of conclusions.

1 Restriction of nutrients or oxygen *in utero* leaves permanent marks on the physiology and structure of the body. As an example, Table 5 shows the blood pressures of the offspring of four groups of pregnant rats given varying amounts of dietary protein [9]. The offspring of the rats given lower-protein diets had raised blood pressure 9 weeks after birth, and this persisted through adult life.

2 Experiments on animals have established that undernutrition at different times in early life has different effects. In early gestation, it leads to proportionate loss of body size, as in the proportionately small newborn human baby. In late gestation, undernutrition leads to disproportionate growth, as in the thin or short human baby. Disproportionate growth rather than small size seems to hold a key to the origins of coronary heart disease. More than 20 years ago McCance and Widdowson showed that undernutrition could effect profound changes in the relative size of the body's organs without any major change in overall body size [2].

3 The rapidly growing baby is more vulnerable to undernutrition. When rickets was common 70 years ago, it was not small babies who got the disease but larger, more rapidly growing ones. Slow growth protects against undernutrition. In some countries such as China, where proportionate intrauterine growth retardation is widespread, coronary heart disease is rare. Growth retardation in China seems to lead to down-regulation of growth in early gestation, which could protect the fetus from the effects of undernutrition later in gestation, and from the development of the disproportion associated with coronary heart disease.

4 Fetal undernutrition, which programmes the body, itself results from inadequate maternal intake of food or from inadequate transport or transfer of nutrients. Studies of the birth weights of families show a strong correlation between the birth weights of people related through their mothers, but not between those of people related only through their fathers. This and other findings suggest that fetal growth is not predominantly

Table 5 Effects of fetal exposure to maternal low-protein diets on systolic blood pressure in adult rats.

Dietary protein (% by weight of food intake)	No. of rats	Mean (s.d.) systolic blood pressure 9 weeks after birth (mmHg)
18	15	137 (± 4)
12	13	152 (± 3)
9	13	153 (± 3)
6	11	159 (± 3)

controlled by the fetal genome but by the supply of nutrients and oxygen from the mother [7]. For a period of 7 months in 1944, there was an embargo on food supplies to the population of western Holland, and people starved. Something is now known about what happened in adulthood to the generation of babies conceived or born during this famine [10]. Girls conceived in the famine but born after liberation by the allies had normal birth weight and grew up to be normal women, but their babies, when they were born, were small. It seems that the ability of these women to deliver nutrients to their babies had been impaired by their own fetal experience. This observation illustrates how fetal nutrition depends not only on what the mother eats during pregnancy but on her physiological and metabolic competence established during her early life, as well as her nutrient stores before pregnancy.

Another aspect of the complex links between maternal and fetal nutrition is shown in Table 6, in which the mean systolic blood pressures of a group of men and women are arranged by four groups of birth weight and four groups of placental weight [11]. As expected from previous findings, those people with a heavier birth weight had lower blood pressure but, unexpectedly, at any birth weight men and women who had had larger placentas had higher blood pressure. From studies in animals, placental enlargement is known to be an adaptation to lack of nutrients including oxygen. In humans, three kinds of baby are known to have disproportionately large placentae: the offspring of mothers who are anaemic in pregnancy, who exercise during pregnancy or who live at high altitude [7]. The fetus seems to attempt to overcome the deficiency in its supply of nutrients or oxygen by increasing the area of its attachment to the mother. A high ratio of placental weight to birth weight is linked to cardiovascular disease, impaired glucose tolerance and raised plasma fibrinogen concentrations in later life as well as to hypertension. The placenta seems to play an important role in programming the baby.

Table 6 Mean systolic blood pressure (mmHg) of men and women aged 46–54 according to placental weight and birth weight.

Birth weight (lb)*	Placental weight (lb)*				
	≤ 1.0	→ 1.25	→ 1.5	> 1.5	All
< 5.5	152 (26)	154 (13)	153 (5)	206 (1)	154 (45)
→ 6.5	147 (16)	151 (54)	150 (28)	166 (8)	151 (106)
→ 7.5	144 (20)	148 (77)	145 (45)	160 (27)	149 (169)
> 7.5	133 (6)	148 (27)	147 (42)	154 (54)	149 (129)
All	147 (68)	149 (171)	147 (120)	157 (90)	150 (449)

Figures in brackets are numbers of subjects.
* See Table 1 for birth weights in kg.

NEW MODEL OF CORONARY HEART DISEASE

A new model for the causation of coronary heart disease is emerging [7]. Under the old model, an inappropriate lifestyle, including cigarette smoking and lack of exercise, leads to accelerated destruction of the body in middle and late life, including the more rapid development of atheroma, raised blood pressure and the development of insulin resistance. Under the new model, coronary heart disease results not primarily from external forces but from the body's self-organization, that is homeostatic settings of enzyme activity, cell receptors and hormone feedback, which are established in response to undernutrition *in utero* and lead eventually to premature death.

REFERENCES

1 Barker DJP, Osmond C. Infant mortality, childhood nutrition, and ischaemic heart disease in England and Wales. *Lancet* 1986;**i**:1977–1981.

2 McCance RA, Widdowson EM. The determinants of growth and form. *Proc R Soc Lond (Ser B: Biol Sci)* 1974;**185**:1–17.

3 Osmond C, Barker DJP, Winter PD, Fall CHD, Simmonds SJ. Early growth and death from cardiovascular disease in women. *Br Med J* 1993;**307**:1519–1524.

4 Barker DJP, Gluckman PD, Godfrey KM *et al*. Fetal nutrition and cardiovascular disease in adult life. *Lancet* 1993;**341**:938–41.

5 Benediktsson R, Lindsay RS, Noble J, Seckl JR, Edwards CRW. Glucocorticoid exposure *in utero*: new model for adult hypertension. *Lancet* 1993;**341**:339–341.

6 Hales CN, Barker DJP, Clark PMS *et al*. Fetal and infant growth and impaired glucose tolerance at age 64. *Br Med J* 1991;**303**:1019–1022.

7 Barker DJP. *Mothers, Babies and Disease in Later Life*. British Medical Journal Books, London, 1994.

8 Barker DJP, Martyn CN, Osmond C *et al*. Growth *in utero* and serum cholesterol concentrations in adult life. *Br Med J* 1993;**307**:1524–1527.

9 Langley SC, Jackson AA. Increased systolic blood pressure in adult rats induced by fetal exposure to maternal low protein diets. *Clin Sci* 1994;**86**:217–222.

10 Lumey LH. Decreased birthweights in infants after maternal *in utero* exposure to the Dutch famine of 1944–45. *Paediatr Perinatal Epidemiol* 1992;**6**:240–253.

11 Barker DJP, Bull AR, Osmond C, Simmonds SJ. Fetal and placental size and risk of hypertension in adult life. *Br Med J* 1990;**30**:259–262.

Glucocorticoids, fetal growth and the programming of hypertension

JONATHAN R. SECKL

Born but to die
    (Alexander Pope, *An Essay on Man.*)
Pope's truism may sound rather prosaic, but is there more than mere poetic licence to link birth and other early life events to the common disorders which contribute to deaths occurring five or more decades later?

LOW BIRTH WEIGHT AND ADULT DISEASE

The major cause of death in our society is ischaemic heart disease. Much current popular, medical and governmental opinion suggests that this heavy cardiovascular mortality and its attendant morbidity are caused by specific elements of our affluent (some would say indolent) western lifestyle, particularly smoking, over-nutrition, lack of exercise and excessive alcohol consumption. These act both directly on the heart and via amplification of other risk factors, such as hypertension, hyperlipidaemia and non-insulin-dependent diabetes mellitus. There is also a well-documented hereditary component to these cardiovascular and metabolic diseases, spawning the currently accepted notion that environmental risk factors act in adult life upon a genetic background to determine disease occurrence.

Recently, however, some provocative epidemiological data, initiated by Professor David Barker and his colleagues in Southampton, have clearly implicated early life or prenatal events as of equal or even greater importance to environmental influences in adult life [1]. These studies, exploiting several independent populations in the UK and elsewhere, have demonstrated that low birth weight (often in association with a large placenta) is closely associated with the development of higher blood pressures in children, adolescents and adults up to late middle age [1–3]. Similar associations with low birth weight have been documented for hyperlipidaemia and syndrome X, insulin resistance and non-insulin-dependent diabetes mellitus and, probably as a consequence of these, ischaemic heart disease. These associations are apparently independent of lifestyle factors, such as adult weight, smoking, alcohol intake or social class, which are additive to the effects of early life [1]. Most importantly, the relationship between birth weight and adult blood pressure is continuous and represents birth weights within the normal range, rather than severely undersized or very premature babies. Indeed, these data should perhaps be less surprising, since it has been known for some time that blood pressure levels track from infancy to adulthood, clearly implicating early events in the determination of blood pressure throughout life [4]. Although it is difficult to distinguish the hereditary components of fetal growth and size in such population studies, it may be noteworthy that hypertension is largely a feature of adults who were born small and showed subsequent catch-up growth in infancy [1,3]. Those born small without later growth acceleration do not later show elevated blood pressures, suggesting that smallness *per se* (presumably in part genetically determined) is not a risk factor, only smallness due to some external growth-restraining influence.

Programming

Although there is still considerable controversy [5] about the explanation of these findings, including dispute about the importance of social class (which also tracks throughout life and from generation to generation), the data have stimulated useful attempts to explain a link between early-life environmental influences and later disease development. Key to these approaches has been the notion that an adverse intrauterine environment may programme or imprint the development and maturation of fetal organs, thus permanently changing tissue responses, causing later disease [6,7]. Such programming has been documented in a variety of organ systems and reflects the ability of a factor (growth factor, hormone, homeotic gene, nuclear transcription factor, etc.) acting during a defined developmental window, to exert permanent organizational effects or hard-wire a response. One of the best-defined examples is the action of endogenous androgens, in many vertebrate species, to programme androgen-metabolizing enzyme expression in the liver, the development of sexually dimorphic structures in the brain and sexual behaviour. These effects can only be exerted during a specific perinatal period, but then persist throughout life, largely irrespective of any subsequent sex steroid manipulations [8].

Clearly, possible biochemical and molecular mechanisms inducing prenatal programming of hypertension (and other disorders) are of considerable interest, both for general scientific understanding and to enable the development of possible preventive strategies. What mechanisms might therefore link modest intrauterine growth retardation and later disease, particularly hypertension? Maternal malnutrition, either generalized or of specific dietary components (e.g. protein or iron deficiency), has been advocated [7]. Much data in a variety of experimental species show that maternal dietary restriction during pregnancy may restrict fetal growth, although any links with later disease are not so clear. In rats, however, dietary protein restriction throughout pregnancy leads to elevated blood pressures in the offspring [9]. Nevertheless, maternal dietary manipulations do not specify the biochemical or molecular pathogenic mechanisms, in the fetus, placenta and/or mother, which produce hypertension and other disorders in later life. Moreover, the importance of maternal nutrition has not yet been established within the normal range of dietary variation (which might be anticipated to vary with social class) pertaining to the human populations which originally stimulated interest in this topic [1]. Indeed, in humans and animals, maternal dietary deprivation may need to be extreme to affect birth weight appreciably [6].

GLUCOCORTICOID EXPOSURE *IN UTERO*

It has been repeatedly shown that fetal exposure to excessive glucocorticoid levels retards fetal growth, both in animal models and humans [10–12]. Glucocorticoids also affect placental size, with the direction and magnitude of change probably dependent upon the dose and timing of exposure [13]. Fetal cortisol levels are elevated in human intrauterine growth retardation [14]. Glucocorticoids also increase blood pressure in adult animals and humans [15], and increase fetal blood pressure directly *in utero*, at least in sheep [16]. Such prenatal hypertensive effects of glucocorticoids appear to persist, since treatment of pregnant rats with the synthetic glucocorticoid dexamethasone, in a modest pharmacological dose which reduces average birth weight by 14%, causes elevated blood pressures in the adult offspring, very many months after exposure to the glucocorticoid *in utero* [17] (Fig. 1).

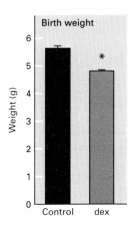
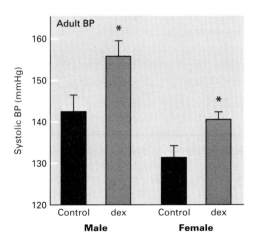

Fig. 1 Treatment of pregnant rats with dexamethasone (dex) reduces birth weight and programmes hypertension in the adult offspring.

Placental 11β-hydroxysteroid dehydrogenase

Dexamethasone is a synthetic glucocorticoid which crosses the placenta fairly readily, but normally the fetus has much lower levels of physiological glucocorticoids (cortisol in humans, corticosterone in rats) than the mother [18,19]. Glucocorticoids are highly lipophilic and readily cross biological membranes and barriers such as the placenta. However, maternal cortisol is clearly excluded from the fetus. This is achieved by placental 11β-hydroxysteroid dehydrogenase (11β-HSD), which catalyses the rapid metabolism of cortisol to the inert 11-dehydro product cortisone (corticosterone to 11-dehydrocorticosterone in rats) [20]. This protective placental enzymic barrier is very efficient, so that almost all maternal cortisol is inactivated when it crosses to the fetus, thus ensuring that about three-quarters of active cortisol in the human fetal circulation at term is derived from the *fetal* adrenal glands [18] (Fig. 2).

Perhaps the best illustration of the potency and importance of 11β-HSD relates to its action around mineralocorticoid receptors in the distal nephron of the kidney [21,22]. Purified or recombinant expressed mineralocorticoid receptors are non-selective for corticosteroid ligands, and bind cortisol (corticosterone) and aldosterone with high and similar affinity *in vitro*. However, it is clear that *in vivo* only aldosterone exerts mineralocorticoid actions (upon sodium and potassium excretion) in the kidney, despite a 100-fold molar excess of circulating cortisol. This

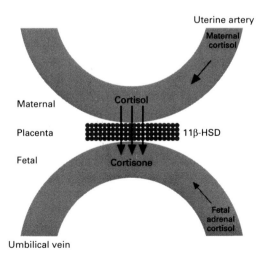

Fig. 2 Placental 11β-hydroxysteroid dehydrogenase (11β-HSD) rapidly inactivates cortisol, thus protecting the fetus from the much higher levels of glucocorticoid in the maternal circulation and ensuring that the majority of cortisol in the fetal circulation comes from the fetal adrenal glands.

selective access of aldosterone *in vivo* is ensured by the action of 11β-HSD, which rapidly inactivates glucocorticoids before they can bind to mineralocorticoid receptors in the distal nephron. When the enzyme is congenitally absent (the rare hypertensive syndrome of apparent mineralocorticoid excess) or is inhibited by liquorice or its derivatives (including the anti-ulcer drug carbenoxolone), then cortisol illicitly occupies and activates renal mineralocorticoid receptors, causing sodium retention, hypokalaemia and hypertension. A very similar or identical enzyme in the placenta is thought to protect the fetus from maternal cortisol.

Recent data in the rat suggest that the efficiency of this placental enzymic barrier to maternal glucocorticoids varies considerably [17]. Intriguingly, the lowest placental 11β-HSD activity, and presumably the highest fetal exposure to maternal glucocorticoids, is seen in the smallest term fetuses with the largest placentae, which, by extrapolation from human studies, are predicted to show the highest adult blood pressures (Fig. 3). Inhibition of 11β-HSD by carbenoxolone treatment during pregnancy also reduces birth weight in rats [23]. The effect of carbenoxolone on birth weight is independent of changes in maternal blood pressure or electrolytes, but requires *maternal* glucocorticoids, suggesting that it is mediated via inhibition of placental 11β-HSD, rather than by less specific actions upon maternal physiology or via direct effects upon the fetus.

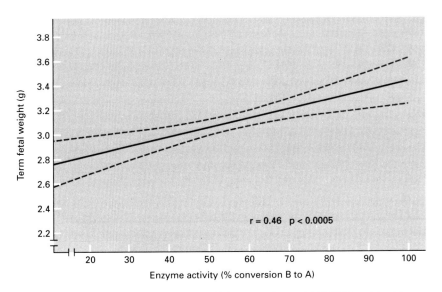

Fig. 3 Relationship (and confidence intervals) between placental 11β-HSD activity (shown as the per cent conversion of active corticosterone (B) to inert 11-dehydrocorticosterone (A) and fetal weight at term in the rat. A similar association between placental 11β-HSD efficiency and birth weight is found in *ex vivo* perfused intact human placenta. (Reproduced with permission from Benediktsson *et al.*, unpublished observations.)

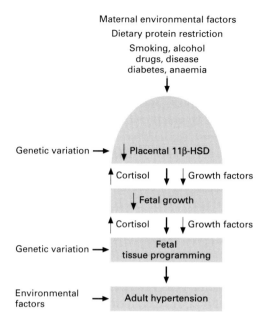

Fig. 4 Possible schema linking maternal environmental factors and genetic influences with fetal growth and the programming of hypertension.

Importantly, the male and female offspring of carbenoxolone-treated pregnancies are hypertensive when adult.

Two additional questions about the rat models immediately occur. First, can overexposure of fetal rats to maternal glucocorticoids model any of the other epidemiological associations in humans? Intriguingly, the answer may be yes, as the offspring of carbenoxolone-treated pregnant rats show basal hyperglycaemia and appear to be insulin-resistant (Lindsay R.S. *et al.* unpublished data). Second, is fetal exposure to excessive maternal glucocorticoids an exceptional or common mechanism affecting intrauterine growth? This point has not yet been resolved, but it is intriguing to note that dietary protein restriction during rat pregnancy, which also reduces birth weight and produces hypertensive offspring [9], markedly reduces placental 11β-HSD activity [24]. Clearly fetoplacental glucocorticoid excess may therefore be a common pathway linking maternal environmental influences to fetal growth retardation (Fig. 4). Moreover, because maternal glucocorticoid levels are much higher than fetal, a relative deficiency of placental 11β-HSD has far greater potential consequences, in terms of the glucocorticoid load upon the fetus, than any alterations in fetal adrenal production.

Placental 11β-HSD in humans

Do any of these results in animal models apply to humans? Measurement of glucocorticoid levels in fetal or cord vessels is technically demanding and complicated by the potential response of plasma cortisol (but not cortisone) to the stress of sampling or labour. In adults, plasma osteocalcin, a protein derived from bone osteoblasts, is very sensitive to longer-term glucocorticoid excess. The fetus also produces osteocalcin which does not appear to cross the placenta and might be a useful and convenient marker of chronic glucocorticoid exposure. Recent data suggest that placental 11β-HSD activity *in vivo*, as assessed by its ability to inactivate cortisol to cortisone across the cord artery to the cord vein (blood going to the fetus), closely correlates with fetal osteocalcin levels [25]. These data are compatible with the notion that the efficiency of the placental enzymic barrier to maternal glucocorticoids is an *important* level of control of fetal glucocorticoid exposure. As far as birth weight, the crucial intermediate phenotype for blood pressure identified in the epidemiological studies, is concerned, this also appears to correlate with placental 11β-HSD. In particular, using an immediate *ex vivo* perfusion system that may closely model the *in vivo* situation at term, we have found that placental 11β-HSD efficiency in humans correlates closely with birth weight [26]. It remains to be determined whether the lower-birth-weight neonates with reduced placental 11β-HSD activity subsequently develop higher blood pressures.

MOLECULAR BIOLOGY OF PLACENTAL 11β-HSD

From the above it is clear that placental 11β-HSD and its regulation are of considerable interest. An enzyme had been purified from rat liver, antisera raised and an encoding complementary DNA (cDNA) isolated. The human, monkey, sheep and mouse cDNA homologues had also been cloned. However, several lines of evidence indicated that this was not the enzyme responsible for protecting the fetus from maternal glucocorticoids [20]. In particular:

1 the affinity of this liver-type 11β-HSD (11β-HSD-1) is too low effectively to exclude glucocorticoids from the fetus;
2 there is a similar protective 11β-HSD in the distal nephron and yet this tissue is devoid of 11β-HSD-1 immunostaining;
3 transcription of the 11β-HSD-1 gene can be almost completely inhibited by high-dose oestrogen and yet placental and renal enzyme activities are increased by oestrogens;
4 transfection of 11β-HSD-1 cDNA into mammalian cells usually produces 11β-reductase activity, which, far from inactivating cortisol, regenerates cortisol from otherwise inert cortisone;
5 there is no apparent defect of the 11β-HSD-1 gene in the syndrome of apparent mineralocorticoid excess.

For these reasons it seemed likely that there were one or more higher-affinity 11β-HSDs in placenta and kidney. Recently, a novel enzyme (11β-HSD-2) has been characterized in human placenta and purified by affinity chromatography [27]. The encoding 11β-HSD-2 cDNA has been isolated and, when transfected into mammalian cells, expresses an exclusive glucocorticoid-inactivating enzyme, with more than 100-fold higher affinity for steroid than 11β-HSD-1 [28]. This is highly expressed in placenta and distal nephron, and is identical to an 11β-HSD-2 cDNA clone isolated from a human kidney library [29]. The gene for 11β-HSD-2 is mutated in the syndrome of apparent mineralocorticoid excess and is an important candidate locus for studies of genetic linkage with blood pressure and birth weight.

REGULATION OF PLACENTAL 11β-HSD

As yet, little is known of the regulation of placental 11β-HSD in animals, and nothing in humans. The variation in activity of the enzyme in humans, and its complex ontogeny in the placenta of non-human primates, suggests that regulatory mechanisms occur. It is conceivable that there is a genetic component to the variation. Environmental factors may also be important. Maternal diet affects placental 11β-HSD, as detailed above [24]. Ethanol, nicotine and other components of tobacco smoke, maternal stress, illness and medication may also have effects, but these remain to be determined.

Oestrogens, synthesized in the placenta from *fetal* adrenal androgens, maintain placental 11β-HSD activity in primates [30]. The control of adrenal androgen release in the fetus is poorly understood. However, intrauterine growth retardation in humans is also associated with reduced fetal adrenal androgen production [14], which may then attenuate placental 11β-HSD activity, increasing maternofetal glucocorticoid transfer. Maternal and/or fetal stress also stimulates placental secretion of corticotrophin-releasing hormone, which is elevated in the neonatal circulation in association with intrauterine growth retardation [14]. This probably stimulates the fetal pituitary–adrenal axis to secrete glucocorticoids, amplifying the fetal glucocorticoid excess. Thus there may be a cascade of effects leading to increased glucocorticoid levels in the growth-retarded fetus. Teleologically, the glucocorticoid excess may produce a short-term benefit by increasing the availability of glucose and other fuel substrates as a result of their catabolic effects. In the longer term, the consequences of such survival measures may be the permanent programming of responses (elevated glucocorticoid levels, higher blood pressure, hyperglycaemia) geared to coping with increased levels of environmental stresses, at the expense of producing disease in later life.

Adrenal androgens may be of more than passing interest for an additional reason. A number of epidemiological studies of ageing human populations have shown that higher circulating levels of adrenal androgens (notably dehydroepiandrosterone and its sulphate) are associated with more successful cardiovascular ageing (i.e. less disease) in humans. In other words, adrenal androgens are higher in those who remain well into grand old age and lower in those who will become ill. Moreover, administration of dehydroepiandrosterone to aged subjects improves well-being and restores declining growth factor levels [31]. Although it is unclear whether adrenal androgen levels *in utero* reflect those in later life, it is tempting to speculate that higher adrenal androgen levels throughout life associate with better cardiovascular and metabolic health. This might be mediated through maximization of placental protection of the fetus from maternal glucocorticoids *in utero* and also the anabolic and antiglucocorticoid effects of adrenal androgens in adult life.

STEROIDS AND PROGRAMMING

By what mechanism(s) might glucocorticoid exposure *in utero* cause later pathology? Steroid hormones have well-characterized programming effects, as described above for androgens. Similarly, neonatal stress or glucocorticoids permanently programme the pattern of hypothalamic–pituitary–adrenal axis responses, effects largely mediated via altered expression of glucocorticoid receptor genes in the brain regions responsible for glucocorticoid feedback [32]. However, the complexity of this system must also be noted. Thus minor stress in the neonatal period (15 minutes of handling of rat pups every day for the first 2 weeks of life) permanently increases glucocorticoid receptors in the brain, increasing sensitivity to feedback and thus keeping glucocorticoid levels low, a state compatible with good adjustment to environmental stress. In contrast, more severe neonatal stress (180 minutes of maternal separation per day, immune challenge or higher-dose glucocorticoid administration) has the opposite effect, programming reduced brain sensitivity to glucocorticoid feedback and hence greater responses to stress throughout life. This may represent a state of poor adjustment of the hypothalamic–pituitary–adrenal axis and associates with adverse 'wear-and-tear' consequences for glucocorticoid target organs. Thus glucocorticoids can programme responses, but what might be the nature of the responses that produce adult hypertension?

TARGETS OF GLUCOCORTICOID PROGRAMMING

The molecular mode of glucocorticoid action is well-defined. Glucocorticoids, like other steroid and thyroid hormones, act by binding to and activating intracellular receptors, which then attach to specific palindromic DNA sequences (glucocorticoid response elements) in the regulatory regions of target genes, affecting transcription. There are two receptor subtypes: type I or mineralocorticoid receptors and type II or glucocorticoid receptors. However, there are numerous potential target genes expressed in most, if not all, cells and the precise genomic targets for glucocorticoid programming of hypertension are obscure. Despite this, several clues are available to guide future studies.

Tissue maturation

In rats, prenatal low-dose dexamethasone affects the maturation of specific organs, including the lungs, heart, vasculature, kidney and brain. Important biochemical effects include permanent induction of the pattern of adrenergic (α and β) receptor expression and potentiation of adenylate cyclase [33]; both might alter subsequent vascular responsivity to vasoconstrictors. In this light, it is interesting that fetal sheep directly infused with cortisol become hypertensive and show increased pressor responses to angiotensin II [16], which is also an important vasoconstrictor in humans. Cardiac development is also programmed by dexamethasone *in utero* [34], as is the pattern of development of the sympathetic innervation of many target organs.

Effects on the brain

As detailed above, stress and glucocorticoids, acting prenatally or in the immediate postnatal period, can programme glucocorticoid receptor expression in the regions of the brain (e.g. hippocampus) responsible for mediating negative feedback upon the hypothalamic–pituitary–adrenal axis. Some preliminary data suggest that prenatal dexamethasone permanently attenuates glucocorticoid receptor expression in the adult brain, reducing sensitivity to feedback and thus programming increased plasma glucocorticoid levels in later life (Levitt N. *et al.* unpublished data). Such chronically elevated plasma glucocorticoid levels might contribute to the hypertension. Indeed, there may be more than coincidence in the morphological similarities between the centripetal obesity that associates with cardiovascular disease and type II diabetes and the truncal adiposity of the Cushing's syndromes. Finally, several reports suggest an association between stress, depression and the occurrence of ischaemic heart disease in humans. At least the first two are also associated with elevated plasma glucocorticoid levels.

Glucocorticoids and growth factors

Of similar or greater importance may be the effects of prenatal glucocorticoids on growth factors produced in the placenta or fetus. In particular, much data indicate a central role for the insulin-like growth factors IGF-1 and IGF-2 in the determination of fetal and placental growth. Both IGFs, their receptors and several IGF-binding proteins are regulated by glucocorticoids in fetal tissues [35,36]. The IGF system is also affected by maternal nutrition and provides a plausible final common pathway whereby a range of maternal or placental factors (including 11β-HSD) might affect fetoplacental development and growth.

Glucocorticoids and glucose–insulin homeostasis

Many hepatic enzymes controlling the production and metabolism of fuels, including phosphoenolpyruvate carboxykinase, the rate-limiting step in gluconeogenesis, are potently regulated by glucocorticoids. Insulin-sensitivity is attenuated by glucocorticoids, which also critically regulate adipose cell biology and adipose distribution. Indeed, it may be more than coincidence that centripetal obesity, which is a documented risk for cardiovascular disease, is very reminiscent of the adipose redistribution in Cushing's syndrome and disease. Prenatal exposure to excess glucocorticoids might programme these systems, leading to subsequent abnormalities in insulin–glucose and fat homeostasis (which in humans associate with low birth weight [37]). Indeed, preliminary evidence in the rat suggests that 11β-HSD inhibition with carbenoxolone during pregnancy leads to induction of phosphoenolpyruvate carboxykinase activity in the livers of offspring at weaning and to insulin resistance when adult (Lindsay R.S. *et al.*, unpublished data).

CLINICAL IMPLICATIONS

Despite the interesting observations in animals, there is surprisingly little clinical literature on the effects of low-dose glucocorticoids *in utero*. Glucocorticoid administration to pregnant animals causes teratogenic effects, but these have not been convincingly observed with modest therapeutic doses in humans [38]. Glucocorticoids also reduce birth weight and alter organ maturation in non-human primates and humans [10,11]. 11β-HSD substrates, such as cortisol (hydrocortisone) and prednisolone, might be anticipated to have little effect, unless the enzyme becomes saturated, which seems unlikely because of its large excess catalytic capacity. Synthetic steroids, which are poorer substrates, are rarely administered, the exception being the treatment of women bearing female fetuses affected by congenital adrenal hyperplasia (usually 21-hydroxy lase deficiency). These subjects often receive dexamethasone from the first trimester in an attempt to suppress fetal adrenocorticotrophic hormone (ACTH) and hence adrenal androgen overproduction which otherwise produces virilization of an affected female baby. No teratogenic effects of low-dose dexamethasone have been noted [39] and birth weight has been reported as normal, although this has not been carefully defined. It should also be recalled that Barker's epidemiological data [37] are based on birth weights within the normal range. Few data on the effects of such therapy on offspring blood pressure or other cardiovascular risk factors have been reported, and in any event, such patients have abnormal adrenal steroid levels throughout life, complicating any interpretation. Moreover, 11β-HSD-2 can metabolize dexamethasone, albeit with lower affinity than for physiological glucocorticoids, and presumably the dose required to produce fetal glucocorticoid excess will be greater than anticipated from regimens in postnatal life. 11β-HSD inhibition (liquorice abuse, carbenoxolone therapy) has rarely been reported in pregnancy and has not been associated with obvious neonatal effects, although reductions in birth weight and subsequent cardiovascular disease have not been sought.

CONCLUSIONS

There is increasing evidence in animal models that relatively modest glucocorticoid excess retards intrauterine growth and programmes subsequent high blood pressure. Physiologically, such increased fetal glucocorticoid exposure may result from relative deficiency of the normal placental enzyme barrier to maternal glucocorticoids. In humans, the efficiency of this placental barrier varies and correlates with birth weight and fetal osteocalcin levels—a possible index of fetal glucocorticoid exposure. Whether environmental or genetic variation in placental 11β-HSD in humans relates to the programming of subsequent disease, and the nature of the crucial biochemical and tissue targets involved in the effects of prenatal glucocorticoid exposure, remain to be determined.

ACKNOWLEDGEMENTS

I am very grateful to Drs Rafn Benedicktsson, Roger Brown and Robbie Lindsay for permission to elude to unpublished data and for helpful discussions. The work from my laboratory described in this chapter is generously supported by a Wellcome Trust senior clinical fellowship and grants from the Wellcome Trust, the Medical Research Council and the Scottish Hospital Endowments Research Trust.

REFERENCES

1 Barker DJP. *Fetal and Infant Origins of Adult Disease*. British Medical Journal, London, 1991.
2 Law CM, de Swiet M, Osmond C *et al*. Initiation of hypertension *in utero* and its amplification throughout life. *Br Med J* 1993;**306**:24–27.
3 Levine RS, Hennekens CH, Jesse MJ. Blood pressure in prospective population based cohort of newborn and infant twins. *Br Med J* 1994;**308**:298–302.
4 Lever AF, Harrap SB. Essential hypertension: a disorder of growth with origins in childhood? *J Hypertens* 1992;**10**:101–120.

5 Bartley M, Power C, Blane D, Davey Smith G, Shipley M. Birth weight and later socioeconomic disadvantage: evidence from the 1958 British cohort study. *Br Med J* 1994;**309**:1475–1478.
6 Edwards CRW, Benediktsson R, Lindsay R, Seckl JR. Dysfunction of the placental glucocorticoid barrier: a link between the foetal environment and adult hypertension? *Lancet* 1993;**341**:355–357.
7 Barker DJP, Gluckman PD, Godfrey KM, Harding JE, Owens JA, Robinson JS. Fetal nutrition and cardiovascular disease in adult life. *Lancet* 1993;**341**:938–941.
8 Arai Y, Gorski RA. Critical exposure time for androgenization of the developing hypothalamus in the female rat. *Endocrinology* 1968;**82**:1010–1014.
9 Langley SC, Jackson AA. Increased systolic blood pressure in adult rats induced by fetal exposure to maternal low protein diets. *Clin Sci* 1994;**86**:217–222.
10 Reinisch JM, Simon NG, Karwo WG *et al*. Prenatal exposure to prednisone in humans and animals retards intra-uterine growth. *Science* 1978;**202**:436–438.
11 Novy MJ, Walsh SW. Dexamethasone and estradiol treatment in pregnant rhesus macaques: effects on gestation length, maternal plasma hormones and fetal growth. *Am J Obstet Gynecol* 1983;**145**:920–930.
12 Mosier Jr HD, Dearden LC, Jansons RA, Roberts RC, Biggs CS. Disproportionate growth of organs and body weight following glucocorticoid treatment of the rat fetus. *Dev Pharmacol Ther* 1982;**4**:89–105.
13 Gunberg DL. Some effects of exogenous hydrocortisone on pregnancy in the rat. *Anat Res* 1957;**129**:133–153.
14 Goland RS, Jozak S, Warren WB, Conwell IM, Stark RI, Tropper PJ. Elevated levels of umbilical cord plasma corticotropin-releasing hormone in growth-retarded fetuses. *J Clin Endocrinol Metab* 1993;**77**:1174–1179.
15 Tonolo G, Fraser R, Connell JMC, Kenyon CJ. Chronic low-dose infusions of dexamethasone in rats: effect on blood pressure, body weight and plasma atrial natriuretic peptide. *J Hypertens* 1988;**6**:25–31.
16 Tangalakis K, Lumbers ER, Moritz KM, Towstoless MK, Wintour EM. Effect of cortisol on blood pressure and vascular reactivity in the ovine fetus. *Exp Physiol* 1992;**77**:709–717.
17 Benediktsson R, Lindsay R, Noble J, Seckl JR, Edwards CRW. Glucocorticoid exposure *in utero*: a new model for adult hypertension. *Lancet* 1993;**341**:339–341.
18 Beitens IZ, Bayard F, Ances IG, Kowarski A, Migeon CJ. The metabolic clearance rate, blood production, interconversion and transplacental passage of cortisol and cortisone in pregnancy near term. *Pediatr Res* 1973;**7**:509–519.
19 Campbell AL, Murphy BEP. The maternal–fetal cortisol gradient during pregnancy and at delivery. *J Clin Endocrinol Metab* 1977;**45**:435–440.
20 Seckl JR. 11β-hydroxysteroid dehydrogenase isoforms and their implications for blood pressure regulation. *Eur J Clin Invest* 1993;**23**:589–601.
21 Edwards CRW, Stewart PM, Burt D *et al*. Localisation of 11β-hydroxysteroid dehydrogenase-tissue specific protector of the mineralocorticoid receptor. *Lancet* 1988;**ii**:986–989.
22 Funder JW, Pearce PT, Smith R, Smith AI. Mineralocorticoid action: target tissue specificity is enzyme, not receptor, mediated. *Science* 1988;**242**:583–585.
23 Lindsay RS, Noble JM, Edwards CRW, Seckl JR. Maternal carbenoxolone treatment reduces birth weight in the rat. *J Endocrinol* 1994;**140**(suppl):P18.
24 Phillips GJ, Langley-Evans SC, Benediktsson R, Seckl JR, Edwards CRW, Jackson AA. The role of dietary protein restriction during pregnancy on the activity of placental 11β-hydroxysteroid dehydrogenase. *Proc Nutr Soc* 1994;**53**:170A.
25 Benediktsson R, Brennand J, Tibi L, Calder AA, Seckl JR, Edwards CRW. Fetal osteocalcin levels are related to placental 11β-hydroxysteroid dehydrogenase activity. *Clin Endocrinol* 1995;**42**:551–555.
26 Benediktsson R, Noble J, Calder AA, Edwards CRW, Seckl JR. 11β-hydroxysteroid dehydrogenase activity in intact dually-perfused fresh human placenta predicts birth weight. *J Endocrinol* 1995;**144**(suppl):P161.
27 Brown RW, Chapman KE, Edwards CRW, Seckl JR. Human placental 11β-hydroxysteroid dehydrogenase: partial purification of and evidence for a distinct NAD-dependent isoform. *Endocrinology* 1993;**132**:2614–2621.

28 Brown RW, Chapman KE, Edwards CRW, Seckl JR. Isolation of 11β-hydroxysteroid dehydrogenase type 2. *J Endocrinol* 1994;**140**(suppl):OC34.

29 Albiston AL, Obeyesekere VR, Smith RE, Krozowski ZS. Cloning and tissue distribution of the human 11β-hydroxysteroid dehydrogenase type 2 enzyme. *Mol Cell Endocrinol* 1994;**105**:R11–R17.

30 Baggia S, Albrecht E, Pepe G. Regulation of 11β-hydroxysteroid dehydrogenase activity in the baboon placenta by estrogen. *Endocrinology* 1990;**126**:2742–2748.

31 Morales AJ, Nolan JJ, Nelson JC, Yen SSC. Effects of replacement dose of dehydroepiandrosterone in men and women of advancing age. *J Clin Endocrinol Metab* 1994;**78**:1360–1367.

32 Meaney MJ, O'Donnell D, Viau V *et al.* Corticosteroid receptors in the rat brain and pituitary during development and hypothalamic–pituitary–adrenal function. In: *Growth Factors and Hormones*, edited by Zagon S, McLaughlin PJ. Chapman and Hall, New York, 1993;163–201.

33 Bian XP, Seidler FJ, Slotkin TA. Promotional role for glucocorticoids in the development of intracellular signalling: enhanced cardiac and renal adenylate cyclase reactivity to β-andrenergic and non-adrenergic stimuli after low-dose fetal dexamethasone exposure. *J Dev Physiol* 1992;**17**:289–297.

34 Bian XP, Seidler FJ, Slotkin TA. Fetal dexamethasone exposure interferes with establishment of cardiac noradrenergic innervation and sympathetic activity. *Teratology* 1993;**47**:109–117.

35 Price WA, Stiles AD, Moats-Staats BM, D'Ercole AJ. Gene expression of the insulin-like growth factors (IGFs), the type 1 IGF receptor, and IGF-binding proteins in dexamethasone-induced fetal growth retardation. *Endocrinology* 1992;**130**:1424–1432.

36 Saunders JC, Gilmour RS, Fowden AL. Insulin-like growth factor-II messenger RNA expression in fetal tissues of the sheep during late gestation: effects of cortisol. *Endocrinology* 1993;**132**:2083–2089.

37 Barker DJP, Hales CN, Fall CHD, Osmond C, Phipps K, Clarke PMS. Type 2 (non-insulin dependent) diabetes mellitus, hypertension and hyperlipidaemia (syndrome X): relation to reduced fetal growth. *Diabetologia* 1993;**36**:62–67.

38 Forest MG, Betuel H, David M. Prenatal treatment in congenital adrenal hyperplasia due to 21-hydroxylase deficiency: update 88 of the French multicentric study. *Endocrinol Res* 1989;**15**:277–301.

39 Forest MG, David M, Morel Y. Prenatal diagnosis and treatment of 21-hydroxylase deficiency. *J Steroid Biochem Mol Biol* 1993;**45**:75–82.

Long-term associations between haemostatic variables and ischaemic heart disease

THOMAS W. MEADE

Recognition of the thrombotic component in ischaemic heart disease (IHD) is now universal, although fairly recent [1,2]. Usually, thrombus is superimposed on pre-existing atheroma. Occasionally, however, coronary artery thrombosis is not associated with atheroma [3], suggesting that characteristics of the circulating blood play a significant part in major clinical episodes of IHD (whether associated with atheroma — as usually — or not). Platelets and fibrin resulting from activation of the coagulation cascade are the two main components of coronary artery thrombi. A growing number of prospective population-based studies now indicate that high levels of some clotting factors, particularly fibrinogen and factor VII, are associated with the incidence of IHD over a period of a few years. More familiar indices of risk such as blood pressure and blood cholesterol levels predict IHD over a matter of decades. But because of the generally large within-person variability in tests of haemostatic function [4], long-term relations between clotting factor levels and IHD may be less easily demonstrable than for lipids or blood pressure. It is now therefore useful to consider whether or not this is so, based on the prospective studies that have followed up their participants for substantial periods.

PLATELETS

While there is no doubt as to the central role of platelets in arterial thrombosis and IHD, attempts to characterize those at risk on account of increased platelet aggregability have so far been few and far between and not very informative so far as associations with first episodes are concerned. One reason may be the particularly large components of within-person and laboratory variability in some tests of platelet function [5]. Another may be that tests so far used do not in fact indicate a biological pathway of any clinical significance and that other, so far untested, measures of platelet function might be more rewarding. A third possibility is that platelets themselves have limited intrinsic properties relevant to thrombogenesis and that they are controlled by plasma influences such as thrombin and fibrinogen — an explanation that in no way diminishes their involvement in thrombosis but accounts for it through these other effects.

In one study, a high total platelet count and rapid aggregability to adenosine diphosphate were significantly associated with an increased risk of IHD over a follow-up period of 13.5 years [6], though the numbers studied were small. On the other hand, the Northwick Park Heart Study (NPHS; MRC Epidemiology and Medical Care Unit, unpublished data) has found no association between either platelet count or platelet aggregability induced by adenosine diphosphate (ADP) or adrenaline over a 10-year follow-up period in a substantially larger number of men.

Two shorter-term studies in survivors of an initial myocardial infarct (MI) have found an association between, in one case, spontaneous platelet aggregation and recurrent IHD [7] and, in another, between platelet volume and recurrent MI [8].

COAGULATION

Many, mostly cross-sectional associations have now been established between clotting factors and IHD (and also between platelet tests and IHD) but in these circumstances it is difficult to distinguish findings that precede the onset of disease from those that are consequential and possibly of limited biological significance. The rest of this review therefore concentrates mainly on prospective findings in which clotting factors have been measured before the onset of clinical disease.

Factor VII activity

Factor VII circulates mainly in an inactive, single-chain form. The two-chain form, VII_a, circulates at a much lower concentration but is many times more active. The direct measurement of VII_a has only recently become possible, so the sensitivity of conventional factor VII assays to VII_a is an important consideration. The most extensive data on factor VII activity and IHD come from the NPHS [9–11], which used an assay sensitive to VII_a [12]. As expected, the association of VII_c with major IHD is clearest for events occurring relatively soon after its measurement [10]. However, VII_c is strongly associated with fatal IHD events over the 16-year follow-up period on which the most recent NPHS results are based [13]. The only other prospective results so far reported on factor VII come from the 6-year Prospective Cardiovascular Münster (PROCAM) follow-up study in Germany [14], in which there is a similar though less marked distinction between fatal and non-fatal events in their association with VII, even though the PROCAM assay for VII activity is less sensitive to VII_a than the NPHS assay. If the suggested contrast in the relation of VII with fatal compared with non-fatal events is indeed true, the explanation may lie in the influence of the VII_a level at the time thrombogenesis is initiated in determining the subsequent size and stability of the occlusive thrombus through the amount of fibrin deposited and through the platelet-aggregating property of thrombin.

Factor VIII activity

NPHS has recently demonstrated an association between VIII activity and IHD [15] and, as with factor VII, the association is strongest for fatal events, the risk of which rises by about 30% for each standard deviation increase in factor VIII activity. Again, the more obvious association with fatal than non-fatal events may be due to the effect of factor VIII activity on thrombin production once coagulation has been initiated. Haemophilic patients experience a significantly reduced incidence of IHD [16] and, since they are not protected against atheroma, any influence of factor VIII on clinical IHD is likely to be through its thrombogenic properties. This conclusion is supported by the probable role of factor VIII in venous thrombosis [17], in which, in the absence of atheroma, the association can with some confidence be attributed to the degree of coagulability.

Fibrinogen

Starting with NPHS [9], 10 or more prospective studies have now shown a generally strong and independent relation between the plasma fibrinogen level and the incidence of both IHD and stroke. The increasing frequency of recent reports means that any overview may quite quickly be outdated, although the main conclusion of one such overview [18] is a fair summary — that those with plasma fibrinogen levels in the upper third of the distribution experience between 2.0 and 2.5 times the incidence of IHD compared with those with values in the lower third. Because the fibrinogen level is also associated with the incidence of stroke, to which the blood cholesterol level is not however strongly related, fibrinogen is likely to prove a valuable index of the risk of major cardiovascular disease defined as the sum of IHD and stroke. Figure 1, from NPHS, shows that the association of fibrinogen with IHD over a 16-year follow-up period is at least as strong as for cholesterol [11]. (The data on fibrinolytic activity are discussed later.) Since fibrinogen and cholesterol are only poorly correlated, the two associations are almost entirely independent, i.e. knowledge of the fibrinogen level adds new information. Figure 2 is from the Caerphilly study, with a follow-up period of 10 years, and makes the important point that fibrinogen levels predict the onset of IHD in non-smokers as well as in smokers. Table 1 summarizes the findings on fibrinogen and stroke from the Göteborg study [20] in which, if anything, fibrinogen was a stronger predictor of stroke than blood pressure during

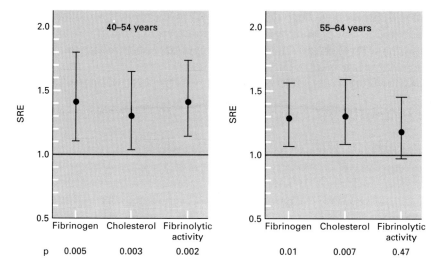

Fig. 1 Standardized regression effects (SRE), 95% confidence intervals and *P* values for relation of variables with incidence of ischaemic heart disease (IHD). SRE is difference in IHD associated with a difference of one standard deviation (I/SD) in variable, i.e. with high fibrinogen and cholesterol levels and with low fibrinolytic activity. Reproduced with permission from [11].

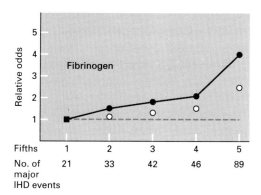

Fig. 2 Relative odds of a major incident of ischaemic heart disease (IHD) event by fifths of fibrinogen adjusted for age (●) and for other risk factors, including smoking (○). Reproduced with permission from [19].

Table 1 Mean plasma fibrinogen levels at entry to the Göteborg study according to subsequent outcome [20].

	Deaths from			
	IHD	Stroke	Other causes	No event
Number	92	37	60	608
Fibrinogen (g/l)	3.56*	3.70*	3.37	3.30

* *P* < 0.01.
IHD, Ischaemic heart disease.

a follow-up of 13.5 years, though it was the combination of both that appeared particularly hazardous.

The PROCAM study in Münster shows an increased risk of IHD with increasing fibrinogen level over a 6-year period. Besides predicting the *onset* of IHD, stroke and also of lower-extremity arterial disease (LEAD) [21], other studies have consistently shown that high fibrinogen levels are associated with the *recurrence* or *progression* of these conditions [22–24].

In summary, therefore, the plasma fibrinogen level provides additional information on the risk of newly developing or of further experiencing IHD, stroke and LEAD. This recognition has led to the establishment of a reference standard [25] to ensure the increasing comparability of results obtained in different laboratories — an important development, bearing in mind that, while the associations of fibrinogen with IHD risk or IHD itself are remarkably consistent from one study to another, absolute fibrinogen levels have so far differed considerably between laboratories as a result of the different methods used.

How should the association between high fibrinogen levels and arterial disease be interpreted? Table 2 summarizes the wide range of personal and other characteristics that apparently influence the fibrinogen level. Whatever the origin of high levels, these predispose to IHD through at least five main pathways — an effect on atherogenesis itself, on whole blood and plasma viscosity, on platelet aggregability, on the amount of fibrin deposited when coagulation is initiated and on clot deformability [26,27]. In addition to the personal characteristics listed, high levels may partly be a result of underlying vessel wall disease, since atheroma has many of the characteristics of an inflammatory response. In this sense,

Table 2 Fibrinogen: determinants and pathways.

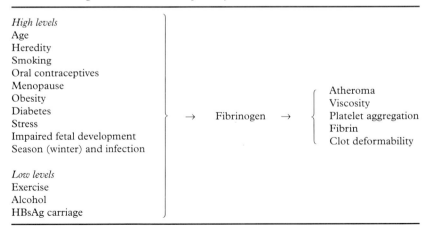

HBsAg, Hepatitis B surface antigen.

high fibrinogen levels are both a marker and a cause of vascular disease. There is some evidence in younger male subjects, presumably free of significant atheroma, that vessel wall pathology may not in fact explain raised fibrinogen levels to any marked extent [28] but even if it does, this component is still likely to be of biological significance and should not be overlooked simply because it may not be entirely independent of the pathogenic process as a whole.

Although many of the well-recognized risk factors for IHD do appear to influence fibrinogen, the obvious omission in Table 2 is diet, the evidence in humans being that no dietary constituents (with the possible but still debatable exception of fish oils) affect it.

It is increasingly clear that infection is associated with an increased risk of both IHD and stroke, relationships of this kind have been demonstrated for a variety of febrile illnessess [29], Chlamydia pneumoniae [30], poor dental health [31] and Helicobacter pylori [32], the last of these also being associated with raised fibrinogen levels [33]. While infection causes many other changes besides a rise in fibrinogen, it is certainly possible that the latter may partly explain the association of infection with increased IHD and stroke mortality, in which case there may be large and significant implications for the prevention and early treatment of infections with a view to reducing the incidence of IHD and stroke.

Elucidating the nature of the association between high fibrinogen levels and arterial events largely depends on trials aimed at preventing them through lowering the fibrinogen level — a question of obvious clinical relevance as well. Whether or not selective fibrinogen-lowering agents become available remains to be seen. Meanwhile, the fibrinogen-lowering effect of most of the fibrates (with the exception of gemfibrozil) is attracting increasing attention. The reduction of 20% or more in the plasma fibrinogen level attributable to bezafibrate [34] would translate into worthwhile reductions in major arterial events, assuming complete reversibility of risk. At least two large trials with IHD or stroke endpoints are now in progress [35] (MRC Epidemiology and Medical Care Unit, in progress). Whether any benefits can be attributed to the effects of lowering fibrinogen levels as distinct from the lipid-modifying effects of bezafibrate largely depends on how far the changes in these two effects are correlated with one another.

Antithrombin III

Most cross-sectional studies of antithrombin III and the risk of arterial disease have established clear associations, although some have been of low levels related to risk while others have been of high levels and increased risk. These apparently contradictory results could be explained by postulating that in some circumstances low antithrombin III levels are of direct causal significance, while in others raised levels represent a compensatory response to increased risk. NPHS has shown what may indeed be a U-shaped relation between antithrombin III and fatal IHD [36].

Fibrinolytic activity

In 1987, Hamsten *et al.* [37] reported that high concentrations of plasminogen activator inhibitor (PAI-1) were associated with an increased risk of recurrence in 109 young survivors of MI. This observation on recurrence in those already affected has now been complemented by the NPHS results summarized earlier in Fig. 1 [11]. NPHS had used the dilute clot lysis time (DCLT) (fibrinolytic activity being defined as 100/ lysis time in hours), since measures of individual components of the fibrinolytic system were not generally available when participants were recruited. Figure 1 shows a strong and largely independent relation of low fibrinolytic activity with IHD over the 16-year follow-up period particularly in younger men. Both PAI-1 and tissue plasminogen activator (tPA) contribute to DCLT, predominantly the former [38]. A nested case-control analysis of samples taken during the US Physicians Health Study showed, counterintuitively, an increasing risk of MI with increasing tPA antigen levels [39]. However, tPA is largely bound to PAI-1 so that antigenic methods for tPA may largely reflect PAI-1 rather than free, active tPA. If so, the NPHS and US Physicians Health Study findings are not incompatible. The Göteborg study [20] found no association with IHD using euglobulin lysis but all the participants in the Göteborg study were aged 54 years at entry, so that the possibility of an association at younger ages, suggested in the Swedish study of recurrent MI [37] and in NPHS [11], could not be assessed.

Within the last few years, a new approach to the coagulation system in IHD has been made possible through assays of the activation peptides of different clotting factors. In particular, the activation peptide of prothrombin, F1.2, indicates the generation of thrombin and the level of fibrinopeptide A (FPA) indicates the extent to which thrombin has acted on fibrinogen in the production of fibrin. Compared with the earlier classical clotting factor assays, these peptides therefore provide a more direct assessment of the activity level of the coagulation system. They have been used to show a state of persistent activation of coagulation in IHD [40]. Thus, levels of F1.2 in patients with unstable angina and MI were raised both on admission to hospital and 6 months later. FPA was also clearly elevated at admission, i.e. in association with the thrombotic episode, but had fallen to normal or near normal levels 6 months later. These patients had therefore maintained a persistent elevation of coagulability, seen as raised F1.2 levels, that carries with it the risk of expression through the action of thrombin and indicated by raised FPA levels at the time of the clinical event. The growing availability of these activation peptide assays will provide many valuable new opportunities for defining the role of coagulability in arterial disease.

Another recent development has been the identification of a mutation in the gene coding for factor V, resulting in resistance to activated protein C and thus to what would be anticipated as an increased risk of thrombosis. While this mutation does indeed predispose to venous thrombosis, it does not, however, appear to be associated with the incidence of IHD or stroke [41].

CONCLUSION

Despite their inherent variability, several components of the haemostatic system are independently associated with the risk of IHD and stroke in the long term about as strongly as cholesterol, for example. The association with IHD and stroke of raised fibrinogen levels, in particular, is at the interface between a research finding and its implementation in clinical practice. The latter depends partly on the growing availability of routine fibrinogen measurements together with their standardization between different laboratories. Even before this has been achieved, however, clinical use can be made of the fibrinogen level, provided each laboratory can interpret the results in terms of the distributions for men and women at different ages established by its own method. Thus, the additional information on risk indicated by the fibrinogen level may be used in deciding whether, for example, to initiate treatment with aspirin in a subject who is at particularly high risk, even though aspirin does not affect the fibrinogen level. Using the fibrinogen level in clinical practice also depends on the value of lowering fibrinogen levels and, until this has been established through the necessary trials, decisions inevitably have to depend on incomplete information. An example where lowering the fibrinogen level might be considered is a patient at high risk on other accounts due, for instance, to a strong family history and perhaps hypertension or hypercholesterolaemia who, in addition, does have an obviously raised fibrinogen level but is a non-smoker. Bezafibrate is likely to lower both fibrinogen and the total cholesterol level so that, coupled with the generally low incidence of significant side-effects with which it is associated, its use could be justified.

REFERENCES

1 DeWood MA, Spores J, Notske R *et al*. Prevalence of total coronary occlusion during the early hours of transmural myocardial infarction. *N Engl J Med* 1980;**303**:897–902.
2 Davies MJ, Thomas A. Thrombosis and acute coronary-artery lesions in sudden cardiac ischemic death. *N Engl J Med* 1984;**310**:1137–1140.

3 El Fawal MA, Berg GA, Wheatley DJ, Harland WA. Sudden coronary death in Glasgow: nature and frequency of acute coronary lesions. *Br Heart J* 1987;**57**:329–335.

4 Thompson SG, Martin JC, Meade TW. Sources of variability in coagulation factor assays. *Thromb Haemostas* 1987;**58**:1073–1077.

5 Vickers MV, Thompson SG. Sources of variability in dose response platelet aggregometry. *Thromb Haemost* 1985;**53**:216–218.

6 Thaulow E, Erikssen J, Sandvik L, Stormorken H, Cohn P. Blood platelet count and function are related to total and cardiovascular death in apparently healthy men. *Circulation* 1991;**84**:613–617.

7 Trip MD, Cats VM, van Capelle FJL, Vreeken J. Platelet hyperreactivity and prognosis in survivors of myocardial infarction. *N Engl J Med* 1990;**322**:1549–1554.

8 Martin JF, Bath PM, Burr ML. Influence of platelet size on outcome after myocardial infarction. *Lancet* 1991;**338**:1409–1411.

9 Meade TW, North WRS, Chakrabarti R *et al.* Haemostatic function and cardiovascular death: early results of a prospective study. *Lancet* 1980;**1**:1050–1054.

10 Meade TW, Mellows S, Brozovic M *et al.* Haemostatic function and ischaemic heart disease: principal results of the Northwick Park Heart Study. *Lancet* 1986;**2**:533–537.

11 Meade TW, Ruddock V, Stirling Y, Chakrabarti R, Miller GJ. Fibrinolytic activity, clotting factors and long term incidence of ischaemic heart disease in the Northwick Park Heart Study. *Lancet* 1993;**342**:1076–1079.

12 Miller GJ, Stirling Y, Esnouf MP *et al.* Factor VII-deficient substrate plasma depleted of protein C raise the sensitivity of the factor VII bio-assay to activated factor VII an international study. *Thromb Haemost* 1994;**71**:38–48.

13 Ruddock V, Meade TW. Factor VII activity and ischaemic heart disease: fatal and non-fatal events. *Q J Med* 1994;**87**:403–406.

14 Heinrich J, Balleisen L, Schulte H, Assmann G, van de Loo J. Fibrinogen and factor VII in the prediction of coronary risk. Results from the PROCAM study in healthy men. *Arterioscler Thromb* 1994;**14**:54–59.

15 Meade TW, Cooper JC, Stirling Y, Howarth DJ, Ruddock V, Miller GJ. Factor VIII, ABO blood group and the incidence of ischaemic heart disease. *Br J Haematol* 1994;**88**:601–607.

16 Rosendaal FR, Varekamp I, Smit C *et al.* Mortality and causes of death in Dutch haemophiliacs, 1973–86. *Br J Haematol* 1989;**71**:71–76.

17 Koster T, Blann AD, Briët E, Vandenbroucke JP, Rosendaal FR. Role of clotting factor VIII in effect on von Willebrand factor on occurrence of deep-vein thrombosis. *Lancet* 1995;**345**:152–155.

18 Ernst E, Ludwig K, Resch L. Fibrinogen as a cardiovascular risk factor: a meta-analysis and review of the literature. *Ann Intern Med* 1993;**118**:956–963.

19 Yarnell JWG, Baker IA, Sweetnam PM *et al.* Fibrinogen, viscosity, and white blood cell count are major risk factors for ischemic heart disease. The Caerphilly and Speedwell Collaborative Heart Disease Studies. *Circulation* 1991;**83**:836–844.

20 Wilhelmsen L, Svardsudd K, Korsan-Bengtsen K, Welin L, Tibblin G. Fibrinogen as a risk factor for stroke and myocardial infarction. *N Engl J Med* 1984;**311**:501–505.

21 Kannel WB. Fibrinogen: a major cardiovascular risk factor. In: *Fibrinogen: A "New" Cardiovascular Risk Factor*, edited by Ernst E, Koenig W, Lowe GDO, Meade TW. Blackwell-MZV, Vienna, 1992:101–109.

22 Haines AP, Howarth D, North WRS *et al.* Haemostatic variables and the outcome of myocardial infarction. *Thromb Haemost* 1983;**50**:800–803.

23 Qizilbash N, Jones L, Warlow C, Mann J. Fibrinogen and lipid concentrations as risk factors for transient ischaemic attacks and minor ischaemic strokes. *Br Med J* 1991;**303**:605–609.

24 Banerjee AK, Pearson J, Gilliland EL *et al.* A six year prospective study of fibrinogen and other risk factors associated with mortality in stable claudicants. *Thromb Haemost* 1992;**68**:261–263.

25 Gaffney PJ, Wong MY. Collaborative study of a proposed international standard for plasma fibrinogen measurement. *Thromb Haemost* 1992;**68**:428–432.

26 Meade TW. The epidemiology of atheroma, thrombosis and ischaemic heart disease. In: *Haemostasis and Thrombosis*, vol. 2, 3rd edn, edited by Bloom AL, Forbes CD, Thomas DP, Tuddenham EGD. Churchill Livingstone, Edinburgh, 1994:1199–1227.

27 Scrutton MC, Ross-Murphy SB, Bennett GM, Stirling Y, Meade TW. Changes in clot deformability — a possible explanation for the epidemiological association between plasma fibrinogen concentration and myocardial infarction. *Blood Coagul Fibrinolysis* 1994;**5**:719–723.

28 Bara L, Nicaud V, Tiret L, Cambien F, Samama MM. Expression of a paternal history of premature myocardial infarction on fibrinogen, factor VIIc and PAI-1 in European offspring — the EARS Study. *Thromb Haemost* 1994;**71**:434–440.

29 Syrjänen J, Valtonen VV, Iivanainen M, Kaste M, Huttunen JK. Preceding infection as an important risk factor for ischaemic brain infarction in young and middle aged patients. *Br Med J* 1988;**296**:1156–1160.

30 Saikku P, Leinonen M, Tenkanen L et al. Chronic *Chlamydia pneumoniae* infection as a risk factor for coronary heart disease in the Helsinki Heart Study. *Ann Intern Med* 1992;**116**:273–278.

31 Mattila KJ, Nieminen MS, Valtonen VV et al. Association between dental health and acute myocardial infarction. *Br Med J* 1989;**298**:779–781.

32 Mendall MA, Goggin PM, Molineaux N et al. Relation of *Helicobacter pylori* infection and coronary heart disease. *Br Heart J* 1994;**71**:437–439.

33 Patel P, Carrington DP, Strachan DP et al. Fibrinogen: a link between chronic infection and coronary heart disease. *Lancet* 1994;**343**:1634–1635.

34 Meade TW. Fibrinogen in ischaemic heart disease. *Eur Heart J* 1995;**16**:31–35.

35 Goldbourt U, Behar S, Reicher-Reiss H et al. Rationale and design of a secondary prevention trial of increasing serum high-density lipoprotein cholesterol and reducing triglycerides in patients with clinically manifest atherosclerotic heart disease (the Bezafibrate Infarction Prevention Trial). *Am J Cardiol* 1993;**71**:909–915.

36 Meade TW, Cooper J, Miller GJ, Howarth DJ, Stirling Y. Antithrombin III and arterial disease. *Lancet* 1991;**337**:850–851.

37 Hamsten A, De Faire U, Walldius G et al. Plasminogen activator inhibitor in plasma: risk factor for recurrent myocardial infarction. *Lancet* 1987;**2**:3–9.

38 Meade TW, Howarth DJ, Cooper J, MacCallum PK, Stirling Y. Fibrinolytic activity and arterial disease. *Lancet* 1994;**343**:1442.

39 Ridker PM, Vaughan DE, Stampfer MJ, Manson JE, Hennekens CH. Endogenous tissue-type plasminogen activator and risk of myocardial infarction. *Lancet* 1993;**341**:1165–1168.

40 Merlini PA, Bauer KA, Oltrona L et al. Persistent activation of coagulation mechanism in unstable angina and myocardial infarction. *Circulation* 1994;**90**:61–68.

41 Ridker PM, Hennekens CH, Lindpaintner K et al. Mutation in the gene coding for coagulation factor V and the risk of myocardial infarction, stroke, and venous thrombosis in apparently healthy men. *N Engl J Med* 1995;**332**:912–917.

Lipids, atherosclerosis and sudden death

ALUN EVANS

It is surprising the controversy that coronary heart disease has generated down the years. Take, for example, the title of a paper in 1957: *Diet and coronary thrombosis: hypothesis and fact* [1] (in this paper the best correlation found between coronary mortality in 15 countries was with the trends in the number of radio and television licences), or the title of an editorial in 1963: *Diet and atherosclerosis: truth and fiction.* The author, Snapper [2], records that as early as 1908, Ignatowsky showed a connection between excessive food intake and arteriosclerosis, which he attributed to excessive protein intake. Anitschkoff's experiments on rabbits in 1913 elucidated the role of cholesterol in the pathogenesis of atherosclerosis. By 1916, De Langen had proved to his satisfaction that the hypocholesterolaemia of the Japanese was due to low cholesterol intake and not to racial characteristics. However, as early as 1819 Dr Samuel Black of Newry, County Down, by dint of meticulous observation, associated [3] angina pectoris with an ossific diathesis (of the coronary arteries) and an accumulation of fat around the heart. He established his credentials as an epidemiologist by attempting to classify those who were *liable* to angina pectoris and those who were *exempt*. He imagined: 'The persons particularly liable are those who are of full and plethoric habits, who live luxuriously, or at least very plentifully, and who do not use a sufficient quantity of exercise'. For such a person he 'should be inclined to propose a regimen of the most abstemious kind, exclusive, in a great measure, of animal food and all fermented drink' but he admitted that experience had taught him 'that it is in vain for men to begin such a system of living, unless they are endowed with a certain firmness and constancy of mind, such as are necessary to enable men to forego Sybaritic gratifications, and to prefer a prospective advantage to a present enjoyment'. The modern American equivalent of this is 'willpower only lasts a fortnight and dissolves in alcohol'.

According to Mann in 1978 [4], the official line from 1950 in the USA was the management of the epidemic of coronary heart disease by means of dietary treatment and that too many Americans 'were wearing the diet/heart hair shirt'. The Americans had contemplated a vast dietary intervention study in middle-aged men who were clinically free of coronary

101

heart disease (CHD). The National Diet Heart Study estimated that a study population of up to 100 000 with a follow-up period of 4–5 years would have been required to detect a 20% reduction in incidence with statistical reliability. Despite much elaborate groundwork, the study never took place — the greatest study never done.

Numerous epidemiological studies established factors which were related to the risk of development of subsequent disease. These were described as 'risk factors' — a term borrowed from the world of insurance and first used in a paper from Framingham in 1957 [5]. Although some would favour referring to these factors as 'risk markers', this is redolent of semantic hair-splitting.

In the early 1980s the World Health Organization (WHO) set up the MONICA project (multinational MONItoring in CArdiovascular diseases). The project drew its inspiration from the fact that many countries were experiencing different trends in CHD mortality — in particular, the USA had shown a decline since the early 1970s and this was debated at a conference called by the National Heart, Lung and Blood Institute in 1978. The MONICA project was established in 40 populations in 26 countries around the world to relate trends in incidence of CHD and stroke (optionally) to trends in the major risk factors of cigarette smoking, raised serum cholesterol and blood pressure over the 10-year study period. Recently published incidence data [6] from 38 MONICA populations in 21 countries showed fairly good agreement between the incidence and the published statutory mortality data (Fig. 1). The Catalonia and Beijing centres had the lowest rates in both men and women. Two Finnish centres, followed by the two UK centres (Belfast and Glasgow), had the highest rates in men and the two UK centres (Belfast and Glasgow) had the highest rates in women. Cholesterol levels, however, in the same age range (35–64 years) were generally high across all the centres, with only Beijing having a median cholesterol level at less than 5.2 mmol/l (Fig. 2). Similarly, in females, Beijing had the lowest cholesterol and Ticino and Stanford, were the only other centres with median levels below 5.2 mmol/l (Fig. 2). A lipid comparison carried out between Belfast and Taiyuan in the People's Republic of China which involved 151 male Chinese subjects and 202 in Belfast showed [8] that the median cholesterol in China was 4.28 mmol/l compared to 6.15 mmol/l in Belfast; 83% of this difference was due to the higher LDL cholesterol in Belfast. Moreover, in China several lipid variables appeared to be favourably affected by specific forms of apolipoprotein (Apo) B and Apo E that are particularly frequent in that population [9].

On the basis of low ischaemic heart disease mortality in the countries with low cholesterol levels, the WHO recommends the shifting of the distribution downwards by 'hygienic' changes in lifestyle (H.L. Mencken once described hygiene as 'the corruption of medicine by morality').

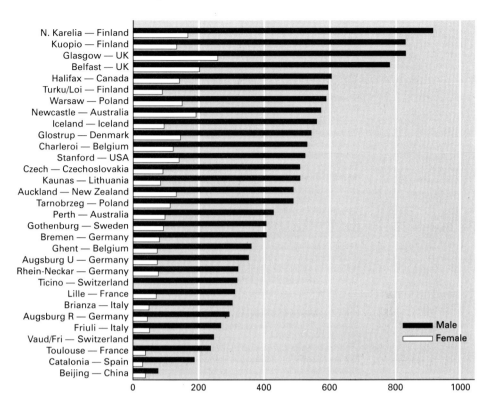

Fig. 1 Age-standardized coronary event annual incidence rates (1985–87; aged 35–64 years). Reproduced with permission from [6].

Evidence of a benefit due to cholesterol lowering has emerged from several studies [10]. What is not clear, however, is the benefit of treating lower levels of cholesterol, treatment in women and treatment in the elderly and there are inconsistent reports on the latter issue. Cholesterol-lowering studies in the primary prevention of CHD, although showing a reduction in coronary events, have not led to a reduction in total mortality due to an unexplained excess of injury, cancer and other non-cardiovascular conditions. This may be because the studies were not large enough to demonstrate this effect, but meta-analyses give conflicting results depending on which studies are included. This has resulted in several hypotheses relating cholesterol levels to murder and accidents. Possibly this could be related to serotonin activity, but the case remains unproven [11].

The Americans have been enthusiastic about the lowering of serum cholesterol in the population and have been running their National Cholesterol Education Programme for several years. Recommendations have been made [12] for a desired cholesterol level of below 5.2 mmol/l,

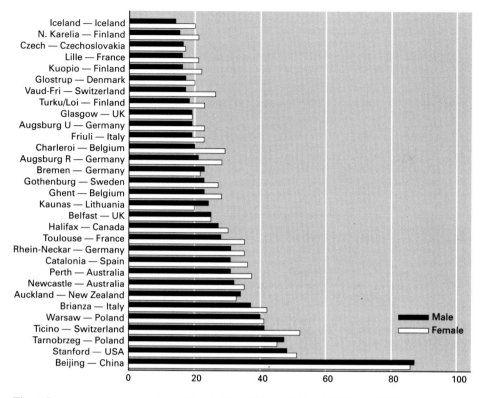

Fig. 2 Percentage of serum cholesterol levels below 5.2 mmol/ĺ (mid 1980s; aged 35–64 years). Reproduced with permission from [7].

with up to 6.2 mmol/l as borderline high cholesterol, and above this level designated high cholesterol. The population is being urged to know 'its cholesterol number' but more recently greater attention has been paid to high-density lipoprotein (HDL) cholesterol with a level of 0.9 mmol/l or below being classified as a major risk factor and a level of 1.6 mmol/l or more being regarded as a negative risk factor. It has even been asked: 'Is knowing your cholesterol number harmful?' and 27 physicians and nine pharmacists in one American university teaching hospital were asked to nominate their preferred way of death after attaining average life expectancy. 'Rapidly fatal cardiac death' was overwhelmingly chosen [13]. However, such preferences ignore the fact that many coronary heart disease sufferers face long periods of illness.

The UK has adopted a more cautious approach, coming out against mass screening for cholesterol, although screening for cholesterol opportunistically is encouraged [14] under the Health Promotion Strategy.

Disappointingly, the Oxford and Collaboration health check (OXCHECK) [15] and the British Family Heart Study, both of which tried to modify risk in general practice, showed only modest changes.

The place of risk factor modification once a heart attack has been sustained is much more encouraging [16]. There are now numerous — admittedly small — regression studies monitored by serial angiography showing non-progression and even regression of plaque in intervention subjects adequately treated with diet and lipid-lowering drugs — clearly those with moderately raised cholesterol benefit. It seems that lipid lowering leads to a stabilization of plaque structure and that this prevents clinical events by selectively depleting lipids or 'regressing' a relatively small subgroup of lipid-rich plaques that are predisposed to plaque fissuring, ulceration and haemorrhage that account for the great majority of clinical events.

The first author of the Scandinavian Simvastatin Survival Study [17], Pedersen, is Norwegian, which is a happy coincidence because a paper by Strøm and Jensen reporting [18] mortality from circulatory diseases in Norway from 1940 to 1945 charted a decline in the disease which mirrored the fall in consumption of fat in the form of butter, milk, cheese and eggs during German occupation — perhaps Hitler's sole benefaction to humanity. The study, carried out in 4444 patients (four-fifths male) with angina pectoris only (one-fifth) or previous myocardial infarction (with or without angina) and a serum cholesterol of 5.5–8.0 mmol/l, employed a lipid-lowering diet and double-blind treatment with simvastatin or placebo. The study had a median follow-up of 5.4 years and brought about a change in total cholesterol of –25%, low-density lipoprotein (LDL) cholesterol by –35% and HDL cholesterol by +8%. Twelve per cent of the placebo group died compared with 8% of the simvastatin group, giving a relative risk of death of 0.70 (95% confidence intervals (CI) 0.58–0.85, $P = 0.0003$). Coronary deaths were much lower in the simvastatin group (relative risk 0.58, 95% CI 0.46–0.73). Non-cardiovascular deaths were similar in the groups. There was also a 37% reduction in the risk of undergoing myocardial revascularization procedures. The drug was well-tolerated and the sustained reduction of total and LDL cholesterol in the simvastatin group was not associated with any serious hazard. It is the first secondary prevention trial to show a benefit in overall survival. Concern had been expressed about the safety of long-term use of hydroxy-methylglutaryl coenzyme A reductase inhibitors and a worry that simvastatin could cross the blood–brain barrier, but perhaps the more challenging task now in the UK is to see that the results of this trial cross the information–brain barrier and become enshrined in clinical practice.

The results of the Scandinavian study are of importance in highlighting the central role of LDL cholesterol, but unfortunately they may not tell us that much about the underlying mechanisms of atherosclerosis. Cardiovascular epidemiology has been dogged, since its inception, by the limitations of what has been measurable. Total cholesterol is quite an unspecific reflection of lipid metabolism and the measurement of its subfractions has become infinitely more sophisticated as it has now been shown that atherogenic lipid profiles [19], lipoprotein (Lp)(a) and dense LDL may define an individual's risk much more accurately. Interest is now focusing on the vessel wall, which is altogether more remote from the point of view of direct measurement and an array of cytokines are under scrutiny.

The smooth-muscle cell is the major cell type in the media of human arteries and plays a major role in atherosclerosis by proliferation and migration from the media to the intima. Lp(a) interferes with fibrinolysis by competing for the plasminogen receptor, increases plasminogen activator inhibitor I and decreases plasminogen-activating (tissue plasminogen activator; tPA) activity [20]. It also inhibits the activation of tissue growth factor-β (TGF-β), which may promote smooth-muscle cell proliferation and migration. When plasmin is lower, i.e. when Lp(a) levels are higher, less TGF-β is activated. Women have higher levels of TGF-β and the association between Lp(a) levels and TGFβ is absent. Grainger and his colleagues have shown [20] that patients with advanced atherosclerosis have only a fifth of the average concentration of TGF-β compared with the normal controls. The use of aspirin correlated with elevated active TGF-β concentration, which hints at a therapeutic opportunity. Measurement of TGF-β may prove to be a useful diagnostic tool. The study was small and prospective data are urgently needed as we get glimpses of interactions between lipid metabolism and thrombosis.

A recent report from WHO, *cardiovascular disease risk factors: new areas for research* [21] covers much familiar ground, confirming that isomeric (*trans*) fatty acids resemble saturated fatty acids in their effects on lipoprotein metabolism. The potential protective effects of antioxidants are also reviewed but the Alpha-tocopherol, Beta-carotene Cancer Prevention Study [22] produced disappointing results because, in the β-carotene group, total mortality was 8% higher in those who took them than among those who did not, primarily due to more deaths from cancer and ischaemic heart disease. Supporters of the antioxidant hypothesis point to the fact that an inappropriate combination of antioxidants was given to the wrong group of subjects and no conclusions on heart disease can be drawn.

At present, properly designed trials in this area are essential. Recently elevated levels of antibodies against oxidized LDL cholesterol have been shown [23] to be predictive for myocardial infarction. The WHO report also covered insulin resistance and the role of homocysteine: 10–25% of those with coronary artery disease in case-control studies have hyperhomocysteinaemia. This is most likely caused by marginal vitamin B deficiency, especially folate, but whether this association is independent of the major antioxidant vitamins, which share common food vehicles, remains to be established.

One major surprise in the report is the lack of space accorded to the genetic influences on heart disease. Apparently an earlier report had dealt with this but 'Because of its great importance, the topic was briefly dealt with here although it was not specifically discussed by the Scientific Group'. Creditably, nutrient–gene interactions were recognized: 'Further research on the genetic basis of the responsiveness of individuals to nutrients that increase cardiovascular risk is urgently needed'. Dr Samuel Black, the Newry physician, had foreseen this and noted:

> We have seen that the disease appears to be connected with a plethoric state of the system and with obesity: that the great majority of the subjects of it have belonged to the better ranks of society, who were in the habit of sitting down everyday to a plentiful table, in the pleasures of which they may have indulged to a greater extent than was suitable to the tendency of their constitution. . . [3]

It is well-accepted that heart disease runs in families. In a study of 136 infants, an association was shown [24] between coronary artery intimal thickening and a family history of coronary artery disease. The authors commented that many genes are involved in lipid metabolism and about 50% can be expected to be polymorphic.

In an important study from the Swedish Twin Registry, 21 004 twins were investigated [25] for the risk of death from coronary heart disease in pairs of those who were monozygotic or dizygotic. Relative hazard estimates were obtained in a multivariate survival analysis. The study assessed the relative hazard of a twin's death from CHD when the other twin had died of CHD before the age of 55 years, as compared with the hazard when the twin had not died before 55 years. The relative hazard in monozygotic twins was roughly double that of dyzygotic twins and, although the effect decreased with age, it persisted into old age. These findings lie rather uneasily with the 'fetal origins of adult cardiovascular disease' hypotheses as they demonstrate the strength of the genetic determinants of adult cardiovascular disease. In any case, in epidemiological family studies the genetic contribution is often underestimated for methodological reasons.

The Etude cas-Témoins de l'Infarctus du Myocarde (ECTIM) study is a large case-control study of myocardial infarction mounted between the MONICA centres in Belfast, Lille, Strasburg and Toulouse; male patients aged 25–64 years were recruited. Despite an almost four times higher level of heart disease in Northern Ireland than in France, classical risk factor levels were very similar. A high-risk profile characterized by a low LpA1 level and high levels of Lp E : B and Lp(a) : B was more frequent in the population of Northern Ireland and a gradient was observed between cases and controls and between Belfast and the French centres [26]. Subsequently, in the ECTIM study a total of 574 cases and 722 controls were available for a comparison of Apo E phenotype and genotype [27].

Competition by Apo B and Apo E for the LDL receptor (the avidity of the receptor being determined genetically) explains the different atherogenic potentials, with ε4 allele being associated with higher levels of LDL cholesterol and consequently a greater susceptibility to atherosclerosis. The ε2 allele favours peripheral LDL catabolism. The relative risk associated between the ε2 and ε4 allele was 0.73 and 1.33 respectively, suggesting that 12% of myocardial infarction might be attributable to this polymorphism. The ε4 allele frequency was 14.3%, 14%, 10.8% and 5.2% in Belfast, Lille, Strasburg and Toulouse, respectively (similarly, the prevalence of ε2 was 10.3%, 11.9%, 8.5% and 5.2%). Recently, it has been shown [28] that the ε4 allele carriers have a several-fold risk of developing Alzheimer's disease and a lesser risk of developing Creutzfeldt–Jakob disease.

The relationship between the D polymorphism of the angiotensin-converting enzyme (ACE) gene and myocardial infarction was detected in the ECTIM study. The I/D (insertion/deletion of 287 base pairs) polymorphism is a marker for the functional variant S/s which is as yet unidentified. It was shown [26] that the prevalence of DD in the cases was 1.34 times that in the controls (26%). Defining a low-risk group in terms of body mass index and Apo B levels, the odds ratios were much higher. Genotype was associated with serum ACE level.

In another paper from the same group, it was found [29] that, although plasma ACE level did not differ between patients and control subjects in those aged more than 54 years, it was higher in patients than in controls in the younger age group. This suggested a differential loss of subjects with high ACE levels and the level depends heavily on the D polymorphism. In addition, ACE level might be a risk factor for myocardial infarction independent of the ACE I/D polymorphism.

Evidence is emerging that the ACE D polymorphism could be a risk factor for sudden death. In the ECTIM study the association of the polymorphism with parental history of fatal myocardial infarction was examined. There was an excess of both DD (odds ratio 2.6, $P = 0.02$) and ID (odds ratio 1.9, $P = 0.08$) genotypes among those having a parental history of MI. To investigate further if the I/D polymorphism might be associated with fatal myocardial infarction, 213 postmortems were studied in Belfast. The ECTIM controls in Belfast were used as the control for this group. The odds ratio for DD versus II was 2.2 ($P < 0.02$), with a stronger relationship observed in older than in younger subjects (2.8 versus 1.9).

More recently, the synergistic effect of ACE polymorphisms and polymorphisms of the angiotensin II type 1 receptor gene has been demonstrated [26] in ECTIM. From the allele frequencies in the control population it was estimated that 15% of individuals carry both the ACE DD and the AGT 1 C allele and 2.5% are double homozygotes. These individuals may be at considerably increased risk. The inconsistent findings concerning the ID polymorphisms in various studies might be explained by this interaction, which has not been taken into account. It is intriguing to speculate whether it is this group (14–28% of the total) which benefits so much in the trials of ACE inhibition in secondary prevention, but as yet this is unknown.

As well as studying people who become ill, the 'new genetics' focus on those who survive. In the UK, if one attains an age of 100 years, the Queen sends a telegram. Apparently, if you attain this prodigious age in France a doctor will come, complete with needle and syringe, to acquire your white cells for the extraction of DNA. A total of 338 subjects were assembled in this way [30], 294 (87%) of whom were women. The ε4 allele was shown to be less common than expected, whereas the DD polymorphism was much more common (39.6% versus 25.6–28.4%) in controls. Polymorphisms which are common must carry advantages in certain individuals at some stage in life — witness the frequency of thalassaemia minor in certain African populations, in which it helps to prevent malaria. Clearly, in this highly selected group of French women it must confer some advantage.

As well as addressing itself to examining several hypotheses relating to lipid and other factors on a case-control basis, the ECTIM study has been used to generate fresh hypotheses by identifying new candidate genes. The understanding of gene interactions will greatly refine treatment in the future, and explain why the classical risk factors are often imprecise in defining an individual's risk. Rare mutations with big effects are disastrous for the individual but have small population impact, whereas common polymorphisms with small effects may together produce common diseases and carry a large population impact.

REFERENCES

1 Yudkin J. Diet and coronary thrombosis: hypothesis and fact. *Lancet* 1957;**ii**:155–162.
2 Snapper I. Diet and atherosclerosis: truth and fiction (editorial). *Am J Cardiol* 1963;**11**:283–289.
3 Black S. *Clinical and Pathological Reports.* Alex Wilkinson, Newry, 1819.
4 Mann GV. Coronary heart disease — the doctor's dilemma (editorial). *Am Heart J* 1978;**96**:569–571.
5 Schoenberger JA, Mann GV. Controversies in cardiology. Proposed: low-dose aspirin should be taken daily after age 40 if total serum cholesterol is greater than 160. *Hosp Pract* 1982;**12**:50A–50M.
6 WHO MONICA Project, prepared by Tunstall-Pedoe H, Kuulasmaa K, Amouyel P, Arveiler D, Rajakangas A-M, Pajak A. Myocardial infarction and coronary deaths in the World Health Organization MONICA project: registration procedures, event rates, and case-fatality rates in 38 populations from 21 countries in 4 continents. *Circulation* 1994;**90**:583–612.
7 World Health Organization MONICA Project Principal Investigators. The WHO MONICA project: a worldwide monitoring system for cardiovascular diseases. *World Health Statistics Annual.* WHO, Geneva, 1989:27–149.

8 Zhang W, Evans AE, Cambien F *et al*. Distribution of lipid variables in subjects in Belfast, Northern Ireland and Taiyuan, P R China. *Atherosclerosis* 1993;**102**:175–180.

9 Evans AE, Zhang W, Moreel JFR *et al*. Polymorphisms of the apolipoprotein B and E genes and their relationship to plasma lipid variables in healthy Chinese men. *Hum Genet* 1993;**92**:191–197.

10 Evans AE. Lipids and cardiovascular disease: ephemeral and elusive receptors. *Q J Med* 1993;**86**:77–79.

11 Santiago JM, Dalen JE. Cholesterol and violent behaviour. *Arch Intern Med* 1994;**154**:1317–1321.

12 Expert Panel. Summary of the second report of the National Cholesterol Education Program (NCEP) expert panel on detection, evaluation, and treatment of high blood cholesterol in adults (adult treatment panel II). *JAMA* 1993;**269**:3015–3023.

13 Reeves RA, Chen E. Who wants to eliminate heart disease? *J Clin Epidemiol* 1994;**47**:667–670.

14 Department of Health. *The Health of the Nation: Key Area Handbook — Coronary Heart Disease and Stroke*. Department of Health, London, 1993.

15 Stott N. Screening for cardiovascular risk in general practice (editorial). *Br Med J* 1994;**308**:285–286.

16 Brown BG, Zhao X-Q, Sacco DE, Albers JJ. Lipid lowering and plaque regression: new insights into prevention of plaque disruption and clinical events in coronary disease. *Circulation* 1993;**87**:1781–1791.

17 Scandinavian Simvastatin Survival Study Group. Randomised trial of cholesterol lowering in 4444 patients with coronary heart disease: the Scandinavian Simvastatin Survial Study (4S). *Lancet* 1994;**344**:1383–1389.

18 Strøm A, Jensen RA. Mortality from circulatory diseases in Norway 1940–1945. *Lancet* 1951;**i**:126–129.

19 Austin MA, King M-C, Vranizan KM, Krauss RM. Atherogenic lipoprotein phenotype: a proposed genetic marker for coronary heart disease risk. *Circulation* 1990;**82**:495–506.

20 Hayden MR, Reidy M. Many roads lead to atheroma. *Nature Med* 1995;**1**:22–23.

21 WHO Scientific Group. *Cardiovascular disease risk factors: new areas for research*. WHO, Geneva, 1994.

22 The Alpha-tocopherol, Beta-carotene Cancer Prevention Study Group. The effect of vitamin E and beta carotene on the incidence of lung cancer and other cancers in male smokers. *N Engl J Med* 1994;**330**:1029–1035.

23 Puurunen M, Manttari M, Manninen V *et al*. Antibody against oxidised low-density lipoprotein predicting myocardial infarction. *Arch Intern Med* 1994;**154**:2605–2609.

24 Kaprio J, Norio R, Pesonen E, Sarna S. Interval thickening of the coronary arteries in infants in relation to family history of coronary artery disease. *Circulation* 1993;**87**:1960–1968.

25 Marenberg ME, Risch N, Berkman LF, Floderus B, de Faire U. Genetic susceptibility to death from coronary heart disease in a study of twins. *N Engl J Med* 1994;**330**:1041–1046.

26 Tiret L, Bonnardeaux A, Poirier O. Synergistic effects of angiotensin-converting enzyme and angiotensin-II type 1 receptor gene polymorphisms on risk of myocardial infarction. *Lancet* 1994;**344**:910–913.

27 Luc G, Bard J-M, Arveiler D *et al*. Impact of apolipoprotein E polymorphism on lipoproteins and risk of myocardial infarction: the ECTIM Study. *Arterioscler Thromb* 1994;**14**:1412–1419.

28 Amouyel P, Vidal O, Launay JA, Laplanche JL for the French research group on epidemiology of human spongiform encephalopathies. The apolipoprotein E alleles as major susceptibility factors for Creutzfeldt-Jakob disease. *Lancet* 1994;**344**:1315–1318.

29 Cambien F, Costerousse O, Tiret L *et al*. Plasma level and gene polymorphism of antiotensin-converting enzyme in relation to myocardial infarction. *Circulation* 1994;**90**:669–676.

30 Schächter F, Faure-Delanef L, Guénot F *et al*. Genetic associations with human longevity at the Apo E and ACE loci. *Nature Genet* 1994;**6**:29–32.

MULTIPLE CHOICE QUESTIONS

1 The US National Diet/Heart Study
- **a** produced inconclusive results
- **b** required 50 000 subjects to be included in it
- **c** required up to 100 000 subjects to be included in it
- **d** required a 4–5-year follow-up
- **e** was designed to detect a 40% reduction in incidence with statistical reliability

2 In the National Cholesterol Education Programme
- **a** the desired level of cholesterol is 6.2 mmol
- **b** HDL cholesterol below 0.9 mmol is classified as a major risk factor
- **c** HDL cholesterol below 1.2 mmol/l is classified as a major risk factor
- **d** HDL cholesterol above 1.4 mmol/l is regarded as a negative risk factor
- **e** HDL cholesterol above 1.6 mmol/l is regarded as a negative risk factor

3 Tissue growth factor-β activity
- **a** is higher in men than women
- **b** is increased by aspirin
- **c** is depressed by lipoprotein a
- **d** is raised in advanced atherosclerosis
- **e** may become a useful diagnostic tool in atherosclerosis

4 The ECTIM study, carried out in the WHO MONICA Centres in Belfast, Lille, Strasburg and Toulouse
- **a** is an example of a prospective study
- **b** is a case-control study
- **c** has identified a high-risk lipid profile characterized by a low LpA1 level and high levels of LPE: B and Lp(a)B
- **d** has established the prevalence of the ACE DD polymorphism in the general population as 39.6%
- **e** has shown that the DD polymorphism is the functional variant

5 In relation to the apolipoprotein E polymorphisms
- **a** the ε2 allele is associated with greater susceptibility to atherosclerosis
- **b** the ε3 allele is associated with Alzheimer's disease
- **c** the ε3 alleles are the most common

d the ε4 allele is associated with higher levels of LDL cholesterol
e together they seem to explain 12% of myocardial infarction at the population level

Answers

1 **a** False
   b False
   c True
   d True
   e False

2 **a** False
   b True
   c False
   d False
   e True

3 **a** False
   b True
   c True
   d False
   e True

4 **a** False
   b True
   c True
   d False
   e False

5 **a** False
   b False
   c True
   d True
   e True

Genetic analysis of essential hypertension

MORRIS J. BROWN

At present, hypertension is divided into essential hypertension and secondary hypertension. The latter refers to ~ 5% of patients in whom an identifiable and sometimes curable cause for their hypertension can be found. Essential hypertension embraces the remainder, with *essential* meaning merely that the cause is currently unknown. However, this distinction between the two classes becomes blurred as we progress to understanding the cause of hypertension in individual patients, and is actually unhelpful in its implication that there is a single known cause of hypertension in secondary hypertensives, and a mixture of factors shared by most essential hypertensives. In hypertension, as elsewhere in medicine, the contribution of molecular genetics to date has been successful in unravelling the nature of a few rare single-gene disorders. But the real prize is to unravel the genetic contribution to one of the commonest *polygenic* disorders. While the existence of a major locus contributing to the disorder in most patients cannot be excluded, it is likely that essential hypertension embraces a number of different genes contributing in different families. The search for these genes should be practically rewarding as well as academically satisfying because it is very likely that the different syndromes will vary both in their optimal treatment and in their prognosis.

SINGLE-GENE DISORDERS

The principal categories of secondary hypertension for which most patients should be screened are renal and adrenal causes, and coarctation. In these classes, presentation with asymptomatic hypertension is most likely due to polycystic kidneys or renovascular disease in the renal class, and to phaeochromocytoma or primary hyperaldosteronism in the adrenal class. Polycystic kidneys are always familial and two genetic loci (APKD1 and 2) described elsewhere in this volume have been identified (see Harris, p. 305). No more will be said here, therefore, except to point out from the perspective of a hypertension specialist that screening for polycystic kidneys, whether by renal ultrasound or by a genetic test, in a patient with normal renal function is of doubtful value. The patient needs good blood pressure

(BP) control, but no other practical treatment exists to affect outcome in the patient or his or her relatives. The downside of screening is the influence on the patient's chances of obtaining life assurance and mortgages.

In the adrenal class, the majority of patients are sporadic, but there are rare familial types of both adrenal disorders, for which the genes have also been recently identified. Primary aldosteronism (Conn's syndrome) is somewhat commoner than phaeochromocytoma if both adrenal adenomas and hyperplasia are included. Operable tumours, however, account for < 1% hypertensives in the case of both Conn's and phaeos, the major difference being that Conn's tumours are always benign, whereas 5–10% of phaeos are malignant. The other difference is that at least 10% of phaeos may be familial in association with either multiple endocrine neoplasia (MEN type 2) or von Hippel–Lindau syndrome, whereas there may be only 50–100 families worldwide with the hereditary form of Conn's, called glucocorticoid remediable aldosteronism (GRA) [1]. The molecular basis for all three of these disorders has been identified in the last 3 years. The tumour syndromes of which phaeo can be a part are due to mutations in either a tumour-suppressor gene (von Hippel–Lindau) or tumour-promoting oncogene (receptor tyrosine kinase (RET)) [2,3]. Not all patients with the disease allele necessarily have a phaeochromocytoma, and their chance of developing it varies with the location of the mutation within the gene. By contrast, patients with the GRA mutation are born with the syndrome, although the phenotype appears to vary even within families. The GRA mutation arises as a chimera between the neighbouring genes for aldosterone synthase and 11β-hydroxylase (in the cortisol synthetic pathway) as a consequence of which aldosterone synthesis is driven by the adrenocorticotrophic hormone (ACTH) promoter to much higher levels than normal. Although GRA can be suspected from an increased 24-hour excretion of 18-OH steroids, this test is neither routinely available nor always abnormal in patients with GRA. The diagnosis of GRA should be considered in any young patient with Conn's due to adrenal hyperplasia, especially when there is either a family history of hypertension or early strokes. An additional clue may arise during the investigations of Conn's syndrome: if dexamethasone is used during the period of the selenium cholesterol isotope scan (to suppress uptake into the zona fasculata) a patient with GRA will be found to have no isotope accumulation in either adrenal.

For phaeochromocytomas, genetic testing is of value in known families in order to determine which members require regular biochemical and radiological follow-up for both phaeos and the other associated tumours. The phaeos are almost always in the adrenal. In patients with MEN, the most sensitive test for early phaeos is plasma adrenaline measurements, since the adrenal gland is the only source of circulating adrenaline but contributes < 2% of circulating noradrenaline [4]. In patients with von

Hippel–Lindau, the phaeo fails to secrete much adrenaline despite arising within the adrenal medulla. These patients may therefore be found to have incidental masses in their adrenal glands (often bilaterally; Fig. 1), and only equivocal evidence of elevated plasma noradrenaline or urinary metabolites. The definitive investigations are a pentolinium suppression test, showing failure to suppress the borderline elevation of plasma noradrenaline (Fig. 2), and selective venous sampling, which shows reversal of the normal predominance of adrenaline in the adrenal veins (Fig. 3).

For GRA, unlike familial phaeo, the best test is molecular screening. Although the chimeric gene which arises from unequal cross-over differs among families, they always create an extra restriction site (for the enzyme BamH1) which is readily detectable on a Southern blot of the patient's DNA extracted from a sample of blood.

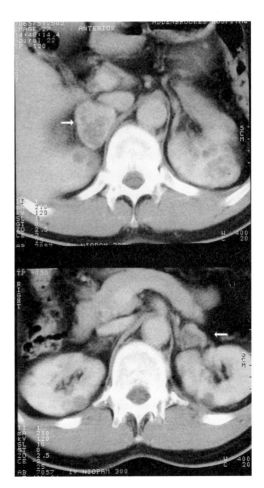

Fig. 1 Computed tomographic (CT) scan of bilateral adrenal phaeochromocytomas in a patient with von Hippel–Lindau syndrome. Arrows show the right and left adrenal tumours in the upper and lower cuts, respectively.

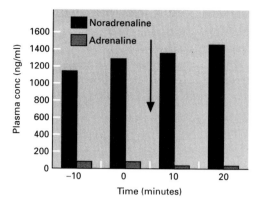

Fig. 2 Pentolinium suppression test in the diagnosis of phaeochromocytoma. The same patient as in Fig. 1 had blood taken for plasma adrenaline and plasma noradrenaline at − 10, 0, + 10 and + 20 minutes relative to a single intravenous bolus of the ganglion-blocking drug pentolinium 2.5 mg. The arrow represents the time of pentolinium administration.

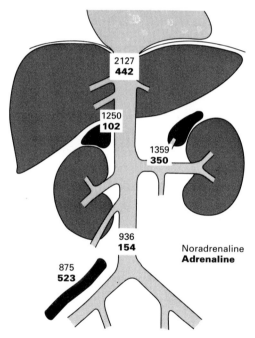

Fig. 3 Selective venous sampling in the diagnosis of phaeo-chromocytoma. Multiple blood samples were drawn from a catheter inserted through the right femoral vein and advanced under screening to the points shown on the map. Blood was analysed for noradrenaline (upper figures) and adrenaline (lower figures) at each site. Both adrenal vein samples showed a reversal of the normal 5–10-fold excess of adrenaline in the adrenal vein.

IS ESSENTIAL HYPERTENSION GENETIC?

Three strands of evidence point to a strong familial component. First are the formal studies of segregation of BP itself within families [5]. Second are twin studies. Third, we have ourselves during the past year questioned over 3000 patients with established hypertension requiring treatment about their families. Approximately 2000 of these know whether their siblings are also receiving treatment, with the answer being positive in one-third. Since our estimate of the incidence of hypertension in the same population (of East Anglia) from which the hypertensives were drawn is less than 10%, our data suggest a surprisingly high familial contribution. If this contribution is mainly genetic, the almost dominant nature of the transmission argues against the need to look within each family for a large number of interacting loci, with the inheritance of either a single or of two linked loci being the simplest explanation.

Why then is hypertension usually considered a polygenic condition, and what is the evidence that familial equals genetic? The argument for the polygenic nature of hypertension derives partly from the shape of BP distribution in the population, and partly from the heterogeneity of physiological, biochemical and pharmacological phenotypes.

Blood pressure distribution

Before a number of good epidemiological studies in the 1950s defined the continuous nature of BP in the population, there was a serious debate — with Platt and Pickering being the main protagonists — as to whether there was a bimodal distribution, with hypertension being categorically different from normal BP. For many years, we have recognized that BP is normally distributed, although with a marked skew to the right side of the distribution. Roughly, the justification for defining hypertension as a discrete entity could be said to be the coincidence of the start of the skew with inflexion in the curve which relates morbidity and mortality with BP.

A recent BP screening study which we performed in 30 000 healthy subjects invited to a 15-minute health screen at their general practice has given us the opportunity to define quite precisely the inflexion point in BP distribution, and also some unexpected support for a stronger genetic contribution to hypertension than suspected from earlier studies of familial segregation of BP in mainly normotensive families. The incidence of undiagnosed hypertension was much lower than in previous studies (5% of subjects with a diastolic blood pressure (DBP) > 90 mmHg, although our general practitioners said they did not treat a DBP < 95 or 100 mmHg in the age groups studied). Whether this finding is evidence of a real fall in the incidence of hypertension is outside the scope of this article. However, we consider that the low incidence does argue for a relatively low contribution to BP from environmental factors in our population. It was therefore of interest to find that, whereas there was very little skew in the distribution of diastolic BP, all age groups showed a pronounced skew in the systolic BP, starting at 140 mmHg in the youngest (Fig. 4). Moreover, whereas a large part of the variance in BP below this value could be explained by variance in age and body mass index, variance in BP above 140 mmHg was not predictable from these parameters. These observations have suggested to us that, in a population where environmental influences on BP may be less marked, truly hypertensive levels of

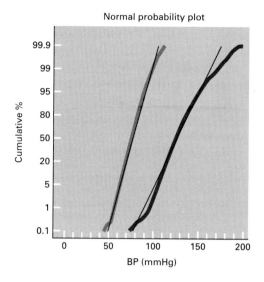

Normal probability plot

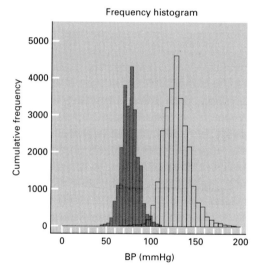

Frequency histogram

Fig. 4 Blood pressure (BP) distribution in 30 000 healthy subjects. The lower panel shows the frequency distribution of systolic (blue) and diastolic (purple) BP. The upper panel shows the probit plots of systolic and diastolic BP, illustrating the greater deviation of systolic than diastolic BP from the straight line of a normal distribution.

BP may not be 'just an extension' of the normal BP distribution, and that we may therefore be better placed to detect the genetic influences on hypertension in such a population.

Blood pressure and birth weight

An invigorating challenge to the orthodox view that familial influences, especially those inferred from twin data, are mainly genetic has come in recent years from the observations of Professor Barker (see p. 69). Since, as will be discussed, the contribution from any one locus to essential hypertension is likely to be small, the endeavour to find these may be misplaced if the overall genetic contribution to hypertension has been overestimated! We have therefore examined our own databases of hypertensive and control subjects to determine whether birth weight differs between these groups when they are matched for other parameters expected to influence BP. Over 1000 patients receiving an average of 1.6 drugs for hypertension (i.e. of moderate severity) and 4500 of the healthy controls who took part in the BP screening described above completed a questionnaire requesting them to find out (if not already known) their birth weight. Such recalled birth weights have been shown to correlate well with actual birth weight records, and in both our groups correlated well with measured heights (Fig. 5). The average birth weight of 7.2 lb

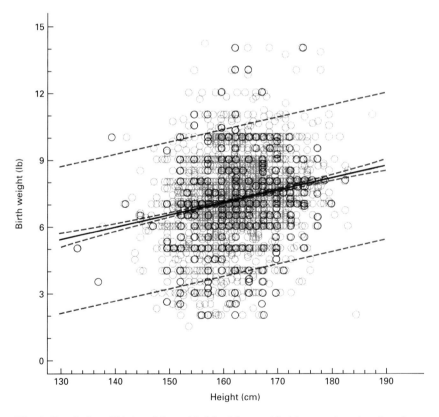

Fig. 5 Correlation of birth weight and height. Measured height was plotted against the recalled birth weight in 4000 healthy subjects (grey circles) and 1000 hypertensive patients (black circles) receiving antihypertensive drugs. Measured height was plotted against the recalled birth weight in 4000 healthy subjects and 1000 hypertensive patients receiving antihypertensive drugs. The regression coefficient was 0.28 ($P < 0.0001$), with no difference in slope between the two groups of patients.

(3.24 kg) in the hypertensives was slightly but significantly less than that of 7.4 lb (3.33 kg) in the controls when compared by a paired *t*-test, but this difference disappeared in a multiple regression analysis that included age, sex, weight and height (Fig. 6). We also asked our hypertensive patients with siblings whether the siblings were smaller or taller than themselves, since siblings provide a secure way of controlling for the genetic and social factors that might confound correlations with birth weight in unrelated subjects.

The birth weight hypothesis would predict that significantly more than 50% of hypertensive patients were of lower birth weight than normotensive siblings. This itself has not yet been tested. However, given the predictive value of birth weight for height, we might have expected hypertensive patients to be generally shorter than normotensive siblings, for which our questionnaires in almost 1500 patients with siblings of the same sex provided no evidence. Obviously these questionnaire data do not challenge the observations leading to the Barker hypothesis, for which placental as

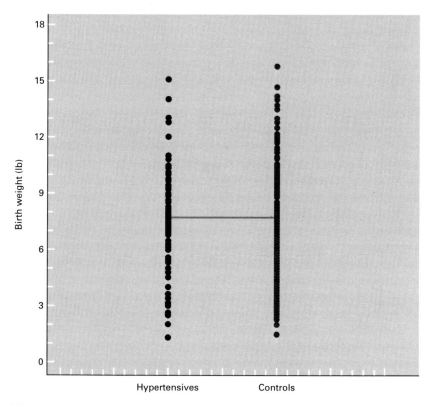

Fig. 6 Comparison of birth weight between hypertensives and controls. The figure shows the individual birth weights for the subjects studied in Fig. 4, after correction for age, sex, weight and height. The mean birth weight was identical in the two groups of subjects.

well as fetal weights have been an important component. All that we would conclude is that, whatever the influence of antenatal programming may be on normal BP development, it seems to be of a different order from its obvious influence on adult height and may be of even less importance in determining actual hypertension.

STRATEGIES FOR FINDING THE GENES FOR ESSENTIAL HYPERTENSION

It is important to emphasize the differences between looking for the gene for single-gene disorders like cystic fibrosis and the multiple genes responsible in part for a disorder like essential hypertension. The latter search suffers from several inevitable consequences of more than one gene being involved.

1 The contribution from individual genetic loci is likely to be small overall.
2 The number of loci to be found is unknown.
3 The loci are only disease-*susceptibility* loci, and the same mutations will be present in healthy subjects who lack either the other interacting loci and/or environmental influences.

On the other hand, the odds against any one genetic locus being one of the responsible loci are clearly lower than for a single-gene disorder. We also do not yet know for any of the polygenic disorders whether they are single disorders requiring most of the contributing loci in each case (family), or whether there are several distinct but overlapping disorders depending on which combination of genetic and environmental influences are involved. My own speculation for essential hypertension, as a result of various theoretical considerations and recent findings, is that the genetic loci do differ to some extent among families, because of the well-described phenotypic variation in hypertension (see later), but that the number of loci per family will be only two to three. Even overall, an alliance of Occam's rasor and combination theory (three loci with biallelic polymorphisms give 2^3 possible phenotypes) suggests that the number of loci need not be large.

Apart from these general problems, the strategy for several of the common polygenic disorders is strongly influenced by their late onset. This means that multigeneration pedigrees are not usually available, since parents of index cases may be dead, and children not yet classifiable.

Linkage versus association studies

Two distinct approaches exist for a molecular genetic analysis of hypertension. For both, it is necessary to understand the nature of the DNA polymorphisms which are used. The term 'polymorphism' refers to a relatively common (> 5%) variation in DNA sequence, the commonest form being a substitution of one of the four bases by another. Such poly-morphisms are estimated to be present every 500 base pairs, but the vast majority occur either outside coding regions, or in the 'wobble' position of codons, not affecting the amino acid expressed. These polymorphisms are called *biallelic* because the substitution gives rise to two different possible genes, or *alleles*. Slightly less common, occurring every few thousand base pairs and only outside the coding regions, are two, three or four nucleotide repeat (*microsatellite*) polymorphisms. Since the number of repeats can be highly variable, the number of alleles may be comparably higher.

It is important to realize that, in both cases, the polymorphism is not usually itself of functional importance, but is useful as a marker. *Association* studies are so called because an association is sought between the marker and the disease by comparing the frequency of the polymorphism between the diseased and control population. Biallelic polymorphisms are preferable for such studies. An association will be found only if the mutation contributing to the disease is so close to the marker polymorphism (within ~ 100 000 base pairs) that the disease allele and one of the marker alleles have not been frequently separated by recombination of chromosomes during the 100s to 1000s of generations that have occurred since the disease mutation first arose. In *linkage* studies, only the meioses of the generations actually studied determine whether the pedigree members with the disease share the same allele of the marker more frequently than expected to occur by chance alone. Microsatellite markers are preferable to reduce the frequency of chance sharing of alleles, and the allele shared by diseased members will vary in different families. Because the marker and disease alleles need to remain linked only for a small number of meioses, the distance between them can be very large (up to 2 million base pairs, which can be many genes apart).

Most studies in human hypertension to date have been association studies, because they can be performed without collection of pedigrees, and are more akin to the descriptive or phenotypic comparisons of hyperten-sives and controls conducted during the last 20–30 years of hypertension research. By the same token, they suffer from the disadvantage that the comparison of two population groups is dependent on the validity of the population definitions, and in particular that the controls differ by nothing other than their BP from the hypertensives. Most hypertensive patients seen in hospital clinics have been selected for referral for reasons not entirely related to severity of hypertension, for example, multiplicity of side-effects, and quite different biases can readily dictate the availability of control subjects. Geneticists also worry, probably needlessly in hy-pertension, about non-random assortment, meaning that hypertensive patients may be more likely to marry each other than expected by chance. Linkage studies rely on mathematical probability analyses within pedigrees, and are in principle immune therefore from confounding effects. Classical linkage studies are almost impossible because of the late onset, mentioned earlier, and therefore the technique of affected pedigree (or sibling) analysis has been utilized. This has the advantage of using only positively diagnosed family members, who may belong to only one generation, but has the great disadvantage that the ratio of observed to expected may be so small (sometimes < 1.1 : 1) that hundreds to thousands of pedigrees need to be studied to establish a significant excess in the ratio. For technical reasons beyond the scope of this paper, the affected pedigree method in the absence of both parents of those studied lacks the mathematical robustness of other linkage techniques because an assumption has to be made (or estimated in a control population) about how often marker alleles would be shared by chance alone. To date there has been only one positive result with a candidate gene studied by linkage analysis in humans, which is the angiotensinogen gene [6]. Although the numbers of siblings studied were relatively small, the finding may be correct since a second, even smaller study confirmed the result. However, the marker for angiotensinogen has not sufficient alleles to permit confident assignment of *identity by descent* to siblings in the absence of parents, and the positive findings in such small samples may have been due to an underestimate of the expected frequency with which siblings would share alleles by chance alone.

Candidate versus anonymous genes

For single-gene disorders, the study of individual candidate genes (for which there is some *a priori* argument for their choice) is viewed as a needle-in-a-haystack approach, at least before positional cloning has narrowed the number of candidates. However, for hypertension, the odds against any one candidate are reduced by the number of genetic loci involved; and if hypertension is due partly to the same loci as influence normal BP, there are a large number of clues from 40 years of physiological research into mechanisms of BP control.

Candidate genes can be studied in either linkage or association studies. The linkage approach seems to have two advantages that outweigh the numbers problem. First, geneticists favour it because of its basis in mathematical theory. Second, it permits the possibility of a systematic search across the whole of the genome, using the random anonymous markers identified during the last few years [7]. In theory, this approach permits the exclusion of most genes which are not contributing to hypertension from further study, and the possible identification of loci which do play a major role. In practice, recruitment of sufficient numbers of pedigrees may limit the whole genome search to identifying one or two regions which are good bets for further study. Whereas high statistical power (and therefore thousands of pedigrees) are required to *exclude* a locus, the value of studying a polygenic condition is that only a low power is required to *include* with reasonable luck at least one of the loci among the positive results. Probably any positive will need to be repeated in an independent study to distinguish it from the false-positives due to the testing of multiple loci without a prior hypothesis. Although, therefore, there is no need to see candidate and anonymous loci as exclusive options, it will be important for the evaluation of progress in the next few years to distinguish studies which have definitively excluded a promising candidate from those which lacked statistical power to exclude one locus, but by good fortune pointed the way at another.

Experimental hypertension

Linkage studies lend themselves well to animal models of hypertension, where several generations can be available. The usual design is to cross a hypertensive strain with a control strain, and then compare BP with genotype in the next generation. Whereas in human studies of one generation polymorphisms need to have large numbers of alleles to minimize the chances of two siblings inheriting the same allele from different parental chromosomes, in animal studies biallelic markers can be used because the investigator knows which of the two alleles originated in the hypertensive strain. Furthermore, all BP readings are in the absence of treatment, allowing use of a technique called *Quantitative trait locus analysis*, which is more powerful than linkage studies where all hypertensive patients are categorized as the same. However, animal studies are of limited value in studying candidate genes, since a negative result in any one model does not exclude that candidate in human hypertension, whilst a positive result also does not prove that the same is true in humans. Of more use would be the finding of novel candidate loci, and this is limited by the lesser availability at present of known microsatellite markers in the rat genome compared to humans.

ASSOCIATION STUDIES IN HUMAN HYPERTENSION

Given the problems of association studies discussed earlier, and the lack of sufficient size of most to date, it is unsurprising that there are no convincing and reproducible results. My view is that no candidate is yet ruled in or out, including renin and angiotensin-converting enzyme (ACE), for which most but not all studies have been negative to date. Yet given the thousands of *families* required for linkage studies compared to the *hundreds* of individual patients required for association studies, the latter have a place in studying polygenic disease. Indeed, they will be essential because of the difference in distance, also discussed earlier, that can exist between a marker polymorphism and disease allele in the two types of study. Whilst the large distance in linkage studies is useful for excluding large areas of genome at a time, the small distance in association means that a positive result indicates that the functional mutation is nearby, and should be accessible by study of the intervening DNA.

To complete this article, I shall now describe how we have approached the search for polymorphisms in candidate genes and the assessment of the biological significance of those that are found. Because association studies are best performed using biallelic polymorphisms, they lend themselves to a powerful but simple technique that detects the usually silent single-base substitutions present every few hundred base pairs in most genes. This technique is based on the polymerase chain reaction (PCR) and is called single-stranded conformation polymorphism (SSCP). It is illustrated in Fig. 7 and is based on the principle that when single-stranded DNA is run in a polyacrylamide gel, it adopts a secondary structure which is critically dependent on every base, and in turn causes perceptible variation in the speed with which the DNA migrates through the gel. Using this technique we have found multiple polymorphisms in several candidate genes for hypertension: nitric oxide synthase, endothelin-1 and its receptors, and the G-protein, $G_{s\alpha}$, which couples β-receptors to adenylyl cyclase in heart and vascular muscle. The PCR product from any sample for which a SSCP is found is purified for DNA sequencing.

Knowledge of the DNA sequence usually permits identification of a commercially available bacterial restriction enzyme which will cut the DNA of one only of the polymorphic alleles. It is then a simple matter to

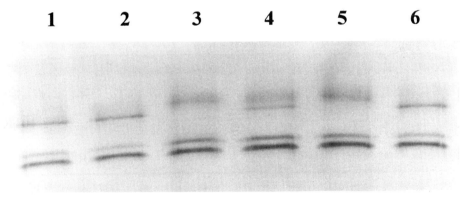

Fig. 7 Single-stranded conformation polymorphism (SSCP) gel, illustrating mutation detection. Polymerase chain reaction (PCR) product for exon 7 of the nitric oxide synthase gene from 6 hypertensive subjects was denatured and analysed. Denatured PCR products (206 bp) were run on a 20% non-denaturing polyacrylamide gel under optimized voltage conditions at 15°C. Bands were visualized by silver staining. Samples from 6 unrelated individuals are shown, demonstrating three SSCP patterns. Lanes 1, 2 and 6 are homozygous for the Glu[298] variant, lanes 3 and 5 homozygous for the Asp[298] variant and lane 4 is a heterozygote. (Courtesy of Dr A. Hingorani.)

compare several hundred samples of hypertensive and control DNA for the presence and absence of the restriction site. For nitric oxide synthase we found no difference in the frequency of a common polymorphism in exon 7 encoding a glutamate to aspartate substitution. However we found a significant excess in hypertensives in the frequency of both a silent polymorphism in exon 5 of $G_{s\alpha}$ and of a polymorphism in the non-coding region of exon 1 of endothelin-1. With such silent polymorphisms, it is likely that the functional mutation is in regulatory regions of the gene affecting the DNA transcription. Since we consider it likely that only some hypertensives will be affected by any one genetic locus, and that different genetic groups of hypertensives may be recognized by their response to different antihypertensive agents, we have tested whether the polymorphisms in some of our candidate genes predict responsiveness. In 230 patients randomized between ACE inhibitors and β-blockers during the last 10 years, we have found that the only predictor of response in a multiple regression analysis that included age, weight and sex was the genotype for angiotensinogen and $G_{s\alpha}$ respectively. Although the prediction was not strong, it illustrates the potential value now of phenotyping patients according to drug response in order to improve the chance of recognizing the different genotypes contributing to essential hypertension.

REFERENCES

1 Lifton RP, Dluhy RG, Powers M. A chimaeric 11 beta-hydroxylase/aldosterone synthase gene causes glucocorticoid remediable aldosteronism and human hypertension. *Nature* 1992;**355**:262–265.
2 Latif F, Tory K, Gnarra J *et al.* Identification of the von Hippel–Lindau disease tumor suppressor gene. *Science* 1993;**260**:1317–1320.
3 Mulligan LM, Kwok JBJ, Healey CS *et al.* Germ-line mutations of the RET proto-oncogene in multiple endocrine neoplasia type 2A. *Nature* 1993;**366**:458–461.
4 Brown MJ, Allison DJ, Jenner DA, Lewis PJ, Dollery CT. Increased sensitivity and accuracy of phaeochromocytoma diagnosis achieved by plasma adrenaline estimations and a pentolinium suppression test. *Lancet* 1981;**II**:174–177.
5 Ward R. Familial aggregation and genetic epidemiology of blood pressure. In: *Hypertension: Pathophysiology, Diagnosis and Management*, edited by Laragh JH, Brenner BM. Raven Press, New York; 1990.
6 Jeunemaitre X, Soubrier F, Kotelevtsev YV, Lifton RP, Williams CS, Charru A. Molecular basis of human hypertension: role of angiotensinogen. *Cell* 1992;**71**:169–180.
7 Davies JL, Kawaguchi Y, Bennett ST *et al.* A genome-wide search for human type I diabetes susceptibility genes. *Nature* 1994;**371**:130–136.

New inhibitors of the renin–angiotensin system

NILESH J. SAMANI

When first introduced in the late 1970s, few people could have fully foreseen the widespread impact that angiotensin-converting enzyme (ACE) inhibitors have had in the treatment of cardiovascular disorders. They have proved to be useful not only in treating hypertension [1], but also in treating symptomatic [2] and asymptomatic [3] left ventricular dysfunction, the post myocardial infarction patient [4–6] and patients with diabetic nephropathy [7]. Some studies [8] have suggested that they are better at reversing left ventricular hypertrophy compared with other antihypertensive drugs. At the same time, we have come to appreciate their side-effects, including the fairly frequent occurrence of an irritating non-productive cough which may be severe enough to require the drug to be stopped [9], the occasional occurrence of renal failure, particularly in subjects with renovascular disease, and the rare occurrence of angioedema [10].

The success of ACE inhibitors has spurred the pharmaceutical industry into the development of novel agents that inhibit the renin–angiotensin at other sites and the last few years has seen the clinical testing of orally active non-peptide renin inhibitors [11] and the evaluation and launch of the first angiotensin receptor antagonist [12]. Will these agents prove just as useful as ACE inhibitors? How will they compare with ACE inhibitors in terms of side-effects? This paper discusses some of these aspects.

THE RENIN–ANGIOTENSIN SYSTEM IN 1996

To help understand the potential differences between the different types of inhibitors it is useful briefly to review our current understanding of the renin–angiotensin system. An updated model of the renin–angiotensin cascade is shown in Fig. 1. Several features that may have a significant impact on the actions of the different agents are worth noting.

1 Despite much research, cleavage of angiotensin I from angiotensinogen still remains the only established function of renin.

2 ACE, in contrast, has a wide range of peptide substrates apart from angiotensin I, including bradykinin, enkephalins, substance P and neurotensin.

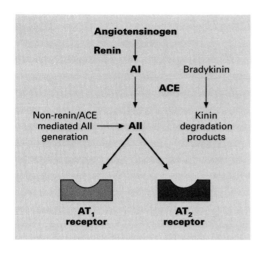

Fig. 1 The renin–angiotensin cascade in 1996.

Thus, ACE inhibition is potentially associated with the accumulation of these substances as well as a decrease in angiotensin II.

3 There is heterogeneity of angiotensin II receptors. On the basis of pharmacological and biochemical properties as well as molecular cloning, at least two distinct subtypes, designated type 1 (AT_1) and type 2 (AT_2), are now known to exist and there may be more subtypes as well as further functional heterogeneity within each of the subtypes [13]. All of the well-established cardiovascular effects of angiotensin II (e.g. vasoconstriction, aldosterone secretion) appear to be mediated through the AT_1 receptor subtype. The functions of the AT_2 receptor subtype remain unclear [13]. The angiotensin antagonists currently being developed are all selectively targeted at the AT_1 receptor [12].

4 Within some tissues, in addition to the classical pathway, there may be biologically important generation of angiotensin II through non-renin and/or ACE-mediated pathways [14]. This proposition remains controversial, although certainly several enzymes have been shown, at least *in vitro*, to be able to cleave either angiotensin I or angiotensin II directly from angiotensinogen and others to convert angiotensin I to angiotensin II [15].

5 The cascade is under tonic feedback regulation. Angiotensin II inhibits renin production and secretion from the kidney through an AT_1 receptor mechanism [16].

THE POTENTIAL IMPACT OF INHIBITING THE RENIN–ANGIOTENSIN SYSTEM AT DIFFERENT LEVELS

Given the above features, a useful way to examine the effects of inhibiting the renin–angiotensin system at different levels — renin inhibition (RI),

ACE inhibition (ACEI) and angiotensin receptor antagonism (AT_1RA) — is to consider the effect of the individual interventions on various key components and examine the resulting consequences. Looked at in this way, four differences emerge which merit discussion (Table 1).

Increase in plasma renin activity (ACEI and AT_1RA) versus decrease (RI)

While all three types of agents will lead to increased renin production and secretion by the kidney [16], plasma renin activity will not increase with RI because the renin will be blocked. At one stage in the 1970s, based on experimental evidence in rats made hypertensive by renal artery clipping, it was proposed that high renin might have a direct vasculotoxic effect independently of angiotensin II generation [17]. However, the now vast clinical evidence with ACE inhibitors [1–6,10] would suggest that, on the contrary, these agents are if anything vasculoprotective and this concern seems unnecessary.

Another possible effect of the feedback increase in plasma renin activity is that it may partly overcome the inhibition or antagonism and thus result in a loss of full efficacy. Certainly, there is evidence that the reactive hyperreninaemia reduces the fall in plasma angiotensin II during chronic ACE inhibition [18]. While both the extensive experience with ACE inhibitors in hypertension [1] and heart failure [2–6] and the more recent experience with AT_1RA in hypertension [12] suggest that these agents maintain efficacy in the long term, whether this is blunted because of the hyperreninaemia is difficult to prove.

Bradykinin increase (ACEI) versus no effect (RI and AT_1RA)

This is potentially a very important difference. Like angiotensin II,

Table 1 Effects of inhibition of the renin–angiotensin system at different sites on some key components of the cascade.

	Renin inhibition	ACEI	AT_1RA
Renin	↓	↑	↑
Angiotensin I	↓	↑	↑
Angiotensin II	↓	↓	↑↑
Bradykinin	↔	↑	↔
Non-renin/ACE AII blocked	No	No	Yes

ACEI, Angiotensin-converting enzyme inhibition; AT_1RA, angiotensin receptor subtype 1 antagonist; ACE, angiotensin-converting enzyme.

bradykinin has diverse effects, including the release of nitric oxide and prostaglandin E_2/I_2 from the endothelium [19]. Recent experimental studies in which a bradykinin antagonist (Hoe 140) was given together with an ACE inhibitor suggest that bradykinin accumulation may play an important role in mediating the effects of ACEI on cardiac function [20], pressure-induced left ventricular hypertrophy [21], neointimal proliferation after vascular injury [22] and insulin sensitivity [23]. Thus, some beneficial effects seen with ACEI may well be blunted with RI or AT_1RA. Sufficient clinical data are simply not available to judge this issue but ongoing trials with the AT_1RA DuP 753 (losartan) in these areas should provide some answers.

On the other hand, it is now also clear that the newer agents do not share some of the side-effects of ACEI linked to bradykinin and in particular the frequent side-effect of cough. This has been elegantly demonstrated recently with respect to AT_1RA in a multicentre study [24] in which subjects who developed a cough on rechallenge with an ACEI were randomized in a double-blind fashion over 8 weeks to either the ACE inhibitor lisinopril, the AT_1RA losartan or a thiazide diuretic. As expected, the majority of patients put on lisinopril — although surprisingly not all for reasons that are not clear — redeveloped the cough, while the majority of those put on losartan did not and the frequency in this group was no higher than that seen with the thiazide diuretic group, which provided a useful treatment control. Similar data are emerging with renin inhibitors [25].

Angiotensin II increase (AT_1RA) versus decrease (ACEI and RI)

The next difference between the agents to consider is the effect on angiotensin II levels — an increase with AT_1RA and a decrease with the other two types (Table 1). The main theoretical concern here is the effect of the stimulation of the unprotected AT_2 receptor subtype by the increased angiotensin II level with the AT_1-selective antagonists. As mentioned earlier, all of the well-described cardiovascular effects of angiotensin II appear to be mediated through the AT_1 subtype receptor. The AT_2 receptor has only recently been cloned and has a structure very different from the AT_1 receptor and other G-protein-coupled receptors [13,26]. The second messenger pathway transducing its signal remains to be fully elucidated, although tyrosine phosphatases may be involved. The distribution of the receptor also shows a distinct pattern with high levels in the reproductive organs, some parts of the brain, the adrenal gland and in the fetus [13]. Interestingly, its expression is also activated in skin wounds and in the neointima following balloon injury. So far no function has been described for the receptor and no side-effect has emerged from the clinical use of losartan that can be attributed to its stimulation. Perhaps none will emerge but, with the likelihood of more widespread use of this class of drugs, it is clearly important that a vigilant eye is kept on more subtle effects.

While the main concern lies with unwanted effects related to stimulation of the AT_2 receptor with selective AT_1 receptor antagonists, somewhat paradoxically, it has been suggested [13] that in some situations such stimulation may actually augment the overall effects of the drug by producing effects analogous to blocking the AT_1 receptor. Thus, in the vascular wall, the AT_2 receptor may mediate an antiproliferative effect [27] and therefore its stimulation may actually enhance the inhibition of neointimal proliferation caused by an AT_1RA through its blockade of the AT_1 receptor. Since ACE inhibitors, despite the experimental evidence, have proved disappointing clinically in preventing restenosis after coronary angioplasty [28], whether AT_1RAs prove to be better, perhaps because of the dual mechanism discussed above, will be interesting to see.

Antagonism of non-renin/ACE-generated angiotensin II (AT_1RA) versus no effect (RI and ACEI)

Finally, there is the issue of non-renin/ACE-mediated tissue angiotensin II generation. There is tremendous controversy at the moment regarding the biological importance of such tissue pathways [14], for example in the heart where a chymase seems to be a major angiotensin II-generating enzyme [29]. Clearly, the AT_1RA antagonists have the potential to block the effects of such angiotensin II, at least at the AT_1 receptor, while renin and ACE inhibitors do not. What clinical impact this may have remains entirely speculative at present but may provide one explanation if significant differences emerge between the agents as experience increases.

FUTURE PERSPECTIVES

Renin inhibition and angiotensin receptor antagonism offer more selective ways of targeting the renin–angiotensin system than is the case with ACEI. Studies to date suggest that they are effective antihypertensive agents which lack some of the side-effects of ACE inhibitors. Whether they share the other beneficial effects of ACE inhibitors or have additional clinically useful properties remains to be determined. This is going to be a difficult task given that ethical considerations may prevent their comparison with placebo or ACEI in situations where ACEI have already been shown to be of benefit. Nevertheless, in the next few years, as clinical experience of these agents increases, their place in the management of cardiovascular diseases should become clearer. It is possible that a case may even emerge for using some of the agents in combination.

REFERENCES

1 Williams GH. Converting enzyme inhibitors in the treatment of hypertension. *N Engl J Med* 1988;**319**:1517–1525.
2 The SOLVD investigators. Effect of enalapril on survival in patients with reduced left ventricular ejection fractions and congestive heart failure. *N Engl J Med* 1991;**325**:293–302.
3 The SOLVD investigators. Effect of enalapril on mortality and the development of heart failure in asymtomatic patients with reduced left ventricular ejection fraction. *N Engl J Med* 1992;**327**:685–691.
4 Pfeffer MA, Braunwald B, Moye LA *et al.*, on behalf of the SAVE investigators. Effect of captopril on mortality and morbidity in patients with left ventricular dysfunction after myocardial infarction. Results of the Survival and Ventricular Enlargement Trial. *N Engl J Med* 1992;**327**:669–677.
5 The Acute Infarction Ramipril Efficacy (AIRE) study investigators. Effect of ramipril on mortality and morbidity of survivors of acute myocardial infarction with clinical evidence of heart failure. *Lancet* 1993;**342**:821–828.
6 ISIS-4 (Fourth International Study of Infarct Survival) collaborative group. ISIS-4: a randomised factorial trial assessing early oral captopril, oral mononitrate and intravenous magnesium sulphate in 58 050 patients with suspected acute myocardial infarction. *Lancet* 1995;**345**:669–685.
7 Bjorck S, Nyberg G, Mulec H, Granerus G, Herlitz H, Aurell M. Beneficial effects of angiotensin converting enzyme inhibition on renal function in patients with diabetic nephropathy. *Br Med J* 1986;**193**:467–470.
8 Dahlof B, Pennert KJ, Hansson L. Reversal of left ventricular hypertrophy in hypertensive subjects: a metaanalysis of 109 treatment studies. *Am J Hypertens* 1992;**5**:95–110.
9 Yeo WW, MacLean D, Richardson PJ, Ramsey LE. Cough and enalapril: assessment by spontaneous reporting and visual analogue scale under double-blind conditions. *Br J Clin Pharmacol* 1991;**31**:356–359.
10 Opie LH. *Angiotensin Converting Enzyme Inhibitors: Scientific Basis for Clinical Use*. Wiley-Liss, New York, 1992.
11 Wood JM, Cumin F, Maibaum J. Pharmacology of renin inhibitors and their application to the treatment of hypertension. *Pharmacol Ther* 1994;**61**:325–344.
12 MacFadyen RJ, Reid JL. Angiotensin receptor antagonists as a treatment for hypertension. *J Hypertens* 1994;**12**:1333–1338.
13 Dzau VJ, Mukoyama M, Pratt RE. Molecular biology of angiotensin receptors: target for drug research? *J Hypertens* 1994;**12**(suppl 2):S1–S5.
14 Samani NJ. Extra-renal renin–angiotensin systems. *In: Textbook of Hypertension*, edited by Swales JD. Blackwell Scientific Publications, Oxford, 1994:253–272.
15 Dzau VJ. Multiple pathways of angiotensin production in the blood vessel wall: evidence, possibilities and hypotheses. *J Hypertens* 1989;**7**:933–936.
16 Samani NJ, Cumin F, Kelly MP, Wood J. Expression of components of the renin–angiotensin system during prolonged blockade at different levels in the marmoset. *Am J Physiol* 1994;**267**:E612–E619.
17 Mohring J. High blood pressure versus humoral factors in the pathogenesis of the vascular lesions of malignant hypertension. *Clin Sci Mol Med* 1977;**52**:113–117.
18 Mooser V, Nussberger J, Juillerat L *et al.* Reactive hyperreninaemia is a major determinant of plasma angiotensin II during ACE inhibition. *J Cardiovasc Pharmacol* 1990;**15**:276–282.
19 De Nucci G, Gryglewski RJ, Warner TD, Vane JR. Receptor-mediated release of endothelium-derived relaxing factor and prostacyclin from bovine aortic endothelial cells is coupled. *Proc Natl Acad Sci USA* 1988;**85**:2334–2338.
20 Gohlke P, Winz W, Scholkens BA *et al.* Angiotensin-converting enzyme inhibition improves cardiac function: role of bradykinin. *Hypertension* 1994;**23**:411–418.
21 Linz W, Scholkens BA. A specific B2-bradykinin receptor antagonist HOE 140 abolishes the antihypertrophic effect of ramipril. *Br J Pharmacol* 1992;**105**:771–772.

22 Farhy RD, Ho K-L, Carretero OA, Scicli AG. Kinins mediate the antiproliferative effect of ramipril in rat carotid artery. *Biochem Biophys Res Commun* 1992;**182**:283–288.

23 Tomiyama H, Kushiro T, Abeta H *et al*. Kinins contribute to the improvement of insulin sensitivity during treatment with angiotensin converting enzyme inhibitor. *Hypertension* 1994;**23**:450–455.

24 Lacourciere Y, Brunner H, Irwin R *et al*. and the Losartan Cough Study Group. Effects of modulators of the renin–angiotensin–aldosterone system on cough. *J Hypertens* 1994;**12**:1387–1394.

25 Nelson DE, Moyse DM, O'Neil JM, Boger RS, Glassman HN, Kleinert HD. Renin inhibitor, Abbott-72517, does not induce characteristic angiotensin converting enzyme inhibitor cough. *Circulation* 1993;**1**:36.

26 Mukoyama M, Nakajima M, Horiuchi M, Sasamura H, Pratt RE, Dzau VJ. Expression cloning of type 2 angiotensin II receptor reveals a unique class of seven-transmembrane receptors. *J Biol Chem* 1993;**268**:24539–24542.

27 Janiak P, Pillon A, Prost JF, Vilaine JP. Role of angiotensin subtype 2 receptor in neointima formation after vascular injury. *Hypertension* 1992;**20**:737–745.

28 MERCATOR Study Group. Does the new angiotensin converting enzyme inhibitor cilazapril prevent restenosis after percutaneous transluminal coronary angioplasty? *Circulation* 1992;**86**:100–110.

29 Urata H, Kinoshita A, Misono KS, Bumpus FM, Husain A. Identification of a highly specific chymase as the major angiotensin II-forming enzyme in the human heart. *J Biol Chem* 1990;**265**:22348–22357.

Vasodilators in chronic heart failure

DAVID P. DE BONO

WHAT IS CHRONIC HEART FAILURE?

Cardiologists have never found it easy to agree on a succinct definition of heart failure. Early definitions have concentrated on inadequacy of cardiac function, but have usually been vague about what 'inadequacy' means. More recent definitions have emphasized measurable features such as left ventricular function, but run the risk of excluding patients with, for example, valvular heart disease who may present with similar symptoms. It may be wisest to accept that what we all recognize as clinical heart failure (Table 1) is one end of a continuum of physiological responses and compensatory mechanisms (Table 2) for which at least the potential exists in normal individuals. The precise point along this continuum at which heart failure is said to exist is arbitrary, and will to some extent depend on the sensitivity of the tools we use to detect it. If we are to manage in the best possible way patients with clinical heart failure, we need to appreciate both the cause of the problem and the extent to which appropriate or inappropriate compensatory mechanisms are being activated.

Causes of chronic heart failure

Data from the Framingham study in the USA suggest that hypertensive heart disease is the commonest cause of clinical chronic heart failure, followed by ischaemic heart disease [1]. More recent UK data suggest that ischaemic heart disease is now the principal cause, at least in this country [2]. In developing countries, chronic rheumatic heart disease, constrictive pericarditis and endocardial fibrosis remain important causes of chronic heart failure.

The clinical history, and in particular, evidence of previous hypertension, myocardial infarction or alcohol abuse, is important in making the diagnosis; echocardiography is the most useful investigation for characterizing ventricular function and the presence or absence of valvular disease.

134

Table 1 Some features of clinical heart failure.

Impaired exercise tolerance/increased muscle fatigue
Dyspnoea
Tachycardia
Fluid retention
  Raised jugular venous pressure
  Ankle oedema
  Pulmonary oedema
  Pleural effusion/ascites
Peripheral vasoconstriction/cyanosis
Features of impaired left ventricular function
  Third sound
  Cardiomegaly
  Dyskinetic apex
Altered diurnal rhythm of diuresis
Increased circulating catecholamines

Table 2 Cardiovascular compensatory mechanisms.

Sympathetic/adrenal medullary activation: Ino/chronotropic

Reduces renal blood flow

Fluid retention

Potentiates renin–angiotensin–aldosterone system activation

Overrides atrial natriuretic peptide

Long-term: down-regulation of β-adrenoceptors

Renin–angiotensin–aldosterone system: sodium and water retention

Increased aldosterone

Vasoconstriction (mainly arteriolar)

Increased fluid intake (via thirst)

Potentiates sympathetic activation

Atrial natriuretic peptide: produced/released in response to atrial stretch

Causes sodium/water excretion

Overrides fluid retention caused by oral steroids

Overridden in heart failure

Antidiuretic hormone (vasopressin): released in response to severe hypotension

Inhibits water diuresis

Selective vasoconstriction

Compensatory mechanisms

It has been suggested that, from an evolutionary perspective, the compensatory mechanisms which come into play in heart failure are those which are acutely involved in adjusting to the demands of exercise, or of sudden loss of circulatory volume. During exercise there is activation of the sympathetic nervous system and of the adrenal medulla, resulting in increased cardiac rate and contractility, together with renal and splanchnic vasoconstriction. Acute blood loss also causes sympathetic activation, together with activation of the renin–angiotensin–aldosterone (RAA) system and increased release of antidiuretic hormone (ADH). The two conventional stimuli to activation of the RAA system are a fall in pulsatile perfusion pressure at the renal glomerulus, and sodium depletion perceived at the macula densa of the glomerulus [3,4]. A major difference between exercise and transient volume depletion on one hand, and heart failure on the other, is the time scale: in heart failure, the compensatory mechanisms are operative over a much more prolonged period. As a result, interactions between the systems become more important: sympathetic activation facilitates renin release, whilst angiotensin II increases noradrenaline release from sympathetic nerve endings [5,6].

In animal models of heart failure produced by vena caval or pulmonary arterial obstruction [7,8] or by rapid pacing [9] there is initial activation of both the sympathetic and the RAA systems, but RAA activation may be transient, particularly if arterial pressure is maintained. This matches, at least to some extent, observations on untreated patients with heart failure: activation of the RAA system is variable, but more common if there is persisting hypotension [10–12].

The atrial natriuretic peptide (ANP) and ADH systems have been less well-characterized. ANP is released by atrial distension and causes increased renal salt and water excretion; it is probably responsible for the 'escape' from aldosterone-induced salt and water retention seen after a few days in animals and human volunteers given aldosterone. This 'escape' does not occur in heart failure, so presumably the natriuretic effect of ANP is fairly easily overridden by other factors [13]. On the other hand, raised plasma ANP levels are a fairly constant feature in patients with clinical heart failure or echo evidence of left ventricular dysfunction, and have been proposed as a biochemical marker for heart failure [14]. ADH may be responsible for the low plasma sodium concentrations seen in heart failure, and may contribute to peripheral vasoconstriction. However, ADH antagonists do not cause a diuresis in heart failure, so their contribution to fluid retention is probably small [15].

Compensatory mechanisms can be profoundly affected by concomitant medication, and this is particularly apparent in respect of diuretics and the RAA system. The initial sodium depletion caused by diuretic therapy causes increased renin release and increased (aldosterone-mediated) distal tubule sodium reabsorption. Sodium homeostasis is restored, but the system is reset at a higher level of RAA activation [16].

THE HISTORY OF VASODILATOR THERAPY FOR HEART FAILURE

Cardiac failure manifesting as fluid retention or dropsy would have been familiar to physicians since before the time of Hippocrates. Treatment would have been with purgatives — presumably with some effect on fluid retenticn, albeit at considerable discomfort and some danger to the patient — or with various herbal diuretics. Squill (*Scilla* spp.) preparations have been used in Mediterranean folk medicine for centuries, and contain digitalis-like glycosides, but the therapeutic margin is narrow and the potential for toxicity large. Withering's studies on digitalis [17] were remarkable as much for his understanding of the principles of clinical pharmacology as for originality in the choice of agent. During the 19th century appreciation of the effects of mercury derivatives as diuretics was to some extent a byproduct of their use in venereal diseases. At the same time the development of *ex vivo* experimental pharmacology shifted emphasis to agents which stimulated the heart, culminating in the discovery of the catecholamine hormones and their derivatives.

Although nitrate vasodilators have been known to be effective in angina since the late 19th century [18], systematic studies of vasodilators in clinical heart failure did not begin until the 1950s, to some extent impelled by the availability of new vasodilator agents to treat hypertension. Clinically, vasodilators for heart failure were also overshadowed by the development of effective orally active diuretics.

HOW VASODILATORS WORK

Conceptually, vasodilators may act as venodilators, general arteriolar vaso-dilators and selective arteriolar vasodilators. The practical value of this classification is limited because agents frequently have effects in more than one category, and the balance of such effects may vary both with time and with clinical conditions. A pure venodilator given to a patient with clinical heart failure produces in effect a pharmacological venesection (Fig. 1). Right atrial pressure falls, right-sided cardiac output falls and so does pulmonary artery pressure. Pulmonary capillary pressure falls, perhaps enough to reverse pulmonary oedema and the associated reflex systemic arteriolar constriction. Left ventricular stroke volume and output also fall, though not necessarily by much, since the Starling curve relating filling pressure and stroke work in a failing ventricle is relatively flat. Acute venodilatation may be helpful in treating acute pulmonary oedema, but is of limited value in chronic heart failure, since over the time course of 2–3 days the body will retain enough fluid to compensate for the venodilatation. Long-term preload reduction (or compensation for

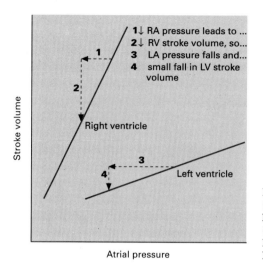

1↓ RA pressure leads to ...
2↓ RV stroke volume, so...
3 LA pressure falls and...
4 small fall in LV stroke
   volume

Right ventricle

Left ventricle

Stroke volume

Atrial pressure

Fig. 1 Effects of venodilatation (or venesection) on haemodynamics in heart failure (adapted & redrawn after Bradley, R, Studies in Acute Heart Failure, Edward Arnold 1978).

excessive fluid retention) is best achieved using diuretics. In practice, there are few drugs which are pure venodilators. Nitrates, including glyceryl trinitrate, isosorbide mononitrate and sodium nitroprusside, initially cause both venodilatation and arteriolar dilatation when given to patients with clinical heart failure, but there is rapid adaptation to the venodilator effect and long-term effects are mediated principally via arteriolar dilatation [19,20].

In contrast, agents such as hydralazine work predominantly as arteriolar dilators. The initial effect is a reduction in systemic vascular resistance and a fall in aortic pressure, hence a reduction in left ventricular afterload [21]. The curve relating left ventricular stroke work to afterload (Fig. 2). is steep in heart failure (contrast the relationship with preload), so even a small afterload reduction causes a marked increase in cardiac output. The increased output is rapidly transmitted to the venous side of the circulation, so there is little, if any, fall in atrial pressure. End-systolic left ventricular volume tends to decrease, and this may help increase cardiac efficiency by Laplace's law. Patients treated with arteriolar vasodilators alone tend in the medium to long term to retain fluid, presumably because the kidney senses a reduced pulsatile perfusion pressure. Indeed, the situation can become analogous to the so-called 'high-output heart failure' seen in patients with peripheral arteriovenous fistulae. α_1-adrenoceptor antagonists such as prazosin also behave as predominant arteriolar vasodilators, but tolerance tends to develop to their action. Other potential vasodilator agents are listed in Table 3.

Angiotensin-converting enzyme (ACE) inhibitors can be described as agents with mixed veno- and arteriolar dilating capacity plus the ability to inhibit the secondary compensatory response of fluid retention by

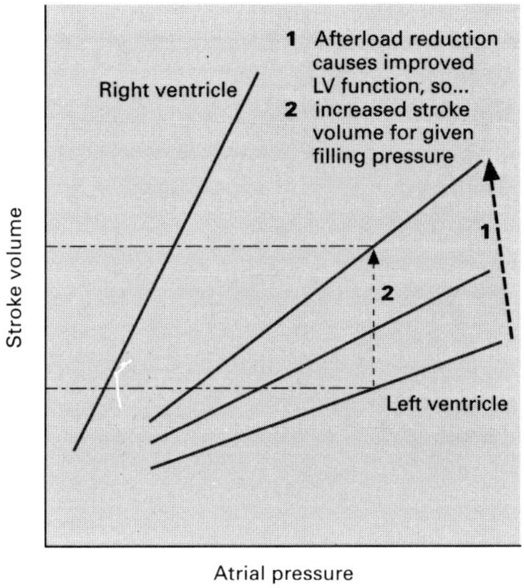

Fig. 2 Effects of arteriolar
dilatation (afterload reduction) on
haemodynamics in heart failure.

blocking angiotensin II-mediated aldosterone release [22–24]. This
however involves a number of important oversimplifications. First, it is
unclear why ACE inhibitors have such a marked venodilator effect, since
angiotensin II has little venoconstrictor activity. Abrupt venodilatation
can cause severe hypotension in patients given excessive initial doses
of ACE inhibitor, particularly if they have previously received large
doses of diuretic. Second, patients given ACE inhibitors may go through
a phase of compensatory fluid retention despite RAA blockade: this
may be due to a reduction in ANP secretion, and is usually self-limiting.
Finally, haemodynamic improvement may continue for several weeks
after initiation of therapy, and seems to correlate poorly with initial or
final indices of RAA system activation. Possible explanations include
effects on extrarenal, organ-specific RAA systems (for example, local renin
production may be important in controlling aldosterone release from the
adrenal cortex), effects on the bradykinin/kallikrein and prostaglandin
systems, and the long-term effects of down-regulating sympathetic nervous
system activation.

ACE inhibitors act to some extent as specific arteriolar vasodilators,
in that they tend specifically to increase renal blood flow in patients with
heart failure (Table 4). Angiotensin II and sympathetic stimulation both
have marked constrictor effects on the afferent arteriole to the glomerulus;
angiotensin II also constricts the efferent arteriole. In patients with bilateral
renal artery stenosis, the fall in blood pressure after ACE inhibitors can
cause distal renal artery pressure to fall below the autoregulation limits
and cause renal failure. In patients with severe heart failure, hypotension
and high sympathetic tone, ACE inhibitors can actually decrease filtration

Table 3 Vasodilators used in heart failure.

Name	Type of effect	Clinical use
ACE inhibitors (captopril, enalapril, quinapril, etc.)	Mixed arteriolar and venous dilators, block aldosterone release, significance of tissue enzyme inhibition uncertain	Improve survival in chronic heart failure and post myocardial infarction
α-Adrenoceptor antagonists (e.g. prazosin)	Arteriolar dilators	So far, disappointing (perhaps because α_2 effects negate benefit)
Calcium-channel blockers (e.g. nifedipine)	Mixed arteriolar and venodilators	Disappointing in chronic heart failure because of negative inotropy (amlodipine and felodipine are likely to be better, but unproven)
Dopamine	Selective renal vasodilator at low doses (higher doses stimulate noradrenaline release)	Acute heart failure, to initiate diuresis in chronic heart failure
Hydralazine	Arteriolar dilator	Increases cardiac output and effort tolerance (with nitrates) in chronic heart failure
Nitrates (e.g. sodium nitroprusside, glyceryl trinitrate, isosorbide mono- and dinitrate)	Complex profile, with predominantly venodilatation early, arteriolar dilatation predominating later	Useful as venodilators in acute left heart failure. With hydralazine, improve cardiac output in chronic heart failure
Phosphodiesterase inhibitors (e.g. milrinone)	Positive inotropes plus arteriolar dilators	In trials improved symptoms but not survival

ACE, Angiotensin-converting enzyme.

pressure by dilating the efferent arteriole — this will be further discussed below. In most patients, however, the maintenance of renal blood flow will enhance the efficacy of diuretics and further contribute to the ease of managing heart failure.

CLINICAL TRIALS OF VASODILATORS IN CHRONIC HEART FAILURE

Because of the complexities of the interactions involved, and the frequency

Table 4 Clinical effects of ACE inhibitors in heart failure (negative or unhelpful effects in brackets).

Effect	Clinical significance
Venodilatation	Reduced PA pressure, less pulmonary oedema (hypotension)
Arteriolar dilatation	Afterload reduction, improved LV function (hypotension)
Renal vasodilatation	Preserved renal function, reduced need for diuretics (high doses may dilate efferent arteriole and inhibit diuresis)
Inhibit aldosterone release	Prevents secondary hyperaldosteronism causing fluid retention (risk of hyperkalaemia with potassium-sparing diuretics)
Reduce sympathetic tone circulating catecholamines	Enhance vasodilator effects, reduce heart rate and cardiac oxygen consumption. Reduce risk of myocardial infarction or sudden death?
Inhibit thirst response to iso-osmotic volume depletion	(Risk of involuntary dehydration)
Alter cough reflex	(Cough as unwanted treatment effect)

ACE, Angiotensin-converting enzyme; PA, pulmonary artery; LV, left ventricular.

with which the long-term effects of antifailure drugs differ from acute or experimental findings, it is essential that management should be guided by the results of large-scale randomized clinical trials (Table 5).

Clinical trials in patients with established clinical heart failure

The Vasodilator Heart Failure Trial I (V-HeFT-1) was the first trial to establish conclusively that vasodilator therapy could improve survival when added to a regimen of diuretic and digitalis in patients with established heart failure [25]. The trial compared placebo, prazosin and isosorbide dinitrate plus hydralazine. The isosorbide dinitrate plus hydralazine arm showed improved survival compared to placebo: the prazosin arm showed no benefit.

The Cooperative North Scandinavian Enalapril Survival Study (CONSENSUS) compared enalapril and placebo as 'add-on' therapy to digitalis and diuretics in patients with severe (New York Heart Association (NYHA) class IV) heart failure symptoms at entry. There was a marked

142 *D.P. de Bono*

Table 5 Major mortality-outcome trials of vasodilators in heart failure.

Trial	Design/outcome	Ref.
V-HeFT-1	Randomized double-blind. Hydralazine + isosorbide dinitrate improved survival compared to prazosin or placebo in patients also receiving digoxin and diuretics	[25]
V-HeFT-2	Randomized double-blind. Enalapril improved survival compared with hydralazine + isosorbide dinitrate. However, the latter combination gave better LV ejection fraction in early visits	[27]
CONSENSUS	Randomized double-blind. Enalapril markedly improved survival compared with placebo in patients initially in NYHA class IV (all patients could have digoxin and diuretics)	[26]
SOLVD	Randomized double-blind. In the treatment arm, patients with initial NYHA class II or III failure showed improved survival with enalapril compared with placebo. In the prevention arm, patients with NYHA class I failure did not show a mortality benefit, but were less likely to be admitted to hospital with worsening failure	[28,29]

V-HeFT-1, Vasodilator Heart Failure Trial 1; CONSENSUS, Cooperative North Scandinavian Enalapril Survival Study; SOLVD, Studies of Left Ventricular Dysfunction; LV, left ventricular; NYHA, New York Heart Association.

survival benefit in the enalapril-treated group, and the study was terminated prematurely [26].

The V-HeFT-2 trial [27] compared enalapril with the isosorbide/hydralazine regimen shown to be effective in V-HeFT-1. At 2 years, there was a clear survival benefit in the ACE inhibitor compared with the isosorbide/hydralazine group. Interestingly, this was largely due to a reduction in the incidence of sudden death in the ACE inhibitor group. Patients treated with isosorbide/hydralazine actually showed a greater improvement in ejection fraction and exercise tolerance, despite their higher mortality rate.

The Studies of Left Ventricular Dysfunction (SOLVD) study was effectively divided into two parts. The SOLVD treatment study compared enalapril and placebo against a background of digitalis and diuretics in patients starting with class II or class III heart failure. The results effectively confirmed CONSENSUS in showing a consistent benefit to ACE inhibitor therapy, albeit in a population with less severe initial symptoms [28].

Clinical trials in asymptomatic patients with impaired left ventricular function

The other part of the SOLVD trial, the SOLVD prevention trial, randomized patients in NYHA class I with left ventricular ejection fractions < 35% to enalapril or placebo. There was no significant reduction in mortality, but the combined endpoint of mortality and hospital admission for heart failure was significantly less common in the ACE inhibitor arm [29]. There was no significant reduction in quality of life in patients randomized to ACE inhibitor [30].

Vasodilators in patients who have had myocardial infarction

Experimental animal studies which suggested that ACE inhibitors could prevent progressive ventricular dilatation after myocardial infarction [31] led to a number of clinical studies. In the CONSENSUS II study [32] enalapril was started early after infarction, and the primary endpoint was cumulative mortality at 180 days. There was no evidence of benefit from ACE inhibition. In the SAVE (Survival and Ventricular Enlargement) study [33] patients with a low ejection fraction (< 40%) were randomized to captopril or placebo. A difference between treated and placebo groups was only apparent after 10 months of follow-up, but thereafter there was a substantial reduction in late mortality in the captopril-treated group. These results were corroborated in the Acute Infarction Ramipril Efficacy (AIRE) trial [34], which had as an entry criterion the simple presence of clinical heart failure at any stage in the early post-infarct period. Again, there was a substantial mortality reduction. Most recently, the Survival of Myocardial Infarction Long-term Evaluation (SMILE) study randomized otherwise unselected post-infarct patients with anterior infarction to receive zofenopril or placebo, and showed a 34% (95% confidence interval (CI) 8–54%) reduction in risk of death or severe congestive failure during the randomized treatment period of 6 weeks, and a 29% (95% CI 6–51%) reduction in risk of mortality at 1 year [35].

Trials unfavourable to vasodilators

The PROMISE (Prospective Randomized Milrinone Survival Evaluation) study with milrinone, a phosphodiesterase inhibitor with both inotropic and vasodilator properties, was stopped because of excess mortality in the group receiving active treatment [36]. A trial of another phosphodiesterase inhibitor, enoximone, suggested a paradoxical effect of increased mortality despite a net improvement in exercise tolerance [37]. Trials of flosequinan, a vasodilator acting via the inosine triphosphate system, also showed increased exercise capacity but also increased hospital admission rates and mortality among patients randomized to the active agent [38].

Unanswered questions

Large-scale trials provide definitive answers, but only to limited numbers of questions. We still lack information about the optimal dose of ACE inhibitor: doses used in some of the trials are larger than those commonly used clinically. We still do not know whether it is rational to combine ACE inhibitor and direct vasodilator therapy: will this combine the survival benefits of ACE inhibition with improved haemodynamic performance, or will it just be an exercise in polypharmacy? At present it seems that ACE inhibitors as a class of agent are beneficial in chronic heart failure, but we lack good comparative trials of different agents.

PRACTICALITIES AND PROBLEMS IN MANAGING CHRONIC HEART FAILURE

On the basis of our present knowledge, it is reasonable to state that every patient who is or has been in clinical heart failure as a consequence of impaired left ventricular systolic function should be considered for long-term vasodilator therapy with an ACE inhibitor [39].

The most appropriate way of approaching this will depend on whether one is starting with a patient already stabilized on diuretics (and perhaps digoxin) or an ill patient with excessive fluid retention.

Stable patients can usually be started on ACE inhibitors on an out-patient or day-case basis. Patients should be examined to ensure they are not fluid-depleted (jugular venous pulsation should be visible). It may be prudent to reduce or withhold diuretics. Baseline plasma urea and electrolyte concentrations should be measured. The initial dose of ACE inhibitor should be small (e.g. 2.5 mg) and the patient allowed to sit or lie under observation for 2–4 hours. A transient, asymptomatic fall in blood pressure is common: severe symptomatic hypotension is very rare with this regimen, but should be treated with intravenous saline if it occurs. Thereafter the dose of ACE inhibitor can be gradually increased, at daily intervals or more slowly, until the doses used in the clinical trials have been achieved.

In patients who have massive oedema when first seen, this author prefers to withhold ACE inhibitors until the patient has been stabilized using low-dose dopamine (2–5 µg/kg per min) and appropriate diuretics, and then to introduce an ACE inhibitor as described above.

Diuretics can usually be maintained at baseline doses for the first 1 or 2 weeks, but may need to be reduced thereafter. It is natural to be cautious about increasing the dose of ACE inhibitor if the patient is found to be hypotensive or complains of dizziness, but in fact these are usually signs that the dose of diuretic needs to be reduced. The eventual aim is the minimum dose of diuretic necessary to control fluid retention. Because ACE inhibitors remove the angiotensin II stimulus to aldosterone production (though sensitivity to potassium remains), potassium-sparing diuretics such as amiloride should be used with caution, and spironolactone should be avoided. On the other hand, patients who need large doses of diuretic to control fluid retention may develop hypokalaemia despite ACE inhibitor therapy, and cautious use of potassium–sparing diuretics here is justified.

A modest but sustained rise in plasma urea and creatinine concentrations is often a price which has to be paid for haemodynamic stability in patients with severe heart failure treated with ACE inhibitors and diuretics. An initial rapid rise in urea and creatinine, particularly if accompanied by oliguria, may indicate unappreciated renal artery stenosis and ACE inhibitor should be withheld until the situation is clarified. In the past we have seen patients apparently well-stabilized on diuretic and ACE inhibitor who suddenly become ill with deteriorating renal function and rising plasma potassium. The precipitating factor has often been dehydration, either in hot weather or following diarrhoea, and we have hypothesized that the central action of ACE inhibitors on hypothalamic thirst perception has blunted the stimulus to increase fluid intake [40]. We now recommend all patients taking ACE inhibitors and diuretics to weigh themselves regularly, and to increase fluid intake and/or reduce diuretic intake if there is a rapid fall in weight of more than 1 kg.

Cough is a well-documented complication of ACE inhibitor therapy [41], but in the author's experience, seldom severe enough to require its discontinuation. Non-steroidal anti-inflammatory agents may suppress the cough, but tend to make heart failure worse and should be avoided. Codeine or other simple cough suppressants may be helpful, as may inhaled disodium chromoglycate.

In patients genuinely unable to tolerate ACE inhibitors, alternative vasodilator therapy with isosorbide mononitrate and hydralazine may be considered. Isosorbide mononitrate should be started at 10–20 mg t.i.d. and progressively increased to at least 60 mg and preferably 100 mg or more daily. Tolerance usually develops to headache, and analgesics such as paracetamol may be helpful. Hydralazine can be started at 25 mg t.i.d. and increased to 75–150 mg daily. These are relatively large doses of hydralazine, and watch must be kept for the hydralazine-associated lupus-like syndrome. Diuretics may need to be reduced if hypertension develops, but in general isosorbide mononitrate plus hydralazine lacks the diuretic-sparing effect of ACE inhibitors.

Table 6 Advice to doctors.

Consider ACE inhibitor for any patient with left ventricular systolic dysfunction

Use diuretics to control fluid balance

Aim for full-dose ACE inhibitor/minimal dose of diuretic

Check urea and electrolytes regularly

Consider hydralazine/nitrates if ACE inhibitor is contraindicated/not tolerated

Consider adding hydralazine to ACE inhibitor

Watch out for:
  Drug interactions
  Sudden dehydration
  Progressive fluid retention
  New events, e.g. diabetes

ACE, Angiotensin-converting enzyme.

Table 7 Advice to patients.

Keep active
Avoid excess salt intake
Avoid unprescribed medication
Maintain fluid intake
Monitor weight:
  Adjust diuretics within agreed limits
  Report excess weight gain or loss

The successful long-term medical management of patients with severely impaired ventricular function is an onerous, if highly rewarding, challenge. By antagonizing inappropriate physiological responses of vasoconstriction and salt and water retention, the clinician and patient take on the responsibilities of long-term manual control of normally automatic functions. For this to be done effectively, the patient must understand what is happening, and continuity of care and meticulous attention to detail must be maintained at both hospital and general practice level. Summarized guidelines for patients and doctors are shown in Tables 6 and 7.

REFERENCES

1 Kannel W. Epidemiological aspects of heart failure. *Cardiol Clin* 1989;7:1–9.
2 Parameshwar J, Poole Wilson PA, Sutton GC. Heart failure in a district general hospital. *J R Coll Phys Lond* 1992;**26**:139–42.
3 Davis JO, Freeman RH. Mechanisms regulating renin release. *Physiol Rev* 1977;**56**:1–56.
4 Reid F. Renin–angiotensin system and body function. *Arch Intern Med* 1985;**145**:1475–1479.

5 Toretti J. Sympathetic control of renin release. *Annu Rev Pharmacol Toxicol* 1982;**22**:167–192.

6 Malik KU, Masjletti A. Facilitation of adrenergic transmission by locally generated angiotensin II in rat mesenteric arteries. *Circ Res* 1976;**40**:422–428.

7 Watkins L, Burton JA, Haber E *et al*. The renin–angiotensin–aldosterone system in congestive failure in conscious dogs. *J Clin Invest* 1976;**57**:1606–1617.

8 Freeman RH, Davis JO, Williams GM, De Forrest JM, Seymour AA, Rowe BP. Effects of the oral converting enzyme inhibitor SQ 14225 in a model of low cardiac output in dogs. *Circ Res* 1979;**45**:540–545.

9 Riegger GAJ. Neurohumoral vasoconstrictor systems in heart failure. *Eur Heart J* 1985;**6**:479–489.

10 Brown JJ, Davies DL, Johnson VW, Lever AF, Robertson JIS. Renin relationships in congestive heart failure, treated and untreated. *Am Heart J* 1970;**980**:329–342.

11 Bayliss J, Norell M, Canepa Anson R, Sutton G, Poole Wilson P. Untreated heart failure: clinical and neuroendocrine effects of introducing diuretics. *Br Heart J* 1987;**57**:17–22.

12 Francis GS, Benedict C, Johnstone DE *et al*. Comparison of neuroendocrine activation in patients with left ventricular dysfunction with and without congestive heart failure. A substudy of the studies of left ventricular dysfunction (SOLVD) trial. *Circulation* 1990;**82**:1724–1729.

13 Miyamori I, Ikeda M, Matsubara T *et al*. Human atrial natriuretic peptide during escape from mineralocorticoid excess in man. *Clin Sci* 1987;**73**:431–436.

14 Struthers AD. Plasma concentrations of brain natriuretic peptide: will this new test reduce the need for cardiac investigations? *Br Heart J* 1993;**70**:397–399.

15 Nicod P, Waeber B, Bussien JP *et al*. Acute haemodynamic effect of a vascular antagonist of vasopressin in patients with congestive heart failure. *Am J Cardiol* 1985;**55**:1043–1047.

16 Francis GS, Rector TS, Cohn JN. Sequential neurohumoral measurements in patients with congestive heart failure. *Am Heart J* 1988;**116**:1464–1468.

17 Withering W. *An Account of the Foxglove and some of its Medical Uses, with Practical Remarks on Dropsy and Other Diseases*. M. Swinney, Birmingham, 1785.

18 Murrell W. Nitro-glycerine as a remedy for angina pectoris. *Lancet* 1879;**I**:80–81.

19 Packer M, Medina N, Yushak M. Contrasting hemodynamic responses in severe heart failure: comparison of captopril and other vasodilator drugs. *Am Heart J* 1982;**104**:1215–1223.

20 Ghio S, Poli A, Ferrario M *et al*. Haemodynamic effects of glyceryl trinitrate during continuous 24 hour infusion in patients with heart failure. *Br Heart J* 1994;**72**:145–149.

21 Schofield PM, Brooks NH, Lawrence GP, Testa HJ, Ward C. Which vasodilator drug in patients with chronic heart failure? A randomised comparison of captopril and hydralazine. *Br J Clin Pharmacol* 1991;**31**:25–32.

22 Packer M, Lee WH, Medina N, Yushak M. Hemodynamic patterns of response during long-term captopril therapy for severe chronic heart failure. *Circulation* 1983;**68**:803–812.

23 Cleland J, Semple P, Hodsman P, Ball S, Ford I, Dargie H. Angiotensin II levels, haemodynamics and sympathoadrenal function after low dose captopril in heart failure. *Am J Med* 1984;**77**:880–886.

24 Creager MA, Massie BM, Faxon DP *et al*. Acute and long term effects of enalapril on the cardiovascular response to exercise and exercise tolerance in patients with congestive heart failure. *J Am Coll Cardiol* 1985;**6**:163–170.

25 Cohn JN, Archibald DG, Ziesche S *et al*. Effect of vasodilator therapy on mortality in chronic congestive heart failure. Results of a Veterans Administration Cooperative Study. *N Engl J Med* 1986;**314**:1547–1552.

26 The CONSENSUS Trial Study Group. Effects of enalapril on mortality in severe congestive heart failure. Results of the Cooperative North Scandinavian Enalapril Survival Study (CONSENSUS). *N Engl J Med* 1987;**316**:1429–1435.

27 Cohn JN, Johnson G, Ziesche S *et al*. A comparison of enalapril with hydralazine–isosorbide dinitrate in the treatment of chronic congestive heart failure. *N Engl J Med* 1991;**325**:303–310.

28 The SOLVD investigators. Effect of enalapril on survival in patients with reduced left

ventricular ejection fractions and congestive heart failure. *N Engl J Med* 1991;**325**:293–302.

29 The SOLVD investigators. Effect of enalapril on mortality and development of heart failure in asymptomatic patients with reduced left ventricular ejection fractions. *N Engl J Med* 1992;**327**:685–691.

30 Rogers WJ, Johnstone DE, Yusuf S *et al.* Quality of life among 5025 patients with left ventricular dysfunction randomised between placebo and enalapril: the studies of left ventricular dysfunction. *J Am Coll Cardiol* 1994;**23**:393–400.

31 Pfeffer JM, Pfeffer MA, Braunwald E. Influence of chronic captopril therapy on the infarcted left ventricle of the rat. *Circ Res* 1985;**57**:84–95.

32 Swedberg K, Held P, Kjeksus J, Rasmussen K, Ryden L, Wedel H on behalf of the CONSENSUS II Study Group. Effects of the early administration of enalapril on mortality in patients with acute myocardial infarction. Results of the Cooperative New Scandinavian Enalapril Survival Study II (CONSENSUS II). *N Engl J Med* 1992;**327**:678–684.

33 Pfeffer MA, Braunwald E, Moye LA *et al.* Effect of captopril on mortality and morbidity in patients with left ventricular dysfunction after myocardial infarction. *N Engl J Med* 1992;**327**:669–677.

34 The Acute Infarction Ramipril Efficacy (AIRE) investigators. Effect of ramipril on mortality and morbidity of survivors of acute myocardial infarction with clinical evidence of heart failure. *Lancet* 1993;**342**:821–827.

35 Ambrosioni E, Borghi C, Magnani B for the survival of myocardial infarction long term evaluation (SMILE) study investigators. The effect of the angiotensin converting enzyme inhibitor Zofenopril on mortality and morbidity after anterior myocardial infarction. *N Engl J Med* 1995;**332**:80–85.

36 Packer M, Carver JR, Rodeheffer RJ *et al.* for the PROMISE Study Research Group. Effect of oral milrinone on mortality in severe chronic heart failure. *N Engl J Med* 1991;**325**:1468–1475.

37 Cowley AJ, Skene AM on behalf of the enoximone investigators. Treatment of severe heart failure: quantity or quality of life? A trial of enoximone. *Br Heart J* 1994;**72**:226–230.

38 Cowley AJ, McEntegart DJ. Placebo controlled trial of flosequinan in moderate heart failure: the possible importance of aetiology and method of analysis in the interpretation of the results of heart failure trials. *Int J Cardiol* 1993;**38**:167–175.

39 Ganong WF. The brain renin–angiotensin system. *Annu Rev Physiol* 1984;**46**:17–31.

40 Baker DW, Konstam MA, Bottorff M, Pitt B. Management of heart failure. I. Pharmacologic treatment. *JAMA* 1994;**272**:1361–1366.

41 Yeo WW, Foster G, Ramsey LE. Prevalence of persistent cough during long-term enalapril treatment: controlled study versus nifedipine. *Q J Med* 1991;**81**:763–770.

MULTIPLE CHOICE QUESTIONS

1 In long-standing severe heart failure due to left ventricular dysfunction treated with diuretics alone, which of the following statements is likely to be true?

a plasma catecholamine levels will be high

b the renin–angiotensin–aldosterone system will be activated

c cardiac muscle is more responsive to β-adrenoceptor agonists

d a small change in left ventricular preload causes a large change in stroke volume

e afterload reduction increases cardiac output

2 **The following are recognized effects of angiotensin-converting enzyme inhibitors in patients with heart failure**
  a mixed arteriolar and venodilatation
  b aldosterone release is blocked in response to sodium and water loss
  c aldosterone release is blocked in response to hyperkalaemia
  d thirst response to volume depletion is inhibited
  e circulating catecholamine levels are reduced

3 **Which of the following statements are true in relation to vasodilator therapy in chronic heart failure?**
  a hydralazine is predominantly a venodilator
  b hydralazine and nitrates increase cardiac output but do not improve survival compared with placebo
  c vasodilators may cause increased fluid retention in patients not taking diuretics
  d effective vasodilator therapy often results in a reduced diuretic requirement
  e non-steroidal anti-inflammatory agents are prone to cause fluid retention in patients on vasodilator therapy

4 **Recognized side-effects of ACE inhibitors include**
  a progressive renal failure in patients with bilateral renal artery stenosis
  b severe hypokalaemia
  c non-productive cough
  d postural hypotension
  e angioneurotic oedema

5 **A patient being treated for chronic heart failure with ACE inhibitor (enalapril 20 mg twice daily) and frusemide (80 mg daily) is admitted to hospital because of breathlessness and increasing ankle oedema. He has recently been prescribed indomethacin 50 mg thrice daily for arthritis. The jugular venous pressure is elevated, blood pressure is 95/60 mmHg, there are bilateral basal lung crepitations. Plasma urea and electrolytes are normal: there is no proteinuria. Which of the following statements is likely to be true?**
  a the dose of ACE inhibitor is inadequate compared with doses used in major trials
  b the non-steroidal anti-inflammatory agent may have precipitated fluid retention

   c low-dose dopamine and temporarily reducing or withdrawing the
      ACE inhibitor will enhance a diuresis
   d adding amiloride or a thiazide to the frusemide will enhance urine
      output
   e renal vein thrombosis is a likely cause of decompensation

Answers

1	a True	2	a True	3	a False
	b True		b True		b False
	c False		c False		c True
	d False		d True		d True
	e True		e True		e True

4	a True	5	a False
	b False		b True
	c True		c True
	d True		d True
	e True		e False

The endothelium in the vascular response to sepsis

NICHOLAS P.CURZEN & TIMOTHY W.EVANS

The endothelium is an intimal layer of simple squamous cells which provides a continuous fluent surface for circulating blood. It is not the passive inert permeability barrier that was once thought, but rather a metabolically and physiologically dynamic tissue. This chapter discusses the clinical syndromes of sepsis and their pathogenesis, concentrating in particular on the central role played by the endothelium in orchestrating and modulating the vascular response to this important clinical problem.

Clinical sepsis syndromes

The clinical syndromes associated with sepsis represent a potentially devastating systemic inflammatory response estimated to occur in around 1% of hospitalized patients, of whom 10–20% die. The mortality in those patients with septic shock is 60–90% [1]. A constellation of typical clinical and haematological features has been identified and used to classify these patients (Table 1). The syndromes are associated with the positive identification of an infecting causative organism in less than 50% of cases. To avoid the requirement for an identifiable infection, the term systemic inflammatory response syndrome (SIRS) is now used to define the resulting clinical state [2]. Sepsis-induced endothelium-mediated circulatory failure is also increasingly recognized in the pathophysiology of multiple organ failure (MOF), which has an especially poor prognosis.

Disruption of the structural and functional integrity of the endothelium resulting in the widespread changes in vascular response seen in adults with sepsis is perhaps most obvious in the acute respiratory distress syndrome (ARDS), which complicates around 25% of cases with SIRS, and has a mortality of about 65% [3]. ARDS represents the most severe end of a clinical spectrum of acute lung injury (ALI), and is characterized by non-hydrostatic pulmonary oedema, elevated pulmonary vascular resistance (PVR) and hypoxaemia due to extensive mismatching between ventilation (V) and perfusion (Q). The elevation in PVR is often manifest as pulmonary hypertension, and results from the combination of both structural (due to thromboemboli and vascular remodelling) and

Table 1 Definitions of sepsis and septic shock.

Sepsis — The systemic response to infection
Includes two or more of the following:
  temperature > 38°C or < 36°C
  heart rate > 90 beats/min
  respiratory rate > 20 breaths/min or $Pa\text{CO}_2$ < 4.3 kPa
  white cell count > 12 000/mm^3 < 4000/mm^3, or > 10% band (immature) forms

Sepsis syndrome — Sepsis with evidence of altered organ perfusion
Altered organ perfusion includes one or more of the following:
  $Pa\text{O}_2/Fi\text{O}_2$ ≤ 280 (without other cardiopulmonary disease)
  elevated lactate level (> upper limit of normal for the lab)
  oliguria < 0.5 ml/kg body weight

Systemic inflammatory response syndrome — The response to a variety of severe clinical insults (not necessarily infective) which is indistinguishable from sepsis

Septic shock — sepsis with hypotension (sustained decrease in systolic blood pressure < 90 mmHg, or drop > 40 mmHg, for at least 1 hour) despite adequate fluid resuscitation, in the presence of perfusion abnormalities that may include, but are not limited to lactic acidosis, oliguria or an acute alteration in mental status Patients who are on inotropic or vasopressor agents may not be hypotensive at the time when perfusion abnormalities are measured

---

functional (due to vasoconstriction) changes in the pulmonary vasculature. At the same time a loss of normal vasoactive mechanisms, and particularly of hypoxic pulmonary vasoconstriction (HPV), contributes to the degree of V/Q mismatch and hypoxaemia [4]. HPV is a beneficial reflex whereby V/Q matching is maintained by vasoconstriction in areas of the lung that are hypoxic due to hypoventilation. As can be seen from detailed examination of the pathogenesis of the septic response, the endothelium is intimately involved in these vascular changes by both direct and indirect mechanisms.

THE PATHOGENESIS OF SEPSIS

Initiation

The initial trigger for the complex cascade of inflammatory pathways that lead to the clinical sepsis syndromes is most frequently endotoxin or another comparable substance derived from yeasts, viruses, fungi or Gram-positive bacteria [5]. Endotoxin is derived from the lipopolysaccharides (LPS) that make up the outermost layer of the cell membrane of all Gram-negative bacteria [6]. LPS is composed of a polysaccharide portion bonded to lipid A, which is responsible for the endotoxic properties of LPS through its ability to interact with both cellular and humoral inflammatory pathways (Fig. 1). Endotoxin can be present in the host circulation either as a result of exogenous bacterial invasion, or by translocation of intestinal flora through the wall of the gastrointestinal tract. Endotoxaemia is frequently

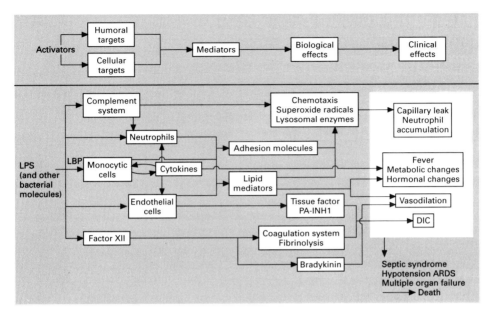

Fig. 1 Activation of cellular and humoral inflammatory pathways by lipopolysaccharide resulting in tissue damage. LPS, lipopolysaccharide; LBP, lipopolysaccharide-binding protein; DIC, disseminated intravascular coagulopathy; ARDS, acute respiratory distress syndrome. Reproduced with permission from [42].

found in patients with septic shock, whether or not blood cultures are positive for a specific pathogen [7]. The evidence that endotoxin is a key initiator of the inflammatory response in sepsis is compelling. In the plasma, endotoxin binds to a 60 kDa acute-phase glycoprotein known as lipopolysaccharide-binding protein (LBP). Animal studies have shown that macrophages and monocytes, which have specific surface proteins (CD14 family) that recognize this LPS–LBP complex can release cytokines, including tumour necrosis factor (TNF), interleukins (IL-1,-6,-8) and platelet-activating factor (PAF) as a result of this activation [8]. In addition, endotoxin leads to the activation and attraction of neutrophils both directly and via the associated production of cytokines, especially TNF. TNF is a 17 kDa peptide whose activation of neutrophils leads to them producing elastases as well as reactive oxygen species such as superoxide and hydrogen peroxide. TNF also activates endothelial cells, and promotes their binding to neutrophils, leading to endothelial damage and destruction. These are the early stages of an amplifying cascade of inflammatory events that ultimately can result in tissue damage and clinical sepsis. Thus, injection of endotoxin causes TNF levels in the blood to rise acutely in both animals and humans, which in turn leads to the characteristic haemodynamic changes of sepsis, including hypotension and increased pulmonary capillary permeability. Indeed, TNF levels are elevated in patients with sepsis, and probably correlate with prognosis.

Platelet activation precipitates the release of numerous vasoactive, chemoattractant and endothelium-damaging substances. Endotoxin is a potent activator of the complement system, and also contributes to the initiation of both intrinsic and extrinsic coagulation pathways. Neutrophil-derived proteases and bradykinin simultaneously stimulate the fibrinolytic systems. All of these mechanisms contribute to the evolving inflammatory crescendo (reviewed in [9]).

The endothelium in sepsis

The endothelium plays an integral role in the acute inflammatory response. The endothelial cell is capable of activation by many of the earliest components of this response, including endotoxin, histamine, bradykinin, cytokines and other products of white cell activation, and responds in several ways. A variable degree of mediator- and cytokine-induced endothelial damage ensues, leading to a loss of function and increased capillary permeability. The latter phenomenon is related to changes in the cytoarchitecture of these cells produced by realignment of intracellular contractile proteins [10].

Endothelial cell activation also facilitates the adherence and subsequent migration from blood to tissue of activated neutrophils. The majority of this migration occurs in postcapillary venules. Initially there is slowing of the white cells with margination, when they can be seen under light microscopy rolling along the vessel wall as a result of loose tethering to the underlying endothelial cells. Subsequently, they become more adherent and change from a spherical to a flatter shape. This facilitates their slow migration between endothelial cells, through the basement membrane, and into the interstitium. This process is now known to be mediated by interaction of specific cell adhesion molecules (CAM) on the surface of both the neutrophil and endothelial cell in a sequence known as the adhesion cascade [11]. Thus, the first phase of the process (slowing and rolling) depends upon the expression of a group of surface glycoprotein molecules, collectively termed selectins. Two such molecules are expressed on the endothelial cell for this process: endothelial-leukocyte adhesion molecule-1 (E-selectin), and granulocyte-associated membrane protein (P-selectin). Endothelial E-selectin expression has been demonstrated in response to cytokines and LPS, and the kinetics of its production in cell cuture imply that it is protein synthesis-dependent. P-selectin is present in the granules of endothelial cells (and platelets), and its expression is stimulated by thrombin and histamine, thereby providing a mechanism by which neutrophil adhesion is initiated very early in the inflammatory response, even before protein synthetic pathways are active. Meanwhile, L-selectin is expressed on neutrophils and is shed from their cell surface during this phase. The use of antibodies directed against these molecules in murine and rat *in vivo* models has demonstrated their importance in the initial phase of neutrophil emigration.

The next phase in the neutrophil–endothelial cell interaction (firm adherence and migration) is dependent on the expression of another set of CAMs, termed integrins, on the neutrophil surface. The most important of these is the CD11/CD18 complex, and increased expression of these molecules on activated neutrophils has been demonstrated in animal models both *in vivo* and *in vitro*. Ligands for these CAMs are present on the endothelial surface, and binding is promoted by cytokines, including TNF, PAF and ILs. The intercellular adhesion molecules (ICAM-1 and -2) are also expressed constitutively by the endothelium, and are therefore available early on for neutrophil binding. In addition, the vascular adhesion molecule, VCAM-1, is expressed by the endothelium in response to the presence of endotoxin and cytokines. The importance of CD11/CD18 molecules in patients with sepsis is gradually emerging; recently an increase in the resting expression of CD11/CD18 on granulocytes from patients with ARDS has been demonstrated and appears to correlate with the hyperadhesiveness of these cells [12]. The actual migration of neutrophils is dependent upon a chemotactic gradient, and probably also upon the expression of platelet-endothelial cell adhesion molecule (PECAM-1) which is mainly situated at the endothelial cell junctions [13]. The adhesion molecule cascade thus provides the machinery for the neutrophil–endo-thelial cell interaction that results in neutrophil migration, and as such represents an attractive set of targets for guided immunotherapy.

The endothelium has other facets of its inflammatory activation. Most importantly, there are other endotoxin-inducible genes besides CAMs, and these result in the expression of messenger RNA coding for a range of proteins, including cyclooxygenase (COX), constitutive and inducible nitric oxide synthase (cNOS and iNOS) and endothelins (see below). It is, to a great extent, the release of these potent vasoactive and inflammatory mediators that allows the endothelium to modulate the vascular response to sepsis. When the inflammatory response is widespread and severe, in-tense activation of the endothelium in some areas and destruction of it in others help to precipitate the overwhelming and devastating clinical syndromes described above.

ENDOTHELIAL MODULATION OF VASCULAR TONE

Nitric oxide

Background

It was in 1980 that the vascular relaxation induced by acetylcholine was shown to be dependent on the presence of intact endothelium and to be mediated via the release of a non-prostanoid, labile vasodilator termed endothelium-derived relaxant factor (EDRF). Overwhelming evidence has since accumulated that the chemical and pharmacological properties of EDRF are shared by nitric oxide (NO). Nitric oxide is synthesized *in vitro* from the semi-essential amino acid, L-arginine, by the membrane-bound enzyme NO synthase (NOS), a process that can be inhibited by L-arginine analogues such as N^G-monomethyl-L-arginine (L-NMMA) [14]. Several distinct NOS genes have been identified, and two forms of NOS exist in the blood-vessel wall: a constitutive calcium- and calmodulin-dependent enzyme (cNOS), and an inducible calcium- and calmodulin-independent enzyme (iNOS) (Table 2). Both forms exist in the vascular endothelium [15].

NO works by activating soluble guanylyl cyclase after binding to its haem moiety, which in turn causes an increase in intracellular cyclic guanosine monophosphate (cGMP), resulting in vascular smooth-muscle relaxation. This mechanism can be demonstrated experimentally. Thus, L-arginine administration has been shown to produce vasodilatation in lambs, and this effect can be blocked by the guanylyl cyclase inhibitor methylene blue or by L-NMMA [16,17]. This vasodilatation can, however, be augmented by a cGMP phosphodiesterase inhibitor, whose ability to raise intracellular cGMP levels has also been shown to produce vasodila-tation in other models. The measurement of cGMP levels in tissue can be used as an indicator of the degree of NOS activity, and this has become a useful tool in experimental studies of sepsis. In addition, the administration of NOS inhibitors has been shown to produce increases in mean arterial

Table 2 Summary of the two different isoforms of nitric oxide synthase (NOS).

NOS isoforms	Type II	Type III
Response in sepsis	Constitutive	Enzyme synthesis induced by LPS and cytokines
	Immediate increase in NO activity	Massive NO production after 2–6 hours
Location	Endothelial cell Membrane-bound	Mainly smooth muscle Cytosolic
Regulation		Induction prevented by corticosteroids and inhibitors of protein synthesis
Activation	Calcium-dependent	Calcium-independent
Non-selective inhibitors	L-arginine analogues (e.g. N^G-monomethyl-L-arginine)	
Selective inhibitors	None known	Aminoguanidine L-canavanine Diphenyleneiodonium

LPS, Lipopolysaccharides; NO, nitric oxide.

blood pressure and decreases in regional blood flow in both animals and humans [18], implying that there is a continuous basal release of NO contributing to vascular tone. The size of the pressor response induced by intravenous L-NMMA in animal models seems to be dependent on basal vascular tone.

Nitric oxide in sepsis

Suprabasal release of NO is known to occur in response to a diverse range of stimuli including endotoxin, cytokines, hypoxia, histamine, thrombin, bradykinin, calcium ionophore, endothelin and substance P (Fig. 2). As a result, increased NO release during the inflammatory response to sepsis is inevitable. Patients and animals with septic shock lose peripheral vascular tone, and the responsiveness of systemic vessels to constrictor agents such as catecholamines is diminished, both *in vitro* and *in vivo*. The incubation of bovine aortic endothelial cells with LPS causes the rapid release of an NO-like factor. Furthermore, the levels of NO metabolites are significantly elevated in patients with septic shock [19], and the administration of NOS inhibitors in these patients [20], or in animal models

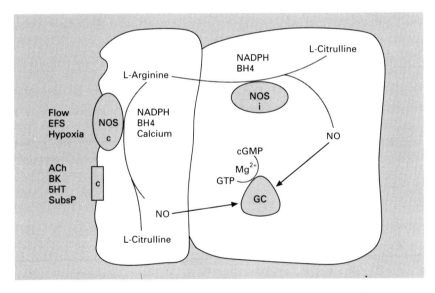

Fig. 2 Synthesis of nitric oxide in the endothelium and smooth muscle, and its mechanism of action. (For simplicity, no inducible nitric oxide synthase is shown in the endothelium, but it does exist in these cells.) NO, nitric oxide; NOSi, inducible nitric oxide synthase; ACh, acetylcholine; BK, bradykinin; 5HT, 5-hydroxytryptamine; SubsP, substance P; NADPH, nicotinamide adenine dinucleotide phosphate; BH4, tetrahydrobiopterin; EFS, electrical field stimulation; R, receptor; cGMP, cyclic guanosine monophosphate; Mg^{2+}, magnesium; GTP, guanine triphosphate; GC, guanylyl cyclase.

of sepsis, can produce reproducible elevations in systemic vascular resistance where other vasoconstrictors are ineffective. In fact, huge quantities of NO are produced in sepsis. Endotoxin leads to the induction of the calcium-independent NOS (iNOS) [21] in both the endothelium and the vascular smooth muscle [22], as well as in the myocardium, where the increase in NO production has been shown to reduce contractility [23]. Other cytokines (TNF, IL-1 and -2) also stimulate iNOS activity in vessel walls.

The time course of the increase in NO release in sepsis is the subject of considerable speculation. In isolated endotoxin-treated rat main pulmonary arteries, NOS inhibitors reverse the vascular hyporesponsiveness to phenylephrine [24], and there is no doubt that in established sepsis NO is largely responsible for this reduced reactivity. The NO-mediated hyporeactivity to noradrenaline starts within 60 minutes in a rat model of sepsis *in vivo* [25], and is therefore probably too rapid to be explained by the induction of iNOS. It therefore seems likely that this early increase in NO release is explained by an elevation in NO production by endothelial cNOS, but this remains controversial. Thus, in one study, although the administration of L-NAME (N-nitro-L-arginine methyl ester) after 1 hour in endotoxin-treated pithed rats did elevate blood pressure and increase vascular responsiveness to catecholamines, this was no greater than in saline-treated controls [26]. This suggests that the early hyporesponsiveness is caused not by NO, but by some other factors. What is clear, however, is that from 3 hours after the endotoxic insult, there is increasing NO production as a result of iNOS activity in the endothelium, and to an even greater extent in the vascular smooth muscle. The endothelium appears to be required for maximal NO response, so that its removal caused a significant delay in the onset of vascular responsiveness (6 compared with 4 hours) and reduced the sensitivity of rat aorta to LPS *in vitro* [27]. The application of the technique of reverse transcription polymerase chain reaction (rt-PCR) has allowed the demonstration of the widespread tissue expression of iNOS messenger RNA in a rat model at 4 hours post LPS injection compared with undetectable expression in control animals [28]. This rise in iNOS messenger RNA expression could be attenuated by pretreatment with dexamethasone (Fig. 3).

NOS inhibitors as therapeutic agents in sepsis

As has already been mentioned, the intravenous administration of L-NMMA (N-nitro-L-arginine) was shown to correct systemic hypotension (temporarily) in 2 patients with septic shock [20]. Another L-arginine analogue that non-specifically blocks NOS, L-NNA, has also been given to critically ill patients with sepsis [29]. This agent did cause a significant increase in both systemic and pulmonary vascular resistance as well as in mean arterial pressure, but with an accompanying reduction in cardiac

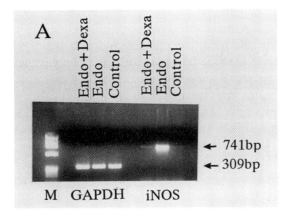

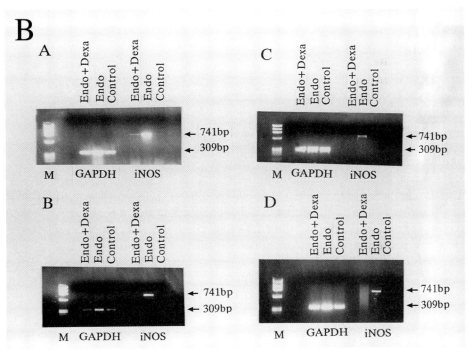

Fig. 3 Gel photographs of polymerase chain reaction (PCR)-amplified inducible nitric oxide synthase (iNOS) and glyceraldehyde-3-phosphate dehydrogenase (GAPDH) complementary DNA derived from iNOS and GAPDH tissue messenger RNA. These gels demonstrate the effects of *in vivo* treatment with lipopolysaccharide (endo) or dexamethasone (dexa) plus lipopolysaccharide on messenger RNA expression in rat tissues. (A) Lung; (B) A = liver; B = spleen; C = kidney; D = skeletal muscle. M = marker size. Arrows indicate expected PCR product size. Reproduced with permission from [28].

index. Further research is underway. The main theoretical objection to using non-specific inhibitors of NOS clinically is that NO is known to contribute to basal vascular tone, and in some organ beds (notably renal, mesenteric and pulmonary) there is frequently an overall reduction in regional blood flow in sepsis which could be amplified by NOS inhibition. Such an appreciation has fuelled investigation into the possibility of the selective blockade of iNOS in sepsis [30]. The theoretical attractions of this as a therapeutic tool are obvious. In comparative studies between L-NMMA and aminoguanidine, the former was found to be at least seven times more potent at inhibiting iNOS. L-NMMA was 15 times more potent at inhibition of the constitutive enzyme than aminoguanidine, however. Recently, evidence has accumulated for aminoguanidine as a selective iNOS inhibitor in sepsis [31]. Thus, aminoguanidine produced a dose-dependent increase in phenylephrine-induced tension in intact and endothelium-denuded pulmonary artery rings from endotoxin-treated rats, but it had no effect on sham-treated controls. The aminoguanidine-precipitated contraction in the endothelium-denuded vessels was abolished by L-arginine or L-NMMA pretreatment, suggesting that its mechanism of action involves the L-arginine/NO axis. Clinical trials on the use of aminoguanidine in septic patients are already underway.

Endothelins

Background

In 1988 an endothelially-derived vasoconstrictor was cloned and sequenced following its isolation from the culture medium of porcine aortic endothelial cells [32]. This substance, termed endothelin (ET), was found to elicit a slow, sustained contraction of isolated arteries from many different species. Three similar but distinct ET-related genomic loci have been identified that encode for three similar but distinct 21-amino-acid ET peptides (ET-1, ET-2, ET-3) [33]. These peptides are produced following cleavage of a prepropeptide via a propeptide. This conversion is mediated by the activity of an endothelin-converting enzyme (ECE). Several types of enzyme with this property have already been demonstrated; two are neutral proteases, one of which is membrane-bound and phosphoramidon-sensitive, and one of which is soluble and insensitive to phosphoramidon.

ET-1 immunoreactivity cannot be demonstrated in homogenates of capillary endothelial cells, and release of ET from cultured endothelial cells can be prevented by the protein synthesis inhibitor cycloheximidine, suggesting that ETs are not stored but synthesized *de novo*. Factors that have been found to be capable of stimulating ET release are diverse and include vessel wall shear stress, hypoxia, endotoxin, TNF, interferon, adrenaline, angiotensin, thrombin, activated platelets and some prostanoids. Local ET release would therefore be expected in response to any form of inflammatory response. ET-induced smooth-muscle contraction occurs due to several secondary messenger pathways whose final common pathway is to increase free intracellular calcium. Phospholipase C activation with increases in inositol triphosphate and diaglycerol synthesis is thought to be the principal effector system, although since staurosporine, a protein kinase C inhibitor, can attenuate ET-1-induced contraction *in vitro*, this system is presumably also involved.

Two ET receptor subtypes have so far been cloned and expressed. ET_A has a higher affinity for ET-1 than ET-2 or -3, and has widespread tissue expression, including vascular smooth muscle, but has not been found on endothelial cells. ET_B is non-selective and binds all three ETs equally avidly so that they are equipotent in their displacement of ^{125}ET-1. ET_B is found on vascular endothelium and also on smooth muscle in some vascular beds. At first it was thought that ET_A receptor stimulation was responsible for the direct constrictor effects of ET and ET_B receptor stimulation resulted in properties such as the release of other vasoactive factors from those cells. ET-1 is certainly a potent vasoconstrictor in humans and animals by direct stimulation of ET_A receptors, and the endothelium can modulate this vascular response to ET via ET_B receptor stimulation, but it has become apparent recently that the situation is complicated by the demonstration of ET_B receptors on some vascular smooth muscle that mediates contraction. Furthermore, ET_A receptors are capable of stimulating prostanoid release [33]. The importance of endothelial ET_B receptors has been demonstrated in several models. First, ET-1-induced contraction of rat pulmonary arteries is enhanced by endothelial removal [34]. Second, there is now clear evidence from both *in vitro* and *in vivo* studies that ETs release NO from the endothelium by ET_B receptor stimulation. This gives rise to the characteristic haemodynamic responses of rats (and other species) to intravenous ET-1, when there is an initial transient fall in systemic blood pressure followed by a sustained pressor response [32]. Only the former can be attenuated by L-NMMA pretreatment, and only the latter can be attenuated by ET_A receptor antagonists such as BQ123. Lastly, there is evidence that at least in some species, and in some vascular beds, ET-1 also stimulates the release of prostacyclin and thromboxane from endothelial cells via ET_B receptors (Fig. 4).

ET-1 is largely cleared in the pulmonary circulation, whilst some is eliminated by the kidneys. The plasma half-life of a bolus of ^{125}ET-1 in anaesthetized rats was 40 seconds in one study, with 82% uptake in the lungs and 10% in the kidneys [35].

Endothelins in sepsis

Taking into account the factors known to stimulate ET release (see above), it is inevitable that this increases during the inflammatory response associated with sepsis. ET release in response to endotoxin has been confirmed by radioimmunoassay *in vitro* and *in vivo*, and in response to

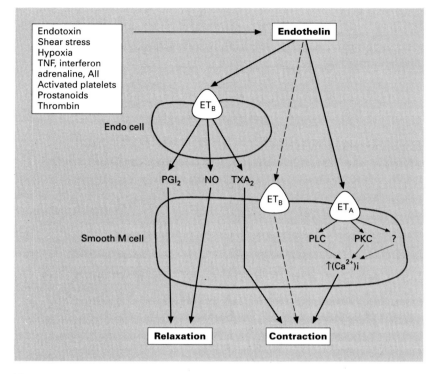

Fig. 4 Endothelins (ETs): release, receptors and intracellular mechanisms. ETs are synthesized *de novo*. They are released in response to many stimuli, making it inevitable that this release will be increased in the presence of local inflammation. Two types of ET receptor have been cloned, although there is emerging evidence that there is at least one further type. ET_A receptors on vascular smooth muscle are responsible for the direct contractile properties of the peptides, via several intracellular pathways, including phospholipase (PLC) and protein kinase C (PKC), which lead to a rise in intracellular free calcium ($[Ca^{2+}]i$). ET_B receptors are present mainly on endothelial cells, where stimulation can result in release of vasoactive and inflammatory mediators such as nitric oxide (NO), prostacyclin (PGI_2) and thromboxane (TXA_2), that can result in the indirect effects of ET. In some tissues, ET_B receptors are present on smooth muscle, and stimulation can also result in direct contraction.

TNF, interferon-γ, IL-1 and free radical species. The level of ET-1 in the plasma is elevated in many animal models, as well as in patients who are critically ill with sepsis, possibly in parallel with indicators of illness severity [36]. It is probable that ET-1 effects on vascular tone are as a result of autocrine and paracrine activity rather than as a circulating hormone, and if this is the case, the level of ET-1 in the blood would only reflect the combination of production rate and breakdown/elimination rate. The expression of ET-1 messenger RNA in several tissues from endotoxin-treated rats (heart, lung, aorta, pulmonary artery) significantly increases when compared with controls, although the time course for this increase varies from tissue to tissue, and no significant increase was seen at all in skeletal muscle from the same animals [37]. This differential tissue expression may reflect the sensitivity of the different tissues to the septic insult and the magnitude of the resultant inflammatory and vascular responses.

Despite potent effects on vascular tone, both direct and indirect, and unequivocal increases in ET-1 production and release in sepsis, the role of these peptides in sepsis remains unclear. As potent vasoconstrictors, it is tempting to speculate that they play a role in the local reductions in regional blood flow seen in certain organ beds such as the gut, kidney and lung. This is an area of intensive investigation, particularly now that the necessary experimental (and potentially therapeutic) tools are becoming available in the form of selective ET_A/ET_B, or combined ET receptor antagonists.

Arachidonic acid metabolites

Background

The endothelium produces prostanoids and thromboxane after the conversion of arachidonic acid by the enzyme cyclooxygenase (COX) [38]. This enzyme exists in two isoforms: COX-1 is constitutive and is responsible for physiological production and COX-2 is cytokine-inducible in inflammatory conditions. Endothelial production of the vasodilator and platelet inhibitor prostacyclin (PGI_2) is important both as an antithrombotic agent and for regulation of basal vascular tone.

COX products in sepsis

Cytokines stimulate prostanoid release both *in vivo* and *in vitro*. During the inflammatory response, this generation of prostanoids and thromboxane (TXA_2) occurs in inflammatory cells such as macrophages as well as in the endothelium. The balance between the local production of vasodilator (PGI_2) and vasoconstrictor (TXA_2 and endoperoxides) agents in this way undoubtedly contributes to the generation of vascular tone in that area [39]. In particular, animal studies suggest that TXA_2 production in the lung is one of the main factors producing the early elevation in the PVR, and possibly also increased vascular permeability following endotoxin challenge. As a result of these findings, several studies have successfully attenuated these changes in pulmonary haemodynamics using COX inhibitors or TXA_2 receptor antagonists with a corresponding improvement in survival [40,41]. TXA_2-mediated increases in PVR are also thought to occur in humans during sepsis, and trials of COX inhibitors in these patients are currently underway in the USA.

SUMMARY

The endothelium is a dynamic cell layer that acts as a selectively permeable barrier between the tissues and the circulation. It is metabolically active, and produces many vasoactive and antithrombotic substances that contribute to physiological vascular tone, although this regulatory role probably varies between different tissue beds. Sepsis syndromes are characterized by clinical features resulting from widespread inflammation whose initiating factor is not always identifiable. It is increasingly recognized that the endothelium plays a central role in both the initiation and amplification of the inflammatory cascade, particularly in the vascular response. Whether the inflammatory response escalates to cause the extensive tissue damage that characterizes conditions such as ARDS, SIRS or MOF probably depends to a great extent on the balance between the endothelially-derived vasoactive and inflammatory factors such as NO, ETs and prostanoids, as well as on the degree of endothelial damage and dysfunction. Current areas of research include the scrutiny of endothelial–inflammatory cell interactions and the role of individual mediators.

ACKNOWLEDGEMENTS

Nicholas Curzen is a Medical Research Council training fellow.

REFERENCES

1 Vincent JL, Bihari D. Sepsis, severe sepsis, or sepsis syndrome: a need for clarification. *Int Care Med* 1992;**18**:255-257.
2 ACCP/SCCM Consensus Conference. Definitions for sepsis and organ failure and guidelines for the use of innovative therapies in sepsis. *Crit Care Med* 1992;**20**:864–874.
3 Macnaughton PD, Evans TW. Management of adult respiratory distress syndrome. *Lancet* 1992;**339**:469–472.
4 Curzen NP, Griffiths MJD, Evans TW. Pulmonary vascular control mechanisms in lung injury. In: *Clinical Pulmonary Hypertension*, edited by Morice AH. Portland Press, London, 1995; Chapter 8; pp. 171–201.
5 Bone RC. The pathogenesis of sepsis. *Ann Intern Med* 1991;**115**:457–469.
6 Sonesson H, Zahringer U, Grimmecke H, Westphal O, Rietschel E. Bacterial endotoxin: chemical structure and biological activity. In: *Endotoxin and the Lungs*, edited by Brigham K. Marcel Dekker, New York, 1994:1–20.
7 Danner RL, Elin RL, Hosseini JM. Endotoxaemia in human septic shock. *Chest* 1991;**99**:169–175.
8 Martin TR, Tobias PS, Mathison JC, Ulevitch RJ. Interactions between endotoxin and endotoxin-binding protein. In: *Endotoxin and the Lungs*, edited by Brigham KL. Marcel Dekker, New York, 1994;45–67.
9 Curzen NP, Griffiths MJD, Evans TW. The role of the endothelium in modulating the vascular response to sepsis. *Clin Sci* 1994;**86**:359–374.
10 Phillips P, Tsan M. Cytoarchitectural aspects of endothelial barrier function in response to oxidants and inflammatory mediators. In: *Lung Vascular Injury*, edited by Johnson A, Ferro TJ. Marcel Dekker, New York, 1992.
11 Albelda SM, Smith CW, Ward PA. Adhesion molecules and inflammatory injury. *Faseb J* 1994;**8**:504–512.

12 Laurent T, Markert M, Fliedner VV *et al.* CD11/CD18 expression, adherence, and chemotaxis of granulocytes in adult respiratory distress syndrome. *Am J Respir Crit Care Med* 1994;**149**:1534–1538.

13 Muller WA, Weigl SA, Deng X, Phillips DM. PECAM-1 is required for transendothelial migration of leukocytes. *J Exp Med* 1993;**178**:449–460.

14 Moncada S, Higgs A. The L-arginine–nitric oxide pathway. *N Engl J Med* (review).1993;**329**:2002–2012.

15 Knowles RG, Moncada S. Nitric oxide synthases in mammals. *Biochem J* 1994;**298**:249–258.

16 Fineman JR, Crowley MR, Heymann MA, Soifer SJ. *In vivo* inhibition of endothelium-dependent pulmonary vasodilatation by methylene blue in the lamb. *J Appl Physiol* 1991;**71**:735–741.

17 Fineman JR, Chang R, Soifer SJ. L-arginine, a precursor of EDRF *in vitro*, produces pulmonary vasodilatation in lambs. *Am J Physiol* 1991;**261**:H1563–H1569.

18 Vallance P, Collier J, Moncada S. Effects of endothelium-derived nitric oxide on peripheral arteriolar tone in man. *Lancet* 1989;**2**:997–1000.

19 Ochoa JB, Udekwu AO, Billiar TR *et al.* Nitrogen oxide levels in patients after trauma and during sepsis. *Ann Surg* 1991;**214**:621–626.

20 Petros A, Bennett D, Vallance P. Effect of nitric oxide synthase inhibitors on hypotension in patients with septic shock. *Lancet* 1991;**338**:1557–1558.

21 Busse R, Mulsch A, Fleming I, Hecker M. Mechanisms of nitric oxide release from the vascular endothelium. *Circulation* 1993;**87**:V18–V25.

22 Fleming I, Gray GA, Schott C, Stoclet JC. Inducible but not constitutive production of nitric oxide by vascular smooth muscle cells. *Eur J Pharmacol* 1991;**200**:375–376.

23 Brady AJ, Poole-Wilson PA, Harding SE, Warren JB. Nitric oxide production within cardiac myocytes reduces their contractility in endotoxemia. *Am J Physiol* 1992;**263**:H1963–H1966.

24 Griffiths MJD, Messent M, Evans TW. The role of nitric oxide in the pulmonary vascular response to sepsis. *Thorax* 1993;**48**:467(abstract).

25 Szabo C, Mitchell JA, Thiemermann C, Vane JR. Nitric oxide-mediated hyporeactivity to noradrenaline precedes the induction of nitric oxide synthase in endotoxin shock. *Br J Pharmacol* 1993;**108**:786–792.

26 Guc MO, Furman BL, Parratt JR. Modification of alpha-adrenoceptor-mediated pressor responses by NG-nitro-L-arginine methyl ester and vasopressin in endotoxin-treated pithed rats. *Eur J Pharmacol* 1992;**224**:63–69.

27 Fleming I, Gray GA, Stoclet JC. Influence of endothelium on induction of the L-arginine–nitric oxide pathway in rat aortas. *Am J Physiol* 1993;**264**:H1200–H1207.

28 Liu S, Adcock IM, Old RW, Barnes PJ, Evans TW. Lipopolysaccharide treatment *in vivo* induces widespread tissue expression of inducible nitric oxide synthase mRNA. *Biochem Biophys Res Commun* 1993;**196**:1208–1213.

29 Gold ME, Wood KS, Byrns RE, Buga GM, Ignarro LJ. L-arginine-dependent vascular smooth muscle relaxation and cGMP formation. *Am J Physiol* 1990;**259**:H1813–H1821.

30 Griffiths MJD, Curzen NP, Sair M, Evans TW. Nitric oxide synthase inhibitors in septic shock: theoretical considerations. *Clin Int Care* 1994;**5**:29–36.

31 Griffiths MJD, Messent M, MacAllister RJ, Evans TW. Aminoguanidine selectively inhibits inducible nitric oxide synthase. *Br J Pharmacol* 1993;**110**:963–968.

32 Yanagisawa M, Kurihara H, Limura S *et al.* A novel potent vasoconstrictor peptide produced by vascular endothelial cells. *Nature* 1988;**332**:411–415.

33 Rubanyi GM, Polokoff MA. Endothelins: molecular biology, biochemistry, pharmacology, physiology, and pathophysiology. *Pharmacol Rev* 1994;**46**:325–415.

34 Bax WA, Saxena PR. The current endothelin receptor classification: time for reconsideration? *TIPS* 1994;**15**:379–386.

35 Sirvio ML, Metsarinne K, Fyhrquist F. Tissue distribution and half-life of ^{125}I-endothelin in the rat: importance of pulmonary clearance. *Biochem Biophys Res Commun* 1990;**167**:1191–1195.

36 Pittet JF, Morel DR, Hemsen A *et al.* Elevated plasma endothelin-1 concentrations are associated with the severity of illness in patients with sepsis. *Ann Surg* 1991;**213**:261–264.

37 Kaddoura S, Curzen N, Firth J, Sugden PH, Poole-Wilson PA, Evans TW. Tissue expression of endothelin-1 expression in endotoxaemia. *Biochem Biophys Res Commun* 1996;**218**:641–647.
38 Mitchell JA, Larkin S, Williams TJ. Cyclooxygenase regulation and relevance in inflammation. *Biochemical Pharmacology* 1995;**50**:1535–1542.
39 Petrak RA, Balk RA, Bone RC. Prostaglandins, cyclo-oxygenase inhibitors, and thromboxane synthetase inhibitors in the pathogenesis of multiple systems organ failure. *Crit Care Clin* 1989;**5**:303–314.
40 Ahmed T, Wasserman MA, Muccitelli R, Tucker S, Gazeroglu H, Marchette B. Endotoxin-induced changes in pulmonary hemodynamics and respiratory mechanics: role of lipoxygenase and cyclooxygenase products. *Am Rev Respir Dis* 1986;**134**:1149–1157.
41 Harlan RWJ, Harker BNL, Hilderbrandt J. Thromboxane A$_2$ mediates lung vasoconstriction but not permeability after endotoxin. *J Clin Invest* 1983;**72**:911–918.
42 Glauser MP, Zanetti G, Baumgartner J-D, Cohen J. Septic shock: pathogenesis. *Lancet* 1991;**338**:732–733.

MULTIPLE CHOICE QUESTIONS

1 Acute respiratory distress syndrome is characterized by
  a diminished right ventricular performance
  b increased permeability of the alveolar capillary membrane
  c a particularly adverse prognosis if precipitated by trauma
  d a loss of hypoxic pulmonary vasoconstriction
  e the fact that it represents only the pulmonary manifestation of a panendothelial insult

2 The endothelium is known to produce a wide variety of vasoactive mediators that modulate both pulmonary and systemic vascular tone. In sepsis
  a there is evidence at a molecular and pharmacological level of increased inducible nitric oxide synthase (iNOS) production
  b a loss of normal vascular control may lead to impaired oxygen uptake in the peripheral microcirculation
  c in all patients with sepsis, an identifiable bacterial or other infective organism can be isolated
  d the endothelins are a family of vasodilator peptides
  e the endogenous vasodilator nitric oxide (NO) has been used successfully to improve ventilation/perfusion matching in the lungs of patients with sepsis complicated by lung injury

Answers

1		2	
a	True	**a**	True
b	True	**b**	True
c	False	**c**	False
d	True	**d**	False
e	True	**e**	True

PART 3
PHARMACOLOGY

Drug discovery and the development of antimigraine drugs

PATRICK P. A. HUMPHREY & HELEN CONNOR

APPROACHES TO DRUG DISCOVERY

At least four different approaches to finding novel medicines can be identified: they are the so-called rational approach, high-volume screening, mimicry and serendipity. The rational approach would seem the most appealing intellectually and has been pioneered by the Nobel Laureate, Sir James Black, with his work on autacoid receptor characterization that led to the development of both the β-adrenoceptor blockers and the histamine H_2-receptor blockers — medicines of great clinical importance [1]. High-volume screening has not been considered an attractive approach until recently, in concert with prejudices against screening in a supposed disease model or 'black-box' which usually provides little, or more likely no, scientific insight despite much resource and effort. However, the revolution in biotechnology, molecular biology and combinatorial chemistry is changing perspectives on screening approaches with much greater chances to identify drug tools and lead compounds, which the chemist can turn into developable medicines [2]. The third approach, mimicry, would seem at first sight unattractive but in some cases may be desirable. For instance, a new drug class exemplified by a prototype drug may provide ample and medically justified scope for therapeutic improvements in terms of selectivity, pharmacokinetic profile, etc. Serendipity cannot really be considered as an approach in its own right but the view expressed by Louis Pasteur in his address given at the inauguration of the Faculty of Science in the University of Lille, in 1854, must be as true today as ever, 'Dans les champs de l'observation le hasard ne favorise que les esprits préparés'. Serendipity will always play its part in innovative research.

The additional benefits to accrue from the rational approach will be exemplified here in relation to the research over the last two decades on cerebrovascular pharmacology which led to the discovery of sumatriptan, a novel medicine for the acute treatment of migraine. Its success in the clinic has generated a large amount of scientific interest, not just in the drug and its possible mechanism(s) of action but the pathophysiology

169

of the disease itself. As a consequence, full-scale clinical trials have now been properly conducted and migraine has finally been recognized as an organic, not a psychosomatic, disease which is amenable to acute drug therapy. The studies on the mechanism of action of sumatriptan have suggested new pathophysiological concepts of the disease and theoretically different approaches to its treatment. Sumatriptan has hopefully helped launch a new era of research on migraine, a debilitating clinical condition which can severely affect the lives and careers of many.

DISCOVERY OF SUMATRIPTAN

Sumatriptan was discovered as a result of applied rational research which focused on the pathophysiology of migraine and the likely chemical mediators involved (see [3,4] for reviews). Such considerations in the mid 1970s led to what was then pioneering research on the pharmacology of intra- and extracranial blood vessels. Since 5-hydroxytryptamine (5-HT) was much implicated in the pathophysiology of migraine, vascular 5-HT receptors were characterized and the novel observation made from animal studies that the cranial blood vessels contained a different, previously unidentified, 5-HT receptor type to that commonly found in peripheral blood vessels. This led to the identification of highly selective agonists, like sumatriptan, for the 'new' 5-HT receptor. These agonists were devoid of marked generalized cardiovascular activity in experimental animals, such as the dog and pig, but had selective vasoconstrictor effects on some, but not all, blood vessels within the head, without affecting cerebral blood flow [5–7]. On the basis of such studies in animals, sumatriptan was developed and evaluated clinically for the acute treatment of migraine [8,9]. It was found to be highly effective in ameliorating the head pain and other associated symptoms [10,11].

PATHOPHYSIOLOGY OF MIGRAINE

Up until the mid 1980s, migraine had been considered to be a vascular disease (for review see [12]). However, the concept that there is a generalized disorder of cephalic blood flow is no longer tenable. Thus, during migraine without aura (or common migraine, as it was known), there are no changes in cerebral blood flow, although a spreading oligaemia is evident in patients with preceding neurological symptoms [13–15]. In some individuals, notably those in early experimental studies, there is an obvious dilatation of the extracranial vasculature, particularly the temporal artery, but this appears not to be common in the migraine population at large [16]. However, there is now good evidence that extracerebral, intracranial vessels may be dilatated and distended — vessels such as the large conducting arteries and those in the meningeal circulation, which are even more difficult to study in humans than the intracranial resistance vessels controlling the blood supply to the brain itself [17].

In support of a neurological rather than a vascular pathophysiology, evidence has been provided for a localized neurological deficit in pain transmission in migraineurs [18]. Migraineurs are more susceptible to pain induced by ingestion of cold substances, such as ice cream, and the pain is frequently felt in a similar unilateral site to the normal migraine headache [19]. Interestingly, patients with intractable pain, who had electrodes implanted into the region of the periaqueductal grey area, experienced severe migraine-like headaches [20]. These observations led to a view that a pathological disturbance within the brain itself could lead to head pain. However, the periaqueductal grey area is close to the dorsal raphé nucleus and vascular changes are likely to have been involved in the headache produced by the electrode implantation [21]. Nevertheless, it is most likely that migraineurs do have a defective (hypersensitive) pain pathway localized to the anatomical location of their migrainous headaches. This is consistent with the well-known observation that reserpine will induce migraine-like headaches in migraineurs but not in normal individuals [22,23].

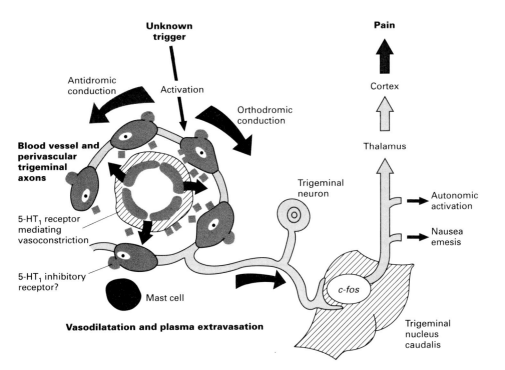

Fig. 1 Pathophysiological mechanisms involved in migraine in relation to the mechanism of action of sumatriptan. Modified from [26] and see [35].

Today, it seems reasonable to propose a unifying hypothesis integrating both neurological and vascular components (Fig. 1). Importantly, the neuroanatomical studies of Moskowitz have clearly implicated the trigeminal (Vth cranial) nerve in the transmission of head pain. Since the afferent terminals of this nerve densely innervate the large intracranial blood vessels, it seems likely that the pain signal originates from a vascular source [24,25]. Thus, a sterile neurogenic inflammatory pathology may occur within the walls of certain intracranial vessels [26]. Since these are located within a fixed structure — the cranium — it seems reasonable to assume that their distension leads to pain, as has been demonstrated experimentally [27,28]. Undoubtedly, however, there must be an as yet unidentified underlying neurological basis for the *initiation* of these pathophysiological events (the so-called migraine generator).

5-HYDROXYTRYPTAMINE AND MIGRAINE

The belief that 5-HT was somehow involved in the pathogenesis of migraine was a key factor behind the discovery of sumatriptan. It was this that led to the systematic characterization of the receptors for 5-HT, particularly those in the vasculature (see above).

5-HT was first implicated in the pathophysiology of migraine by Sicuteri *et al.* [29], who showed that its metabolite, 5-hydroxyindoleacetic acid (5-HIAA), was increased in amount in the urine during the period of a migraine headache. Furthermore, reserpine-induced migraine-like headaches in migraineurs, like spontaneous attacks, were correlated with a fall in plasma (platelet) 5-HT content [22,30]. Another observation which linked 5-HT and migraine was the clinical study of Lance and colleagues [31] investigating a number of 5-HT receptor antagonists in the prophylaxis of migraine. They concluded that methysergide was markedly superior and this led to a focus on the pharmacology of methysergide in relation to 5-HT receptors, which in turn led to the discovery of the novel sumatriptan receptor in intracranial blood vessels [3,4].

Another essential pointer in the literature was that 5-HT administered intravenously could abort a migrainous headache, whether it be a spontaneous attack or reserpine-induced [22]. This was an important confirmation of an earlier observation that intravenous 5-HT had a beneficial effect in treating spontaneous migrainous headache [32]. It seemed likely that 5-HT was acting as a vasoconstrictor to ameliorate the headache, as is the case for ergotamine, noradrenaline and other vasoactive agents [3,33]. It was therefore argued that an agent which would mimic the desirable effects of 5-HT (possible carotid vasoconstriction) but not mimic the undesirable effects (including generalized vasoconstriction, bronchoconstriction, platelet aggregation) would be of benefit in the acute treatment of migraine [8]. It was speculated that a full agonist at the novel receptor (later called

5-HT$_1$) identified from studies with methysergide (a weak partial agonist) might be such an agent. This idea became particularly attractive as evidence from animal studies indicated that this receptor mainly occurred in some but not all cranial vessels. The concept also had some appeal in that such an agonist could be thought of as a replacement for the abnormally reduced plasma levels of circulating 5-HT, but no reliance was placed on this consideration. It was simply speculated that a 5-HT$_1$ receptor agonist would produce selective vasoconstriction of those particular vessels distended and dilatated during the headache period. This is conceptually analogous to the anti-asthma drug salbutamol, which mimics the desirable effects (bronchodilatation) of the natural hormone, adrenaline, without mimicking its undesirable effects on the heart, by *selectively* activating β_2-adrenoceptors. However, in the same way that falls in plasma adrenaline levels are not responsible for asthma, so changes in plasma levels of 5-HT are unlikely to be causative in migraine [16,34].

MECHANISMS OF ACTION OF SUMATRIPTAN

The mechanism of action of sumatriptan in migraine has been the subject of debate [26,35–37]. This has focused on whether vasoconstriction or neuronal inhibition is the primary mechanism by which sumatriptan alleviates the symptoms of a migraine attack.

The ability of sumatriptan to produce vasoconstriction within the human cranial vascular bed is now well established. Thus, sumatriptan contracts human isolated basilar, middle cerebral and middle meningeal arteries via activation of vascular 5-HT$_1$ receptors [38,39]. Recent clinical studies have also demonstrated a vasoconstrictor action of sumatriptan in the cranial circulation of migraineurs. Friberg et al. [17] found an increased blood flow velocity in the middle cerebral artery during a migraine attack on the headache side following sumatriptan (2 mg intravenously), with no change in regional cerebral blood flow. An increase in blood flow velocity, without a change in regional blood flow, is indicative of large artery vasoconstriction. No significant change in middle cerebral artery blood flow velocity was found on the non-headache side, or on either side outside the migraine attack. In a larger, placebo-controlled study, Caekebeke et al. [40] found that sumatriptan caused a dose-dependent increase in blood flow velocity in the middle cerebral and internal carotid arteries on both headache and non-headache sides, both during and outside a migraine attack. However, sumatriptan had no effect on blood flow velocity in the external and common carotid arteries. This suggests that the vasoconstrictor effect of sumatriptan occurs in the internal but not external carotid artery bed. Interestingly, in this study those patients who obtained the best headache relief appeared to be those having the greatest increase in blood flow velocity. Hence, the data suggest that sumatriptan produces a rapid-onset vasoconstrictor effect on large cerebral arteries and that the timescale of headache relief parallels this vasoconstrictor effect.

The meningeal circulation, with its dense sensory innervation and sensitivity to painful stimuli, is thought to be particularly important in the pathophysiology of a migraine headache. Although sumatriptan constricts the human isolated meningeal vascular bed [38], clinical studies to examine the effects of sumatriptan on this vascular bed during a migraine attack cannot be readily performed, principally because of the more invasive procedures required. However, a single case report has recently been described [36] where an arteriography of the external carotid circulation, including the meningeal vessels, was performed in a patient before and after sumatriptan (6 mg subcutaneously (s.c.)). Following sumatriptan, the diameters of the middle meningeal and external carotid arteries were reduced by 11% and 21% at 10 minutes, and by 26% and 37% at 20 minutes, respectively. This finding supports the *in vitro* data and suggests that sumatriptan can rapidly constrict meningeal blood vessels in migraineurs.

An action of sumatriptan on trigeminal perivascular nerve terminals to cause a decrease in the release of pro-inflammatory neurotransmitters, substance P and calcitonin gene-related peptide (CGRP), was first proposed by Buzzi and Moskowitz [41]. This stemmed from animal studies where sumatriptan inhibited neurogenically mediated plasma protein extravasation in the dura of anaesthetized rats and guinea-pigs. However, sumatriptan had no effect on either dural plasma protein extravasation induced by exogenously administered substance P or neurogenic plasma protein extravasation in extracranial vascular beds [41]. These data suggested therefore that sumatriptan has an inhibitory effect on trigeminal nerve terminals and furthermore that this effect is selective for the dural vascular bed [26]. The clinical relevance of this animal neurogenic inflammation model to migraine has been questioned [36] and furthermore, it remains difficult to exclude the possibility that vasoconstriction contributes, at least in part, to the inhibitory effects of sumatriptan in this animal model [37].

Animal studies have revealed that sumatriptan only very poorly penetrates into the brain [42,43] and the compound, even at very high doses, fails to show analgesic activity in a range of animal tests [44]. Together, these data suggest that a central action is unlikely to account for the antimigraine effects of sumatriptan in humans. It could be that local disruption of the blood–brain barrier may occur during migraine headache and that, under these conditions, sumatriptan may then gain greater access to central sites in the brain. Could an action on central neuronal pathways then contribute to its clinical efficacy? Whilst such a possibility cannot totally be discounted, it remains unlikely. Interestingly, recent animal studies with GR46611, a compound having a similar pharmacological profile to sumatriptan but with high lipophilicity (log P = 3.9 compared to log P of 1.1 sumatriptan) and which is known to penetrate readily into the central nervous system (CNS) [45], failed, like sumatriptan, to produce any analgesic effects in animal models (our unpublished data). This suggests that even when access to the CNS readily occurs, this class of compound does not inhibit central pain pathways.

FUTURE CLINICAL RESEARCH ON MIGRAINE

Further studies on the cerebrovascular actions of sumatriptan in humans during migraine and other types of headache may well provide useful clinical insight into the underlying pathological mechanisms. For example, the influence of sumatriptan on nitrate-induced headache is currently under investigation [46,47]. The ability to provoke migraine-like headache in susceptible individuals (e.g. nitroglycerin, red wine, etc.) allows the monitoring of specific cerebrovascular parameters, for example regional cerebral blood flow and blood velocity, before and during headache and then following sumatriptan. The ability of sumatriptan (6 mg s.c.) effectively and rapidly to alleviate single attacks of cluster headache has been established in placebo-controlled clinical trials [48]. More recent studies have investigated the effect of sumatriptan on other headaches. For example, in chronic tension-type headache, sumatriptan (2 and 4 mg s.c.) caused only a modest relief of headache, although this was significantly superior to placebo [49]. This would support suggestions that tension-type headache has a primary pathophysiology different from that of migraine, but that some overlap may occur [14].

When evidence from clinical studies is considered, vasoconstriction seems the most likely primary mechanism by which sumatriptan alleviates the symptoms of a migraine attack (see above and [37]). However, it remains possible that both vasoconstriction and neuronal inhibition may contribute to the antimigraine effects of sumatriptan. The observation that CGRP plasma levels sampled from the external jugular vein are raised during a migraine headache, and that sumatriptan attenuates this increase and relieves headache (Fig. 2; [50]), is an important clinical observation that supports the suggestion that sumatriptan interacts with the trigemino-vascular system to cause headache relief. Interestingly, a single patient who did not have an elevation in CGRP levels during headache also did not respond to sumatriptan [51]. However, either a vasoconstrictor or neuronal inhibitory action of sumatriptan could account for its effect on CGRP plasma levels in migraine patients. Thus, CGRP release may merely reflect trigeminal nerve activation, which itself is the cause of the migraine headache. Alleviation of the head pain by whatever mechanism would be expected to result in cessation of activation of trigeminal nerve activity and consequent cessation of release of neuropeptides from its

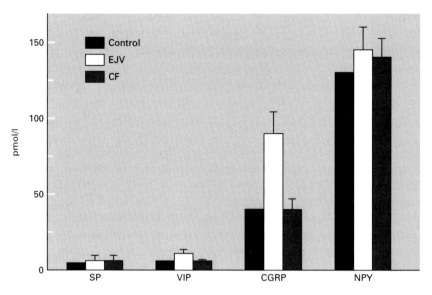

Fig. 2 Measurement of concentrations of various neuropeptides in migraineur plasma, sampled from the cubital fossa (CF) and external jugular vein (EJV) ipsilateral to the headache. The peptides measured were substance P (SP), vasoactive intestinal polypeptide (VIP), calcitonin gene-related peptide (CGRP) and neuropeptide Y (NPY). Data from [50,51].

nerve terminals. Ultimately, the clinical importance of trigeminal neuronal inhibition *per se* will only be determined when compounds that cause neuronal inhibition, but lack vasoconstrictor activity, are clinically evaluated in migraine patients. Preliminary data on one such compound, CP-122,288, have been described but no clinical data are yet available.

CP-122,288 is an analogue of sumatriptan which very potently inhibits neurogenically mediated plasma protein extravasation in the dura of anaesthetized guinea-pigs [52] and rats [53]. This effect of CP-122,288 is seen at doses at least 2000-fold lower than those needed for sumatriptan, and importantly, at these very low doses, CP-122,288 has no vasoconstrictor effects. Hence, CP-122,288 appears to be a compound which selectively inhibits trigeminal neurons. The specific receptor mechanism involved in this effect is unclear, and indeed, an action at any of the known 5-HT receptor subtypes can probably be ruled out [53]. However, the clinical testing of compounds like CP-122,288 will provide valuable information on whether inhibition of trigeminal nerve activity alone will confer antimigraine efficacy. The dose at which CP-122,288, or similar compound, shows clinical efficacy will be crucial to this question. Will this be at low doses which, on the basis of animal data, would be expected selectively to inhibit trigeminal nerve activity, or are higher doses required which, like sumatriptan, cause cranial vasoconstriction? The results of such studies are awaited with interest.

CONSIDERATIONS ON NOVEL TREATMENTS FOR MIGRAINE

The current theories of migraine pathophysiology focus on the involvement of the trigeminal nervous system in the development of migraine headache and, specifically, on the role of the trigeminal neurotransmitter neuro-peptides, substance P and CGRP, in this process [54]. However, whilst levels of CGRP are increased in plasma samples taken from the external jugular vein during a migraine attack, compared to controls, no such increase in plasma levels of substance P was detected [50], although this may reflect the more labile nature of substance P in plasma [46,55]. Undoubtedly, neurogenic inflammation within cranial blood vessels, mediated via the trigeminal nerve, is an attractive theory for explaining the various features of migraine headache, but neurogenic inflammation has not yet been shown clinically to occur during migraine.

The potential role of the trigeminal neurotransmitter neuropeptides, substance P and CGRP, in the development of neurogenic inflammation within intracranial blood vessels and hence the development of migraine headache, leads to the possibility that drugs which block the actions of substance P and CGRP will have antimigraine activity. Substance P causes vasodilatation and oedema formation within the cranial circulation via activation of endothelial neurokinin NK_1 receptors [56–58]. Hence the clinical efficacy of an NK_1 receptor antagonist in migraine would be worth determining to gain a better understanding of the pathological mechanisms involved. CGRP acts directly on cerebrovascular smooth muscle to cause marked vasodilatation [59] and furthermore, in peripheral tissues, has been shown to potentiate the inflammatory actions of substance P [60]. It is therefore possible that a CGRP receptor antagonist would have a beneficial effect in migraine.

It could also be argued that substance P or CGRP might function as neurotransmitters at the central terminals of the trigeminal nerve, in the trigeminal nucleus caudalis within the hind brain [61]. This could provide an attractive mechanism by which an NK_1 or CGRP receptor antagonist might alleviate the headache of migraine, regardless of peripheral mediators involved, by blocking activation of second-order neurons in the nucleus caudalis, and hence preventing activation of central pain pathways. Alter-natively, a peripherally acting agonist (e.g. somatostatin) to selectively inhibit neuronal firing of the trigeminal ganglia and its sensory projections might provide a broad-spectrum analgesic for head pain [34,62].

REFERENCES

1 Humphrey PPA, Spedding M,Vanhoutte PM. Receptor classification and nomenclature: the revolution and the resolution. *Trends Pharmacol Sci* 1994;**15**:203–204.
2 Alper J. Drug discovery on the assembly line. *Science* 1994;**264**:1399–1401.
3 Humphrey PPA, Feniuk W, Perren MJ. 5-HT in migraine: evidence from 5-HT$_1$-like receptor agonists for a vascular aetiology. In: *Migraine: A Spectrum of Ideas*, edited by Sandler M, Collins GM, Oxford University Press, Oxford, 1990:147–172.
4 Humphrey PPA, Apperley E, FeniukW, Perren MJ. A rational approach to identifying a fundamentally new drug for the treatment of migraine. In: *Cardiovascular Pharmacology of 5-Hydroxytryptamine*, edited by Saxena PR, Wallis DI, Wouters W, Bevan P. Kluwer Academic Publishers, Dordrecht, 1990:417–431.
5 Humphrey PPA, Feniuk W, Perren MJ *et al.* GR43175, a selective agonist for the 5-HT$_1$-like receptor in dog isolated saphenous vein. *Br J Pharmacol* 1988;**94**:1123–1132.
6 Feniuk W, Humphrey PPA, Perren MJ. The selective carotid arterial vasoconstrictor action of GR43175 in anaesthetized dogs. *Br J Pharmacol* 1989;**96**:83–90.
7 den Boer MO, Villalón CM, Heiligers JPC, Humphrey PPA, Saxena PR. Role of 5-HT$_1$-like receptors in the reduction of porcine cranial arteriovenous anastomotic shunting by sumatriptan. *Br J Pharmacol* 1991;**102**:323–330.
8 Humphrey PPA, FeniukW, Perren MJ, Connor HE, Oxford AW. The pharmacology of the novel 5-HT$_1$-like receptor agonist GR43175. *Cephalalgia* 1989;**9**(suppl. 9):23–33.
9 Humphrey PPA, FeniukW, Perren MJ, Oxford AW, Britain RT. Sumatriptan succinate. *Drugs of the Future* 1989;**14**:35–39.
10 Connor HE, FeniukW, Lloyd K, Humphrey PPA. Migraine, serotonin and sumatriptan. *Vasc Med Rev* 1992;**3**:95–108.
11 Tansey MJB, Pilgrim AJ, Lloyd K. Sumatriptan in the acute treatment of migraine. *J Neuro Sci* 1993;**114**:109–116.
12 Wolff HS. *Headache and Other Head Pain*. Oxford University Press, Oxford, 1963.
13 Olesen J, Tfelt-Hansen P, Henriksen L, Larsen B. The common migraine attack may not be initiated by cerebral ischaemia. *Lancet* 1981;**ii**:438–440.
14 Olesen J. Clinical and pathophysiological observations in migraine and tension-type headache explained by integration of vascular, supraspinal and myofacial inputs. *Pain* 1991;**46**:125–132.
15 Olesen J. Migraine and regional cerebral blood flow. *Trends Neurosci* 1985;**8**:318–320.
16 Humphrey PPA. 5-Hydroxytryptamine and the pathophysiology of migraine. *J Neurol* 1991;**238**:S38–S44.
17 Friberg L, Olesen J, Iversen HK, Sperling B. Migraine pain associated with middle cerebral artery dilatation: reversal by sumatriptan. *Lancet* 1991;**338**:13–17.
18 Raskin NH. Pharmacology of migraine. *Annu Rev Pharmacol Toxicol* 1981;**21**:463–478.
19 Raskin NH, Knittle SC. Ice cream headache and orthostatic symptoms in patients with migraine. *Headache* 1976;**16**:222–225.
20 Raskin NH, Hosobuchi Y, Lamb S. Headache may arise from perturbation of brain. *Headache* 1987;**27**:416–420.
21 Goadsby PJ, Piper RD, Lambert GA, Lance JW. The effect of activation of the nucleus raphé dorsalis on carotid blood flow. *Am J Physiol* 1985;**248**:R257–262.
22 Anthony M, Hinterberger H, Lance JW. The possible relationships of serotonin to the migraine syndrome. *Res Clin Studies Headache* 1969;**2**:29–59.
23 Lance JW, Lambert GA, Goadsby PJ, Zagami AS. 5-Hydroxytryptamine and its putative aetiological involvement in migraine. *Cephalalgia* 1989;**9**(supp 9):7–13.
24 Moskowitz MA, Reinhard JF, Romero J, Pettibone DJ. Neurotransmitters and the fifth cranial nerve: is there a relation to headache phase of migraine? *Lancet* 1979;**ii**:883–885.
25 Moskowitz MA, Henrikson BM, Markowitz S. Experimental studies on the sensory innervation of the cerebral blood vessels. *Cephalalgia* 1986;**7**(suppl. 4):63–66.
26 Moskowitz MA. Neurogenic versus vascular mechanisms of sumatriptan and ergot extravasation in dura mater: proposed action in vascular headaches. *Trends Pharmacol Sci* 1992;**13**:307–311.

27 Ray BS, Wolff HG. Experimental studies on headache: pain-sensitive structures of the head and their significance in headache. *Arch Surg* 1940;**41**:813–856.
28 Nichols FT, Mawad M, Mohr JP, Stein B, Hilal S, Michelsen WJ. Focal headache during balloon inflation in the internal carotid and middle cerebral arteries. *Stroke* 1990;**21**:555–559.
29 Sicuteri F, Testi A, Anselmi B. Biochemical investigations in headache: increase in the hydroxyindole acetic acid excretion during migraine attacks. *Int Arch Allergy* 1961;**19**:55–58.
30 Curran DA, Hinterberger H, Lance JW. Total plasma serotonin 5-hydroxyindoleacetic acid and *p*-hydroxy-*m*-methoxymandelic acid excretion in normal and migrainous subjects. *Brain* 1965;**88**:997–1008.
31 Lance JW, Anthony M, Somerville B. Comparative trials of serotonin antagonists in the management of migraine. *Br Med J* 1970;**2**:327–330.
32 Kimball RW, Friedman AP, Vallejo E. Effect of serotonin in migraine patients. *Neurology* 1960;**10**:107–111.
33 Lance JW. *The Mechanism and Management of Headache*, 2nd edn. Butterworth, London, 1973.
34 Humphrey PPA, Feniuk W, Perren MJ, Oxford AW. Serotonin, sumatriptan and migraine. In: *Science and Practice in Clinical Neurology: Reviews in Pathophysiology, Diagnosis and Management*, edited by Gandevia SC, Burke D, Anthony M. Cambridge University Press, London, 1993:323–333.
35 Humphrey PPA, Feniuk W. The mode of action of the anti-migraine drug, sumatriptan. *Trends Pharmacol Sci* 1991;**12**:444–446.
36 Ferrari MD, Saxena PR. On serotonin and migraine: a clinical and pharmacological review. *Cephalalgia* 1993;**13**:151–165.
37 Humphrey PPA, Goadsby PJ. The mode of action of sumatriptan is vascular? A debate. *Cephalalgia* 1994;**14**:401–410.
38 Humphrey PPA, Feniuk W, Motevalian M *et al.* The vasoconstrictor action of sumatriptan on human isolated dura mater. In: *Serotonin: Molecular Biology, Receptors and Functional Effects*, edited by Fozard JR, Saxena PR, Birkhauser Verlag, Basel, 1991:421–429.
39 Parsons AA, Whalley ET, Feniuk W, Connor HE, Humphrey PPA. 5-HT$_1$-like receptors mediate 5-hydroxytryptamine-induced contraction of human isolated basilar artery. *Br J Pharmacol* 1989;**96**:434–449.
40 Caekebeke JF, Ferrari MD, Zwetsloot CP, Jansen I, Saxena PR. Anti-migraine drug sumatriptan increases blood flow velocity in large cerebral arteries during migraine attacks. *Neurology* 1992;**42**:1522–1526.
41 Buzzi MG, Moskowitz MA. The antimigraine drug, sumatriptan (GR43175), selectively blocks neurogenic plasma extravasation from blood vessels in dura mater. *Br J Pharmacol* 1990;**99**:202–206.
42 Humphrey PPA, Feniuk W, Perren MJ, Beresford IJM, Skingle, M. Serotonin and migraine. *Ann NY Acad Sci* 1990;**600**:587–600.
43 Sleight AJ, Cervenka A, Peroutka SJ. *In vivo* effects of sumatriptan (GR43175) on extracellular levels of 5-HT in the guinea-pig. *Neuropharmacology*, 1990;**29**:511–513.
44 Skingle M, Birch PJ, Leighton GE, Humphrey PPA. Lack of antinociceptive activity of sumatriptan in rodents. *Cephalalgia* 1990;**10**:207–212.
45 Skingle M, Higgins GA, Feniuk W. Stimulation of central 5-HT$_{1D}$ receptors causes hypothermia in the guinea-pig. *J Psychopharmacol* 1994.
46 Fanciullacci M, Alessandri M, Figini M, Geppetti P, Michelacci S. Increase in plasma calcitonin gene-related peptide from the extracerebral circulation during nitroglycerin-induced cluster headache attack. *Pain* 1995;**60**:119–123.
47 Iversen HK, Thomsen LL. Nitroglycerin-induced headache. In: *Experimental Headache Models, Frontiers in Headache Research*, vol 5, edited by Olsen J, Moskowitz MA. Raven Press, New York, 1995:251–258.
48 The sumatriptan cluster headache study group. Treatment of acute cluster headache with sumatriptan. *N Eng J Med* 1991;**325**:322–326.
49 Brennum J, Kjeldsen M, Olesen J. The 5-HT$_1$-like agonist sumatriptan has a significant effect in chronic tension-type headache. *Cephalalgia* 1992;**12**:375–379.

50 Goadsby PJ, Edvinsson L, Ekman R. Vasoactive peptide release in the extracerebral circulation of humans during migraine headache. *Ann Neurol* 1990;**28**:183–187.

51 Goadsby PJ, Edvinsson L. The trigeminovascular system and migraine: studies characterising cerebrovascular and neuropeptide changes seen in humans and cats. *Ann Neurol* 1993;**50**:48–56.

52 Lee WS, Moskowitz MA. Conformationally restricted sumatriptan analogues, CP-122,288 and CP-122,738, exhibit enhanced potency against neurogenic inflammation in dura mater. *Brain Res* 1993;**626**:303–305.

53 Beattie DT, Connor HE. The pre- and postjunctional activity of CP-122,288, a conformationally restricted analogue of sumatriptan. *Eur J Pharmacol* 1995;**276**:271–276.

54 Moskowitz MA, Buzzi MG, Sakas DE, Kinnik MD. Pain mechanisms underlying vascular headaches. *Rev Neurol (Paris)* 1989;**145**:181–193.

55 Katayama M, Nadel JA, Bunnet NW, Marla GU, Haxhlo M, Borson DB. Catabolism of calcitonin gene-related peptide and substance P by neutral endopeptidase. *Peptides* 1991;**12**:563–567.

56 Stubbs CM, Waldron GJ, Connor HE, Feniuk W. Characterization of neurokinin receptors mediating relaxation to substance P in canine middle cerebral artery: no evidence for involvement of substance P in neurogenically mediated relaxation. *Br J Pharmacol* 1992;**105**:875–880.

57 Beattie DT, Stubbs CM, Connor HE, Feniuk W. Neurokinin-induced changes in pial artery diameter in the anaesthetized guinea-pig. *Br J Pharmacol* 1993;**108**:146–149.

58 Shepheard SL, Williamson DJ, Hill RG, Hardgreaves RJ. The non-peptide neurokinin NK₁ receptor antagonist, RP67580, blocks neurogenic plasma extravasation in the dura mater of rats. *Br J Pharmacol* 1993;**108**:11–12.

59 McCulloch J, Uddman R, Kingman TA, Edvinsson L. Calcitonin gene-related peptide: functional role in cerebrovascular regulation. *Proc Natl Acad Sci* 1986;**83**:5731–5735.

60 Brain SD, Williams TJ. Inflammatory oedema induced by synergism between CGRP and mediators of increased vascular permeability. *Br J Pharmacol* 1985;**86**:855–860.

61 Shepheard SL, Williamson DJ, Williams J, Hill RG, Hardgreaves RJ. Comparison of the effects of sumatriptan and the NK₁ antagonist CP-99,994 on plasma extravasation in dura mater and c-*fos* mRNA expression in trigeminal nucleus caudalis of rats. *Neuropharmacology* 1995;**34**(3):255–261.

62 Humphrey PPA, McKeen ES, Feniuk W. Somatostatin and the regulation of pain. In: *Experimental Headache Models, Frontiers in Headache Research*, vol. 5, edited by Olesen J, Moskowitz MA. Raven Press, New York, 1995:135–141.

MULTIPLE CHOICE QUESTIONS

1 5-Hydroxytryptamine (5-HT) appears to be involved in the pathophysiology of migraine

a 5-HT is an endogenous neurotransmitter

b a migraine attack is associated with a low plasma concentration of 5-HT

c reserpine alleviates the pain of migraine by release of 5-HT from platelets

d urinary 5-hydroxyindoleacetic acid (5-HIAA), a metabolite of 5-HT, is excreted in decreased amounts during a migraine headache

e intravenous 5-HT has been shown to alleviate migraine headache experimentally

2 **Novel drug discovery is important for patient care and frequently, but not always, involves significant advances in medical science**
   a β-adrenoceptor blocking drugs were discovered by accident
   b the clinical efficacy of sumatriptan confirms the hypothetical involvement of 5-HT in the pathophysiology of migraine
   c the precise mechanism of action of sumatriptan is still not known
   d possible antimigraine drugs of the future could include substance P receptor antagonists, somatostatin receptor agonists, calcitonin gene-related peptide (CGRP) receptor antagonists
   e sumatriptan activates a 5-HT_1 receptor in some, but not all, blood vessel walls

3 **The pain of migraine arises from the cephalic vasculature**
   a mainly extracranial blood vessels are involved
   b cerebral blood flow is not changed in a migraine attack without aura
   c transcranial Doppler flow measurements indicate that vasodilatation of intracranial large cerebral vessels occurs during a migraine attack
   d sumatriptan administered subcutaneously to migraineurs reduces cerebral blood flow
   e a localized cerebral oligaemia has been demonstrated clinically in migraine attacks with aura

4 **Various neuropeptides have been implicated in the pathophysiology of migraine**
   a they include substance P and CGRP
   b substance P and CGRP can be released from the terminals of the trigeminal nerve when the nerve is activated
   c substance P levels have been shown to be increased in jugular venous blood during a migraine attack
   d the concentration of CGRP is raised in cubital fossa venous plasma during a migraine attack
   e CGRP is a potent vasodilator and may contribute to localized extravasation when released from sensory nerve terminals

5 **There is still controversy about whether migraine is a 'vascular' or 'neuronal' disease**
   a modern theories on the pathophysiology involve both vascular and neuronal elements
   b it is most likely that the pain of migraine arises from within the walls of cranial blood vessels
   c CGRP is thought to activate trigeminal nerve endings

d the pain of migraine has been shown to arise from abnormal firing within the periaqueductal grey area of the brain

e cephalic vascular distension has been shown to cause pain

Answers

1 a True
  b True
  c False
  d False
  e True

2 a False
  b False
  c True
  d True
  e True

3 a False
  b True
  c True
  d False
  e True

4 a True
  b True
  c False
  d False
  e True

5 a True
  b True
  c False
  d False
  e True

Vitamin D and its analogues: classic and novel applications

HUIBERT A. P. POLS, TRUDY VINK-VAN WIJNGAARDEN, JAN C. BIRKENHÄGER & JOHANNES P. T. M. VAN LEEUWEN

The name 'vitamin D' is a misnomer and in fact vitamin D has to be considered as a prohormone. Vitamin D_3 is generated in the skin by ultraviolet irradiation or is absorbed from the diet. Subsequently, vitamin D_3 is metabolized in the liver to 25-hydroxyvitamin D_3 and then in the kidney to the active metabolite 1,25-dihydroxyvitamin D_3 (1,25-$(OH)_2D_3$). This active compound acts through binding to a specific receptor, the vitamin D receptor (VDR), which is a member of the steroid hormone family [1–4].

Regulation of bone mineral homeostasis, principally through actions on calcium and phosphate handling by bone, intestine and kidney, has for a long time been regarded as the only physiological activity of vitamin D. During the past decade a number of tissues have been found to contain the VDR and to respond to 1,25-$(OH)_2D_3$ with a change in function. The classic target tissues — intestine, kidney and bone — are now only part of a list, together with a wide variety of tissues not related to calcium homeostasis, including various elements of the haematopoietic and immune system, cardiac, skeletal and smooth muscle, breast, skin and several endocrine glands. Furthermore, malignancies developing within these tissues may also contain VDRs and several *in vitro* studies indicate that cell lines derived from these tumours respond to 1,25-$(OH)_2D_3$ [4,5].

Although the response of the different target tissues may vary considerably, the non-classical actions of 1,25-$(OH)_2D_3$ can broadly be separated in to two sorts:

1 modulation or regulation of the synthesis and secretion of different hormones (e.g. parathyroid hormone, insulin, prolactin) and cytokines (e.g. interleukin-2 and tumour necrosis factor);
2 regulation of cellular differentiation and proliferation [4–6].

These two themes also underlie the interest in the potential clinical application of 1,25-$(OH)_2D_3$ for non-classical indications, like psoriasis, cancer and autoimmune disease.

The major problem for the clinician to manipulate the newly recognized actions is that supraphysiological doses of systematically administered 1,25-$(OH)_2D_3$ are required. Thus, doses optimal in terms of preventing tumour growth will inevitably result in complications, like hypercalcaemia, hyper-calciuria and soft-tissue calcifications. These severe complications have prompted the development of vitamin D analogues in an attempt to separate the calcaemic activity from the antiproliferative and cell differentiation stimulatory activity [4,6].

This paper will focus on the recent progress towards the understanding of 1,25-(OH)$_2$D$_3$ actions in hyperproliferative disorders and discuss the development of vitamin D analogues.

1,25-DIHYDROXYVITAMIN D$_3$ MODULATES CELLULAR PROLIFERATION AND DIFFERENTIATION: THE BASIS OF NEW CLINICAL APPLICATIONS

Haematopoietic cells

A role of 1,25-(OH)$_2$D$_3$ in the differentiation of haematopoietic stem cells was demonstrated for the first time in 1981 by Abe *et al.* [7]. They showed that, after exposure to 1,25-(OH)$_2$D$_3$, immature mouse myeloid leu-kaemia cells differentiated towards mature macrophage-like cells. This differentiation process was accompanied by a reduced growth rate. Sub-sequently these studies were extended to human leukaemic cell lines, and currently the HL60 and U937 cell lines are frequently used to study the effect of vitamin D$_3$ and its analogues on haematopoietic differentiation and proliferation [4–6]. The suggestion from *in vitro* studies that 1,25-(OH)$_2$D$_3$ may be of clinical use in the treatment of leukaemia is further supported by animal studies. Honma *et al.* [8] observed for the first time that treatment with 1,25-(OH)$_2$D$_3$ may indeed be operative *in vivo*: the survival of athymic mice that had been inoculated with mouse myeloid leukaemia cells was significantly prolonged after the administration of 1α-hydroxyvitamin D$_3$.

In addition to regulating growth and differentiation, 1,25-(OH)$_2$D$_3$ affects a wide range of specific functions of haematopoietic cells, such as regulation of cytokine and antibody production, 1,25-(OH)$_2$D$_3$ inhibits T-lymphocyte activation *in vitro* and also in animal models immuno-suppressive activity has been observed [9]. The immunomodulatory properties of 1,25-(OH)$_2$D$_3$ may form the basis of new clinical applica-tions of the hormone in the treatment of autoimmune diseases or in transplantation.

Epidermal differentiation

The skin as well as cultures of human epidermal keratinocytes contain the VDR. 1,25-(OH)$_2$D$_3$ causes a decrease in proliferation and an increase in differentiation (as assessed on the basis of morphological and biochemical criteria) of cultured keratinocytes [10]. The potential clinical application of treatment with the active form of vitamin D became clear when a woman treated with 1α-hydroxyvitamin D_3 for osteoporosis had a dramatic remission of her psoriasis [11]. The mode of action of 1,25-$(OH)_2D_3$ in psoriasis may involve different mechanisms. Apart from reversing hyperproliferation and promoting epidermal differentiation, 1,25-$(OH)_2D_3$ may have effects on the immunological and inflammatory processes [11].

Cancer cells

Receptors for 1,25-$(OH)_2D_3$ are also present in a variety of non-leukaemia cancer cell lines [2,4,6]. Analogous to its antiproliferative activity on leukaemic cell lines, 1,25-$(OH)_2D_3$ induces differentiation and/or inhibits the proliferation of a wide variety of cell lines that have been established from solid tumours, including breast, colon, prostate and melanoma. Several *in vivo* studies have confirmed the antiproliferative action observed *in vitro* and shown that 1,25-$(OH)_2D_3$ exerts tumour suppressive activity. Table 1 summarizes a number of studies on the effects of 1,25-$(OH_2)D_3$ on tumour growth in animal models for cancer.

DEVELOPMENT OF NEW VITAMIN D_3 ANALOGUES

The use of 1,25-$(OH)_2D_3$ as an antiproliferative or an immunosuppressive agent is restricted by a considerable risk of severe complications, like hypercalcaemia, hypercalciuria and soft-tissue calcification. However, at present vitamin D analogues are available that have antiproliferative and/or immunosuppressive effects, whereas the effects on calcium and bone metabolism appear to be reduced [6,8,9].

In vitro and *in vivo* testing of new vitamin D_3 analogues

The majority of the new vitamin D_3 analogues synthesized are based on side-chain modifications of the 1,25-$(OH)_2D_3$ molecule [12]. The *in vitro* growth-inhibitory and differentiation-inducing potential of the main analogues have extensively been compared to the native compound 1,25-$(OH)_2D_3$. Although the maximum inhibition of these analogues is not dramatically increased, the median effective concentrations (EC_{50}) of the analogues are sometimes several orders of magnitude lower.

The calcaemic activity of new analogues is mostly tested by measuring serum calcium levels and/or urinary calcium excretion of rats treated with an analogue. The analogues that have an increased antiproliferative effect *in vitro*, but a similar or even reduced calcaemic activity compared to

Table 1 *In vivo* effects of vitamin D_3 on animal models for cancer.

Tumour	Model	Administration*	Effect	Ref.
Breast	NMU-induced breast cancer in rats	$1\alpha(OH)D_3$, i.p.	Tumour suppression	[23]
Breast	DMBA-induced breast cancer in rats	$1\alpha(OH)D_3$, orally	Tumour suppression	[24]
Colon	Human colon cell line implanted into nude mice	$1,25(OH)_2D_3$, i.p.	Tumour suppression	[25]
Colon	DMH-induced colon cancer in rats	$1,25(OH)_2D_3$, s.c.	Reduction of the incidence of colon adenocarcinomas	[26]
Leydig tumour	Leydig cell tumour implanted into rats	$1,25(OH)_2D_3$, osmotic minipumps	Tumour suppression	[18]
Lung	Implantation of lung carcinoma cells	$1,25(OH)_2D_3$, i.p.	Reduction in the number of metastases	[27]
Melanoma	Human melanoma cells implanted in nude mice	$1,25(OH)_2D_3$, i.p.	Tumour suppressions	[25]
Osteosarcoma	Human osteosarcoma cells implanted into nude mice	$1\alpha(OH)D_3$, i.p.	Tumour suppression	[28]

* The dosage duration of treatment, diet, and effects on serum/urinary calcium vary between the studies.
NMU, nitrosomethylurea; DMBA, 7,12-dimethylbenz[a]anthracene: DMH, 1,2-dimethylhydrazine dihydrochloride.

$1,25\text{-}(OH)_2D_3$, offer promise for clinical applications [4,6]. Ultimately, these analogues have to be tested in animal models and in clinical studies to investigate whether the analogues also inhibit tumour growth *in vivo*. Very few analogues have advanced to this stage.

The compound 1,25-dihydroxy-16-ene-23-yne-vitamin D_3 increased the survival time of mice inoculated with leukaemic cells without the development of hypercalcaemia [13]. Topical application of the anti-psoriatic analogue calcipotriol (MC903) was effective in reducing the size of treated lesions of some patients with advanced breast cancer [14]. The analogues 22-oxa-calcitriol (OCT) [15] EB1089 [16,17], and CB966 [16] have shown promising results after systemic treatment in rat mammary tumour models. These analogues suppressed the tumour growth without the development of hypercalcaemia. Furthermore, it was shown that EB1089 prolonged the survival time of rats implanted with Leydig tumours [18]. Finally, the analogue 1α,25-dihydroxy-16-ene-23-yne-26,27-hexa-fluorocholecalciferol (Ro24-5531) inhibited rat mammary carcinogenesis induced by *N*-nitroso-*N*-methylurea [19].

POSSIBLE MECHANISMS FOR THE SELECTIVE ACTIONS OF VITAMIN D_3 ANALOGUES

The mechanism behind the increased *in vitro* antiproliferative and differentiation-inducing effects of new vitamin D_3 analogues is largely unknown. Also, the selectivity between antitumour and calcium-related effects of new vitamin D_3 analogues *in vivo* is not well-understood [4].

For the selective action on the different target organs the pharmacological differences between the analogues and $1,25-(OH)_2D_3$ are believed to play an important role. A decreased binding to the major carrier of vitamin D, vitamin D-binding protein, has been observed for the majority of analogues. This may result in a rapid clearance of the analogue and consequently a decreased biological activity. On the other hand, low binding may result, at least initially, in a higher proportion of the free active form. The transport of analogues (22-oxa-calcitriol) may also proceed via different carrier proteins (e.g. lipoproteins), which may influence the biological half-life and the uptake by the cells or tissues. In addition, the time of exposure required to trigger a biological response may vary between target tissues. Thereby, the mode of delivery may result in a target tissue or response-selective action of vitamin D analogues. Also at the cellular level, an altered metabolism may play a role in the differences between $1,25-(OH)_2D_3$ and its analogues. Modifications in the side chain influence the catabolism of the molecule because the side chain is sensitive to oxidation (Fig. 1). Alternatively, intracellular metabolism of an analogue may lead to an accumulation of active metabolites in the target cell.

In addition, VDR binding may play an important role in the selectivity of the action of the analogues. An increased binding affinity to the VDR could theoretically result in an increased activity. However, up to now all analogues tested have a similar or reduced affinity for the VDR compared to $1,25-(OH)_2D_3$. In other words, there is no direct correlation between receptor binding and the biological activity of the analogues. Still, a complete failure to bind to the VDR is accompanied by a loss of cell-regulating activity. A selective action via different tissue or cell-specific VDRs is unlikely because it is currently accepted that VDRs are identical in all cell types. Binding of an analogue to the VDR may induce conformational changes of the receptor. This may lead to alterations in DNA binding, dimerization of the VDR and phosphorylation and/or intracellular clearance of the receptor complex. All these changes may result in cell- and response-specific transcriptional activation and may alter the magnitude of the biological response. Finally, the intracellular signalling via non-genomic mechanisms may vary between cell types and the ability to activate non-genomic mechanisms may vary between the analogues [4,6].

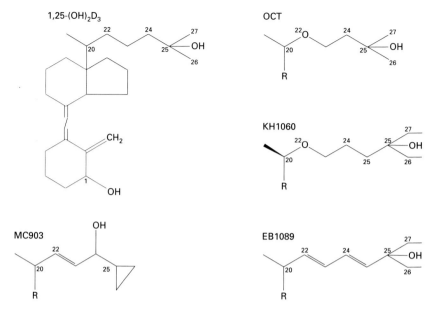

Fig. 1 Examples of side chain modifications of 1,25-dihydroxyvitamin D_3 (1,25-$(OH)_2D_3$). The analogues shown are some of those discussed in the text.

Taken together, the mechanisms mentioned in this paragraph are at the moment the possible candidates to explain the response-specificity of the analogues. Probably all these mechanisms contribute to the differential action of the analogues but a definite answer still needs further research.

CONCLUSIONS

The non-classical effects of 1,25-$(OH)_2D_3$ and its analogues have opened a new field of basic and clinical research. To date this has already resulted in an approved clinical application of a vitamin D analogue (calcipotriol) for the treatment of psoriasis. Recently also, phase 1 clinical studies have been initiated to evaluate some promising new vitamin D analogues in the treatment of breast cancer. In the case of breast cancer, special attention has to be given to the potential additive or even synergistic antiproliferative effect of the combination of tamoxifen and a vitamin D analogue [20,21]. This approach might have an important additional advantage, namely the inhibition of bone resorption induced by analogues [22].

As the number of vitamin D analogues still grows, it becomes increasingly difficult to select the most promising candidates. It is therefore essential to expand our knowledge of the actions of the different analogues, both at the basal level, but also in clinical research.

REFERENCES

1 Haussler MR. Vitamin D receptor: nature and function. *Annu Rev Nutr* 1986;**6**:527–562.
2 Reichel H, Koeffler HP, Norman AW. The role of the vitamin D endocrine system in health and disease. *N Engl J Med* 1989;**320**:980–991.
3 Pike JW. Vitamin D_3 receptors: structure and function in transcription. *Annu Rev Nutr* 1991;**11**:189–216.
4 Pols HAP, Birkenhäger JC, Van Leeuwen JPTM. Vitamin D analogues: from molecule to clinical application. *Clin Endocrinol* 1994;**40**:285–291.
5 Walters MR. Newly identified actions of the vitamin D endocrine system. *Endocrine Rev* 1992;**13**:719–764.
6 Bikle DD. Clinical counterpoint: vitamin D: new actions, new analogs, new therapeutic potential. *Endocrine Rev* 1992;**13**:765–784.
7 Abe E, Miyaura C, Sakagami H *et al.* Differentiation of mouse myeloid leukemia cells induced by 1α,25-dihydroxyvitamin D_3. *Proc Natl Acad Sci USA* 1981;**78**:4990–4994.
8 Honma Y, Hozumi M, Abe E *et al.* 1α,25-dihydroxyvitamin D_3 and 1α-hydroxyvitamin D_3 prolong the survival time of mice inoculated with myeloid leukemia cells. *Proc Natl Acad Sci USA* 1983;**80**:201–204.
9 Binderup L. Immunological properties of vitamin D analogues and metabolites. *Biochem Pharmacol* 1992;**43**:1885–1892.
10 Bikle DD, Pillai S. Vitamin D, calcium and epidermal differentiation. *Endocrine Rev* 1993;**14**:3–19.
11 Morimoto S, Kumahara Y. A patient with psoriasis cured by 1α-hydroxyvitamin D_3. *Med J Osaka Univ* 1985;**35**:51–54.
12 Calverley MJ, Jones G. Vitamin D. In: *Antitumor Steroids* edited by Blickenstaff RF. Academic Press, New York, 1992:93–270.
13 Zhou JY, Norman AW, Chen DL, Sun GW, Uskokovic M, Koeffler HP. 1,25-dihydroxy-16-ene-23-yne-vitamin D_3 prolongs survival time of leukemic mice. *Proc Natl Acad Sci USA* 1990;**87**:3929–3932.
14 Bower M, Colston KW, Stein RC *et al.* Topical calcipotriol treatment in advanced breast cancer. *Lancet* 1991;**337**:701–702.
15 Abe J, Nakano T, Nishii Y, Matsumoto T, Ogata E, Ikeda K. A novel vitamin D_3 analog, 22-oxa-1,25-dihydroxyvitamin D_3, inhibits the growth of human breast cancer *in vitro* and *in vivo* without causing hypercalcemia. *Endocrinology* 1991;**129**:832–837.
16 Colston KW, Mackay AG, Chandler S, Binderup L, Coombes RC. Novel vitamin D analogues suppress tumour growth *in vivo*. In: *Vitamin D: Gene Regulation, Structure-function Analysis and Clinical Application*, edited by Norman AW, Bouillon R, Thomasset M. Walter de Gruyter, Berlin, 1991:465–466.
17 Colston KW, Mackay AG, James SY, Binderup L. EB1089: a new vitamin D analogue that inhibits the growth of breast cancer cells *in vivo* and *in vitro*. *Biochem Pharmacol* 1992;**44**:2273–2280.
18 Haq M, Kremer R, Goltzman D, Rabbani SA. A vitamin D analogue (EB1089) inhibits parathyroid hormone-related peptide production and prevents the development of malignancy-associated hypercalcemia *in vivo*. *J Clin Invest* 1993;**91**:2416–2422.
19 Anzano MA, Smith JM, Uskokovic MR *et al.* 1α,25-dihydroxy-16-ene-23-yne-26,27-hexafluorocholecalciferol (Ro24-5531), a new deltanoid (vitamin D analogue) for prevention of breast cancer in the rat. *Cancer Res* 1994;**54**:1653–1656.
20 Vink-van Wijngaarden T, Pols HAP, Buurman CJ, Birkenhäger JC, Leeuwen van JPTM. Combined effects of 1,25-dihydroxyvitamin D_3 and tamoxifen on the growth MCF-7 and ZR-75.1 human breast cancer cells. *Breast Cancer Res Treat* 1993;**29**:161–168.
21 Vink-van Wijngaarden T, Pols HAP, Binderup L *et al.* Synergistic inhibition of breast cancer cell growth by combined treatment with vitamin D_3 analogues and tamoxifen. *Cancer Res* 1994;**54**:5711–5717.
22 Vink-van Wijngaarden T, Birkenhäger JC, Kleinekoort WMC, Bemd van den GJCM, Pols HAP, Leeuwen van JPTM. Antiestrogens inhibit *in vitro* bone resorption stimulated by 1,25-dihydroxyvitamin D_3 and the vitamin D_3 analogs EB1089 and KH1060. *Endocrinology* 1995;**136**:812–815.

23 Colston KW, Berger U, Coombes RC. Possible role for vitamin D in controlling breast cancer cell proliferation. *Lancet* 1989;1:188–191.

24 Lino Y, Yoshida M, Sugamata N *et al.* 1α-Hydroxyvitamin D₃, hypercalcemia, and growth suppression of 7,12-dimethylbenzanthracene-induced rat mammary tumors. *Breast Cancer Res Treat* 1992;22:133–140.

25 Eisman JA, Barkla DH Tutton PJM. Suppression of *in vivo* growth of human cancer solid tumor xenografts by 1,25-dihydroxyvitamin D₃. *Cancer Res* 1987;47:21–25.

26 Belleli A, Shany S, Levy J, Guberman R, Lamprecht SA. A protective role of 1,25-dihydroxyvitamin D₃ in chemically induced rat colon carcinogenesis. *Carcinogenesis* 1992;13:2293–2298.

27 Young MRI, Halpin J, Hussain R *et al.* Inhibition of tumor production of granulocyte-macrophage colony-stimulating factor by 1α,25-dihydroxyvitamin D₃ reduces tumor motility and metastasis. *Invasion Metastasis* 1993;13:169–177.

28 Tsuchiya H, Morishita H, Tomita K, Ueda Y, Tanaka M. Differentiating and antitumor activities of 1α,25-dihydroxyvitamin D₃ *in vitro* and 1α-hydroxyvitamin D₃ *in vivo* on human osteosarcoma. *J Orthopaedic Res* 1993;11:122–130.

MULTIPLE CHOICE QUESTIONS

1 The active metabolite of vitamin D₃, 1,25-dihydroxyvitamin D₃

a stimulates intestinal calcium absorption

b regulates cellular differentiation and proliferation

c is a cofactor in the synthesis of calcitonin

d inhibits parathyroid hormone synthesis

2 Vitamin D analogues

a are developed to have a reduced calcaemic effect

b are useless in the treatment of psoriasis

c can inhibit growth of breast cancer cells

d always have a high affinity for the vitamin D receptor

3 A possible mechanism for the selective action of vitamin D analogues is

a conversion to 1,25-dihydroxyvitamin D₃

b different binding to vitamin D carrier proteins

c altered metabolism compared to 1,25-dihydroxyvitamin D₃

d activation of non-genomic mechanisms

4 The actions of vitamin D analogues have been widely studied in

a vitamin D-deficient individuals

b cancer patients

c haematopoietic cell lines

d in cultures of human epidermal keratinocytes

5 The vitamin D receptor

a is found in tissues not directly related to calcium homeostasis

b only binds 25-hydroxyvitamin D_3
c needs to be present for the action of vitamin D analogues
d belongs to the superfamily of steroid hormone receptors

Answers

1	a True	2	a True	3	a False
	b True		b False		b True
	c False		c True		c True
	d True		d False		d True

4	a False	5	a True
	b False		b False
	c True		c True
	d True		d True

PART 4
RESPIRATORY DISEASE

Breathing and breathlessness — update 1995

ABRAHAM GUZ

BASIC NEURAL STRUCTURES OF BREATHING

The objective of this presentation is to review recent experimental evidence in humans on two separate but related subjects: (i) mechanisms underlying voluntary or behavioural control of breathing; and (ii) mechanisms underlying the sensation of breathlessness. In order to understand the story, it is necessary to examine Fig. 1 with some care! Few readers will be professional neuroanatomists; the diagrammatic representation of the neurology underlying breathing is intended for the broadly based medical reader.

Automatic breathing originates in the pontomedullary respiratory oscillator from which a descending bulbospinal projection synapses with the anterior horn cells in the cervical and thoracic spinal cord with projections to the respiratory muscles to cause rhythmic breathing. We now know from studies in the isolated brainstem/high cervical cord preparation from the guinea-pig that the pontomedullary respirator oscillator genuinely oscillates automatically and can function without any peripheral feedback but only in the presence of a normal $P\text{CO}_2$ and pH — provided the preparation is kept well-oxygenated. This automatic breathing is what we see in humans asleep (especially in the deep non-rapid-eye-movement (REM) state) or anaesthetized. Proprioceptive afferent input from the lungs via the vagus nerve with a synapse in the nucleus of the tractus solitarius can either inhibit or excite the respiratory oscillator, but there is very little evidence that this system, thoroughly studied over the last century [1], controls breathing in humans with normal lungs and at rest. Vagal input does become significant in driving breathing, particularly respiratory frequency, when the lobes of the lungs are the seat of either inflammation at alveolar level or collapsed. There is also little evidence that afferent input from the diaphragm and intercostal muscles has any influence on breathing in normal humans at rest. Afferent input from the carotid body (and to a minimal extent, the aortic body) excited by hypoxia, hypercapnia

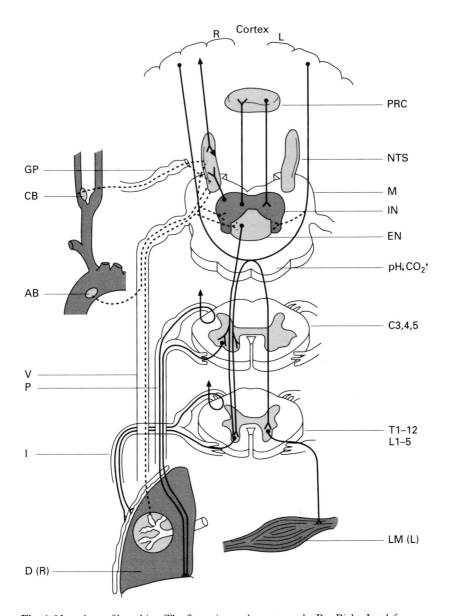

Fig. 1 Neurology of breathing. The figure is not drawn to scale. R = Right; L = left;
GP = glossopharyngeal nerve; CB = carotid body; AB = aortic body; V = vagus nerve;
P = phrenic; I = intercostal nerves; D = diaphragm; LM = leg muscle; pH
CO_2 = medullary chemosensitivity to H^+ and CO_2; IN and EN = inspiratory and
expiratory neuronal pools constituting pontomedullary respiratory oscillator;
M = medulla; NTS = nucleus of tractus solitarius; PRC = pontine respiratory complex.
Two corticospinal tracts are shown: right: descending tract crosses pyramidal decussation
to synapse in anterior horn cells of left L_{1-5} controlling leg movement; dotted lines to
medullary respiratory oscillator symbolically represent irradiation from impulse traffic in
the corticospinal tract; left: descending corticospinal tract decussates to synapse on to
anterior horn cells of C_{3-5} and T_{1-12} controlling voluntary or behavioural inspiration and
expiration; dotted line to the medullary respiratory oscillator represents a probable input
from this corticospinal tract.

or acidosis acts via synapses in the nucleus of the tractus solitarius to excite or inhibit the respiratory oscillator. Significant chemical control on the oscillator is also exerted at the medulla both via its ventral surfaces or deep within its structure.

ANATOMY AND PHYSIOLOGY UNDERLYING VOLUNTARY/BEHAVIOURAL BREATHING

The schematic outline so far does not explain how humans can take a breath *at will*, nor how expiratory air flow can be perfectly controlled to produce phonation. It also does not explain how emotions can affect breathing. Most importantly, it does not explain how breathing increases the 'right amount' during exercise where there would appear to be no error signal to regulate breathing, in the absence of metabolic acidosis with more severe exercise. Such failure to explain essentially error-free regulation of a bodily function such as the cardiorespiratory response to exercise is now clear after intensive investigation over the last 25 years [2]. As a result, concepts such as 'central command' in physiological studies, or 'feed forward' in bioengineering studies, have arisen.

Figure 1 shows a descending corticospinal tract on the left side making synapses with the anterior horn cells of the right diaphragm and intercostals. Evidence for this tract has been obtained in animals since 1958 [3–5] by stimulating the frontal lobes and recording an output from the contralateral phrenic motoneurones with a short latency. Evidence in humans was obtained as long ago as 1936 by Foerster [6]; stimulation of the exposed motor cortex in humans during neurosurgery under local anaesthesia localized a spot anterior to the 'chest' area of Foerster's homunculus where stimulation resulted in a hiccup! More recently, transcranial electrical stimulation at the vertex in conscious humans [7] elicited diaphragmatic contractions with compound action potentials occurring approximately 14 ms after stimulation.

Further studies by our own group [7] with transcranial magnetic stimulation using a coil with some focusing facility over a motor cortex have shown that compound action potentials recorded over the contralateral diaphragm were maximal when the centre of the coil (where the highest magnetic flux was present) was placed 2–3 cm anterior to the interauricular plane and 3 cm to one side of the midline; this is approximately where Foerster found stimulation effective. The compound action potential was predominantly contralateral, although a small response was seen on the ipsilateral side; ultrasonic techniques confirmed that the diaphragmatic twitch occurred contralaterally and not ipsilaterally. This result generates a question about how the two diaphragms move together. Does the integration occur within the cervical cord or via the corpus callosum?

IMAGING THE BRAIN TO ELUCIDATE NEURONAL AREAS CONCERNED WITH VOLUNTARY/BEHAVIOURAL BREATHING

Positron emission tomography (PET) allows the non-invasive measurement of regional cerebral blood flow and has been used to define areas of increased neural activity associated with specific motor tasks in conscious humans. Our group [9] has used this technique to identify areas of neuronal activation associated with volitional inspiration. Such areas were found: (i) bilaterally in the primary motor cortex — superolaterally (where Foerster [6] and we [8] had previously found optimal sites of stimulation for the diaphragm); (ii) in the right premotor cortex and in the supplementary motor area; and (iii) in the cerebellum. These results are analogous to the results of similar imaging studies on voluntary limb movement.

We have further defined areas of neuronal activation with volitional expiration [10]. Similar areas were activated, as was found in the study on volitional inspiration, with one notable addition; the right and left primary motor cortices showed increases in regional cerebral blood flow over large areas ventrolaterally well down towards the Sylvian fissure. It is of extraordinary interest that vocalization (or speech arrest) was obtained by Penfield and Rasmussen [11] over this same large area. Vocalization or speech arrest requires active expiratory air flow or cessation of such air flow. These additional excitations with active expiration require much further study.

THE 'CURSE OF ONDINE' AND THE 'LOCKED-IN SYNDROME': CLINICAL LESSONS

These studies provide some physiological basis for the voluntary aspects of breathing as opposed to the automatic pontomedullary breathing. Figure 1 shows a dotted line from the corticospinal tract for volitional breathing, which represents a probable input into the respiratory oscillator. Experiments in the cat [12,13] suggest that voluntary or behavioural influences are integrated within the brainstem areas that house the automatic pontomedullary oscillator. In humans, evidence comes from clinical studies of patients with defined brainstem lesions [14] or very high cervical cord lesions [15,16]. The syndrome of particular interest is that of 'Ondine's curse'; these patients lack automatic breathing when drowsy or asleep, but breathe apparently normally when awake and can breathe normally to command. Evidence strongly suggests that bulbospinal fibres run separately and more anterolaterally in the cord than the relevant corticospinal fibres. There is, however, no evidence in humans about integration of corticospinal control with bulbospinal control at the brainstem level. What happens to the pontomedullary respiratory oscillator when a person takes a breath without changing the arterial P_{CO_2}?

The congenital Ondine's curse syndrome has now been well-studied in children. These patients have ineffective chemical regulation of breathing and either severely hypoventilate or do not breathe at all during sleep. Awake, the level of spontaneous breathing is adequate and during steady-state moderate exercise — below the level of lactate accumulation — ventilation is raised appropriately so that the prevailing level of P_{CO_2} is maintained [17]. We do not know why this happens! What is the meaning of needing to be awake to breathe? Are these children breathing when awake, at rest or while exercising, with their corticospinal tracts?

Breathing at rest has a considerable degree of variability from moment to moment. A lesion in the ventral pons and lower midbrain involving motor tracts to the rest of the body will remove all voluntary control of muscle movement, except for elevation of the eyes; this is the 'locked-in syndrome' [18]. Sensation is intact. Breathing is normal but very regular, maintaining a normal P_{CO_2}; voluntary effort to change breathing has no effect but emotion will disrupt breathing. Our own group has confirmed this finding.

Maintenance of emotional influences on breathing in the absence of voluntary control shows that emotional (presumably limbic) pathways to the brainstem are anatomically separate from the corticobulbar pathways. Such patients give us the opportunity to study the function of the 'isolated' pontomedullary oscillator and its intact bulbospinal tract to the muscles of breathing. Ventilatory sensitivity to inhaled carbon dioxide is normal, with associated breathlessness (see below). However, if resting P_{CO_2} is lowered (with mechanical ventilation) by as little as 1–3 mmHg, breathing ceases. This does not occur in intact humans awake [22], but does occur during deep non-REM sleep [23]. Do these findings imply that higher-centre (?cortical) input into the brainstem oscillator is occurring normally when awake at rest to keep breathing stable but irregular? Is this the wakefulness 'drive to breathe' [22]?

CORTICAL INVOLVEMENT IN BREATHING CONTROL DURING EXERCISE

This question takes us back to the proposal of Krogh and Lindhard [19] that motor cortical activation to exercising muscles might induce increases in breathing via irradiation of either brainstem respiratory centres (Fig. 1; see dotted lines from right corticospinal tract to pontomedullary oscillator) or of cortical areas controlling respiratory muscles. Could these cortical areas described above be shown to be active during exercise? Recently [20,21] we have been able to show, with modest leg exercise in normal adult subjects lying with their heads in a PET scanner, that there is indeed evidence of activation in the left and right superolateral primary motor cortices in areas previously shown to be associated with volitional breathing (Plate 1). Such results have suggested motor cortical involvement in exercise-related hyperpnoea. Is this one of the forms of irradiation — at cortical level — suggested by Krogh and Lindhard [18]? Or is this a learned response providing an appropriate amount of central command?

THE SENSATION OF BREATHLESSNESS; FOCUS ON 'AIR HUNGER'

An up-to-date review of this subject is being published as a multiauthor volume in 1996 [24]. It would not be appropriate to summarize this here. Breathlessness is not a uniform sensation; it has many different qualities [25]. I shall focus on the sensation of 'air hunger' or the 'urge to breathe'. This sensation typically occurs in subjects given carbon dioxide to breathe or made to exercise when breathing discomfort is further described by such phrases as 'could not breathe fast or deep enough' or 'could not get enough air' or 'suffocating'. There would appear to be an enhanced respiratory drive normally manifested by an increase in neural output to the muscles of breathing.

Increasing clinical evidence over the last few years suggests that it is not the neural output to the muscles of breathing that is particularly relevant to the genesis of the air hunger sensation. The key requirement would appear to be an intact brainstem automatic respiratory controller that can respond to stimulation. The evidence is shown below.

1 Totally curarized unsedated subjects have been mechanically ventilated while end-tidal (alveolar) P_{CO_2} has been varied by changing the inspired P_{CO_2} [26]. When the end-tidal P_{CO_2} was raised from a median of 35 mmHg, at which the subjects were comfortable, to a median of 44 mmHg, all reported severe air hunger. The subjects reported no fundamental difference in the sensation during paralysis or, as a control, before paralysis; both experiment and control were done while ventilation was kept constant with a mechanical ventilator.

2 Ventilator-dependent quadriplegics with the lesion as high as C_{1-2} could sense the typical 'air hunger' when the end-tidal carbon dioxide was raised as in the paralysis study above [27]. Here, the brainstem respiratory oscillator is presumably intact, but its activity, at rest or when stimulated, cannot be transmitted via the bulbospinal fibres to the anterior horn cells of the respiratory musculature.

3 Children with the congenital central hypoventilation syndrome (curse of Ondine — see above) neither have a ventilatory response to hypercapnia nor experience any air hunger sensation [28]. It should be noted that the entire brain, including the sensory cortex, is experiencing hypercapnia — but there are no respiratory sensations. These children

can also voluntarily hold their breath for an inordinate length of time without any apparent urge to breathe.

4 A patient with the locked-in syndrome (see above) with intact and regular automatic breathing has a normal ventilatory response to the inhalation of carbon dioxide with the normal associated air hunger. The sensory pathways are intact.

Although this clinical evidence is weighty, it is essential to ask how the activation of an intact pontomedullary respiratory oscillator can be sensed. Recent work in the cat [29] has shown respiratory-associated firing of both midbrain hypothalamic and thalamic neurons related to respiratory drive and entirely dependent on an intact connection with the medulla. There may therefore be an afferent pathway from the oscillator up to the sensory cortex — but this has not yet been demonstrated.

A very recent PET (see above) study [30] has now identified areas of probable neuronal activation extending from the upper brainstem, up through the midbrain, hypothalamus and thalamus in humans, while breathless as a result of elevated end-tidal $P\text{CO}_2$ raised from 40 to 50 mmHg. In addition, activation of the limbic system (cingulate gyrus, parahippocampus, hippocampus, fusiform gyrus and insula) was present; this may be relevant to the unpleasantness of the air hunger sensation.

We are at a very early stage in trying to understand how higher brain centres can both control breathing and experience breathlessness in humans. New methods have now made these studies possible.

REFERENCES

1 Ullmann E. The two original papers by Hering and Breuer submitted by Hering to the K.K. Akademie der Wissenschaften ZV Wien in 1868. In: *Breathing: Hering-Breuer Centenary Symposium CIBA Foundation*, edited by Porter R. Churchill, London, 1970:357–394.
2 Somjen GG. The missing error signal-regulation beyond negative feedback. *News Physiol Sci* 1992;7:184–185.
3 Colle J, Massion J. Effet de la stimulation du cortex moteur sur l'activite electrique des nerfs phreniques et medians. *Arch Int Physiol Biochem* 1958;66:496–514.
4 Aminoff MJ, Sears TA. Spinal integration of segmental, cortical and breathing inputs to thoracic respiratory motoneurones. *J Physiol* 1971;215:557–575.
5 Planche D. Effets de la stimulation du cortex cerebral sur l'activité du nerf phrenique. *J Physiol* 1972;64:51–56.
6 Foerster O. Motorische Felder und Bahen. In: *Handbook der Neurologie*, edited by Bumke O, Foerster O. Springer, Berlin, 1936:50–51.
7 Gandevia SC, Rothwell JC. Activation of the human diaphragm from the motor cortex. *J Physiol* 1987;384:109–118.
8 Maskill D, Murphy K, Mier A, Owen M, Guz A. Motor cortical representation of the diaphragm in man. *J Physiol* 1991;443:105–121.
9 Colebatch JG, Adams L, Murphy K *et al*. Regional cerebral blood flow during volitional breathing in man. *J Physiol* 1991;443:91–103.
10 Ramsay SC, Adams L, Murphy K *et al*. Regional cerebral blood flow during volitional expiration in man. *J Physiol* 1993;461:85–101.
11 Penfield W, Rasmussen T. Vocalization and speech arrest. In: *The Cerebral Cortex of Man. A Clinical Study of Localization of Function*. Macmillan, New York, 1950:88–108.

12 Orem J, Nettick A. Behavioural control of breathing in the cat. *Brain Res* 1986;366:238–253.

13 Orem J. Neural basis of behavioural and state-dependent control of breathing. In: *Clinical Physiology of Sleep*, edited by Lydic R, Biebuy KJF. American Physiological Society, Bethesda, Maryland, 1988:78–96.

14 Plum F, Leigh RJ. Abnormalities of central mechanisms. In: *Regulation of Breathing*, Part II, Vol. 17. *Lung Biology in Health and Disease*, edited by Hornbeim TF. Marcel Dekker, New York, 1981:989–1067.

15 Lahuerta J, Buxton P, Lipton S, Bowsher D. The location and function of respiratory fibres in the second cervical spinal cord segment: respiratory dysfunction syndrome after cervical cordotomy. *J Neurol Neurosurg Psychiatry* 1992;55:1142–1145.

16 Severinghaus JW, Mitchell RA. Ondine's curse — failure of respiratory centre automaticity while asleep. *Clin Res* 1962;10:122.

17 Shea SA, Andres LP, Shannon DC, Banzett RB. Ventilatory responses to exercise in humans lacking ventilatory chemosensitivity. *J Physiol* 1993;468:623–640.

18 Munschauer FE, Mador MJ, Ahuja A, Jacobs L. Selective paralysis of voluntary but not limbically influenced automatic respiration. *Arch Neurol* 1990;48:1190–1192.

19 Krogh A, Lindhard J. The regulation of respiration and circulation during the initial stages of muscular work. *J Physiol* 1913;47:112–136.

20 Fink G, Adams L, Watson JDG. *et al*. Motor cortical activation in exercise-induced hyperpnoea in man; evidence for involvement of supra-brainstem structures in control of breathing. *J Physiol* 1993;473:58P.

21 Fink G, Adams L, Watson JDG *et al*. Hyperpnoea during and immediately after exercise in man: evidence of motor cortical involvement. *J Physiol* 1995; 489(3):663–675.

22 Fink BR. Influence of cerebral activity in wakefulness on regulation of breathing. *J Appl Physiol* 1961;16:15–20.

23 Datta AK, Shea SA, Horner RL, Guz A. The influence of induced hypocapnoea and sleep on the endogenous respiratory rhythm in humans. *J Physiol* 1991;440:17–33.

24 Adams L, Guz A. (eds) *Respiratory Sensation*, vol. 90. *Lung Biology in Health and Disease*. Marcel Dekker, New York, 1996.

25 Simon PM. Schwartsztein RM, Weiss JW, Fencl V, Teghtsoonian M, Weinberger SE. Distinguishable types of dyspnoea in patients with shortness of breath. *Am Rev Respir Dis* 1990;142:1009–1014.

26 Banzett RB, Lansing RW, Brown R *et al*. 'Air hunger' from increased P_{CO_2} persists after complete neuromuscular block in humans. *Respir Physiol* 1990;80:1–18.

27 Banzett RB, Lansing RW, Reid MB, Adams L, Brown R. Air hunger arising from increased P_{CO_2} in mechanically ventilated quadriplegics. *Respir Physiol* 1989;76:53–67.

28 Shea SA, Andres LP, Shannon DC, Guz A, Banzett RB. Respiratory sensations in subjects who lack a ventilatory response to CO_2. *Respir Physiol* 1993;93:203–219.

29 Chen Z, Eldridge FL, Wagner PG. Respiratory-associated thalamic activity is related to level of respiratory drive. *Respir Physiol* 1992;90:99–113.

30 Corfield DR, Fink JR, Ramsay SC *et al*. Evidence for limbic system activation during CO_2-stimulated breathing in man. *J Physiol* 1995;488(1):77–84.

Nitric oxide and the lung

TIM W. HIGENBOTTAM

The discovery of nitric oxide (NO·) and the L-arginine–citrulline pathway is one of the more remarkable and unexpected advances in biological science of recent times. The importance of the discovery of endothelial-derived relaxing factor (EDRF) by Robert Furchgott [1] was not realized in the 1980s until it became evident that EDRF was NO· [2,3].

Far from being limited to the endothelial cell the enzyme which elaborates NO·, called nitric oxide synthase (NOS), has been found in most cells of the body [4]. Subsequently NO· has been found to subserve many different physiological roles, and has a very early representation in animal evolution [5].

Three isoforms of NOS have been identified. Each has a separate gene and each is located on a different chromosome (see Table 1) [4]. These isoforms also differ in their need for Ca^{2+}. The Ca^{2+}-independent isoform, previously called inducible or iNOS has been found in most cells. Its expression can be induced by cytokines, but the same also appears true, although to a lesser degree, of the Ca^{2+}-dependent isoforms of NOS. The neural isoform of the enzyme is Ca^{2+}-dependent; it is abreviated to ncNOS. This was first identified in nerve cells but has now been found in epithelial and muscle cells. The endothelial isoform of the enzyme is also Ca^{2+}-dependent — ecNOS. It has also been found in other cell types (see Table 1).

The lungs, as with other organs, have a complex network of NO·-producing cells (Fig. 1). They differ in having an aqueous layer covering the lung epithelial surface, which has an enormous surface area. This surface is in contact with air. As NO· is a gas, it will partition across a gas–liquid interface. This provides a unique opportunity to measure NO· in the exhaled air. Also NO· can be delivered to the lung surface in the inhaled air. Unlike other organs, as a result of measurements of NO· in the exhaled air, the output of NO· from the various NOS-containing cells of the lungs can be assessed directly. Potentially inhaled NO· can be used as a treatment for certain lung diseases.

Table 1 Nitric oxide synthase nomenclature: c denotes dependence on Ca^{2+} whilst i denotes independence of elevated Ca^{2+}.

Number of isoform	Description	Definition	Location on the chromosomes	Tissue location
I	ncNOS	Ca^{2+}-dependent	12q24.2	Muscle Epithelium Neutrophils
II	iNOS	Ca^{2+}-independent	17cen–q12	All cells?
III	ecNOS	Ca^{2+}-dependent	7q35–36	Endothelium Neurons

THE PHYSICAL AND CHEMICAL PROPERTIES OF NITRIC OXIDE

Solubility

The partitioning of the gas between the liquid and gas phase depends upon the physical properties of the gas and the liquid. Therefore the behaviour of NO· in the lungs depends on its physical and chemical properties. NO· shares a similar degree of insolubility in water to oxygen (O_2; Table 2), being fourfold less soluble than carbon dioxide (CO_2) [6]. To understand the partitioning of NO· between lung tissue and the air spaces it is necessary to consider Henry's law, which states that the amount of gas in solution is proportional to the pressure of the gas above the liquid [7]. The Henry's constants for a number of physiological gases and water are shown in Table 3. In order to dissolve all the gaseous NO· in water, a pressure of over 33 000 atm is required. Normally only 1 atm is applied to the air space gases of the lungs. Under these conditions, only 3% of the NO· is likely to remain in an aqueous solution. The remaining 97% partitions to the gas phase.

As a small molecule, NO· is highly diffusible. The NO· diffusivity is proportional to the water-solubility divided by the square root of the molecular weight. It exceeds the diffusivity of CO by 1.8. Also NO· is relatively soluble in lipid — a property it shares with O_2 [8]. These properties allow NO· to pass easily through lung tissue.

Any NO· formed close to the air–liquid interface of the lungs is likely to enter the air space. Only a small amount will remain in the tissue or in solution in the aqueous liquid which lines the surfaces of the lungs. This makes it possible to detect NO· in the exhaled air. The concentration and rate of release of NO· into the exhaled air should reflect the amounts of NO· produced locally within the lungs.

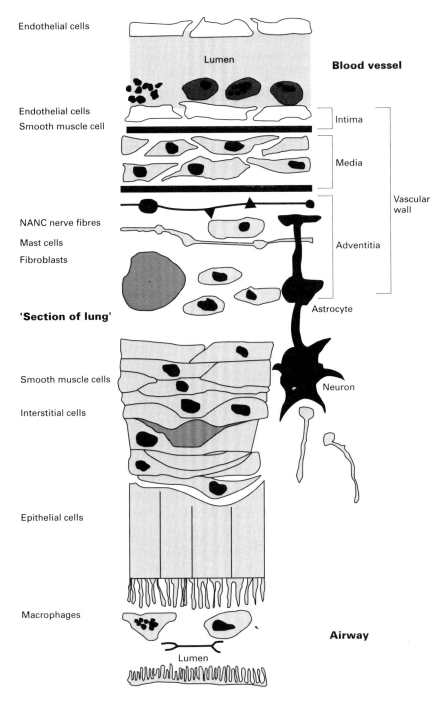

Fig. 1 Representation of the many different types of cell which potentially release nitric oxide in the lungs. NANC = Non-adrenergic non-cholinergic.

Table 2 The solubilities — Ostwald coefficients — of the gases of physiological interest in water at a close to normal temperature.

Temperature	CO_2	NO·	O_2	CO
35°C	0.6659	0.0420	0.0277	0.0211

Table 3 Henry's constant for common respiratory gases in the atmosphere.

Temperature	CO_2	NO·	O_2	CO
35°C	2096	33 200	50 301	66 269

Reaction with haemoglobin

A further property of NO· which determines its behaviour in the lungs is its affinity for haemoglobin (Hb). This property results from the ability of NO· to react with transitional metals such as iron II and iron III. With Hb, NO· combines with the iron II atom of the porphyrin ring of Hb. NO· has the fastest rate of reaction of all the ligands of Hb [9]. When it combines with HbO_2 there is no back-reaction. The products of this reaction are methaemoglobin (MetHb) and nitrate [10]. This contrasts with O_2 and carbon monoxide (CO), where the products of their reaction with haemoglobin, HbO_2 and COHb, are capable of dissociation back to the gas and haemoglobin. Compared with O_2, NO· has a sixfold greater affinity for Hb (Table 4).

The solubility of the gas NO· in physiological solutions can be studied with head-space equipment [11]. This approach has clearly illustrated the relative insolubility of NO· in water and in a crystalloid solution such as Krebs buffer. By contrast, NO· has greatly enhanced solubility in aqueus solutions which contain free Hb or red blood cells [12]. The rate of uptake of NO· from the gas phase of the head space into the blood or Hb solutions is fast, with a half-time of only 9 minutes, whilst little or no uptake occurs into aqueous solutions alone; half-times are in excess of 45 minutes [12].

From these observations it is possible to predict the behaviour of NO· in the air spaces of the lungs. NO· will not be greatly taken up from the airways into the aqueous lining fluid of the airway surface liquid. But

Table 4 The high affinity of nitric oxide (NO·) for the haemoglobin reflects in part the absence of a back-reaction by comparison with carbon monoxide (CO) and oxygen (O_2).

NO·	3×10^{-9} mol/l
CO	2×10^{-7} mol/l
O_2	6×10^{-4} mol/l

from those airspaces in close proximity to cells containing Hb, NO· will be rapidly taken up, for example, from the alveolar spaces into the capillaries containing circulating red blood cells. It is possible to predict that preferentially NO· will only minimally pass into the airway walls and will largely pass into the alveolar capillaries.

An alternative site of uptake in the lungs would be into those cells containing other haem-associated proteins. An example of this would be the reaction of NO· with the haem moiety of the soluble gaunylate cyclase enzyme of vascular smooth-muscle cells [13]. Soluble guanylate cyclase is activated by NO· to increase the intracellular concentration of cyclic guanosine monophosphate (cGMP). The second messenger cGMP causes relaxation and reduction of tone in the smooth-muscle cell [14]. The precapillary resistance arteries, which have muscular walls, are found in the region of the respiratory bronchioli and alveoli. The smooth-muscle cells of these arteries are within the same short diffusion distance for NO· as the alveolar capillaries.

Some years ago we were interested in exploiting the high affinity of NO· for Hb to measure gas diffusion in the lungs. It should be an equivalent to CO as a measure of transfer factor of the lung for CO (TLCO) but the greater affinity for Hb offers certain advantages. Like CO, NO· shares a high-affinity Hb and relative insolubility in the aqueous surface liquid of the airways [9]. The selective uptake of NO· in the alveoli was tested in humans by the inhalation of volumes of a gas mixture containing low concentrations of both NO· (80 parts per million (p.p.m.)) and CO (0.2%). We found that NO· and CO were absorbed in the lungs only when volumes of the gas mixture in excess of the volume of the physiological dead space were inhaled. That is, both gases were taken up close to the region of the alveoli when over a litre of the gas mixture was inhaled. It was found that, following a full inhalation of the gas mixture, the rate of uptake of NO· into the alveolar capillaries was 4.5 times faster than the uptake of CO [8,15]. These observations provided the basis for the first medical use of inhaled NO· as a measurement of TLNO, an equivalent measure of gas diffusion to the TLCO.

Oxidation of nitric oxide

Nitric oxide is a radical with an odd number of electrons (hence the NO· abreviation). The presence of an unpaired electron of NO· renders it susceptible to oxidation. Oxygen reacts with NO· to form nitrogen dioxide (NO_2) either in solution or in air at a rate dependent upon the concentration of NO·. It is a first-order reaction with respect to NO· [16]. This means that, at low concentrations of NO·, such as might be encountered in the body, either pico- or nanomolar, it is relatively unreactive. This is important when considering the use of inhaled NO· as a treatment, particularly as NO· is so insoluble in aqueous solutions. Even in higher concentrations of 80 p.p.m. in air, the half-time to produce 5 p.p.m. of NO_2 [17] is over 5 minutes. During quiet breathing the inhaled gases reside in the lungs for less than 4 seconds [18]. This allows insufficient time for oxidation of NO· at these concentrations.

THE NITRIC OXIDE PRODUCTION BY PULMONARY VASCULAR ENDOTHELIUM

The complexity of the network of NO·-producing cells in the lungs

The lung has a network of NO·-producing cells. It is difficult to separate to the individual role of the NO· produced by each cell type. The studies have required an integrated approach involving molecular and cellular biology, together with whole-organ physiology. A starting point has been the measurement of exhaled NO·.

Exhaled nitric oxide

Nitric oxide can be measured in the exhaled breath of both animals and humans [19,20]. Indeed, with a combination of a mass spectrometer and gas chromatography, the NO· molecule has been characterized in the exhaled breath [21]. In most studies NO· is measured by chemiluminescence [22]. This is a specific measurement and depends on the oxidation of NO· by ozone. The NO_2 so formed is in an excited electronic state which emits radiation (hv) between 600 and 300 nm and can be detected by a photomultiplier. The chemiluminescence measurement is sensitive down to concentrations as low as parts per billion (p.p.b.), equivalent to picomolar concentrations. The disadvantage of the currently available devices is their slowness of response — as slow as 2.5 seconds for a full-scale deflection in commonly used machines. This has effectively precluded in early work concurrent measurement of NO· concentration during breathing. Samples of exhaled gas need to be collected and then separately analysed [12].

Despite these limitations, it has proved possible to measure the rate of production of NO· in the lungs and to combine these measurements with studies of the effects of stimulating and inhibiting production of NO· in the pulmonary vascular bed.

The pulmonary vascular source of exhaled nitric oxide

There is now convincing evidence that pulmonary NO· is in part derived from the pulmonary vascular endothelium. The evidence is from the isolated perfused and ventilated lungs preparation. Large mammalian lungs can be so studied [23], including human lungs from transplant patients as well as lungs from sheep, pig and dog. The pulmonary circulation can be studied in isolation of the systemic circulation and separate from the cells of the upper airway and nose, which are also important sources of NO·.

The pulmonary vascular responses to a variety of vasoactive agents can be specifically studied by adding them to the perfusate solution of the isolated lung preparation, which flows only through the pulmonary circulation. The thromboxane analogue U46689 elevates the pulmonary vascular resistance (PVR) in all the mammalian species studied. Inhibition of the NOS of the endothelium is achieved by adding to the perfusate one of a number of analogues for L-arginine [24]. A popular one is L^G-nitroarginine methyl ester (L-NAME), used at a concentration of 10^{-7} mol/l. The Ca^{2+}-dependent NOS in endothelial cells is stimulated by acetylcholine (ACh), which acts on a muscarinic M_1 receptor found on the endothelial cell membrane. Concentrations of 10^{-7} mol/l in the perfusate are known to elicit NO·-dependent relaxation. These agents are added to the lung perfusate and so act only upon the vascular endothelium of pulmonary arteries, capillaries and veins.

Inhibition of endothelial NOS results in a fall in the exhaled NO· and a rise in the PVR (Table 5) [25]. The thromboxane analogue increases the PVR but fails to alter exhaled NO·. Subsequent addition of ACh (10^{-7} mol/l) to the perfusate dramatically increased the exhaled NO· and

Table 5 Exhaled nitric oxide (NO·) in isolated lungs — vasorelaxation and constriction.

n = 8	Baseline	Hypoxia	Baseline	U46619 (10^{-9} mol/l)	Acetylcholine (10^{-6} mol/l)
NO· concentration (p.p.b.)	5.8 ± 1.8	3.6 ± 1.8	5.9 ± 2.0	5.1 ± 1.9	7.0 ± 2.0
Molar rate of production of NO· (nmol/min)	1.81 ± 0.6	1.12 ± 0.6	1.84 ± 0.6	1.59 ± 0.6	2.18 ± 0.6
Pulmonary vascular resistance (mmHg/ml per kg per min)	0.39 ± 1.8	0.60 ± 0.1	0.26 ± 0.1	0.92 ± 0.2	0.64 ± 0.1

The results are shown for 8 pig lungs expressed as mean ± standard error. The exhaled concentration of NO· is given in parts per billion (p.p.b.) and the molar rate of production is expressed as nmol/min. Pulmonary vascular resistance is expressed as mmHg/ml per kg per min. All but the hypoxic ventilation, where fractional inspired oxygen concentration (Fio_2) was 5%, were studied at an Fio_2 of 21%.

lowered the PVR. This closely associates the production of NO· as measured in the exhaled NO· with the endothelium of the pulmonary vasculature. Changes in the PVR themselves do not affect NO· release.

The effects of alveolar hypoxia and blood perfusate on the exhaled nitric oxide

When the isolated lungs are ventilated with a fractional inspired O_2 concentration (Fio_2) of 10% (the normal value in air is 21%), there are changes in both exhaled NO· and the PVR. The increase of PVR is associated with a fall of the concentration of NO· in exhaled air from the lungs (Table 6). Exchanging a colloidal perfusate for one containing blood at a haematocrit of 9% reduced the exhaled NO· concentration in the exhaled air but left the PVR unchanged [25]. These data confirm that NO· is formed by the vascular endothelium. They suggest that NO· release by the pulmonary endothelial cells is also sensitive to the alveolar O_2 concentration. This may have particular importance to the regulation of blood flow in the lungs as the fall in NO· release with a low O_2 concentration, unlike that with a blood perfusate, was associated with a rise in the PVR.

Species differences in the role of pulmonary endothelial nitric oxide

It is unlikely that the role of NO· in the pulmonary vascular bed is the same in different mammalian species. Certainly, inhibition of NOS in the

Table 6 Action of inhibitors of nitric oxide (NO·) synthesis and action on exhaled NO·.

	A ($n = 4$)		B ($n = 4$)	
	Baseline	L-NAME (10^{-5} mol/l)	Baseline	Erythrocytes ($9 = 1\%$)
NO· concentration (p.p.b.)	5.5 ± 2.0	1.5 ± 1.0	5.6 ± 0.6	2.7 ± 0.5
Molar rate of production of NO· (nmol/min)	1.72 ± 0.3	0.47 ± 0.3	1.75 ± 0.1	0.84 ± 0.1
Pulmonary vascular resistance (mmHg/ml per kg per min)	0.25 ± 0.1	1.25 ± 0.2	0.28 ± 0.1	0.32 ± 0.1

The results are shown for A, the addition of NO· synthase inhibitor N^G-nitro-L-arginine methyl ester (L-NAME) in 4 lungs and B, the addition of autologous blood in 4 lungs. All were ventilated with a fractional inspired concentration (Fio_2) of 21%. The mean $\pm$ standard deviations are given. NO· is expressed in parts per billion (p.p.b.); molar rate of production is expressed as nmol/min and pulmonary vascular resistance is expressed in mmHg/ml per min per kg.

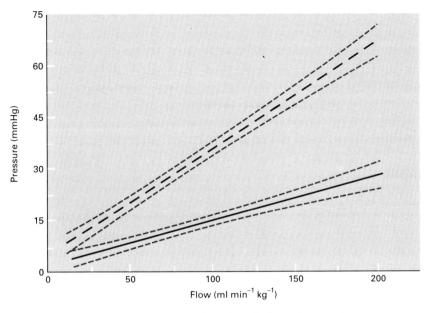

Fig. 2 Changes in pressure–flow relationships after L^G-nitroarginine methyl ester (L-NAME) in isolated human donor lungs ($n = 4$) perfused with Krebs–dextran solution. Mean pressure–flow lines in isolated lungs before (solid line) and after (dashed line) L-NAME (10^{-5} mol/l). Dotted lines show 95% confidence limits.

pulmonary vasculature has varying effects in the different species [23]. In humans (Fig. 2), pigs (Fig. 3) and sheep (Fig. 4), the addition of L-NAME to the perfusate of isolated lungs increases PVR, as shown by a change in the relationship between pressure and flow. In the dog lung (Fig. 5) this is not the case; the relationship between pulmonary blood flow and perfusion pressure is unchanged. The same has also been reported in the rat [26]. There is no physiological explanation for these differences in the role of pulmonary endothelium NO· but it is likely to be a result of differences in the adaptation of the pulmonary circulation to increased blood flow.

The nitric oxide release in pulmonary hypertension

Studies making use of the dissected pulmonary arteries in an organ bath have shown that arteries from patients with hypoxic lung disease have impairment of the stimulated release of NO· with agents such as ACh [27]. This is not the result of substrate deficiency of the endothelial NOS [28]. Again, making use of explanted lungs from patients undergoing heart–lung transplantation and the isolated perfused and ventilated lung assembly, it has proved possible to show that the same is true in the whole lung [29].

First the PVR was elevated by addition of the thromboxane analogue A46689 to the perfusate. ACh was then added until a maximal relaxation

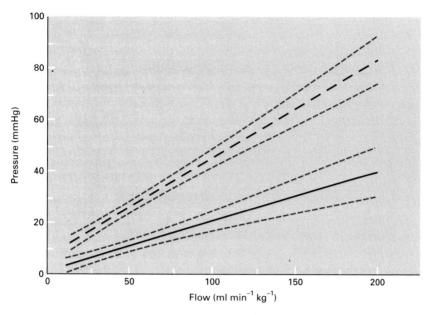

Fig. 3 Changes in pressure–flow relationships after L^G-nitroarginine methyl ester (L-NAME) in isolated pig lungs (*n* = 6) perfused with Krebs-dextran solution. Symbols as in Fig. 2.

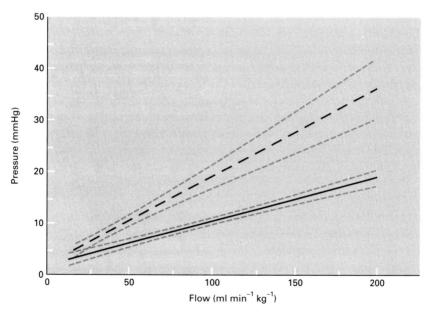

Fig. 4 Changes in pressure–flow relationships after L^G-nitroarginine methyl ester (L-NAME) in isolated sheep lungs (*n* = 4) perfused with Krebs-dextran solution. Symbols as in Fig. 2.

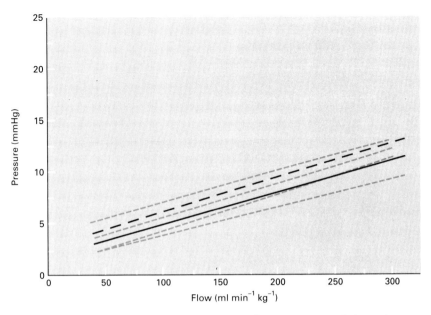

Fig. 5 Changes in pressure–flow relationships after L^G-nitroarginine methyl ester (L-NAME) in isolated dog lungs ($n = 3$) perfused with Krebs-dextran solution. Symbols as in Fig. 2.

was achieved. The degree of relaxation was less in the lungs from the patients with chronic obstructed lung disease and hypoxia than in lungs which were relatively normal. The latter were donor lungs not used in transplantation. Lungs from patients with severe pulmonary hypertension also responded to ACh, but not so well as the normal lungs (Fig. 6).

At present there is no mechanism to account for this impairment of stimulated release of NO· but there may be parallels with the effects of acute hypoxia on the activity of NOS. This will be described later when the mechanism of hypoxic vasoconstriction is discussed.

Whilst there is evidence that chronic hypoxia can impair the stimulated release of NO· from the pulmonary endothelium, the basal release of NO· appears normal in pulmonary hypertension.

When L-NAME (10^{-5} mol/l) was added to the perfusate of the isolated lungs under basal conditions, the PVR rose by a similar amount in the lungs from hypoxaemic patients, those with severe pulmonary hypertension as well as those from normal donor lungs (Fig. 7).

The regional differences in endothelial production of nitric oxide in the lungs

The functional production of NO· by pulmonary endothelium shows large regional differences. The study of this has been difficult and to date has

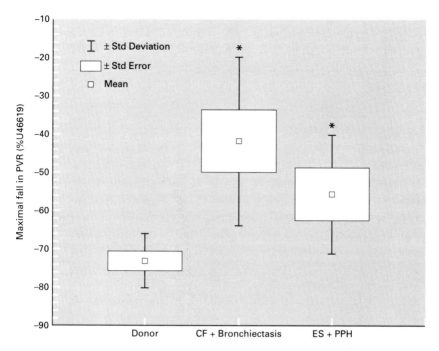

Fig. 6 The maximal change in pulmonary vascular resistance (PVR) after treatment with acetylcholine (10^{-9} to 10^{-5} mol/l) in lungs from donors. CF/bronchiectasis and primary pulmonary hypertension/ES patients perfused with Krebs-dextran solution and preconstricted with U46619.

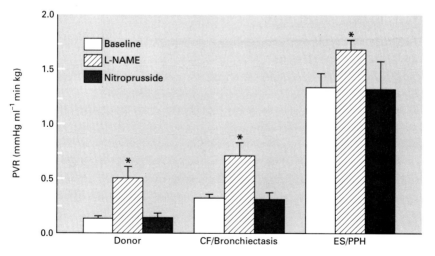

Fig. 7 The maximal change in pulmonary vascular resistance (PVR) in lungs from donors, cystic fibrosis (CF)/bronchiectasis and primary pulmonary hypertension/ES patients perfused with Krebs–dextran solution and treated with U46619 (10^{-5} mol/l) and subsequently with sodium nitroprusside 10^{-5} mol/l. * Significant difference from initial level.

largely depended on demonstrating that inhibition of endothelial NOS causes a non-uniform change in the resistance of flow and the compliance of the pulmonary circulation. Again, the isolated lung preparation has been utilized, but with the addition of a further technique — the arterial, venous and double occlusion technique which was first described by Hakim et al. in the dog [30]. From the records of the changes in pressure after occlusion it proved possible to determine the resistance of different segments of the pulmonary circulation. From this it is possible to measure the resistance of pulmonary arteries, pulmonary veins and from the pre- and postcapillary vessels.

Inhibition of endothelial NOS causes a rise in resistance only in the arterial and precapillary arteries (Fig. 8) [31]. Little or no change occurs in the resistance to flow in the venous segments. These effects can be reversed by addition of sodium nitroprusside (10^{-7} mol/l) to the perfusate. Inhalation of a gas mixture containing 40 p.p.m. of $NO\cdot$ reverses the effects of inhibition of NOS in the pulmonary arteries. This supports the notion that inhaled $NO\cdot$ not only is taken up into the alveolar capillaries but enters the vascular smooth-muscle cells to cause relaxation. The overall view is that only the endothelium of the arterial segments of the pulmonary circulation is producing $NO\cdot$ in functionally active levels.

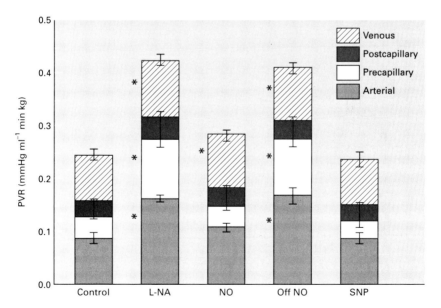

Fig. 8 Effect of N^G-nitro-L-arginine (10^{-5} mol/l) and subsequent inhaled nitric oxide (NO; 80 p.p.m.) and sodium nitroprusside (SRIP) on the segmental pulmonary vascular resistance measured by occlusion technique. After termination of ventilation with NO, resistance returned to the elevated levels caused by N^G-nitro-L-arginine, and this was taken as a second baseline. * Significant differences from control.

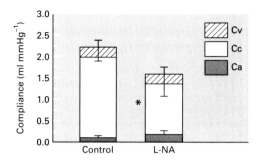

Fig. 9 Effect of N^G-nitro-L-arginine (L-NA; 10^{-5} mol/l) on the compliance of the arterial (Ca), capillary (Cc) and venous (Cv) compartments estimated by non-linear regression according to the 2R3C model. * Significant differences from control.

The distribution of perfusion of the capillary bed of the lungs is determined not only by the resistance of flow in the arteries but also by the compliance of the alveolar capillaries [32]. The occlusion technique of measurement can be applied to study the compliance of arteries, veins and the central segment, made up principally by the alveolar capillaries and the pre-capillary arteries and postcapillary veins [33]. Addition of the NOS inhibitor again showed inhomogeneity in the changes in compliance. Strikingly, the compliance of the central segment, including the alveolar capillaries falls to a greater degree than the other segments (Fig. 9).

This offers a further insight into the potential role of endothelial NO· in the lung. Pulmonary NO· production falls with alveolar hypoxia (Table 6). The change in PVR is principally achieved in the resistance arteries, pulmonary muscular arteries and the precapillary arteries. These are precisely the vessels concerned with the distribution of pulmonary perfusion. The fall in NO· production is likely also to reduce the compliance of the capillaries. A powerful mechanism is therefore provided which responds to hypoxia and can divert blood flow away from such a region. In other words, the endothelial NO· system of the lungs offers a complementary system to hypoxic vasoconstriction in ensuring the matching of the distribution of ventilation and perfusion (V_A/Q).

Hypoxic pulmonary vasoconstriction

In order to understand the relationship between a potential mechanism of NO· regulation of V_A/Q matching and hypoxic vasoconstriction, it is necessary to consider in detail the cellular effects of a reduction of alveolar O_2 tension. Characteristically, a low alveolar O_2 affects only the small pulmonary arteries of diameters of less than 300 μm. These arteries undergo constriction with hypoxia [34]. Larger pulmonary arteries and systemic arteries vasodilate as the O_2 tension falls. There is again no uniformity in the hypoxic pulmonary vasoconstriction in the different animal species. Dogs show the least vasoconstriction whilst ferrets show the most [35].

In the isolated porcine lung preparation alveolar hypoxia causes increased resistance mainly in the precapillary arteries; larger arteries and veins do not undergo vasoconstriction (Fig. 10). The same is true in other species. Presently it is thought that the low partial pressure of O_2 acts directly on the vascular smooth-muscle cell. There is now evidence that the Ca^{2+}-dependent K^+ channel of the smooth-muscle cell is inhibited by hypoxia. This in turn causes depolarization of the cell membrane and subsequent smooth-muscle contraction [36]. This effect is quite separate from the action of hypoxia on pulmonary endothelial NOS. Both arterial and precapillary arterial segments of the pulmonary circulation are affected by a low alveolar O_2 tension. The resistance to flow increases in both these segments, whereas only the precapillary segment is affected by hypoxia alone. The difference in the location of the effects of NO· mechanism and the direct hypoxia effects suggest potentially separate roles for these two systems.

A further observation which draws a parallel between the pulmonary endothelial NO· system and the hypoxic vasoconstriction mechanism is that NO· also acts on the Ca^{2+}-dependent K^+ channel of vascular smooth-muscle cells. NO· opens this channel, causing vasorelaxation by a separate mechanism from the activation of soluble guanylate cyclase [37].

There is still some uncertainty as to the molecular mechanism by which hypoxia affects the endothelial NOS. The effects of hypoxia on NOS are not confined to the lungs. Hypoxia causes a fall in NO· production by cultured endothelial cells [38]. In the corpus cavernosum hypoxia causes a marked fall in NO· release [39]. Penile erection depends upon an increased release of NO·, leading to blood filling the corpus cavernosum and consequent increased turgor [40]. To prevent sustained erection and priapism the increased release of NO· needs to be reduced. Hypoxia is probably the release mechanism; in static blood the O_2 tension falls and this is associated with a fall in NO· release.

The rate of production of messenger RNA for the endothelial NOS is not reduced in culture by hypoxia [41]. It is more probable that hypoxia exerts its effect through an alteration in the activity of the enzyme. One

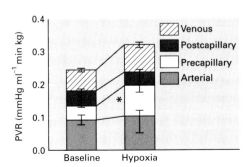

Fig. 10 Effect of ventilation with 5% oxygen, 90% nitrogen and 5% carbon dioxide on the segmental pulmonary vascular resistance measured by the occlusion technique. * Significant differences from control.

potential mechanism is the energy-dependent phosphorylation of the inactive form of NOS, which allows endothelial NOS to be activated through calcium-calmodulin [42].

INHALED NITRIC OXIDE TREATMENT

Cigarette smoking and inhaled NO·

Since the 1880s a significant proportion of the population have been inhaling quantities of NO·. In the UK cigarettes contain up to 200 p.p.m. of NO· per puff of smoke [43]. Cigarettes containing tobacco leaves with high nitrate content deliver much higher concentrations of NO· in the smoke compared with UK cigarettes; some USA brands may have levels as high as 1000 p.p.m.

The NO· yields of cigarettes appear not to contribute significantly to the excess mortality seen in cigarette smokers for diseases like carcinoma of the lung, chronic obstructive bronchitis and ischaemic heart disease. The UK, which has lower cigarette yields of NO· than the USA and France, has by far the higher mortality rates for these diseases [43]. More likely candidates to cause disease in cigarette smoke are the polycyclic aromatic hydrocarbons and possibly other volatiles in the smoke.

Inhaled cigarette smoke has been shown to be able to reduce the PVR in smokers with lung disease. This has been shown to be the result of the NO· in the cigarette smoke [44].

Inhaled nitric oxide — early observations on toxicology

When inhaled in concentrations as low as 40–80 p.p.m., little or none of the gas is taken up by the lung until it reaches the small airways [8,15]. At these concentrations long-term exposure studies reveal no evidence of lung injury [45]. Indeed, it would appear that the NO· is taken up largely by its reaction with HbO_2. MetHb is the main product, with nitrate formation [10]. The rapid rate of uptake in the region of the alveoli and bronchioli, together with the short residence time of inhaled gases during quiet breathing, precludes significant formation of NO_2. As described earlier, the rate of oxidation of NO· by O_2 depends upon the concentration of NO·. As a result the reaction for low concentration of NO· proceeds very slowly, even in high O_2 concentrations.

Inhaled nitric oxide — a selective vasodilator

The first study of the effects of inhaled NO· was undertaken in normal subjects and studies of the haemodynamics were performed in patients with cardiac disease and patients with severe primary pulmonary hypertension (PPH). A comparison was made between the inhalation of low

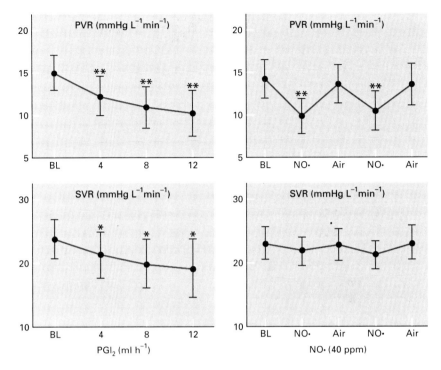

Fig. 11 The haemodynamic effects of infused prostacyclin (PGI_2) and inhaled nitric oxide (NO·). Comparison of the effects on pulmonary (PVR) and systemic vascular resistance (SVR) of an intravenous infusion of PGI_2 (0.5 mg in 250 ml) at rates of 4, 8, 12 ml/h, and the inhalation of NO· (40 p.p.m. in air) with baseline (BL) values in 8 patients with pulmonary hypertension. Means and s.e.m. are shown. * $P < 0.05$; ** $P < 0.01$. With permission from [47].

concentrations of 80 p.p.m. of NO· in air and an intravenous infusion of prostacyclin (PGI_2), a powerful short-acting vasodilator [46].

It was found that NO· acted as a selective pulmonary vasodilator [47]. There was in the PPH patients a significant fall in the PVR, equivalent to the effects of the maximum dose of PGI_2 (Fig. 11). By contrast to PGI_2, there was no fall in systemic vascular resistance. It is inferred that any NO· not acting on the vascular smooth muscle of resistance pulmonary arteries will be taken up in the alveolar capillaries to react with HbO_2. The MetHb so formed no longer has any capacity to cause vasorelaxation in the systemic circulation, so confining the effects of inhaled NO· to the pulmonary circulation.

Clinical uses of inhaled nitric oxide

Given the apparent absence of toxicity of inhaled NO· (in low concentrations) and the selective nature of the vasodilation it causes, clinical use rapidly followed the early experimental observations.

Infantile pulmonary hypertension has a poor prognosis and many patients are currently managed with extracorporeal membrane oxygenation (ECMO). Inhaled NO· was tried in severely afflicted patients [48]. Not only was the PVR reduced but there was also a marked improvement in the arterial O_2 tension. This was affected through the reduction of right-to-left shunting through the patent ductus arteriosus associated with the fall in PVR. Further studies have confirmed these findings and as a result ECMO is no longer considered unless inhaled NO· has failed. This has led to substantive cost savings in the care of these severely ill patients. Other groups of infants with pulmonary hypertension have also benefited from inhaled NO·, for example, those who have undergone cardiac surgery and are susceptible to highly variable PVR in the postoperative period.

Acute respiratory distress syndrome (ARDS) can also be associated with an elevated PVR. More importantly, there is often a marked mismatch of the distribution of V_A/Q. There are large areas of the lung with right-to-left shunting of pulmonary blood flow and in others there are areas of low V_A/Q. In theory, inhaled NO· will not reach these areas of the lungs. It will be distributed to the well-ventilated areas and in these, perfusion will increase. The shunt fraction is then reduced by what is thought to be a steal phenomenon [49]. An early study of ARDS has confirmed this and has led to enhanced survival of the treated patients [61]. Large-scale randomized controlled studies are now in progress to assess the relative efficacy of inhaled NO· compared with standard treatments.

Besides acting on the vascular smooth-muscle cells, inhaled NO· has been shown to reduce experimentally induced bronchoconstriction [50]. In humans NO· has some bronchodilating actions [51]. This is a further area where inhaled NO· may have a role in treatment. However, inhaled NO· can lead to a fall in the arterial O_2 in some patients with chronic obstructive lung disease [52]. Further experimental work is needed before inhaled NO· is advised for patients with airways disease.

AIRWAY PRODUCTION OF NITRIC OXIDE

The focus of this review has been the pulmonary vasculature. However, the other cellular sources of NO· are also very important in pulmonary function in health and disease.

Nitric oxide production by cells of the airways

There is strong experimental evidence that airway nerve cells produce NO·. This NO· is considered important in lowering airway smooth-muscle tone. Diseases such as viral bronchitis reduce airway NO· production. This has been suggested as a cause of the enhanced bronchial hyper-reactivity in these conditions [53]. It is not known whether this is true in humans. But there is certainly non-adrenergic non-cholinergic (NANC) nerves in human airways which release NO· [54].

Asthma patients have been shown to have inducible, Ca^{2+}-independent NOS, expressed in the airway epithelial cells [55]. This may be allergen-induced NOS expression [56].

Perhaps of greater importance for the physiology of the NO· system in the lung is the observation that it contributes to the regulation of bronchial blood flow. The increase in blood flow to the tracheal mucosa which occurs when the epithelial surface is exposed to hypertonic saline can be blocked by the NOS inhibitor L-NAME [57]. It has been proposed that the bronchial blood flow is similarly regulated, through a signalling pathway from epithelium to the NO· producing cells. This may have considerable importance in determining airway responses to inhaled irritants.

Nasal production of nitric oxide

Measurement of exhaled NO· in asthmatics and in patients on assisted ventilation has shown that the nose produces larger amounts of NO· than the lower airways [58,59], although certain bacteria, including *Pseudomonas aeroginosa*, contain the denitrificans enzymes which reduce nitrates and nitrites to NO· [60].

However the nasal NO· production is reduced by topical application of the NOS inhibitor L-NAME to nasal mucosa [61]. The role of this NO· released by the nasal mucosa is not known, but could represent a regulating system akin to the bronchial mucosal blood flow. The nasal turbinates swell intermittently to regulate the process of humidification and warming of the inhaled air. Other workers have suggested that iNOS is responsible for nasal NO· [62]. There is still much to learn in this important area of physiology.

CONCLUSION

An integreted approach to the NO·-producing cells of the lungs, involving standard physiological methods, cellular studies and molecular techniques, has uncovered a surprising number of roles for NO· in the lungs. Uniquely, a new treatment of lung disease has emerged from these studies — inhaled NO·. Potentially, others are sure to emerge, as we learn more about the cellular mechanisms of control of NO· production.

REFERENCES

1 Furchgott RF, Zawadski JV. The obligatory role of endothelial cells in the relaxation of arterial smooth muscle by acetylcholine. *Nature* 1980;**288**:373–376.
2 Palmer RM, Ferrige AG, Moncada S. Nitric oxide release accounts for the biological activity of endothelium-derived relaxing factor. *Nature* 1987;**327**:524–526.

3 Feelisch M, te-Poel M, Zamra R et al. Understanding the controversy over the identity of EDRF. Nature 1994;**368**:62–65.

4 Nathan C, Xie Q-W. Nitric oxide synthases: roles, tolls and controls. Cell 1994;**78**:915–918.

5 Gelperin A. Nitric oxide mediates network oscillations of the olfactory interneurons in a terrestrial mollusc. Nature 1994;**369**:61–63.

6 Steward A, Allott PR, Cowles AL, Mapleson WW. Solubility coefficients for inhaled anaesthetics for water, oil and biological media. Br J Anaesth 1973;**45**:282–293.

7 Gerrard W. Gas Solubilities: Widespread Applications. Pergamon Press, Oxford, 1980:347.

8 Borland CDR, Higenbottam TW. A simultaneous single breath measurement of pulmonary diffusing capacity with nitric oxide and carbon monoxide. Eur Respir J 1989;**2**:56–63.

9 Olsen JS. Stopped-flow, rapid mixing measurements of ligand binding to haemoglobin and red cells. Methods Enzymol 1981;**76**:631–704.

10 Wennmalm A, Benthin G, Petersson A-S. Dependence of the metabolism of nitric oxide (NO) in healthy human whole blood on the oxygenation of its red cell haemoglobin. Br J Pharmacol 1992;**106**:507–508.

11 Chung S-J, Fun H-L. Identification of the subcellular site for nitroglycerin metabolism to nitric oxide in bovine coronary smooth muscle cells. J Pharmacol Exp Ther 1990;**253**:614–619.

12 Demoncheaux EAG, Maniscalo M, Roe S, Cremona G, Higenbottam T. Exhaled NO, ideas on its origin and physiological meaning. In: Nitric Oxide and Oxygen Radicals in the Pulmonary Vasculature, edited by Weir EK, Archer S, Reeves J. Fortuna, New York, 1995.

13 Ignarro LJ, Harbison RG, Wood KS, Kadowitz PJ. Activation of purified soluble guanylate cyclase by endothelium-derived relaxing factor from intrapulmonary artery and vein: stimulation by acetylcholine, bradykinin and arachidonic acid. J Pharmacol Exp Ther 1986;**237**:893–900.

14 Ignarro LJ. Haem-dependent activation of guanylate cyclase and cyclic GMP formation by endogenous nitric oxide: a unique transduction mechanism for transcellular signaling. Pharmacol Toxicol 1990;**67**:1–7.

15 Moinard J, Guenard H. Determination of lung capillary blood volume and membrane diffusing capacity in patients with COLD using the NO-CO method. Eur Respir J 1990;**3**:318–322.

16 Wink DA, Darbyshire JF, Nims RW, Saavedra JE, Ford PC. Reactions of the bioregulatory agent nitric oxide in oxygenated aqueous media. Chem Res Toxicol 1993;**6**:23–27.

17 Centers for Disease Control. Recommendations for occupational safety and health standard. MMWR 1988;**37**:(suppl):21.

18 Lugliana R, Whipp BJ, Seard C, Wasserman K. Effects of carotid body resection on the ventilatory control at rest and during exercise in man N Engl J Med 1971;**285**:1105–1111.

19 Gustafsson LE, Leone AM, Persson MG et al. Endogenous NO is present in the exhaled air of rabbits, guinea pigs and humans. Biochem Biophys Res Commun 1991;**181**:852–857.

20 Borland C, Cox Y, Higenbottam T. Measurement of exhaled nitric oxide in man. Thorax 1993;**48**:1160–1162.

21 Leone AM, Gustafsson LE, Francis PL et al. Nitric oxide is present in exhaled breath in humans: direct gc-ms confirmation. Biochem Biophys Res Commun 1994;**201**:883–887.

22 Clyne MAA, Thrush BA, Wayne RP. Kinetics of the chemiluminescent reaction between nitric oxide and ozone. Trans Faraday Soc 1964;**60**:359–370.

23 Cremona G, Wood AM, Hall LW, Bower LW, Higenbottam T. Effects of inhibitors of nitric oxide release and actions on vascular tone in isolated lungs. J Physiol 1994;**48**:185–195.

24 Rees DD, Palmer RM, Schultz R, Hodson HF, Moncada S. Characteristics of three inhibitors of endothelial nitric oxide synthase in vitro and in vivo. Br J Pharmacol 1990;**101**:746–752.

25 Cremona G, Higenbottam TW, Takao M, Hall L, Bower E. Exhaled nitric oxide in isolated pig lung. J Appl Physiol 1995;**78**:59–63.

26 Barer G, Emery C, Stewart A, Bee D, Howard P. Endothelial control of the pulmonary circulation in normal and chronically hypoxic rats. *J Physiol* 1993;**463**:1–16.

27 Dinh Xaun AT, Higenbottam TW, Clelland CA *et al.* Impairment of endothelium-dependent relaxation in chronic obstructive lung disease. *N Engl J Med* 1991;**324**:1539–1547.

28 Dinh Xaun AT, Pepke-Zaba J, Butt AY, Cremona G, Higenbottam TW. Impairment of pulmonary artery endothelium-dependent relaxation in chronic obstructive lung disease is not due to dysfunction of the endothelial cell membrane receptors nor to L-arginine deficiency. *Br J Pharmacol* 1993;**109**:587–591.

29 Cremona G, Higenbottam TW, Wood AM *et al.* Pulmonary endothelial nitric oxide release in isolated human lungs. *Am J Respir Crit Care* 1996; (in press).

30 Hakim TS, Michel RP, Chang HK. Partitioning of pulmonary vascular resistance by arterial and venous occlusion. *J Appl Physiol* 1982;**52**:710–715.

31 Cremona G, Takao M, Bower EA, Hall LW, Higenbottam T. The effects of hypoxia, inhaled nitric oxide and endothelial nitric oxide on the total and segmental vascular resistance of isolated pig lungs. *J Appl Physiol* 1996; (in press).

32 Overholser KA, Lomongino NA, Parker RE, Pou NA, Harris TR. Pulmonary vascular resistance distribution and the recruitment of microvascular surface area. *J Appl Physiol* 1994;**77**:845–855.

33 Linehan JH, Dawson CA, Rickaby DA. Distribution of vascular resistance and compliance in a dog lung lobe. *J Appl Physiol* 1982;**53**:158–168.

34 Madden JA, Dawson CA, Harden DR. Hypoxia-induced activation in small isolated pulmonary arteries from the cat. *J Appl Physiol* 1985;**59**:113–118.

35 Peake MD, Harabin AL, Brennan NJ, Sylvester JT. Steady-state vascular responses to graded hypoxia in isolated lungs of five species. *J Appl Physiol* 1981;**51**:1214–1219.

36 Post JM, Hume JR, Archer SL, Wier EK. Direct role for potassium channel inhibition in hypoxic pulmonary vasoconstriction. *Am J Physiol* 1992;**262**:C882–C892.

37 Bolotina VM, Najibi S, Palacino PJ, Cohen RA. Nitric oxide directly activates calcium-dependent potassium channels in vascular smooth muscle. *Nature* 1994;**368**:850–853.

38 Shaul PW, Wells LB. Oxygen modulates nitric oxide production selectively in fetal pulmonary endothelial cells. *Am J Respir Cell Mol Biol* 1994;**11**:432–438.

39 Kim N, Vardi Y, Padma-Nathan H, Daley J, Goldstein I, Saenz de Tejada I. Oxygen tension regulates the nitric oxide pathway. *J Clin Invest* 1993;**91**:437–442.

40 Rajfer J, Aronson WJ, Bush PA, Dorey FJ, Ignarro LJ. Nitric oxide as a mediator of relaxation of the corpus cavernosum in response to nonadrenergic, noncholinergic neurotransmission. *N Engl J Med* 1992;**326**:90–94.

41 Smith APL, Higenbottam TW, Pepke-Zaba J, Ahmed I, Kealey T. Chronic hypoxia appears not to reduce the expression of mRNA for endothelial nitric oxide synthase (cNOS). *Am J Respir Crit Care Med* 1994;**149**:A26.

42 Michel T, Li GK, Busconi L. Phosphorylation and subcellular translocation of endothelial nitric oxide synthase. *Proc Natl Acad Sci* 1993;**90**:6252–6256.

43 Borland C, Higenbottam TW. Nitric oxide yields of contemporary UK, US and French cigarettes. *Int J Epidemiol* 1987;**16**:31–34.

44 Skwarski KM, Gorecka D, Sliwinski P, Hogg J, Macnee W. The effects of cigarette smoking on pulmonary hemodynamics. *Chest* 1993;**103**:1166–1172.

45 Hugod C. Effects of exposure to 43 ppm nitric oxide and 3.6 ppm nitrogen dioxide on rabbit lung. *Int Arch Occup Health* 1979;**42**:159–167.

46 Higenbottam TW, Spiegelhalter D, Scott JP *et al.* The value of prostacyclin (epoprostenol) and heart–lung transplantation as a treatment for severe pulmonary hypertension. *Br Heart J* 1993;**70**:366–370.

47 Pepke-Zaba J, Higenbottam TW, Dinh-Xaun AT *et al.* Inhaled nitric oxide as a cause of selective pulmonary vasodilatation in pulmonary hypertension. *Lancet* 1991;**338**:1173–1174.

48 Kinsella JP, Neish SR, Shaffer E, Abman SH. Low-dose inhalational nitric oxide in persistent pulmonary hypertension of the new born. *Lancet* 1992;**340**:819–820.

49 Rossiant R, Falke KJ, Lopez F, Slama K, Pison U, Zapol WM. Inhaled nitric oxide for the adult respiratory distress syndrome. *N Engl J Med* 1993;**328**:399–405.

50 Dupuy PM, Shore SA, Drazen JM, Frostell C, Hill WA, Zapol WM. Bronchodilator action of inhaled nitric oxide in guinea pigs. *J Clin Invest* 1992;**90**:421–428.

51 Sanna A, Kurtansky A, Veriter C, Stanescu D. Bronchodilator effect of inhaled nitric oxide in healthy man. *Am J Respir Crit Care Med* 1994;**150**:1702–1713.

52 Katyama Y, Atuara MJ, Cremona G *et al.* The effect of inhaled nitric oxide on gas exchange in patients with chronic obstructive disease and severe pulmonary hypertension. *Am J Respir Crit Care Med* 1995;**151**:A784.

53 Folkerts G, van der Linde H, Nijkamps FP. Nitric oxide deficiency and virus-induced airway hyperresponsiveness in guinea pigs. *Eur Respir J* 1994;**7**(suppl 18):157s.

54 Belvisi MG, Streetton CD, Yacoub M, Barnes PJ. Nitric oxide is the endogenous neurotransmitter of bronchodilator nerves in humans. *Eur J Pharmacol* 1992;**210**:221–222.

55 Hamid Q, Springall DR, Riveros-mereno V *et al.* Induction of nitric oxide synthase in asthma. *Lancet* 1993;**342**:1510–1513.

56 Persson MG, Gustafsson LE. Allergen-induced airway obstruction in guinea-pig is associated with changes in nitric oxide levels in exhaled air. *Acta Physiol Scand* 1993;**149**:461–466.

57 Smith TL, Prazma J, Coleman CC *et al.* Control of mucosal microcirculation in the upper respiratory tract. *Oto Laryngol Head Neck Surg* 1993;**109**:646–652.

58 Lundberg JON, Weitzberg E, Nordvall SL *et al.* Primary nasal origin of exhaled nitric oxide and absence in Kartagener's syndrome. *Eur Respir J* 1994;**7**:1501–1504.

59 Gerlach H, Rossiant R, Pappert D *et al.* Auto-inhalation of nitric oxide after endogenous synthesis in the nasopharynx. *Lancet* 1994;**343**:518–519.

60 Cannons AC, Barber MJ, Solomonson LP. Expression and characterisation of the heme-binding domain of chlorella nitrate reductase. *J Biol Chem* 1993;**268**:3268–3271.

61 Maniscalco M, Roe S, Chaquoat A, Demoncheaux E, Higenbottam T. Nitric oxide production in the nasal cavity-reversible inhibition by L-NAME. *Am J Respir Crit Care Med* 1995;**151**:A103.

62 Lundberg JON, Rinder J, Weitzberg E, Lundberg JM. Nitric oxide found in the nasal cavity air is produced in the paranasal sinuses. *Am J Respir Crit Care Med* 1995;**151**:A127.

Asthma: a disease of inflammation and repair

STEPHEN T. HOLGATE

THE HEALTH AND ECONOMIC BURDEN OF ASTHMA

Statistics worldwide indicate that the prevalence of asthma continues to increase and the UK is no exception. However, the major health burden of asthma relates to severe, chronic and relapsing disease. The recent World Health Organization (WHO)/National Heart, Lung and Blood Institute (NHLBI) *Technical Report on a Global Strategy for Asthma* describes severe persistent asthma as frequent or continuous daily symptoms despite treatment; frequent sleep disturbance on account of asthma; severe physical and other lifestyle limitations; peak expiratory flow (PEF) or forced expiratory volume in 1 second (FEV_1) < 60% predicted and within- and between-day variability of PEF > 30% [1]. Much of the mortality and some of the morbidity of asthma results from underestimation of disease severity by patient and doctor, inadequate action at the onset of deterioration and undertreatment. However, there remain many patients who receive antiasthma drugs in large doses and yet remain symptomatic. The clinical phenotype of such patients is often complex and varied, with no single pattern dominating.

Cost of illness for adult asthma analysed by disease severity reveals a disproportionate use of medical resources by patients with severe disease. In Canada, severe asthma comprised 10% of the asthma population and accounted for 51% of all direct medical care costs and 54% of total asthma costs [2]. Patients with severe disease were three times more likely to consult an asthma specialist, 15 times more likely to use an accident and emergency department and 19 times more likely to require hospitalization. In Australia, severe asthma comprises 6% of the adult asthma population and consumes 47% of the total annual costs for this disease — an estimate similar to that for the UK. Thus, on the grounds of unsatisfactory treatment, life quality and health economics, there is a strong case for focusing attention on this group of asthma patients.

CYTOKINE AND MEDIATOR NETWORKS AS THE BASIS OF ASTHMA

Asthma is a multifactorial disease that spans the full spectrum of activity from mild seasonal symptoms to being severe and intractable. When classifying asthma by severity, the majority falls into the mild-to-moderate range and can be managed well with currently available drugs. It is also this end of the disease spectrum and in those with atopy that most of our understanding of inflammatory and mediator mechanisms of asthma has been based. Application of immunohistochemistry (IHC), *in situ* hybridization (ISH) and reverse transcription polymerase chain reaction (rt-PCR) to lavage cells, mucosal biopsies and T cells from the airways of such patients reveals up-regulation of the interleukin-4 (IL-4) gene cluster (IL-4, IL-13, IL5, IL-3, IL-6, granulocyte-macrophage colony-stimulating factor (GM-CSF), IL-9) in T cells, mast cells and eosinophils. These cytokines are of crucial importance in the initiation and maintenance of the allergic inflammatory response through isotype switching of B cells to immunoglobulin E (IgE) synthesis (IL-4, IL-13), the selective maturation of Th2-like CD4$^+$ T cells expressing the IL-4 gene cluster (IL-4), growth, maturation and activation of eosinophils and basophils (IL-3, IL-5, GM-CSF) and maturation of mast cells (stem cell factor (SCF), IL-6, IL-9; Fig. 1). The expression of a counterregulatory signal provided by interferon-γ (IFN-γ; from Th-1 cells) and macrophage/monocyte-derived IL-12 which induces its synthesis becomes reduced. This has led to the concept that cytokines from the Th-2 subtype of T cell dominate over those of the Th-1 subtype, leading to expression of the eosinophilic bronchitis characteristic of asthma. While far less is known of the cytokine networks in asthma, other than that associated with atopy, the therapeutic efficacy of disease-modifying drugs, and especially corticosteroids, is likely to be the consequence of transcription factor-mediated down-regulation of cytokine production and the pro-inflammatory pathways that these signalling molecules influence.

MECHANISMS OF ASTHMA SEVERITY AND CHRONICITY

There is overwhelming evidence to indicate that airway inflammation underlies the pathophysiology of asthma, but its relationship to disease severity is less clear. While the presence of eosinophils in the sputum, a persistent blood eosinophilia and increased circulating levels of eosinophil granule proteins broadly relate to disease severity, these measures are too variable to provide clinically useful markers to predict the level of airway inflammation.

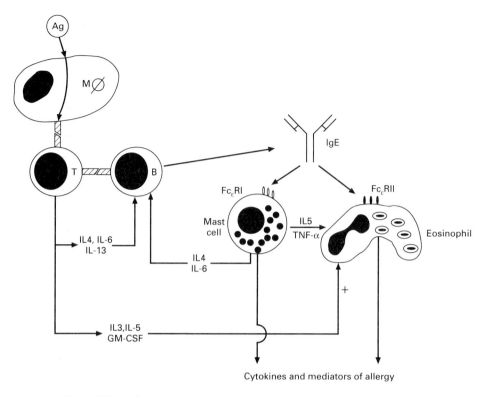

Fig. 1 Schematic representation of the key cytokine involved in the regulation of allergic inflammation.

The selective recruitment of cells from the microvasculature underlies the ongoing inflammation in severe and chronic disease. Increased mast cell, eosinophil and T-cell survival through cytokine-mediated inhibition of apoptosis is also important. Lung transplantation has shown that alone, with its lymphoid tissue, the lung is able to sustain ongoing asthma, also emphasizing the importance of local factors [3]. From a therapeutic standpoint the wide variation observed in these biomarkers in relation to the complexity of the clinical phenotypes suggests complex cellular and mediator mechanisms.

Corticosteroids are highly effective antiasthma drugs acting to reduce the inflammatory response. However, there are many patients in whom only partial relief is achieved, even with high doses. In a well-defined population of corticosteroid-resistant asthmatics with preservation of β_2-agonist bronchodilation, abnormalities of circulating monocyte and T-cell cytokine function have been described [4]. However, such patients represent only a minority of the 'difficult-to-control' asthmatics.

The majority of asthma occurs in association with atopy — the predisposition to generate IgE to common environmental allergens through a Th-2-cell-dependent mechanism. Ongoing allergen-specific IgE production in severe disease provides the rationale for allergen avoidance and high-altitude treatment. However, environmental interventions have no effect on non-allergic asthma and many patients with severe atopic disease only partially respond or fail to respond. Irrespective of atopy, powerful epidemiological studies have linked the total serum IgE to the presence of asthma and the level to disease progression [5]. There have been very few long-term studies but what evidence does exist suggests that severe and poorly controlled asthma progresses to an increasing irreversible component [6]. Severe and prolonged inflammation is almost always accompanied by tissue remodelling. The airways are no exception; however, the mechanisms involved and their contribution to the overall pathophysiology of severe and chronic asthma have not been evaluated.

It follows that the severity and chronicity of asthma result from the dysregulation of cytokine networks leading to persistent inflammation in structurally altered airways which becomes refractory to treatment. The responsibility for disease progression does not lie with any single cellular element but embraces T- and B-cells, mast cells, eosinophils, endothelial cells, epithelial cells and myofibroblasts acting cooperatively with each other and with formed elements of the airways, including smooth muscle and nerves, leading to the variable phenotype characteristic of severe disease. This integrated view of asthma as a chronic disease of ongoing inflammation and repair leads us to incriminate a number of effector cells.

Continuous T-cell activation

Severe disease increasingly engages airway T-cells, leading to their oligoclonal expansion, activation with a mixed pattern of cytokine expression and failure of normal counterregulatory mechanisms.

T-cell activation and expression of messenger RNA for cytokines is a common feature of all types of asthma. In mild disease, the level of T-cell involvement in the airways is low, but there is ample evidence for mast cell and eosinophil activation and this may explain why cromone-like drugs are more efficacious at this end of the asthma spectrum. By contrast, our biopsy and lavage study of patients admitted to the Dutch Asthma Centre in Davos [7], together with observations of severely symptomatic asthmatic patients in the UK taking high doses of inhaled corticosteroids [8], indicates that activated T-cells drive the ongoing inflammatory process in severe disease by mechanisms in addition to eosinophil recruitment and activation. While 24 hours post allergen challenge, we and others have shown increased IL-5 transcription in relation to T-cell recruitment and activation supporting the Th2 hypothesis, however, our T-cell cloning studies have shown that lavage T-cells from asthmatics of differing disease severity exhibit considerable heterogeneity of cytokine expression [9]. At baseline, T-cells from atopic asthmatic airways show strong expression of messenger RNA for IL-13, GM-CSF, IFN-γ and tumour necrosis factor (TNF-α), whereas with allergen instillation there was a cytokine shift in favour of IL-3, IL-4, IL-5 and IL-13 and away from IFN-γ and TNF-α. These data support the recent T-cell cloning studies that recognize the existence of Th-2-like cells that are allergen-responsive, while the majority of activated airway T-cells in the airways serve other functions [10].

Using monensin to inhibit Golgi-mediated cytokine transport and flow cytometry applied to permeabilized cells, we have evaluated the cytokine protein production by airway T-cells. Confirming our observations on airway T-cell clones, a high proportion of asthmatic broncho alveolar lavage (BAL) T-cells produced IFN-γ and/or IL-2 and only a few accumulated IL-4 or IL-5 [11]. Even more surprising was the finding in asthma when compared to normal controls of a significantly greater production of IFN-γ but not IL-2. During acute exacerbations of asthma there is evidence for T-cell up-regulation in the peripheral circulation accompanied by enhanced IL-5 gene expression. However, during acute episodes in the UK we have shown that proliferative T-cell responses to house dust mite allergen, when compared to responses before or 8 weeks after the episode, decreased rather than increased, indicating that factors influencing T-cells other than allergens are important in directing the immune response during exacerbations. It is clear that little is known about T-cell cytokine responses influencing disease chronicity and severity in asthma and how they may escape corticosteroid suppression.

Based on the lung transplant experiments and bronchoscopy studies in mild-to-moderate disease, an important aspect of T-cell involvement local expression, studying the T-cell receptor (TcR) V-gene usage will shed light on factors that shape the airways' T-cell repertoire. In normal subjects, the peripheral TcR repertoire is diverse, resulting from use of different variable domain (VD) and junctional (J) segments in forming the α and β chain and as a consequence non-specific recruitment would result in a heterogeneous TcR repertoire at the inflammatory site, reflecting populations in blood. The exciting observation that atopy (and asthma) is associated with linkage to specific polymorphisms of the Vα repertoire on chromosome 14 indicates that genetic determinants involving allergen recognition are an important component of T-cell selection [12]. Specific stimulation of T-cells would modify the Vα and Vβ repertoire so that allergen-driven responses would result in dominant oligoclonal T-cell interaction, whereas superantigens would select a single dominant TcR Vα or Vβ family, but with random use of DJ segments. In preliminary experiments we have amplified the TcR repertoire in airways by PCR of complementary DNA prepared from BAL and blood lymphocytes of the same subjects and have found that TcR Vβ selection in favour of V_H5 is a feature of airway T-cells in atopic asthma, supporting a role for superantigens in driving the immune response [13]. These promising initial experiments need to be expanded to embrace more exaggerated forms of the disease in the presence and absence of atopy.

Mast cells and eosinophils

The mast cell and eosinophil contribute to the maintenance of mucosal inflammation through their release of proinflammatory cytokines and mediators.

Mast cell subtypes

The mast cell has long been regarded as an important effector cell of asthma through its capacity to respond to IgE-dependent activation with release of both preformed and newly generated mediators. This function has found wide acceptance as the cause of acute allergen- and exercise-induced bronchoconstriction. We believe that, as a constituent cell of the airway, the mast cell also plays a key role in maintaining chronicity of the inflammatory response. Of the two types of mast cell phenotyped through their granule neutral protease content, it is that containing only the unique four-chained neutral protease, tryptase, that dominates (MC_T), although tryptase- and chymase-containing cells (MC_{TC}) are found in relation to the submucous glands and microvasculature. Both MC_T and MC_{TC} require SCF (c-*kit* ligand) for survival, MC_T cells are under the influence of T-cell cytokines (IL-6, IL-9) while the MC_{TC} phenotype is determined by fibroblast-derived growth factors. The relevance of mast cell products to asthma has been revealed in a large study of 151 patients with different types of asthma in BAL fluid; the products of mast cell activation, tryptase, histamine and prostaglandin D_2 were all present in higher concentrations than in normal subjects with levels that correlated positively with albumin as a marker of microvascular permeability ($P < 0.01$) and negatively with FEV_1, suggesting an important link to disease activity.

Mast cell cytokines

The importance of IL-4 and IL-5 in the pathogenesis of asthma is well-established but, until recently, it was thought that their major source was the Th2-like helper T-cell. As an alternative source, we have shown that human mast cells are an important source of IL-4, IL-5, IL-6, IL-8 and TNF-α [14,15]. Both by IHC and immunoelectronmicroscopy we are the first to show that human mast cells contain granule-associated IL-4,

IL-5, IL-6 and TNF-α and that these are differentially expressed between the two mast cell subtypes [16]. In purified lung mast cells, messenger RNA for all of these cytokines is induced by IgE-dependent activation and is followed by protein secretion for up to 48 hours [17]. The inducing stimuli for secretion appear to be different, IL-4 and IL-5 being more dependent upon $Fc_\varepsilon R_1$ receptor signalling, while SCF initiates TNF-α production. Both IL-6 and IL-8 messenger RNA is constitutively expressed at a high level, although IL-6 transcription could be further enhanced with SCF. Our recent finding that in severe atopic disease a proportion of MC_T cells also contain preformed SCF provides an autocrine mechanism for local mast cell survival and activation. Since every mast cell, but perhaps only 1 in 300–5000 airway T-cells, is antigen-specific, we hypothesize that cytokine release from airway mast cells initiated by allergen or other stimuli is pivotal in the induction and maintenance of the inflammatory response, through up-regulation of IgE (IL-4, IL-6), Th2-like T-cell (IL-4), mast cell (IL-6, SCF) eosinophil (IL-5, IL-8) and vascular adhesion molecule (TNF-α, IL-4) functions.

The use of monoclonal antibodies (MoAbs) directed to different epitopes of IL-4 in GMA sections of biopsies and free mast cells has allowed us to differentiate preformed (MoAb4D9) from the secreted (MoAb3H4) form of the cytokine [15]. In both atopic and non-atopic asthma the proportion of bronchial mast cells demonstrating ring staining with 3H4 is considerably greater than in normal subjects, indicating ongoing cytokine release in the absence of specific challenge. Seasonal exposure to allergen increases [18], whereas treatment with inhaled corticosteroids decreases, [19] the number of 3H4+ mast cells without altering the overall number of cells staining with 4D9 for the preformed cytokine, indicating that IL-4 secretion is sensitive to changes in the microenvironment. Recent evidence shows that IL-4 binds strongly to the GAG side chains of heparin [20] — a property it shares with IL-8 and TNF-α. Since heparin is a unique product of human mast cells, its secretion on to the mast cell surface is likely to provide a pericellular environment in which these cytokines are present in high concentrations, to mediate local signalling effects pertinent to ongoing inflammation.

Mast cell proteases

Tryptase, chymase, carboxypeptidase A and a capthepsin G-like enzyme are also tightly bound to heparin, which serves to preserve integrity and direct the specificity of the enzymes. Tryptase is the major secretory component of mast cells and comprises in excess of 20% of the total granule content of protein. Elevated concentrations have been detected in BAL fluid collected from patients with chronic severe asthma as well as from milder cases of atopic asthma. Evidence is emerging that this serine protease may act as a key mediator of disease. Tryptase is capable of participating in tissue remodelling in being able to cleave several components of the extracellular matrix (e.g. collagen VI, fibronectin), in addition to activating matrix metalloproteases (stromelysin). The generation of kinins by tryptase may have important consequences and this enzyme can also degrade certain neuropeptides postulated to have a regulatory role in asthma (vasoactive intestinal polypeptide (VIP), calcitonin G-related peptide (CGRP)). Interacting directly with the cell surface, we have shown that tryptase can also enhance proliferation of epithelial cells, fibroblasts and smooth-muscle cells, up-regulate expression of intracellular adhesion molecule 1 (ICAM-1), stimulate IL-8 release and induce eosinophil chemotaxis and activation — all of which are dependent upon preservation of the enzyme's catalytic site [21–23] (Fig. 2).

Chymase, a protease co-released with tryptase by MC_{TC}, can also cleave several structural proteins and activate other tissue-degrading proteases (stromelysin, gelatinase A) as well as degrade selective cytokines. In addition, chymase is one of the most potent secretagogues of mucus-secreting cells to have been described when injected into laboratory animals [24]. We have shown that both tryptase and chymase induce microvascular leakage and granulocyte accumulation (Fig. 3).

Despite their potential importance as mediators, relatively little is known of the expression of proteases in mast cells of the respiratory tract

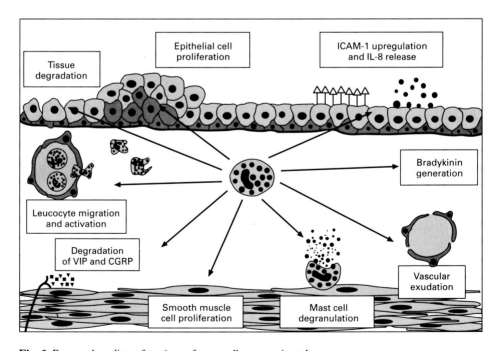

Fig. 2 Proposed mediator functions of mast cell tryptase in asthma.

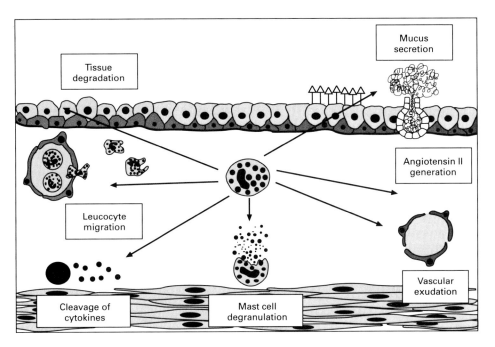

Fig. 3 Proposed mediator functions of mast cell chymase in asthma.

of asthmatic patients. Numbers of mast cells in bronchial tissue (as revealed by immunostaining for tryptase) are not greatly altered in asthma, though the elevated concentrations of tryptase in BAL fluid suggest that the mast cells are in a more activated state. The process of protease synthesis and the kinetics of release from mast cells are not well-understood. Multiple complementary DNAs have been cloned for tryptase, but the significance of this variation is not known. Sequences have also been derived for complementary DNA for chymase, and for other proteases which have been detected in mast cells, including carboxypeptidase and cathepsin G. These advances now permit new approaches to be applied to answer basic questions of the biology of mast cell proteases and better to understand their roles in bronchial asthma.

Triggering role of IgE

Cytokine-induced IgE leads to disease progression by shifting specificity from external to other antigens, including autoantigens, and through the formation of autoantibodies against IgE.

Although the ability of IgE to bind to mast cells, and to mediate antigen-induced degranulation is clear, its role in maintaining chronic asthma is not fully understood. However, patients with chronic disease have raised

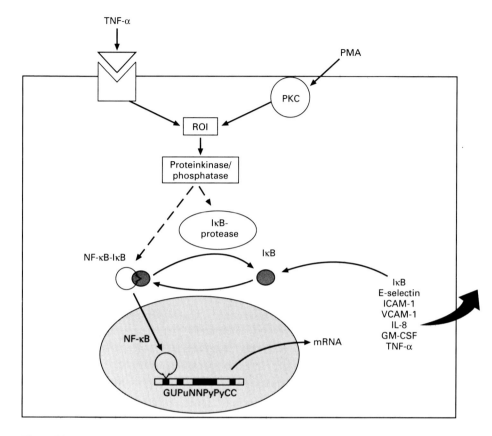

Fig. 4 The mechanisms of NF-κB transcription factor activation and function.

levels of allergen-specific IgE in serum and IgE, particularly in complex form, is capable of mediating the release of a range of cytokines via $Fc_\varepsilon R_1$ and $Fc_\varepsilon R_2$ (CD23). Since both high- and low-affinity IgE receptors are up-regulated on eosinophils, and bronchial epithelial cells in asthma, the opportunities for IgE to contribute to local inflammatory processes are numerous.

The question raised is whether the IgE is specific for allergens, or whether the spectrum of recognition widens during disease progression, to include viral antigens and autoantigens, as recently described in chronic urticaria. Past analysis of IgE specificities has been limited to serological investigation of mixed IgE but the new technology will allow investigation of individual IgE molecules. It will also be feasible to compare the molecular range of IgE found at the local sites of inflammation to that in the blood. Methods for amplifying the variable-region genes used to encode IgE have been developed and already reveal an unexpected asymmetric usage of immunoglobulin V_H genes in patients with asthma. In the inflammatory environment, where there may be local release of cytokines, possibly exacerbated by viral infection, it is conceivable that autoantigens may be released. IgE antibodies could therefore be generated against allergens, viral antigens or autoantigens. The high levels of IgE characteristic of chronic asthma could also induce autoantibodies against IgE itself [25]. These could have an important additional role in inflammation, either by cross-linking IgE on the mast cell surface, or by generating immune complexes, which stimulate mononuclear phagocytes to release cytokines.

The endothelial–leukocyte recruitment

Cytokine-driven activation of the microvasculature leads to increased expression of vascular adhesion molecules, mediators and chemokines to promote leukocyte activation and recruitment.

The recruitment of leukocytes to sites of inflammation involves a well-coordinated and dynamic sequence of events in which several cell adhesion molecules (CAMs) and chemotactic cytokines play an active role [26]. *In vitro* lines of evidence predict a multistep model involving: (i) initial low-affinity selectin molecule-dependent 'vascular rolling' (margination); (ii) leukocyte activation by endothelial-derived chemoattractants (e.g. IL-8, MCP-1) and (iii) a transition to β_2-integrin-dependent high-affinity leukocyte adherence cytokine-mediated up-regulation of the Ig superfamily of adhesion proteins, ICAMs and vascular adhesion molecules (VCAMs) followed by (IV) transendothelial migration involving combinations of CAMs.

In asthma the presence of eosinophils and mononuclear cells in the bronchial mucosa involves initial recruitment from the microvasculature. We have shown that within 6 hours of segmental allergen challenge of sensitized asthmatic airways there occurs marked endothelial up-regulation of E-selectin and ICAM-1, accompanied by an influx of lymphocyte function antigen (LFA)-1 + leukocytes comprising neutrophils and eosinophils [27]. By 24 hours there was a marked increase in activated T-cells and eosinophils present in BAL with variable expression of VCAM-1, an adhesion molecule not normally constitutively expressed. Because leukocyte recruitment occurs so rapidly, we suggest that the first step involves up-regulation of P-selectin (by histamine) and E-selectin (by TNF-α) released from activated mast cells which mediate rolling through a lectin interaction with the ligand sialyl Lewis x on the leukocyte surface. The IgE-dependent secretion of newly formed TNF-α would increase ICAM-1 expression, while its interaction with mast cell-derived IL-4 induces VCAM-1 expression. These CAMs interact with the integrins LFA-1 and very late antigen (VLA)-4 selectively to recruit T-cells and eosinophils.

Preliminary IHC studies on biopsies from severe asthmatics from the National Dutch Asthma Hospital in Davos have revealed a marked up-regulation of ICAM-1 and VCAM-1 in the absence of allergen exposure and while taking high doses of corticosteroids [25]. We suggest that in severe asthma there is continued expression of endothelial CAMs to promote ongoing leukocyte recruitment and activation. Such a mechanism would explain the finding of elevated circulating and BAL levels of soluble CAMs in symptomatic asthma [28].

The expression of E-selectin, ICAM-1 and VCAM-1 is controlled by the nuclear transcription factor nuclear factor (NF)-κB, a heterodimer p50/p65, of which both subunits contain the 300-amino acid NF-κB/rel/dorsal (NRD) domain. The N-terminal end of NRD is involved in specific binding to DNA, while the C-terminal end contains the nuclear location signal (NLS), a cluster of positively charged amino acids necessary for translocation of NF-κB across the nuclear membrane. NF-κB binds to the decameric DNA sequence $5'-GG^A_GNN^C_T{}^C_TCC-3'$, found in the promoters of a number of genes that are up-regulated in inflammation, especially the CAMs and specific cytokines (IL-2, IL-6, IL-8, members of the IL-4 gene cluster and TNF-α; Fig. 4).

Within the E-selectin promoter there are three closely spaced binding sites for NF-κB clustered within a 40 base pair segment and two additional regulatory elements NF-E-selectin-1 and NF-E-selectin-2, the latter recognizing members of the cyclic adenosine monophosphate (cAMP)-independent ATF-CREB family of transcription factors and the former involved in the repression of the basal NF-κB enhancer in quiescent cells. Following cytokine exposure all three NF-κB sites are essential for maximal promoter activity. The promoter for the human ICAM-1 gene contains binding sites for Sp-1, AP-1, AP-2, AP-3, NF-κB and a putative silencer, whereas NF-κB alone mediates VCAM-1 expression.

A range of factors have been shown to initiate activation of NF-κB, including TNF-α, IL-1, IL-2, leukotriene B_4 (LTB_4) and viruses. Endothelial cells express a cytoplasmic inhibitor of NF-κB activity, IκBα, the over-expression of which inhibits E-selectin and VCAM-1 transcription. IκBα binds selectively to NF-κB heterodimers and prevents its nuclear uptake by binding to the NLS. A pathway of NF-κB activation has been proposed that sequentially involves phosphorylation of IκBα, followed by its specific chymotryptic proteolysis which reveals the previously masked NLS site and nuclear translocation. The activation is only transient, since NF-κB is also able to induce IkB messenger RNA transcription, resulting in reaccumulation of IκBα and its functional inhibition of cytoplasmic NF-κB. Reactive oxygen intermediates (ROIs) serve as second messengers of NF-κB activation, redox changes leading to activation of chymotryptic IκBα protease through modification of intracellular serpins. These intra-cellular events provide unique opportunities to investigate NF-κB activation in severe asthma as it relates to increased CAM and cytokine expression and to investigate pharmacological intervention with potential therapeutic significance.

The epithelium as a source of proinflammatory products

There is persistent epithelial activation with production and secretion of mediators and cytokines resulting in enhanced cell recruitment, broncho-constriction and airway wall remodelling.

The bronchial epithelium has been viewed traditionally as a passive barrier which serves as a target for the inflammatory response; however, it is also an important source of inflammatory products, including arachidonic acid products, endothelin, nitric oxide (NO) and cytokines. In asthma, the increased expression of ICAM-1, human leukocyte antigen (HLA)-DR and CD44 demonstrates the capacity of the epithelium to participate directly in inflammatory cell recruitment and activation.

Arachidonic acid metabolism

We and others have shown that the epithelium is a major source of 15-HETE and, although expression of immunoreactive 15-lypoxygenase is unaltered [29], Shannon et al. showed increased enzyme activity in severe disease [30]. Although 15-hydroxyeicosa-tetraenoic (HETE) and 15-dihydroxy acids exhibit some mediator functions, more active oxidate products of arachidonic acid are prostaglandins E_2 and $F_{2\alpha}$ with their opposing actions in bronchial smooth muscle. We have recently shown that in mild-to-moderate asthma epithelial expression of the inducible form of cyclooxygenase (COX2) is enhanced over the constitutive form (COX1), a change that is suppressed by corticosteroid treatment in parallel with their clinical efficacy [31]. In asthma poorly controlled with corticosteroids, COX2 up-regulation might be expected to persist.

Endothelin

Human endothelin comprises three structurally distinct 21-amino acid peptides, ET-1, ET-2 and ET-3, encoded on separate genes. In addition to its potent vasoconstrictor property, ET-1 is a powerful contractor of airway smooth muscle, mediated through the ET_B receptor subtype, whereas ET-2 and ET-3 have lower binding affinities for ET_B receptors. ET-1 is a mitogen for airway smooth muscle and in fibroblasts is chemo-attractant and mitogenic and provides an activating signal for collagen synthesis, largely mediated through ET_B receptors. ET-1 induces collagenase production and is important in myofibroblast-mediated contraction of granulation tissue.

Human bronchial epithelial cells cultured from the airways of asthmatics secrete increased amounts of ET-1, which is sensitive to inhibition with corticosteroids [32]. ET-1 immunoreactivity *in vivo* is also increased in the epithelium [33]. In BAL levels of ET-1 are increased in proportion to the resting level of air flow obstruction [34]. The importance of ET-1 as a novel bronchoconstrictor is revealed by its capacity to reduce FEV_1 by $\geq 20\%$ of baseline at inhaled concentrations of $10^{-10}-10^{-12}$ mol/l. With effective corticosteroid treatment of asthma, both lavage ET-1 levels and ET-1 expression in the epithelium return to those found in normal subjects.

Nitric oxide

NO is a short-lived, highly soluble free radical which plays a major role in cell–cell communication. It is generated enzymatically from L-arginine by NO synthase which exists in both constitutive and inducible isoforms (iNOS). Both enzymes require NADPH as cofactor and are inhibited by L-arginine analogues such as N^G-nitro-L-arginine (L-NNA) and N^G-monomethyl-L-arginine (L-NMMA) while the inducible form is selectively inhibited by aminoguanidine. We have recently shown that iNOS immunolocalizes strongly to the bronchial epithelium in bronchial biopsies from asthmatics but only rarely in those from normal controls [35]. Consistent with enhanced NO generation in airway mucosal inflammation is the increased NO detected in exhaled air active asthma and rhinitis. *In vitro* iNOS is induced in response to IFN-γ, IL-1β and TNF-α and is inhibited by corticosteroids. We have evidence that in corticosteroid-responsive asthma iNOS in the epithelium is down-regulated, associated with a reduction in exhaled NO. Whilst NO generated by iNOS also contributes to vasodilatation, when up-regulated this enzyme has greater synthetic capacity than the constitutive enzymes in producing nanomolar concentrations of NO, which are cytotoxic through formation of peroxynitrite and hydroxyl radicals and nitrosylation of key mitochondrial enzymes. In severe asthma, the epithelium is likely to be a major source of toxic levels of NO and as such may provide a novel surrogate marker of disease activity and response to treatment.

Cytokines

Human bronchial epithelial cells *in vitro* constitutively synthesize and release IL-1β, IL-6, IL-8 and GM-CSF with greatly enhanced production occurring on exposure to IL-1β or TNF-α. Enhanced release of these cytokines has also been reported in asthmatic epithelial cells *in vitro*. Application of IHC shows that the bronchial epithelium in asthma is a particularly rich source of IL-1β, IL-8 and GM-CSF.

IL-8, a member of the α (C-x-C) chemokine family, is particularly important in the expression of chronic and severe disease, although it is usually regarded as a neutrophil chemoattractant. We have shown that IL-8 can induce human eosinophils from asthmatic subjects to secrete IL-3, IL-5 and GM-CSF. In an explant model of nasal polyp tissue, repeated allergen exposure produces a supernatant, exhibiting a markedly enhanced eosinophil survival property. The explant supernatant contains IL-2, IL-3 and IL-5 and particularly high amounts of GM-CSF and IL-8 [36]. Using a range of blocking MoAbs, the eosinophil survival properties imparted by the explant medium were shown to be IL-8 and GM-CSF. These findings help explain why in atopic but not in non-atopic subjects we were able to show that instillation of human recombinant (hr) IL-8 into the nasal cavity produced a marked eosinophil in addition to neutral influx.

IL-8 in bronchial biopsies from asthmatics and in the peripheral circulation binds strongly to IgA [37]. Thus, despite clear immunostaining for IL-8 in the epithelium, no free IL-8 can be detected in detergent-extracted homogenates; however, IL-8–IgA complexes can be readily detected, with significantly more being presented in the allergic asthmatics. In patients with chronic severe asthma, both free and complexed forms of IL-8 are present in mucosal tissue and in serum. Thus, although IL-8 can be formed by many cells in asthma, our studies point to the bronchial epithelium being the major site of production and concentration of this chemokine. Of particular importance is that IL-8 co-localizes with a secretory IgA in the epithelium, since secretory but not serum IgA is able markedly to up-regulate the eosinophil chemotactic response to IL-8, reaching optimum levels at 10^{-10} mol/l, whereas under the same conditions the neutrophil response was inhibited. IL-8 is also known to complex with the glycosaminoglycan side chains of proteoglycans, an interaction that we have taken advantage of when purifying the cytokine from asthmatic BAL. The eosinophil-specific properties of IL-8 are greatly enhanced when it is complexed to cell-bound matrix. These include the secretory piece of IgA containing up to 20% N-linked oligosaccharide and proteoglycans such as the granule products of mast cells and eosinophils and CD44, which is expressed in greater amounts in the asthmatic epithelium. We hypothesize that IL-8 binding regulates the activity of and changes the target-cell specificity for this cytokine, rendering it a potent attractant and activator of eosinophils. In contrast to ET-1 and iNOS, corticosteroids only partially inhibit IL-8 transcription by epithelial cells *in vitro* and have no effect on BAL free or complexed IL-8 levels. That this chemokine is regulated by NF-κB and is markedly increased in proportion to asthma severity increases its importance among the chemokines as a prominent contributor to disease chronicity.

Epithelial repair

Epithelial damage results in persistent activation of repair mechanisms, abnormal epithelial–mesenchymal interactions and detrimental remodelling of the airway.

Epithelial cell biology

Epithelial damage is a key feature of asthma, with the extent of damage being related to disease. A recent study has shown that impaired detection of bronchial obstruction, a characteristic feature of severe disease, closely relates to the level of eosinophil infiltration and extent of epithelial damage when assessed in bronchial biopsies. We have provided evidence that the major structural site of damage is between the columnar and basal cells and between adjacent columnar cells, implicating disruption to the desmosomes. The cause of increased epithelial dysfunction in asthma is not understood, although the arginine-rich basic proteins of the eosinophil and active radicals are considered to be important. The level of damage may reflect either increased fragility or increased insult to the epithelium. To understand the importance of epithelial disruption in severe and chronic asthma, there is a need to understand the processes of damage, repair and regeneration of the epithelium and which normal functions of the epithelium are compromised.

On the basis of our preliminary work and studies by others, we propose the following steps in epithelial damage and repair.

1 *Immediate damage and effects* — selective cell loss due to injury with loss of barrier function.

2 *Immediate response* — epithelial cells adjacent to areas of damage reduce cell-substrate adhesion, increase cell migration and form a temporary squamous barrier.

3 *Proliferative response* — division, differentiation and remodelling lead to reformation of fully functional differentiated epithelium.

4 *Ongoing damage* in asthma occurring during the above processes may further compromise epithelial integrity. Lack of appropriate down-regulation of the normal response may produce a similar effect.

Eosinophil–epithelial interactions

Cytokines. Eosinophils are a newly recognized source of cytokines, including IL-3, IL-4, IL-5, GM-CSF, IL-6, IL-8, TNF-α, monocyte/macrophage inhibitory peptide (MIP)-1α, transforming growth factor-α (TGF-α) and TGF-β [38]. Important among these for eosinophil survival are IL-3, IL-5 and GM-CSF, indicating an autocrine function. Eosinophils exposed to these cytokines have their life expectancy extended from days to weeks and are also more responsive to chemoattractant and mediator-secreting stimuli. Additionally, since the three eosinophilopoietins antagonize the accelerating effect of corticosteroids on eosinophil apoptosis, their sustained production would serve to render the cells functionally corticosteroid-resistant.

The use of blocking antibodies in our organ culture model has clearly shown that IL-8 is important as an effector of eosinophil survival by stimulating the release of IL-3, IL-5 and GM-CSF. Within the limitations of available enzyme-linked immunosorbent assay (ELISA) techniques, these cytokines were not released but remained cell-associated. Eosinophils also synthesize and release IL-8 in response to platelet-activating factor (PAF) and other stimuli, indicating that within the inflammatory focus eosinophil survival and activation are supported by a cytokine network dependent upon paracrine and autocrine loops. We now wish to extend these observations in relation to asthma chronicity by investigating the expression, intracellular localization and mechanisms of release of IL-8, IL-5 and GM-CSF. Our hypothesis is that the expression of eosinophil survival cytokines is increased in bronchial tissue in proportion to disease severity and that the intracellular cytokines are presented as a complex with proteoglycans of the eosinophil granules similar to the role of mast cell heparin in presenting IL-4. We propose that cytokine release is dependent upon activation of cell-surface immunoglobulin receptors.

Secretory IgA has been suggested to be the principal immunoglobulin mediating eosinophil function at mucosal surfaces [37]. Eosinophil basic proteins are released in response to secretory IgA via a mechanism which is enhanced by IL-3, IL-5 and GM-CSF. Functional effects of secretory IgA are most probably mediated by binding to either $Fc_\alpha R$, whose expression on eosinophils is increased in asthma, or to specific receptors for the secretory component (SC). We have shown that in asthma peripheral blood eosinophils carry both IgA and SC bound to the cell surface. Unexpectedly, the concentrations of SC on asthmatic blood eosinophils was greater than in a cultured epithelial cell line known to generate SC. We interpret this as the recirculation of eosinophils from the mucosal site — a phenomenon previously suggested but never proven. We have also noted strong synergism between secretory IgA and IL-8-induced eosinophil migration *in vitro*.

Although it is likely that enzymes of the 5-lipoxygenase (LO) pathway are up-regulated in eosinophils in asthma, this has not yet been investigated. If accompanied by a decrease in prostaglandin E_2 production, then the unimportant autocrine cAMP-mediated inhibitory effect of this mediator on a number of eosinophil responses is removed, including the secretory IgA-induced release of basic granule proteins and presumably cytokines. We have observed that eosinophils in culture secrete prostaglandin E_2 which is increased in the presence of PAF or IL-5. Over 90% of the prostaglandin E_2 is released into the fluid phase and available for mediating negative feedback. In non-steroidal anti-inflammatory drug-induced asthma, removal of prostaglandin E_2 inhibition of mast cell and eosinophil leukotriene C_4 (LTC_4) production has been suggested.

Eosinophils isolated from the airways are spontaneously cytotoxic towards alveolar epithelial cells. However, in the airways of asthmatics viable columnar cells are shed from their basal cell attachments but will remain firmly fixed to the membrane via hemidesmosomes utilizing both $\alpha_6\beta_4$ and fibronectin–integrin adhesion. Using a bovine bronchial epithelial explant, we suggest that activated eosinophils mediate epithelial detachment via a cognate interaction involving ICAM-1 and the subsequent release of: (i) metalloendoproteases; (ii) oxidants; and (iii) arginine-rich proteins [37].

Metalloendoproteases. In BAL from patients with asthma we have shown increased concentrations of the 92 kDa gelatinase metalloproteinase along with a range of other metalloendoproteases. Eosinophils are an important source of the 92 kDa gelatinase, which has a broad substrate specificity in being able to degrade both basement membrane collagen type IV and interstitial matrix molecules [39]. Because of the extensive eosinophil infiltrate in severe asthma, this enzyme is likely to be important in both cell migration and tissue remodelling; however, other than describing its existence, little is known about its expression and regulation.

Oxidants. The tissue-damaging effect of the products of eosinophil peroxidase (EPO) are indicated by the effectiveness of antioxidants to inhibit eosinophil-mediated injury to lung epithelial cells and interstitial matrix *in vitro*. EPO is released asynchronously with eosinophil cationic protein (ECP) or major basic protein (MBP) 1 and, as with many highly charged proteins, largely remains cell-associated. Thus, in line with our hypothesis that eosinophil–epithelial cell contact is required for effective epithelial disruption, we will investigate the hypothesis that EPO, along with reactive oxygen, increases epithelial fragility through pericellular proteglycan and adhesion glycoprotein degradation. A close-coupled mechanism would serve to exclude naturally occurring antioxidants such as GSH, vitamin E or albumin, and concentrate the delivery of the oxidant injury.

Basic proteins. Considerable evidence exists for the disruptive effects of eosinophil cationic proteins (MBP, ECP, EDN) on epithelial integrity in asthma. Their extreme cationicity renders matrix proteoglycans as susceptible targets. A number of proinflammatory cytokines, including IL-4, IL-8, IFN-γ and basic fibroblast growth factor (bFGF) are tightly bound to GAG side chains of highly *O*-sulphated proteoglycans — an association which stabilizes the cytokine, localizes its activity and deter-mines its specificity. Using IHC we suggest that IL-8 and IFN-γ localize to interepithelial clefts on account of their association with the GAGs of CD44 and *N*-sulphated carbohydrate moities' secretory IgA. Similarly, IL-4 binds to heparin on mast cells, together with bFGF heparin SO_4 in basement membranes and TGF-β to decarin. Levels of IL-8, TGF-β and bFGF are elevated in BAL from asthmatics, with further increases occurring with allergen challenge [40–42]. We suggest that an interaction of the eosinophil basic proteins with cytokine binding sites on matrix molecules results in release of free cytokine so that a wider range of activity is achieved in severe disease. An additional possibility is that MBP and ECP interact with the highly alkaline-sensitive Ser-O-GAG linkage of proteoglycans to produce non-enzymatic hydrolysis further to effect tissue cytokine localization and activity.

Epithelial–mast cell–epithelial interactions

In mucosal biopsies mast cells aggregate both within the epithelium and in relation to the connective tissue elements of the basement membrane and associated myofibroblasts. We have recently shown that, when assessed by flow cytometry on an H292 epithelial cell line, human mast cell tryptase is able to up-regulate the cell surface expression of ICAM-1 to a similar extent as TNF-α. A small increase in P-selectin and an apparent down-regulation of N-cadherin expression were also observed as the activity of tryptase was increased. Tryptase also stimulated DNA synthesis in epithelial cells measured by ^{3}H-thymidine incorporation and produced a dose-related release of IL-8. Inhibition of tryptase with leupeptin or benzamidine HCI prevented these actions of tryptase, indicating the obligatory requirement for an active catalytic site [17]. These studies suggest an important role for mast cells in epithelial repair, in the recruit-ment of granulocytes and in rendering the lower respiratory tract vulnerable to human rhinovirus infection, since the major type of human rhinovirus utilizes ICAM-1 to gain access to epithelial cells and up-regulate cytokine production.

Epithelial cell–myofibroblast interactions

We have shown that the apparent thickening of the subepithelial basement membrane in asthma is due to the deposition of collagen types II and V and fibronectin [43] and that produced by proliferating myofibroblasts. The presence of tenascin in the lamina reticulosa indicates that this is a site of high matrix turnover and cell migration, towards which both epithelial cells and myofibroblasts contribute. In addition to their capacity to secrete matrix proteins, we have recently shown that cultures of human

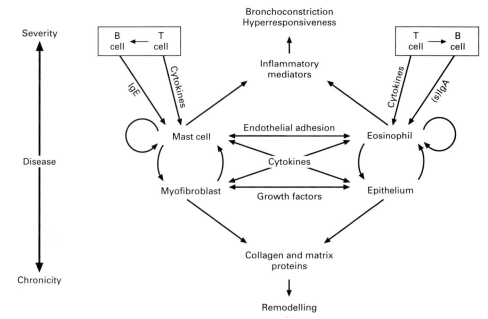

Fig. 5 Proposed interrelationship between airway inflammation and repair in asthma, highlighting the important role of cytokines.

bronchial subepithelial myofibroblasts produce GM-CSF, IL-6, IL-8 and SCF constitutively and that the supernatant from cultures could greatly extend eosinophil survival [44]. GM-CSF transcription demonstrated by RNase protection assay was greatly up-regulated in the presence of TNF-α and was accompanied by secretion of GM-CSF, which accounted for the majority of the eosinophil survival capacity of the supernatants. The enhancement of GM-CSF production by TNF-α was inhibited in a dose-dependent manner by prednisolone, but maximum inhibition was not achieved until 1 mmol/l — a concentration far beyond that achieved therapeutically. These findings suggest that human myofibroblasts located beneath the bronchial epithelium establish close contact with eosinophils and mast cells and as such play a critical role in up-regulating mucosal inflammation, especially in chronic disease.

AN INTEGRATED MODEL OF ASTHMA

The complexities of human asthma as an inflammatory disorder are only just being appreciated. We have passed through the eras of believing that the disease is one of smooth muscle, or mast cells, or eosinophils or T-cells, to a picture where all these and other cells are involved in a cooperative fashion. Figure 5 attempts to demonstrate this by showing a close interrelationship between those factors responsible for inflammatory events and those involved in repair. Implicit in this model is an interdependence between the classical cells of inflammation and the formed elements of the airway. Varying contributions from each of these processes provide a rational basis for the variable clinical phenotype and responses to therapeutic interventions.

ACKNOWLEDGEMENTS

This paper has also been published in slightly altered form in *Allergology International* 1996.

REFERENCES

1 World Health Organization and National Heart, Lung and Blood Institute. *Technical Report on a Global Strategy for Asthma*. Global strategy for asthma management and prevention workshop report. 1995; Publ. No. 95–3659.

2 Weiss KB, Gergen PJ, Hodgson TA. An economic evaluation of asthma in the US. *N Engl J Med* 1992;**326**:862–866.

3 Corris PA, Dark JH. Aetiology of asthma: lessons from lung transplantation. *Lancet* 1993;**341**:1377–1378.

4 Cypcar D, Busse WW. Steroid-resistant asthma. *J Allergy Clin Immunol* 1993;**92**:362–372.

5 Burrows B, Martinez FD, Halonen M, Barbee RA, Cline MG. Association of asthma with serum IgE levels and skin test reactivity to allergens. *N Engl J Med* 1989;**320**:271–277.

6 Burrows B, Lebowitz MD, Barbee RA, Cline MG. Findings before diagnoses of asthma among the elderly in a longitudinal study of a general population sample. *J Allergy Clin Immunol* 1991;**88**:870–877.

7 Djukanovic R, Howarth P, Vrugt B *et al*. Determinants of asthma severity. *Int Arch Allergy Immunol* 1995;**107**(No 1–3):389.

8 Frew AJ, Teran LM, Madden J *et al*. Cellular changes 24 hours after endobronchial challenge in asthma. *Int Arch Allergy Immunol* 1995;**107**(No 1–3):576–577.

9 Krug N, Madden J, Redington AE *et al*. Intracellular cytokine staining of T cells obtained from human asthmatic airways. *Am J Respir Cell Mol Biol* 1996 (in press).

10 Bodey KJ, Semper AE, Redington AE *et al*. Phenotype and cytokine profile of T-cell clones derived after local allergen challenge of asthmatic airways. *J Allergy Clin Immunol* 1996 (in press).

11 Holt P. Developmental immunology and host defence. Kinetics of postnatal maturation of immune competence as a potential etiologic factor in early childhood asthma. *Am J Respir Crit Care Med* 1995;**151**:S11–S13.

12 Moffatt MF, Hill MR, Cornelis F *et al*. Genetic linkage of T cell receptor α/δ complex to specific IgE responses. *Lancet* 1994;**343**:1597–1600.

13 Herman A, Kappler JW, Marrack P, Pullen AM. Superantigens: mechanism of T cell stimulation and role in immune responses. *Am Rev Immunol* 1991;**9**:745–772.

14 Bradding P, Feather IH, Wilson S *et al*. Immunolocalisation of cytokines in the nasal mucosa of normal and perennial rhinitic subjects: the mast cell as a source of IL-4, IL-5 and IL-6 in human allergic mucosal inflammation. *J Immunol* 1993;**151**:3853–3865.

15 Bradding P, Roberts JA, Britten KM *et al*. Interleukin-4, -5, -6 and TNFα in normal and asthmatic airways: evidence for the human mast cell as an important source of these cytokines. *Am J Respir Cell Mol Biol* 1994;**10**:471–480.

16 Bradding P, Okayama Y, Church MK, Holgate ST. Heterogeneity of human mast cells based on their cytokine content. *J Immunol* 1995;**155**:297–307.

17 Okayama Y, Petit-Frére C, Kassel O *et al*. Expression of messenger RNA for IL-4 and

IL-5 in human lung and skin mast cells in response to FCε receptor cross-linkage and the presence of stem cell factor. *J Immunol* 1995;**155**:1796–1808.

18 Djukanović R, Feather I, Gratziou C *et al*. The effects of natural allergen exposure during the grass pollen season on airways inflammatory cells in asthma symptoms. *Am J Respir Crit Care Med* 1996; (in press).

19 Howarth PH, Feather I, Montefort S, Underwood J, Holgate ST. The influence of the inhaled corticosteroid fluticasone propionate on airway cytokine immunoreactivity in asthma. *Am J Respir Crit Care Med* 1995;**4**(part 2):A40(abstract).

20 Jones CA, Williams KA, Finlay-Jones J, Hart PH. Interleukin-4 production by human amnion epithelial cells and regulation of its activity by glycosaminoglycan binding. *Biol Reproduct* 1995;**52**:839–847.

21 Walls AF, He S, Teran L *et al*. Granulocyte recruitment by human mast cell tryptase. *Int Arch Allergy Immunol* 1995;**107**(No 1–3):372–373.

22 Cairns JA, Walls AF. Mast cell tryptase is a mitogen for epithelial cells. Stimulation of IL-8 production and ICAM-1 expression. *J Immunol* 1996;**156**:275–283.

23 Walls AF, He S, Teran L, Holgate ST. Mast cell proteases as mediators of vascular leakage and cell accumulation. *J Allergy Clin Immunol* 1993;**91**:256.

24 Sommerhoff CP, Caughey GH, Finkbeiner WE, Lazarus SC, Basbaum CB, Nadel JA. Mast cell chymase. A potent secretagogue for airway gland serous cells. *J Immunol* 1989;**142**:2450–2456.

25 Shakib F, Sihoe J, Smith SJ, Wilding P, Clark MM, Knox A. Circulating levels of IgG and IgG₄ anti-IgE antibodies and asthma severity. *Allergy* 1994;**49**:192–195.

26 Manning AM, Anderson DC, Bristol JA. (eds) *Annual Reports in Medicinal Chemistry*. Academic Press, San Diego; 1994:pp.235–244.

27 Montefort S, Gratziou C, Goulding D *et al*. Bronchial biopsy evidence for leucocyte infiltration and upregulation of leucocyte endothelial cell adhesion molecules 6 hours after local allergen challenge of sensitised asthmatic airway. *J Clin Invest* 1994;**93**:1411–1421.

28 Montefort S, Lai CKW, Kapahi P *et al*. Circulating adhesion molecules in asthma. *Am J Respir Crit Care Med* 1994;**149**:1149–1153.

29 Bradding P, Redington AE, Djukanović R, Conrad DJ, Holgate ST. 15-lipoxygenase immunoreactivity in normal and asthmatic airways. *Am J Respir Crit Care Med* 1995;**151**:1201–1204.

30 Shannon VR, Chanez P, Bousquet J, Holtzman MJ. Histochemical evidence for induction of arachidonate 15-lipoxygenase in airway disease. *Am Rev Respir Dis* 1993;**147**:1024–1028.

31 Springall DR, Meng Q-H, Redington AE, Howarth PH, Polak JM. Inflammatory genes in asthmatic airway epithelium: suppression by corticosteroids. *Eur Respir J* 1995;**8**(suppl 19):44s (abstract).

32 Mattoli S, Mezzetti M, Riva G, Allegra L, Fasoli A. Specific binding of endothelin on human bronchial smooth muscle cells in culture and secretion of endothelin-like material from bronchial epithelial cells. *Am J Respir Cell Mol Biol* 1990;**3**:145–151.

33 Springall DR, Howarth PH, Counihan H, Djukanovic R, Holgate ST, Polak JM. Endothelin immunoreactivity of airway epithelium in asthmatic patients. *Lancet* 1991;**337**:697–701.

34 Redington AE, Springall DR, Ghatei MA *et al*. Endothelin in bronchoalveolar lavage fluid and its relationship to airflow obstruction in asthma. *Am Rev Respir Crit Care Med* 1995;**151**:1034–9.

35 Hamid Q, Springall DR, Riveros-Moreno V *et al*. Induction of nitric oxide synthase in asthma. *Lancet* 1993;**342**:1510–1513.

36 Park H-S, Jung K-S, Shute J *et al*. GM-CSF is the predominant cytokine which enhances eosinophil survival in nasal polyp tissue cultures with allergen. *Am J Respir Crit Care Med* 1995;**151**(No 4):A240 (abstract).

37 Shute JK, Lindley I, Piechl P, Holgate ST, Church MK, Djukanović R. Mucosal IgA is an important moderator of eosinophil responses to tissue derived chemoattractants. *Int Arch All Appl Immunol* 1995;**107**(No 1–3):340–1.

38 Herbert CA, Edwards D, Boot JR, Robinson C. *In vitro* modulation of the eosinophil dependent enhancement of the eosinophil dependent enhancement of the permeability. *Br J Pharmacol* 1993;**104**:391–397.

39 Stahle-Backdahl M, Parks WC. 92-kd gelatinase is actively expressed by eosinophils and stored by neutrophils in squamous cell carcinoma. *Am J Pathol* 1993;**142**:995–1000.

40 Teran LM, Carroll M, Frew AJ *et al.* The role of interleukin-8 in neutrophil and eosinophil recruitment into asthmatic airways following local bronchial allergen or saline challenge. *Am J Respir Crit Care Med* 1996; (in press).

41 Redington AE, Madden J, Djukanović R, Roche WR, Howarth PH, Holgate ST. Transforming growth factor-beta levels in bronchoalveolar lavage are increased in asthma. *J Allergy Clin Immunol* 1995;**95**:377.

42 Redington AE, Madden J, Frew AJ *et al.* Basic fibroblast growth factor in asthma: immunolocalisation in bronchial biopsies and measurement in bronchoalveolar lavage fluid at baseline and following allergen challenge. *Am J Respir Crit Care Med* 1995;**15**(No 4):A702 (abstract).

43 Brewster CEP, Howarth PH, Djukanović R, Wilson J, Holgate ST, Roche WR. Myofibroblasts and sub-epithelial fibrosis in bronchial asthma. *Am Rev Respir Cell Mol Biol* 1990;**3**:507–511.

44 Zhang S, Howarth PH, Roche WR. Cytokine production by cultured bronchial subepithelial myofibroblasts. *Eur Respir J* 1996; (in press).

MULTIPLE CHOICE QUESTIONS

1 Which of the following cytokines are considered important in the pathogenesis of allergic asthma?

a interferon-α

b tumour necrosis factor-β

c interleukin-12

d interleukin-5

e transforming growth factor-β

2 Which adhesion molecules are considered critical for eosinophilic infiltration in asthma?

a very late antigen-2 (VLA-2)

b vascular cell adhesion molecule-1 (VCAM-1)

c intercellular adhesion molecule-1 (ICAM-1)

d L-selectin

e lymphocyte function antigen-1 (LFA-1)

3 Which proteolytic enzymes are stored within the secretory granules of human mast cells?

a carboxypeptidase C

b trypsin

c chymase

d neutral endopeptidase

e stromolysin

4 Mediators of inflammation that are secreted by the asthmatic epithelium are
a nitric oxide
b endothelin-1
c interleukin-4
d granulocyte-macrophage colony-stimulating factor (GM-CSF)
e prostaglandin D_2

5 The nuclear transcription factor NF-κB
a is a homer–dimer p50/p50
b is activated by removal of a specific inhibitor
c is involved in the regulation of vascular adhesion molecule expression
d is restricted to endothelial cells
e binds to a nuclear DNA consensus containing 25 bases

6 The generation of immunoglobulin E by B cells
a requires the presence of IL-4 or IL-13
b may occur both systematically and at mucosal surfaces
c binds to only a single Fc_ε receptor subtype
d requires the presence of stem cell factor for optimal synthesis
e is inhibited by corticosteroids

Answers

1 a False	2 a False	3 a False
b False	b True	b False
c False	c True	c True
d True	d False	d False
e True	e True	e False

4 a True	5 a False	6 a True
b True	b True	b True
c False	c True	c False
d True	d False	d False
e False	e False	e False

The genetic model of cystic fibrosis: accuracy and application

RICHARD A. KNIGHT

The purpose of this paper is to review the present state of knowledge of the molecular genetics of cystic fibrosis (CF) and to assess the predictive value of a molecular genetic hypothesis of the clinical disease. The application of molecular genetics to the clinical management of CF has begun, and this review also attempts to highlight problems — real and incipient — which have already arisen and where further research is needed.

CLINICAL EXPRESSION OF CYSTIC FIBROSIS

CF is a multisystem genetic disease in which the pattern and severity of organ involvement vary widely from patient to patient. The clinical prognosis is largely determined, however, by the degree of lung pathology. The lungs become colonized from an early age, commonly with *Staphylococcus aureus*, which is later replaced as a pathogen by *Pseudomonas aeruginosa*. In older patients, this latter organism grows as large mucoid macrocolonies, probably as an adaptation to the particular environment in the CF airway. The chronic bacterial colonization leads to chronic inflammation, mostly neutrophil-mediated, although the concentration of other inflammatory cells in CF lavage fluid is also increased. Neutrophils normally die by apoptosis, where a rigid protein polymer envelope is formed around the dying cell, preventing the release of intracellular contents. For reasons unknown, this process would seem to be ineffective in CF airways, and large amounts of neutrophil enzymes, such as elastase and myeloperoxidase, are released into the airways. The inability of neutrophils to phagocytose the large bacterial macrocolonies also accentuates chronic neutrophil enzyme release, as a result of the process of 'frustrated phagocytosis'. Furthermore, the major natural inhibitor of neutrophil elastase, α_1-antitrypsin, is proteolytically degraded, probably secondary to oxidative inactivation. This means that there are not only high concentrations of neutrophil elastase in CF airways, but also high levels of elastase activity. Neutrophil elastase, as well as digesting elastin fibres within the lung parenchyma, also damages cell surface receptors and thereby compromises local immunity. It is also a potent secretagogue, increasing the mucus load, and recruits still more neutrophils to the lung by its induction of interleukin-8 (IL-8). It therefore appears that much of the lung damage in CF is immune-inflicted secondary to chronic infection, rather than being directly caused by the genetic abnormality itself (reviewed in [1]).

In roughly 85% of CF patients, there is a failure of exocrine pancreatic function from early life, such that patients present in childhood with malabsorption and failure to thrive. In the remaining 15% of pancreas-sufficient (PS) patients, there are no gastrointestinal problems. Exocrine pancreatic function may, however, continue to decline with age in PS patients, and individual PS patients may become pancreas-insufficient (PI) in later life once 85–90% of their exocrine pancreas has been destroyed. As median survival in CF improves, diabetes mellitus, as a consequence of endocrine pancreatic failure, is also becoming more common. Both pancreatic dysfunctions, however, can be successfully treated with replacement therapies, either of exocrine pancreatic enzymes or with insulin.

In approximately 5% of patients, hepatic involvement is the dominant clinical phenotype. The liver disease can be expressed with or without pancreatic insufficiency and with different degrees of pulmonary severity. Patients may also suffer from various forms of arthropathy and from vasculitis.

BASIC AND MOLECULAR GENETICS

It has been known for many years that CF is inherited as an autosomal recessive disease, with heterozygous carriers being asymptomatic. It is the most common lethal recessive genetic disease in the white population, with a carrier frequency of 4–5%. Linkage analysis had established, by 1985, that the gene was localized on the long arm of chromosome 7 (7q22–7q31.1) [2]. Only 4 years later, intense reverse genetic studies had identified the gene itself and its most common mutation [3,4]. The gene spans some 250 kb of genomic DNA, divided into 27 exons. It is transcribed as a 6.5 kb messenger RNA, which, in turn, is translated into a protein of 1480 amino acids, and which, in its mature glycosylated form, has an apparent molecular weight of 170 kDa. The protein (called the cystic fibrosis transmembrane conductance regulator, CFTR) is a member of a pro- and eukaryotic superfamily of membrane transport proteins. These have a basic two-domain structure, one being a hydrophobic transmembrane region and the other a nucleotide-binding domain. Most eukaryotic members are duplexes of the two-domain structure, but in CFTR, uniquely, the two halves of the duplex are separated by an R domain, which binds phosphokinase enzymes [5]. The CFTR functions as a chloride channel, and the defect in CF involves a failure of the channel to open in response to cyclic adenosine monophosphate (cAMP). It is unclear whether CFTR has additional functions, such as macromolecular transport or the regulation of other channel proteins. This failure of activated chloride flux is reflected in elevated concentrations of chloride and sodium in the sweat and in an abnormally electronegative potential difference across epithelia [6].

The mutation originally identified involves the deletion of an effectively in-frame triplet of nucleotides, corresponding to the deletion (Δ) of a phenylalanine residue (for which the single-letter code is F) at position 508 of the amino acid sequence. This ΔF508 mutation accounts for some 70% of CF chromosomes in Northern European and North American patients, but a lower proportion in other populations. Currently (July 1995), 546 mutations, together with over 100 phenotypically silent polymorphisms, have been identified (Cystic Fibrosis Genetic Analysis Consortium, personal communication). These affect all regions of the gene, including some intron sequences, and include nucleotide substitutions and additions as well as deletions. Definitive evidence that CFTR is the correct gene derives from transfection studies showing that wild-type CFTR complementary DNA corrects the abnormal potential difference in cultured CF cells [7].

A consequence of many, but not all, CFTR mutations is the misfolding and degradation of the mutant protein in the endoplasmic reticulum and its failure to be expressed not only on the plasma membrane, but in the membrane of intracellular organelles [8]. Lowering the temperature of expression, for example, by transfecting mutant CFTR complementary DNA into insect cells, allows much higher levels of cell-surface CFTR and this is associated with essentially normal chloride-channel activity [9].

THE GENOTYPE–PHENOTYPE RELATIONSHIP

With such a wide clinical spectrum and such a large number of mutations, it is tempting to speculate that particular mutant alleles are associated with distinct clinical phenotypes. Is this true in practice?

With the pancreas, the situation is clear-cut. There are different groups of mutations associated with PI and with PS, and PS mutations are genetically dominant over PI mutations [4,10,11]. Being homozygous for PI mutations such as ΔF508 results in a PI phenotype. Inheriting ΔF508 and a PS mutation results in a PS phenotype.

The situation is different in relation to the clinically more important lung involvement. We identified two extreme cohorts of patients from our adult CF population — one with very mild, the other with severe lung disease. There were similar numbers of patients in both groups, who were of similar mean ages and sex distribution. The mild group had a mean forced expiratory volume in 1 second (FEV_1) of 95% predicted with no or only minimal changes on chest X-ray. The severe patients had a mean FEV_1 of 23% predicted and all showed widespread bronchiectatic changes on the chest radiograph. The frequency of patients homozygous for ΔF508 was not significantly different in the two groups, nor from the frequency in the overall CF population. Similarly, there was no difference in ΔF508 allele frequency [12]. Although doing similar studies on allele–lung phenotype relationships with the less common mutations requires collaborative multicentre studies, with their disadvantages of lack of standardization of clinical parameters and patient segregation, such an international study on patients carrying the fifth most common N1303K mutation similarly revealed no concordance between inheritance of one or two copies of this allele and the severity of lung disease [13].

Analysis of ΔF508 frequency in the smaller group of patients in whom hepatic involvement is the principal clinical feature also showed no difference from the frequency in patients without clinical evidence of liver disease [14]. Apart from the pancreas, therefore, which is not a major determinant of morbidity and mortality, there is little association between genotype and phenotype in CF.

There are several possible interpretations for this disparity. The lung is an open system and environmental factors may be expected to play a role in the determination of the pulmonary phenotype. In our own mild and severe lung disease cohorts, there was a greater frequency of PS patients and a lower frequency of those chronically colonized with *P. aeruginosa* in the mild group. Nevertheless, the mild group still contained a majority who were PI and roughly half had harboured *P. aeruginosa* for the preceding 5 years. As far as we could tell, from a retrospective analysis, there were no other consistent environmental factors discriminating the mild and severe groups.

Other genetic factors can be invoked to explain genotype–phenotype disparity, though few of the possibilities have been systematically explored in CF. In both normal individuals and CF patients, a proportion of CFTR transcripts are aberrantly spliced, with one or more exons missing from the messenger RNA [15]. It has been postulated that truncated transcripts, lacking the mutant exon, may function better than full-length mutant transcripts. However, there is no evidence that the proportion and type of misspliced transcripts differ consistently between patients with different clinical phenotypes [16].

Another possibility is the involvement of other genes outside the CFTR locus (epistatic effects). We have recently obtained preliminary evidence in our own patients that a mild pulmonary phenotype may segregate with particular immune-response gene alleles, although studies with other patients with mild and severe pulmonary profiles have so far failed to confirm this [17]. Several other candidate epistatic genes await investigation, such as those coding for mucins and for α_1-antitrypsin.

GENETIC SCREENING

A fundamental question in any genetic screening programme is to whom screening should be offered. Irrespective of the chosen target group, however, several issues bear on the effectiveness of a screening programme. Among these are the real information screening can provide (and what it cannot), the avoidance of stigmatization, from an employment and insurance as well as from a psychosocial standpoint, the rates of uptake and the cost–benefit implications.

In CF, the real information that screening can provide is limited by the factors discussed above. Clearly, it is impracticable for any genetics laboratory to be able to detect over 500 mutations, and even screening for the 20 most common in a Northern European population will only detect 80% of mutant chromosomes. In a CF family, where both mutations in the index case are known, these alleles can be tracked through siblings and both maternal and paternal relatives and carriers identified. If only one mutant allele has been characterized, only maternal or paternal carrier relatives can be detected. The problem is greater in a random population. Here, by excluding, say, the 20 most common mutations, the relative risk of being a carrier can be reduced, but screening cannot say definitively that any one negative individual is or is not a heterozygote. Moreover, since particular mutations are not predictive of clinical course, screening and prenatal diagnosis cannot predict prognosis.

Uptake of an available screening programme appears partly to reflect perceived self-interest and convenience. In a highly motivated group like pregnant mothers, uptake rates of 90% have been reported [18]. With a more random population, uptake appears to reflect personal convenience. Patients waiting in a general practitioner's surgery were given a face-to-face interview about the nature of CF, and the genetic basis for the disease was explained. They were offered genetic screening and told that the test was non-invasive. Seventy per cent of those offered an immediate test accepted; for patients told that they would have to make another appointment and return later for the test, the uptake rate was only 25% [19]. Indirect approaches, such as wall posters or leaflets, appear to excite little response: even in members of a hospital genetics department approached in this way, uptake was again only around 20%.

One problem, particularly screening subjects who have no direct personal experience of CF, and little genetic background is, therefore, the time and labour required to be certain that consent for the investigation is genuinely informed. This becomes still more important with newly identified carriers, in whom much of the information given at first interview was misunderstood or had been forgotten after 3 months, and repeat counselling was necessary [19]. It is difficult to quantify the additional costs of providing the labour-intensive information and counselling services required, although clearly these are important factors in determining the overall cost–benefit implications of genetic screening.

GENE THERAPY

A number of studies have begun, aimed at finding whether a single installation of wild-type CFTR complementary DNA in a suitable vector, either in the nostril or applied to the airway through a bronchoscope, can correct the electrophysiological abnormality in CF. They are, therefore, not strictly trials of gene therapy, but preliminary *in vivo* experiments to assess its likely efficacy. The current philosophy is to design mechanisms for delivering gene therapy to the lung by inhalation.

Two vector systems have been used in these early studies. In one, replication-defective adenovirus is used not simply to carry the complementary DNA, but, by incorporating the sequence which determines the respiratory tropism of the adenovirus, to target the complementary DNA to the respiratory epithelium. The other system uses cationic liposomes. Both vector systems have been shown, at least in a proportion of patients, to deliver translatable complementary DNA that temporarily reverses the potential difference abnormality across the respiratory epithelium [20,21]. Clearly, both forms of delivery are effective on a one-off basis, though for therapy repeated treatments will be necessary.

The problems to be overcome in the implementation of true gene replacement therapy will partly depend on the age at which treatment can be started. Ideally, gene therapy should be initiated directly after birth and before pulmonary disease is evident. However, there are thousands of older patients with varying degrees of pulmonary pathology from whom it would be unethical to withhold treatment, but in whom additional problems of delivery may be anticipated. In these older patients, genetic replacement will, at best, arrest the progress of the lung disease, but cannot be expected to reverse pathological changes that have already occurred.

Some difficulties may arise irrespective of the age at which treatment is started. For example, it would seem likely that inhalation of large numbers of DNA-containing liposomes into the airway would lead to their rapid removal by resident phagocytic cells within the lung, such as alveolar macrophages. It may prove possible to swamp this barrier by increasing liposome dose, but resident phagocytic cells satiated with liposomes may show compromised antibacterial functions. This could predispose neonatal patients to infection and accentuate bacterial colonization in older patients.

A further potential immunological problem is inherent in gene and protein replacement therapy for genetic disease. The immune system of the affected subject matures in the context of the mutant protein, which it regards as self and to which it does not respond. The wild-type protein may, therefore, be recognized as a foreign antigen, and an immune response generated to it. This may be more likely if self/non-self discrimination has been learned in an environment of some mutant proteins (say deletions) rather than others (say substitutions), and if the wild-type sequence is expressed in a particularly immunogenic form in antigen-presenting cells such as the alveolar macrophage/dendritic cell system within the lung.

Roughly 10% of all upper respiratory tract infections are due to adenovirus, and many adult patients have antiadenoviral antibodies. Not surprisingly, the titres of these increase following experimental adenovirus-complementary DNA exposure, and this may limit the suitability of adenovirus vectors for repeated treatments [22]. It is unclear how immunogenic adenovirus vectors would be in the neonate. In older infected patients, also, the viscous mucus may prevent passage of inhaled vectors into the airway cells in the same way as it hinders effective delivery of other drugs to the airway epithelium. Recent studies have, however, shown that rhDNase reduces mucus viscosity and improves pulmonary function in CF [23], and this may allow more effective penetration of the vector.

CONCLUSION

The tone of this review has intentionally been cautious. Rightly, we regard the rapid progress over the last 10 years from the genomic localization of the CFTR gene to its complete sequence, the identification of over 500 mutations and the beginnings of genetic therapy as an impressive achievement. But we also need to be clear about what we don't understand and where, therefore, further research is required.

Apart from the pancreas, there is no direct mutant allele–phenotypic concordance in CF. Why do some 25-year-old patients have essentially normal lungs, whereas others are in respiratory failure? It would seem that both environmental and non-CFTR genetic factors contribute, and defining what these are and how they interact with each other and with particular CFTR mutations to produce a particular phenotype may lead to a better understanding of polygenic disease in general. It may also help us to identify risk factors specific for individual patients, which we can advise them to avoid.

Genetic carrier screening, particularly of random populations, may only lead to a statistical reduction of risk. Family members of affected patients, who have some knowledge of the disease and who may be more highly motivated than a general population, would seem the most suitable candidates for screening, especially where one or both mutations in the affected case are known. Even here, there is a need for skilled professional counselling, whose costs should not be forgotten in any overall assessment of the cost–benefit implications of a screening programme.

Genetic correction, at least at the electrophysiological level, is clearly possible. How readily, using the current delivery systems, this can be developed into effective repeated aerosolized therapy is unclear. It may therefore be prudent also to encourage the parallel development of more conventional forms of treatment, such as a purely pharmacological approach to reversing the abnormality of CFTR function, and towards selective anti-inflammatory therapies such as elastase inhibitors.

REFERENCES

1 Doring G, Bellon G, Knight R. Immunology of cystic fibrosis. In: *Cystic Fibrosis*, edited by Hodson ME, Geddes DM. Chapman & Hall, London, 1995:99–129.
2 Tsui L-C, Buchwald M, Barker JC *et al.* Cystic fibrosis locus defined by a genetically linked polymorphic DNA marker. *Science* 1985;**230**:1054–1057.
3 Riordan JR, Rommens JM, Kerem B *et al.* Identification of the cystic fibrosis gene: cloning and characterisation of complementary DNA. *Science* 1989;**245**:1066–1073.
4 Kerem B, Rommens JM, Buchanan JA *et al.* Identification of the cystic fibrosis gene: genetic analysis. *Science* 1989;**245**:1073–1080.
5 Hyde SC, Emsley P, Hartshorn MJ *et al.* Structural model of ATP-binding proteins associated with cystic fibrosis, multidrug resistance and bacterial transport. *Nature* 1990;**346**:362–365.
6 Knowles M, Gatzy J, Boucher R. Increased bioelectric potential difference across respiratory epithelia in cystic fibrosis. *N Engl J Med* 1981;**305**:1489–1495.
7 Drumm ML, Pope HA, Cliff WH. Correction of the cystic fibrosis defect *in vitro* by retrovirus-mediated gene transfer. *Cell* 1990;**62**:1227–1233.
8 Cheng SH, Gregory RJ, Marshall J *et al.* Defective intracellular transport and processing of CFTR is the molecular basis of most cystic fibrosis. *Cell* 1990;**63**:827–834.
9 Kartner N, Hanrahan JW, Jensen TJ *et al.* Expression of the cystic fibrosis gene in non-epithelial invertebrate cells produces a regulated anion conductance. *Cell* 1991;**64**:681–689.
10 Santis G, Osborne LA, Knight RA, Hodson ME. Independent genetic determinants of pancreatic and pulmonary status in cystic fibrosis. *Lancet* 1990;**336**:1081–1084.
11 Krisitides P, Bozon D, Corey M *et al.* Genetic determination of exocrine pancreatic function in cystic fibrosis. *Am J Hum Genet* 1992;**50**:1178–1184.
12 Santis G, Osborne LA, Knight RA, Hodson ME. Linked marker haplotypes and the Δ F508 mutation in adult patients with mild pulmonary disease and cystic fibrosis. *Lancet* 1990;**335**:1426–1429.
13 Osborne L, Santis G, Schwarz M *et al.* Incidence and expression of the N1303K mutation of the cystic fibrosis (CFTR) gene. *Hum Genet* 1992;**89**:653–658.
14 Duthie A, Doherty DG, Williams C *et al.* Genotype analysis for Δ F508, G551D and R553X mutations in children and young adults with cystic fibrosis with and without chronic liver disease. *Hepatology* 1992;**18**:660–664.
15 Chu CS, Trapnell BC, Murtagh JJ *et al.* Variable deletion of exon 9 coding sequences in cystic fibrosis transmembrane conductance regulator gene mRNA transcripts in normal bronchial epithelium. *EMBO J* 1991;**10**:1355–1363.
16 Chu CS, Trapnell BC, Curristin SM *et al.* Extensive posttranscriptional deletion of the coding sequence for part of nucleotide binding fold 1 in respiratory epithelial mRNA transcripts of the cystic fibrosis transmembrane conductance regulator gene is not associated with the clinical manifestations of cystic fibrosis. *J Clin Invest* 1992;**90**:785–790.
17 Dean M, Osborne L, Santis G, Knight R. Association of HLA and IL1RA alleles with pulmonary disease severity. *Pediatr Pulm* 1994;**s10**:212.
18 Harris H, Scotcher D, Hartley N, Wallace A, Craufurd D, Harris R. Cystic fibrosis carrier testing in early pregnancy by general practitioners. *Br Med J* 1993;**306**:1580–1583.
19 Bekker H, Modell M, Denniss G *et al.* Uptake of cystic fibrosis testing in primary care: supply push or demand pull? *Br Med J* 1993;**306**:1584–1586.

20 Zabner J, Couture LA, Gregory RJ, Graham SM, Smith AE, Welsh MJ. Adenovirus-mediated gene transfer transiently corrects the chloride transport defect in nasal epithelia of patients with cystic fibrosis. *Cell* 1993;75:207–216.
21 Caplen NJ, Alton EWFW, Middleton PG *et al*. Liposome-mediated CFTR gene transfer to the nasal epithelium of patients with cystic fibrosis. *Nature Med* 1995;1:39–46.
22 Yei S, Mittereder N, Tang K, O'Sullivan C, Trapnell BC. Adenovirus-mediated gene transfer for cystic fibrosis: quantitative evaluation of repeated *in vivo* vector administration to the lung. *Gene Ther* 1994;1:192–200.
23 Ranasinha C, Assoufi B, Shak S *et al*. Efficacy and safety of short-term administration of aerosolised recombinant human DNase 1 in adults with stable stage cystic fibrosis. *Lancet* 1993;342:199–202.

MULTIPLE CHOICE QUESTIONS

1 The abnormal gene responsible for cystic fibrosis
a is inherited as an autosomal recessive character
b is associated with some disease, even if inherited in a heterozygous form
c shows only a single mutation associated with the disease
d codes for a chloride channel
e is associated with an abnormal potential difference across airway epithelia

2 The lung disease in cystic fibrosis
a is directly due to the genetic abnormality
b is associated with chronic bacterial infection
c tends to be more severe in patients with pancreatic sufficiency
d is related to the release of neutrophil proteolytic enzymes
e has been corrected by gene therapy

3 Particular genetic mutations are predictive of
a overall survival
b severity of lung involvement
c severity of pancreatic involvement
d incidence of liver involvement
e aberrant messenger RNA splicing

4 Genetic screening for cystic fibrosis
a can identify all heterozygous carriers
b can predict overall prognosis in any homozygote
c has a higher uptake if subjects receive face-to-face interview
d may have social and psychological consequences
e has been shown to be financially justified

5 Gene therapy for cystic fibrosis
a has been delivered by liposomes
b is being delivered systemically

c can correct the abnormal potential difference across airway epithelia
d has been shown to arrest the progress of lung disease
e has been shown not to be associated with immunological problems

Answers

1	a	True	2	a	False	3	a	False
	b	False		b	True		b	False
	c	False		c	False		c	True
	d	True		d	True		d	False
	e	True		e	False		e	False

4	a	False	5	a	True
	b	False		b	False
	c	True		c	True
	d	True		d	False
	e	False		e	False

PART 5
GROWTH FACTORS

Growth factors:
new insights — new opportunities

JEFF M. P. HOLLY

Over the last couple of decades it has become clear that there are a large number of peptide growth factors. These growth factors can be broadly classified into six families of closely related peptides (Table 1). Some of these are large families with numerous different growth factors, indeed there are so many transforming growth factor-β (TGF-β)-like growth factors that this is now referred to as the TGF-β superfamily, whilst other families are numerically relatively small; the insulin-like growth factors (IGFs) comprise just two peptides, IGF-I and IGF-II. Until recently it was considered that these peptide growth factors differed from classical peptide hormones due to their more ubiquitous sites of production. Locally produced peptides which acted on neighbouring cells (paracrine actions) or even on their own cells of origin (autocrine actions) appeared to be quite distinct from peptides produced within specialized glands with endocrine actions on distant target tissues. This distinction has gradually been eroded by the increasing awareness that many traditional peptide hormones are produced in many tissues other than their traditional endocrine gland. However, it has also become apparent that there may be other much more fundamental differences which distinguish the way in which growth factors are used as cell regulators.

Hormonal activity is tightly regulated, normally by precise control of secretion of the hormone from large stores held in secretory granules within the cells of the endocrine glands. The sites of hormone action are also well-defined by the cell-specific expression of the relevant cell receptors. In contrast, many growth factors and their receptors are constitutively expressed widely throughout most tissues. As the growth factor is slowly secreted as it is produced, no intracellular stores are built up. However, mechanisms have evolved to interrupt the signal, preventing the growth factors from immediately interacting with their ubiquitous receptors and enabling extracellular stores of the growth factor to be maintained. This is accomplished in various ways with the different growth factors; they are either secreted in an inactive proform or bind to other components which hold them in latent complexes. The important regulatory stage is then the control of the activation or the mobilization of the growth factor

Table 1 Peptide growth factor families.

Epidermal growth factor (EGF)
Transforming growth Factor-β (TGF-β)
Platelet-derived growth factor (PDGF)
Fibroblast growth factor (FGF)
Insulin-like growth factor (IGF)
Neurotrophic growth factor (NGF)

---

from the extracellular store. It has also become apparent that many of the growth factors are not just mitogens but have a pluripotential nature and can stimulate many aspects of the function of their target cells [1]. These growth factors are therefore produced in most tissues where they can affect most aspects of tissue function.

The critical questions now being addressed are how specificity is conferred on these growth factors, enabling them to play important regulatory roles according to developmental stage and according to the local setting. With a number of growth factors this appears to be accomplished by the growth factor being part of a complex system comprising multiple components which control its availability and cellular actions. These components are generally independently regulated and their interactions presumably confer specificity, enabling the growth factor actions to be controlled in a manner most appropriate according to the local situation.

STORAGE OF GROWTH FACTORS

One of the first storage sites for growth factors to become apparent was the platelets, which not only provide a store of platelet-derived growth factor (PDGF) but also a number of other growth factors, including TGF-β and IGFs. This provides an obvious source of growth factor which can be targeted to appropriate sites of action which are particularly important for tissue injury and the wound-healing response. However, it has become apparent that this is just one of many systems which enable large stores of growth factors to be maintained throughout the body. The fibroblast growth factors (FGFs) associate with high affinity to glycosaminoglycans which enable stores of FGFs to be maintained on cell surfaces and in particular on the extracellular matrix (ECM) [2]. Basic and acidic FGFs (FGF-1 and FGF-2) are expressed without signal peptide sequences to direct them for secretion from the cell. How these FGFs are externalized from cells is not clear but may involve their association with glycosaminoglycans within the cell and then being externalized with the glycosaminoglycan. Binding to the glycosaminoglycans enables the FGF to be held in a latent form within the tissues ready for activation when needed.

The ECM in many tissues holds a large reservoir of a number of growth factors, including not only FGFs and other heparin-binding growth factors but also members of the TGF-β superfamily and IGFs. The TGF-β isoforms are expressed as propeptides which are heavily glycosylated and cleaved to form the mature growth factors and a corresponding amino-terminal glycopeptide. The amino-terminal glycopeptide remains non-covalently associated with the growth factor and is called the latency-associated peptide (LAP); the TGF-β along with the LAP then dimerizes to form the latent TGF-β complex which is secreted [3]. This latent complex then becomes associated with matrix components either directly or after association with a specific binding protein which binds to LAP.

The IGFs appear to be secreted as mature active growth factors but immediately associate with specific high-affinity binding proteins (IGFBPs) which are generally present in excess, such that virtually all IGFs are present in complexed forms. It is now apparent that there are at least six distinct IGFBPs which form a family of closely related peptides, sharing a number of structural features but having very distinct patterns of expression, regulation and functional properties [4]. The IGFs bind to these IGFBPs with affinities generally greater than that with which they bind to the IGF-I cell receptor, which mediates most cell actions, and therefore the IGFBPs again hold these growth factors in an apparently latent form. A number of the IGFBPs have proteoglycan binding sequences and can bind to components of the ECM and maintain IGFs immobilized on the matrix; two (IGFBP-1 and IGFBP-2) have RGD (-arg -gly -asp-, tripeptide) sequences which can bind to cell-surface intergrin receptors and target or localize IGFs to cells which express the appropriate receptor. In addition, IGFBP-3 binds specifically to a further peptide known as the acid-labile subunit (ALS), forming a soluble complex which appears to maintain a large reservoir of IGF within the circulation [5]. Very high levels of IGFs are found in the circulation where this complex appears to form a circulating store of IGF.

There are therefore a variety of mechanisms which maintain high levels of growth factors throughout the body in latent reservoirs. The cells are therefore generally surrounded by a ready source of many growth factors held in latent forms within the pericellular environment.

MOBILIZATION/ACTIVATION OF GROWTH FACTORS

In many tissues the levels of growth factors in the extracellular stores exceeds that required for maximal stimulation of the cells and the control of availability of these latent reservoirs is tightly regulated according to tissue requirements. The liberation of growth factors from platelets at sites of tissue damage has long been acknowledged as a specific delivery system to target growth factors to sites of specific acute need. Over the last few years it has become apparent that there are many other mechanisms for controlling the mobilization and activation of growth factors from their stores. This generally involves specific enzymatic modification of the growth factor or of the component with which they are bound. This can be by small modifications such as phosphorylations or by proteolytic cleavage. Basic FGF can be phosphorylated by a protein kinase on the surface of target cells increasing its availability for its high-affinity receptors [6]. A number of the IGFBPs exist in differentially phosphorylated states which can alter the affinity with which they bind IGFs [7]. There are many matrix-degrading enzymes with well-characterized roles in processes from embryo implantation to tissue remodelling, wound repair and neoplastic growth; these enzymes can obviously also affect the storage of growth factors held on the matrix. Many enzymes are involved in these processes, including the plasmin system, matrix metalloproteinases and cathepsins; indeed, in most circumstances activation of one enzyme leads to a cascade with sequential activation of other proenzymes to degrade the many different components of the matrix. A number of enzymes which degrade components of the ECM result in the mobilization of FGFs attached to soluble glycosaminoglycan fragments; indeed, binding to such glycosaminoglycans appears to be necessary for the FGF to be presented to its high-affinity cell receptor [8].

Binding molecules involved in storage of other growth factors also appear to play a role in either the presentation of the growth factor to cell receptors or modulating receptor interaction and/or signalling. A number of the IGFBPs which interact with cell surfaces can enhance IGF actions. There have also been several reports that IGFBPs can alter cell function independently of their ability to bind IGFs. This can be due to interaction with cell-surface integrin receptors via RGD sequences in IGFBP-1 and IGFBP-2 or due to other IGFBPs interacting with specific cell-surface proteoglycans [7]. The proteoglycan betaglycan binds TGF-β on cell surfaces and can present the growth factor to its signalling receptors.

A number of the general extracellular proteases which participate in matrix breakdown are also involved in activation of other latent growth factors. For example, plasmin activity can activate latent TGF-β and plasmin, cathepsins and metalloproteinases can all fragment IGFBPs, resulting in mobilization of the IGFs they carry. These mechanisms may have many important implications. It has recently been shown that the cardiovascular risk factor apolipoprotein a is a homologue of plasminogen and can inhibit the conversion of plasminogen to active plasmin. In mice transgenic for overexpression of apolipoprotein a the conversion of plasminogen to plasmin in aortic wall was considerably reduced and as a result there was much less activation of TGF-β, despite total TGF-β levels being unaltered [9]. As TGF-β is an inhibitor of smooth-muscle proliferation, a decrease in its activity could obviously contribute to vascular lesions. In addition to these non-specific proteases there appear to be specific proteases for a number of individual IGFBPs and these are regulated in different situations, presumably to modulate IGF activity [10].

GROWTH FACTOR ACTIONS

Most peptide growth factors can regulate the function of many cells throughout the body. The names of specific growth factor families are only of historical significance; for example, the FGFs can stimulate many non-fibroblastic cells and indeed appear to be particularly potent angiogenic factors stimulating vascular endothelial cells. It has also gradually become apparent that most of the peptide growth factors are not just mitogens but can have many actions on cell function. The IGFs are growth stimulators, they have metabolic actions due to their insulin-like nature, they can be potent cell survival factors delaying programmed cell death, they can induce the differentiation of undifferentiated cells and they promote the differentiated function of many cells. Many of the other growth factors are similarly also pluripotenital cell regulators [1]. Indeed, a number can both stimulate and inhibit cell proliferation depending on the target cell type and on the circumstances or context in which the signal is received. An example of this is TGF-β which stimulates proliferation of most fibroblast-like cells but has antiproliferative effects on epithelial cells [3].

GROWTH FACTOR INTERACTIONS

Cells *in vivo* are generally exposed to many growth factors simultaneously and it appears that these signals are integrated to determine cell function. There are many levels at which the different growth factors can interact. A number of growth factors can directly alter the receptors or cell sensitivity to another growth factor — processes termed transmodulation. For example, PDGF can decrease the affinity of the epidermal growth factor (EGF) receptor for its ligand. Other more complex interactions may also be present between the different growth factors. The activation of the latent TGF-β complex in some tissues may be facilitated by its binding to the IGF-II receptor via mannose-6-phosphate binding sites present on this multifunctional receptor [11]. The IGF-II receptor is itself regulated by insulin, which does not bind to the receptor but dynamically controls its redistribution from cytoplasmic sites to the cell surface [12]. The proliferative effects of TGF-β can be mediated through PDGF pathways [13] and the antiproliferative effects of TGF-β on other cells may be mediated through its effects on IGFBP-3 [14].

In addition to all these complex means of direct cross-talk, there are also many other ways in which growth factors can affect the critical control mechanisms which regulate the availability and activity of other growth factors. As outlined above, many growth factors interact with either cell surfaces or the EMC and regulators which alter the production or proteolytic processing of these structures can therefore have important effects on the storage and mobilization of such growth factors. The production of matrix components is stimulated by TGF-β which also decreases the production of matrix-degrading enzymes such as metalloproteinases and increases production of their inhibitors [15]. TGF-β also potently increases the production of IGFBP-3 from a number of cell types which can inhibit IGF activity and possibly has other inhibitory actions [14]. All of these actions of TGF-β can affect the sequestration, mobilization and actions of a number of other growth factors. The IGF-II receptor, via its ability to bind mannose-6-phosphate groups, can bind procathepsins, the latent secreted form of these enzymes. This may lead to activation of the cathepsin which in turn can activate further latent enzymes such as metalloproteinases and thus initiate a cascade, resulting in proteolysis of matrix and activation and mobilization of a variety of growth factors. Such a sequence of events appears to be active in some neoplastic growths such as in certain breast cancers, where an association between the IGF-II receptor and cathepsin D has been described [16].

SUMMARY

The peptide growth factors form a complex component of the language used by cells to communicate with each other within the body. These growth factors are pluripotential regulators affecting many aspects of cell function. It is becoming clear that there are a number of mechanisms whereby specificity is conferred on these ubiquitous signals. Many of the growth factors are part of complex systems involving many interrelated components which interact to determine cellular activity. For example, there are at least seven distinct FGFs which bind with high affinity to components of the ECM, cell surfaces and at least four specific cell receptors. This provides the opportunity for a variety of components to interact variably and confer specificity according to local circumstances. Similarly, the IGF system comprises many interacting components (Fig. 1) which are all independently regulated, enabling specificity to be conferred such that IGF actions are elaborated in the most appropriate manner according to circumstances. In addition to the complexity within each growth factor system, it is becoming increasingly clear that there is much cross-talk between the different growth factors and indeed with other cytokines. This enables cells to respond to a growth factor according to the context in which it receives the signal; so the same growth factor could stimulate a cell within certain conditions but inhibit the same cell

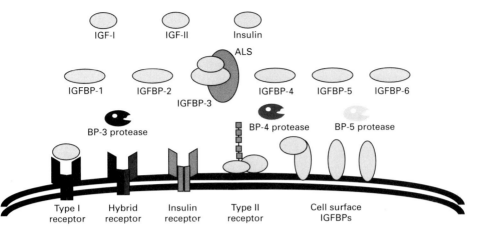

Fig. 1 The numerous components of the insulin-like growth factor (IGF) system which are now known to interact to control the activity of these growth factors at the cellular level.

under different conditions. The new understanding of how these signalling systems operate provides new opportunities for understanding how systems may go wrong. This may also lead to the design of novel strategies for intervention either to mobilize latent growth factors or to prevent their activation.

REFERENCES

1 Sporn MB, Roberts AB. Peptide growth factors are multifunctional. *Nature* 1988;**332**:217–219.
2 Baird A, Bohlen P. Fibroblast growth factors. In *Peptide Growth Factors and their Receptors*, edited by Sporn MB, Roberts AB. Springer-Verlag, Berlin, 1990:369–418.
3 Lyons RM, Moses HL. Transforming growth factors and the regulation of cell proliferation. *Eur J Biochem* 1990;**187**:467–473.
4 Kiefer MC, Schmid C, Waldvogel M *et al*. Characterization of recombinant human insulin-like growth factor binding proteins 4, 5, and 6 produced in yeast. *J Biol Chem* 1992;**267**:12692–12699.
5 Baxter RC. Physiological roles of IGF binding proteins. In: *Modern Concepts of Insulin-like Growth Factors*, edited by Spencer EM. Elsevier Science, New York, 1991:371–380.
6 Vilgrain I, Baird A. Phosphorylation of basic fibroblast growth factor by a protein kinase associated with the outer surface of a target cell. *Mol Endocrinol* 1991;**5**:1003–1012.
7 Clemmons DR, Camacho-Hubner C, Jones JI, McCusker RH, Busby WH. Insulin-like growth factor binding proteins: mechanisms of action at the cellular level. In: *Modern Concepts of Insulin-like Growth Factors*, edited by Spencer EM. Elsevier Science, New York, 1991:475–486.
8 Yayon A, Klagsbrun M, Esko JD, Leder P, Ornitz DM. Cell surface, heparin-like molecules are required for binding of basic fibroblast growth factor to its high affinity receptor. *Cell* 1991;**64**:841–848.
9 Dennis PA, Rifkin DB. Cellular activation of latent transforming growth factor beta

requires binding to the action-independent mannose 6-phosphate/insulin-like growth factor II receptor. *Proc Natl Acad Sci USA*. 1991;**88**:580–584.

10 Grainger DJ, Kemp PR, Liu AC, Lawn RM, Metcalfe JC. Activation of transforming growth factor-β is inhibited in transgenic apolipoprotein(a) mice. *Nature* 1994;**370**:460–462.

11 Holly JMP, Claffey DCP, Cwyfan-Hughes SC, Frost VJ, Yateman ME. Proteases acting on IGFBPs; their occurrence and physiological significance. *Growth Regul* 1993;**3**:88–91.

12 Appell KC, Simpson IA, Cushman SW. Characterization of the stimulatory action of insulin on insulin-like growth factor II binding to rat adipose cells. *J Biol Chem* 1988;**263**:10824–10829.

13 Seifert RA, Coats SA, Raines EW, Ross R, Bowen-Pope DF. Platelet-derived growth factor (PDGF) receptor alpha-subunit mutant and reconstituted cell lines demonstrate that transforming growth factor-beta can be mitogenic through PDGF A-chain dependent and -independent pathways. *J Biol Chem* 1994;**269**:13951–13955.

14 Yateman ME, Claffey DC, Cwyfan-Hughes SC, Frost VJ, Wass JAH, Holly JMP. Cytokines modulate the sensitivity of human fibroblasts to stimulation with IGF-I by altering endogenous IGFBP-3 production. *J Endocrinol* 1993;**137**:151–159.

15 Roberts AB, Sporn MB. The transforming growth factor-βs. In: *Peptide Growth Factors and their Receptors*, edited by *Sporn MB, Roberts AB*. Springer-Verlag, Berlin, 1990:419–472.

16 Zhao Y, Escot C, Maudelonde T, Puech C, Rouanet P, Rochefort H. Correlation between mannose 6-phosphate/IGF-II receptor and cathepsin D RNA levels by *in situ* hybridization in benign and malignant mammary tumours. *Cancer Res* 1993;**53**:2901–2905.

MULTIPLE CHOICE QUESTIONS

1 Are peptide growth factors generally stored
a in secretory granules within specific cell types?
b within most cells?
c within specific tissues?
d outside cells, on matrix or in solution?
e nowhere in the body?

2 Do peptide growth factors
a stimulate mitogenesis?
b prevent programmed cell death?
c stimulate cell differentiation?
d stimulate the differentiated function of cells?
e do all of the above?

3 In general, is the activity of peptide growth factors acutely regulated by
a induction of the production of new growth factor?
b mobilization or activation of growth factors from extracellular stores?
c secretion of growth factor from cellular stores?
d acute changes in cell-surface receptors?
e all of the above?

4 Do specific families of peptide growth factors
  a differ in the cell types from which they are produced?
  b differ in the cell types on which they act?
  c interact to regulate most cell types?
  d act only within specific tissues?
  e do none of the above?

5 How is specificity thought to be conferred on the general peptide growth factors?
  a by the context within which a signal is seen in relation to the other signals which the cell also receives?
  b by their specific site of expression?
  c by the site of expression of specific receptors?
  d by the specific activation/mobilization of the growth factor at certain sites or times?

Answers

1			2			3		
	a	False		**a**	False		**a**	False
	b	False		**b**	False		**b**	True
	c	False		**c**	False		**c**	False
	d	True		**d**	False		**d**	False
	e	False		**e**	True		**e**	False

4			5		
	a	False		**a**	True
	b	False		**b**	False
	c	True		**c**	False
	d	False		**d**	False
	e	False			

Growth factors in breast cancer. The role of TNF-α: implications for prognosis and possible strategies for intervention

CLAIRE E. LEWIS & JAMES O'D. McGEE

Solid human tumours consist of a heterogeneous population of cells comprising the malignant cell population and such stromal cells as macrophages, lymphocytes, natural killer (NK) cells, neutrophils, fibroblasts and endothelial cells [1,2]. These cell types communicate with one another by a complex network of extracellular signals, including many cytokines and their soluble receptors. Intratumoral cytokines are usually polypeptides produced by cells within the tumour to act locally in an autocrine, paracrine and/or juxtacrine manner [3,4]. Plate 2 summarizes the last 10 years of research into the cellular sources and effects of individual cytokines within solid human tumours. It illustrates the complex, interactive network of communication formed by such molecules. Although the net effect of these pleiotropic cytokines within the tumour microenvironment has yet to be fully elucidated, they appear from a plethora of *in vitro* studies to be capable of regulating: (i) the proliferation and metastatic activity of malignant cells; (ii) the tumoricidal activity of infiltrating immune cells; and (iii) the establishment of the stromal compartment by stimulating both the deposition of matrix components and the development of a new blood supply for the tumour [1,3,4].

There is growing evidence for the involvement of the cytokine 'tumour necrosis factor-α (TNF-α)' in the progression of breast cancer. This form of tumour comprises a considerable number of mononuclear-infiltrating cells which are predominantly T lymphocytes, NK cells and macrophages [5–7]. These cell types, when activated, produce and secrete TNF-α *in vitro* and may therefore be a potential source of this cytokine *in vivo*. Indeed, it has been demonstrated that tumour-infiltrating lymphocytes isolated from breast cancer biopsies secrete TNF-α when challenged with autologous tumour cells in the presence of interleukin-2 *in vitro* [8,9]. More recently, we have shown that individual immunophenotyped macrophages derived from enzymatically dispersed primary breast cancers secrete TNF-α *ex vivo* [10]. Moreover, direct evidence for the *in situ* production of TNF-α in the microenvironment of breast tumours has been provided by the demonstration of messenger RNA for TNF-α in such tumours [11,12].

The potential biological consequences of the presence of TNF-α in the microenvironment of breast cancer are numerous. TNF-α may restrict the growth of neoplastic cells in several ways. It may be directly cytotoxic or cytostatic and/or augment the immune response against tumour cells by recruiting infiltrating cells to the tumour site and stimulating their cytotoxic activity [13–16]. TNF-α may also induce haemorrhagic necrosis within tumours by its procoagulant and thrombotic activity on endothelial cells [17,18]. Under certain circumstances, it is also conceivable that TNF-α may promote tumour growth. TNF-α has been demonstrated to be angiogenic in experimental systems (reviewed by us in [1], and has also been shown to enhance the metastatic potential of ovarian carcinoma cells in rodent tumour models [19–21]).

Two separate receptors for TNF-α have been cloned and designated TNF-R p55 and TNF-R p75 respectively [22,23]. The extracellular ligand-binding domains of the two receptors show some homology but their intracellular domains differ. The cellular distribution of the two types of TNF receptors appears to be distinct, although in some cases it may overlap [24,25]. It has been suggested that the two receptors mediate different biological effects of TNF-α [26].

In a recent study [27], we compared the cellular distribution of TNF-α with that of its two distinct TNF receptors, TNF-R p55 and p75, by immunohistochemistry on frozen sections of human breast cancer biopsies. The expression of this cytokine and its receptors was also examined in a small number of reduction mammoplasty specimens (i.e. normal breast tissue).

TNF-α was expressed focally in 50% of the tumours studied, being largely localized to macrophage-like cells in the stroma. TNF-R p55 was expressed by a population of stromal cells in all the tumours examined, and a varying proportion of neoplastic cells and endothelial cells in 75% of these tissues. TNF-R p75 was detected in about 70% of the tumours, immunoreactivity being confined mainly to leukocytes in the stroma (Plate 3). Expression of TNF-α or TNF-R p75 was not detectable in normal breast tissue or in non-malignant breast tissue adjacent to the tumours. By contrast, TNF-R p55 was expressed by occasional stromal cells in normal tissue (not shown).

Taken together, these results demonstrate that TNF-α and its receptors are up-regulated in breast cancer, although the cytokine itself is not present in all breast tumours and even then only in a minority of tumour-infiltrating macrophages. There may be a number of reasons for this. First, this may reflect the relative absence of activated leukocytes in the tumour micro-environment due either to the escape of neoplastic cells from immune recognition or to the presence of immune-suppressor activity [28,29]. Second, such an expression pattern may reflect the existence of permanent, spatially localized cytokine 'hot spots' within the tissue. Several reports have indicated that cytokines, though scarce, are not entirely absent from human breast tumours. Interleukins-1,-2 and -6, interferon-α, and TNF-α are expressed focally in many tumours, indicating that heterogeneity exists with respect to cytokine production, and possibly secretion, within the tumour microenvironment [11,12,30,31]. Such putative cytokine hot spots may have biological significance by providing an environmental force which drives phenotypic changes in adjacent neoplastic and stromal cells. This is based on the presumption (yet to be proven) that TNF-α is produced and secreted at sufficiently high concentrations and duration to induce phenotypic changes in adjacent cells. Such hot spots of TNF-α expression may contribute to the genesis of phenotypic heterogeneity amongst individual neoplastic and/or stromal cells within breast tumours. For example, in theory, spontaneous TNF-resistant clones may arise in such locations due to exposure to high local concentrations of TNF-α for sufficiently prolonged periods. Such clones could subsequently expand. It is worth noting that a TNF-α-resistant phenotype also confers resistance to certain chemotherapeutic drugs *in vitro* [30]. Indeed, indirect evidence for the existence of similar cross-resistance *in vivo* was provided by experiments on short-term primary cultures of breast cancers. A positive correlation between sensitivity to TNF-α and doxorubicin was reported on neoplastic mammary epithelial cells in these experiments [32].

Third, the limited intracellular storage of such cytokines as TNF-α and the transient nature of their production by activated cells in the tumour may limit their immunodetection. Technical aspects of the present study, such as potential limitations in the sensitivity of the immunocytochemical method applied, may also have contributed to the limited number of cells which were immunoreactive for this cytokine. However, many of the results of this study have recently been confirmed by the similar findings of Balkwill's group using *in situ* hybridization and immunocytochemistry to localize the messenger RNA and protein respectively for these molecules in a larger number of frozen breast biopsies [12].

Immunoreactivity for TNF-R p55 protein was evident both in stromal cells (including tumour-infiltrating leukocytes and vascular endothelial cells) and neoplastic cells in breast tumours. This contrasts with the recent findings of Naylor and his colleagues who used *in situ* hybridization (ISH) to demonstrate the absence of expression of messenger RNA for TNF-R p55 by stromal macrophages in ovarian cancer [33]. This discrepancy may mean that the low levels of TNF-α expressed by macrophages in ovarian tumours are not detectable by the ISH technique used in the latter study, or that this cell type simply does not perform this function in ovarian cancer.

The physiological significance, if any, of the up-regulated and heterogeneous expression of TNF-R p55 and p75 in malignant compared to normal breast tissue is unclear at the present time. It is not unexpected in light of the fact that virtually all breast cell lines bind TNF-α *in vitro*. Furthermore, Dolbaum and colleagues demonstrated that the majority of primary breast cancer cultures were inhibited by TNF-α, whilst normal mammary epithelial cells were relatively resistant to this effect of TNF-α [32].

To assess the possible contribution of TNF-α to the biology and progression of breast cancer, we compared the expression of TNF-α and its receptors with the following biological parameters of the same tumours: (i) proliferative activity (assessed by Ki67 expression); (ii) neovascularization (assessed by CD31 expression); (iii) metastatic potential (indicated. by the lymph node status); and (iv) degree of lymphoid infiltration (estimated by the presence of cells expressing the leukocyte common antigen, CD45) [27].

There was no significant association between the expression of TNF-α and its receptors and any of these tumour parameters, although a larger number of tumours (i.e. than the 28 included in this study) should be evaluated for this to be assessed accurately for the disease as a whole. Furthermore, the present study has focused on clinically manifest and therefore, by definition, quite advanced tumours. The possibility of a more prominent role for TNF-α and its receptors at an early (preclinical) stage in the progression of breast cancer cannot be excluded.

However, even with such a small group size, there was a significant correlation between the expression of TNF-R p55 by blood vessels and the number of infiltrating leukocytes present. This suggests that the expression of this receptor by vascular endothelial cells may facilitate migration of immunocompetent cells into the tumour site. Such an effect is anticipated from the reported activities of TNF-α *in vitro*, particularly the ability of this cytokine to induce the expression of selectins on endothelial cells (which have ligands on certain leukocytes) [3,4,34]. Alternatively, it might represent an endothelial reaction to the presence of mononuclear inflammatory cells and/or neoplastic cells infiltrating the tissue.

Recent studies have indicated that increased levels of soluble TNF receptors of both type may be detected in the serum of patients with advanced breast cancer [35]. The origin of these soluble receptors is unclear. Since there is increasing evidence that these proteins are derived from the cell-surface receptors by proteolytic cleavage [36], our results, and those of others, suggest that neoplastic and stromal cells in breast tumours may be a source of receptor shedding. Although this suggests that such tumours may, indeed, be a source of TNF-α receptor release into the blood stream, a direct correlation of TNF-α receptor expression by breast tumour cells with the levels of soluble TNF receptors in the serum of the same patients has yet to be established.

The possible biological function of soluble TNF-α receptors is not known at present. Soluble TNF receptors may neutralize TNF-α bioactivity by mopping up TNF-α and protecting various target-cell types from this cytokine. They may also serve to provide local and systemic reservoirs of cytokine. The sera of the patients studied by Aderka *et al.* [35] had a marked inhibitory effect on the *in vitro* activities of TNF-α; moreover, this inhibition could be abolished by the exposure of the sera to anti-TNF-α receptor antibodies, suggesting an active suppressive role for circulating TNF receptors. It is noteworthy that in the present study the expression/release of TNF-α was not correlated with that of either form of TNF-α receptor. It appears, therefore, that the production of immunoreactive TNF-α may not be tightly coupled to that of its receptors in breast tumours.

Using a highly sensitive single-cell cytokine assay called the reverse haemolytic plaque assay (or RHPA), in which each individual producer cell can be identified, we screened 40 invasive breast carcinomas for production of TNF-α [10]. Of these, 17.5% (7 of 40) were seen to secrete detectable levels of this cytokine, the producer cells being mainly CD68-positive macrophages (Plate 4) and occasional malignant epithelial cells. Tumours secreting TNF-α expressed significantly ($P < 0.05$) lower levels of both epidermal growth factor receptors (EGF-R: 17.7 ± 2.6 fmol/mg) and oestrogen receptors (ER: 6.9 ± 2.9 fmol/mg) than non-TNF-α-secreting tumours (45.1 ± 4.9 and 59.35 ± 5.2 fmol/mg respectively). These data accord well, in part, with a recent study published by a group at the National Cancer Institute, Bethesda, in which the authors reported the inhibition of ER on breast cancer cells by their *in vitro* exposure to TNF-α [37]. However, they represent an interesting contrast to the report of Sedlak *et al.* [38], demonstrating the up-regulation of EGF-R expression by the breast cancer cell line, BT-20, by TNF-α *in vitro*. Either the effect of TNF-α varies between different forms of breast cancer cells (e.g. cell lines versus *in situ* cells) or the lower levels of EGF-R seen in TNF-α-secreting tumours may represent the long-term, down-regulating response of breast cancer cells to prolonged TNF-α stimulation *in situ*.

A possible correlation of TNF-α *release* with angiogenesis (as assessed by quantifying CD31 expression on vessels) in these tumours is currently under investigation in one of our laboratories, although it is unlikely that levels of a single cytokine such as TNF-α will correlate directly with such an important prognostic parameter as it works in a complex, highly context-specific manner within the tumour microenvironment. However, in a collaborative study with Harris's group [39], we have recently demonstrated the prognostic significance of macrophage numbers in over 100 breast cancer patients and a significant correlation of this parameter with angiogenesis. Whether this is linked to the production of TNF-α by these cells in breast tumours and/or a number of alternative macrophage-derived factors, such as other cytokines and matrix-degrading enzymes, has yet to be elucidated.

Various studies have implicated macrophages in the regulation of intratumoral angiogenesis [1]. That tissue hypoxia, such as that present in certain stages of developing tumours, may stimulate, in part, intra-tumoral macrophages to make TNF-α has been confirmed by the finding that experimentally induced hypoxia stimulates the release of this cytokine by human monocytes *in vitro* [40]. Moreover, we have recently described the use of dual immunohistochemistry (indirect peroxidase and ABC-alkaline phosphatase) simultaneously to localize TNF-α in tumour macrophages and CD31 blood vessels [10]. We are currently using this method to investigate the effect of hypoxia *in situ* on TNF-α production by macrophages in solid tumours (i.e. investigate the production of this cytokine in vascular versus avascular sites in sections of breast carcinomas, to see whether relatively hypoxic areas stimulate macrophages to produce TNF-α *in situ*). We are also examining the effects of experimentally induced hypoxia on the release of TNF-α by tumour macrophages *ex vivo* in the RHPA. This experimental approach will facilitate the visualization of the response of *individual* intratumoral macrophages in short-term cultures, and to investigate the role of specific signal transduction pathways in mediating the effect of hypoxia on angiogenic cytokine secretion.

As TNF-α is also known to modulate the growth of some cell types *in vitro*, we examined its effects on the growth and DNA synthesis of the human breast cell line, T47D [41]. A dose-dependent, reversible inhibition of thymidine incorporation and cell growth was observed in the range of 0.1–100 ng/ml of TNF-α. Cell viability was not impaired in any of the experiments (data not shown). On the other hand, the tumour promoter and protein kinase C (PKC) agonist, phorbol-12-myristate-13-acetate (PMA) was seen to enhance thymidine incorporation by these cells (Fig. 1). Flow-cytometric DNA analysis demonstrated that after 24 hours of exposure to TNF-α, T47D cells accumulated in the G1 phase of the cell cycle, and were depleted in the G2/M and S phases, suggesting a block in the progression of the G1/S transition (Fig. 2). The involvement of protein kinases (PK) and protein phosphatases in TNF-α-induced signal transduction was also investigated. A transient and rapid two-fold increase in total cellular PKC activity was detected within 10 minutes of exposure to TNF-α (Fig. 3). To study the role of the observed PKC activation in the cytostatic effect of TNF-α, T47D cells were exposed to the cytokine in the presence of the potent PKC inhibitor, H7. The inhibitory effect of TNF-α on thymidine incorporation was not affected by exposure to H7 at concentrations sufficient to block the stimulation of thymidine uptake induced by PMA (data not shown). The involvement of other signalling pathways was addressed using the cyclic nucleotide-dependent PK in-hibitor, 118, the calmodulin-dependent PK inhibitor, W7, and the inhibitor of protein phosphatases, PP1 and PP2B okadaic acid. Exposure of T47D cells to these enzyme inhibitors failed to antagonize the inhibition of

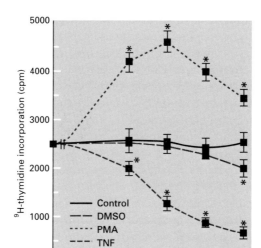

Fig. 1 Effects of tumour necrosis factor-α (TNF-α) and phorbol-12-myristate-13-acetate (PMA) on thymidine incorporation by T47D cells. Cells were exposed to TNF-α or PMA for 24 hours. The effects of the corresponding dilutions of dimethylsulphoxide (DMSO) are also shown (diluent for PMA). Data are presented as the mean of triplicate measurements ± s.d. *P < 0.05 compared to corresponding control group. Reproduced with permission from [27].

thymidine incorporation by TNF-α. Taken together, these results indicate that the cytostatic effect of TNF-α on T47D cells occurs at the G1/S transition of the cell cycle, and is mediated by an intracellular pathway which does not involve the activity of protein kinases C and A, nor protein phosphatases PP1 and PP2B.

Our observation that malignant epithelial cells in breast tumours express TNF-R p55 (Plate 3) is particularly interesting in view of our recent finding that this type of TNF R mediates the cytostatic/cytotoxic effect of TNF-α on breast cancer cell lines *in vitro* [42] and may therefore play a part in regulating the growth and viability of malignant cells *in vivo*.

As mentioned earlier, such cytokines as TNF-α do not work in isolation within the tumour microenvironment, but rather within a complex interactive network of protein signals [3,4]. We therefore decided to investigate the effect of three prominent growth factors produced in breast tumours — epidermal growth factor (EGF), basic fibroblast growth factor (bFGF) and insulin-like growth factor-1 (IGF-1) on the cytostatic activity of TNF-α on breast cancer cells [3,4,43]. TNF-α completely blocked the potent growth-promoting activity of all three factors on T47D cells. EGF, bFGF and IGF-1 augmented the growth of these cells *in vitro* when working

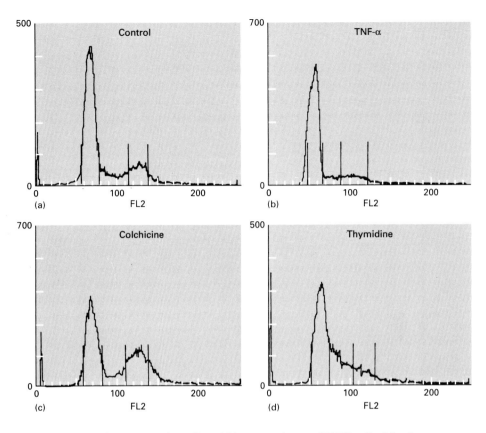

Fig. 2 Flow-cytometric profiles of (a) untreated, control T47D cells; (b) cells synchronized by tumour necrosis factor-α (TNF-α; 10 ng/ml); (c) cells treated with colchicine (50 μg/ml); and (d) a single thymidine pulse (2 nm). The fluorescence intensity is plotted on the x axis against the relative cell number on the y-axis. The gates for diploid, tetraploid and S-phase cells were set manually as indicated. Reproduced with permission from [27].

Fig. 3 Protein kinase C (PKC) activity (represented by 32P incorporation into specific substrate peptide) after 10 minutes of exposure to tumour necrosis factor-α (TNF-α) or phorbol-12-myristate-13-acetate (PMA; 10 ng/ml) was measured in total cellular extracts eluted from a DEAE column. Substrate phosphorylation in the presence of a PKC inhibitor (pseudosubstrate PKC 129–36) is also shown. Data are presented as the mean of triplicate measurements ± s.d. *$P < 0.05$ compared to baseline PKC activity detected in exponentially growing T47D cells. Reproduced with permission from [27].

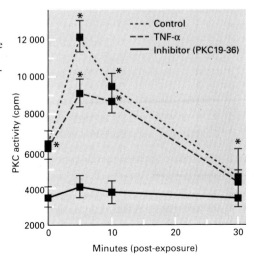

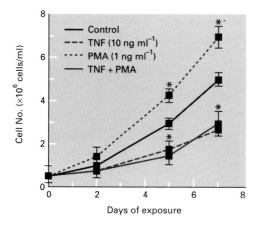

Fig. 4 Effect of epidermal growth factor (EGF; 10 ng/ml), insulin-like growth factor (IGF-1; 10 ng/ml), basal fibroblast growth factor (bFGF; 10 ng/ml) and tumour necrosis factor-α (TNF-α; 10 ng/ml) on the growth of T47D cells. Reproduced with permission from [43].

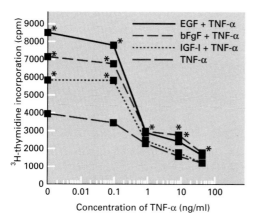

Fig. 5 Effects of epidermal growth factor (EGF; 10 ng/ml), insulin-like growth factor (IGF-1; 10 ng/ml) and basal fibroblast growth factor (bFGF; 10 ng/ml) on the growth of T47D cells in the presence of increasing concentrations of tumour necrosis factor-α (TNF-α). Reproduced with permission from [43].

alone, and antagonized the inhibition of cell growth and thymidine incorporation induced by TNF-α (Figs 4 and 5). These data suggest that the growth of such breast cancer cells *in vivo* may be regulated, in part, by the antagonistic interaction between the cytostatic effect of TNF-α and the growth-promoting activity of factors such as EGF, IGF-1 and bFGF.

CONCLUDING REMARKS

Adoptive immunotherapy for cancer involving cytokine manipulation of host immune cells has gained considerable momentum in the past few years [44]. One approach, currently employed in clinical trials, is to transfect tumour-infiltrating lymphocytes with genes for such cytokines as TNF-α and then to reintroduce these cells into the circulation of the patient [45].

Tumour-infiltrating lymphocytes have been shown to localize within the tumour and it is postulated that they may mount an immune-boosting/ antiproliferative effect on solid tumours, mediated partly by their enhanced secretion of TNF-α. However, the use of anticancer therapies involving TNF-α (as a single agent, as part of a combined chemotherapy regimen, or in such new gene therapy protocols) has met with only limited success in recent years. With regard to the treatment of breast cancer, this may have been due, in part, to the marked differences in and between such carcinomas in their expression of TNF-R p55 and p75, and thus the lack of uniformity in the multiple and complex effects of TNF-α on this type of solid tumour. Indeed, our data suggest that the study of any given single cytokine (e.g. TNF-α) is meaningless if conducted in isolation from the complex, multisignal milieu in which it operates within a tumour. As this is likely to vary between individual tumours, it may be that the analysis of a number of important intratumoral cytokines, rather than individual ones, is of greatest relevance to the future design of new cytokine-based anticancer therapies.

Our studies indicate that the effective future utilization of the TNF-α/ TNF-α receptor system for the purposes of prognosis or therapeutic manipulation in breast cancer patients awaits further studies to elucidate: (i) the differential effects of TNF-α on the multiple cell types bearing one or both types of TNF-α receptor in solid tumours; (ii) the modulating effect on these TNF-α actions of other cytokines and signals present in the tumour microenvironment; and (iii) the local and systemic effects of soluble TNF-R p55 and TNF-R p75 in cancer patients.

REFERENCES

1 Leek R, Harris AL, Lewis CE. Cytokine networks in solid human tumours: regulation of angiogenesis. *J Leuk Biol* 1994;**56**:423–435.
2 O'Sullivan C, Lewis CE. Tumour-associated leukocytes: friends or foes in breast carcinomas. *J Pathol* 1994;**172**:229–235.
3 Pusztai L, Lewis CE, Lorenzen J, McGee JO'D. Growth factors: regulation of normal and neoplastic growth. *J Pathol* 1993;**169**:191–201.
4 Lewis CE. Cytokines in neoplasia. In: *The Oxford Textbook of Pathology*, edited by McGee JO'D, Wright NA, Isaacson PG. Oxford University Press, Oxford, 1992;709–714.
5 Naukkarinen A, Ssyajanem KJ. Quantitative immunohistochemical analysis of mononuclear infiltrates in breast carcinomas — correlation with tumour differentiation. *J Pathol* 1990;**16**:217–222.
6 Whitwel HL, Hughes HPA, Moore M, Ahmed A. Expression of major histocompatibility antigenes and leucocyte infiltration in benign and malignant human breast disease. *Br J Cancer* 1984;**49**:161–172.
7 Kelly PMA, Davis RS, Bliss E, McGee JO'D. Macrophages in human breast disease: a quantitative immunohistochemical study. *Br J Cancer* 1988;**57**:174–177.
8 Rubbert A, Manger B, Lang N, Kalden JR, Platzer E. Functional characterization of tumour-infiltrating lymphocytes, lymph-node lymphocytes, and peripheral lymphocytes. *Int J Cancer* 1991;**49**:25–31.
9 Schwartzentruber DJ, Topalian SL, Mancini M, Rosenberg SA. Specific release of

granulocyte-monocyte colony stimulating factor tumour necrosis-factor alpha and interferon-gamma by human tumour infiltrating lymphocytes after autologous tumour stimulation. *J Immunol* 1991;**146**:3674–3681.

10 Lewis CE, Leek RD, Harris AL, McGee JO'D. Cytokines regulation of angiogenesis in breast cancer: the role of tumor-associated macrophages. *J Leuk Biol* 1995;**57**:747–751.

11 Vitolo D, Zerbe T, Kanbour A, Dahl C, Herberman RB, Whiteside TL. Expression of mRNA for cytokines in tumour-infiltrating mononuclear cells in ovarian adenocarcinoma and invasive breast cancer. *Int J Cancer* 1992;**51**:573–580.

12 Miles DW, Happerfield LC, Naylor MS, Bobrow LG, Rubens LD, Balkwill FR. Detection of tumour necrosis factor in primary breast cancer by *in situ* hybridization and immunohystochemistry. *Int J Cancer* 1994;**56**:777–782.

13 Sugamen BJ, Aggarwal BB, Hass PE, Figari IS, Pallidino MA, Shepard HM. Recombinant human tumour necrosis factor-alpha: effects on proliferation of normal and transformed cells *in vitro*. *Science* 1985;**230**:943–945.

14 Ostesen M, Thielle D, Lipsky P. Tumour necrosis factor-α enhances cytolytic activity of human natural killer cells. *J Immunol* 1987;**138**:4185–4191.

15 Wang JM, Walter S, Mantovani A. Re-evaluation of the chemotactic activity of tumour necrosis factor for monocytes. *Immunology* 1990;**71**:364–367.

16 Scheurich P, Thom B, Ucer U, Pfizenmaier K. Immunoregulatory activity of recombinant human tumour necrosis factor-α: induction of human TNF receptors on human T cells and TNF-α mediated enhancement of T cell responses. *J Immunol* 1987;**138**:1786–1790.

17 Schuger L, Varani J, Marks RM, Kunkel SJ, Johnson KJ, Ward PA. Cytotoxicity of tumour necrosis factor-α for human umbilical vein endothelial cells. *Lab Invest* 1989;**61**:62–69.

18 van Der Poll T, Buller HR, Cate H *et al.* Activation of coagulation after administration of tumour necrosis factor to normal subjects. *N Engl J Med* 1990;**322**:1622–1627.

19 Frater-schroder M, Risaul W, Hallmann R, Gautschi P, Bohlen P. Tumour necrosis factor-α, a potent inhibitor of endothelial cell growth *in vitro*, is angiogenic *in vivo*. *Proc Natl Acad Sci USA* 1987;**84**:5277–5281.

20 Malik STA, Naylor MS, Oliff A, Balkwill FR. Cells secreting tumour necrosis factor show enhanced metastases in nude mice. *Eur J Cancer* 1990;**26**:1031–1034.

21 Fajardo LF, Kwan HH, Kowalski J, Prinoas SD, Allison AC. Dual role of tumour necrosis factor-α in angiogenesis. *Am J Pathol* 1992;**140**:539–544.

22 Loetscher H, Pan YCA, Lahm HW *et al.* Molecular cloning and expression of the human p55 kd tumour necrosis factor receptor. *Cell* 1990;**61**:351–359.

23 Schall TJ, Lewis M, Koller KJ, Lee A, Rice GC, Wong GHW. Molecular cloning and expression of a receptor for human tumour necrosis factor. *Cell* 1990;**61**:361–370.

24 Brockhaus M, Schoenfield H-J, Schlaeger E-J, Hunziker W, Lesslauer W, Loetscher H. Identification of two types of tumour necrosis factor receptors on human cell lines by monoclonal antibodies. *Proc Natl Acad Sci USA* 1990;**87**:3127–3131.

25 Ryffel B, Brockhaus M, Dermuller U, Gudat F. Tumour necrosis factor receptors in lymphoid tissues and lymphomas. *Am J Pathol* 1991;**139**:7–15.

26 Tartaglia LA, Weber RF, Figari IS, Reynolds C, Palladino MA, Goeddel DV. The two different receptors for tumour necrosis factor mediate distinct cellular responses. *Proc Natl Acad Sci USA* 1991;**88**:9292–9296.

27 Pusztai L, Clover LM, Cooper K, Starkey PM, Lewis CE, McGee JO'D. Expression of tumour necrosis factor α and its receptors in breast carcinoma *Br J Cancer* 1994;**70**:289–292.

28 Al-Sumidaie AM, Leinster SJ, Webster DJ, Jenkins SA. Alterations in monocyte function in patients with breast cancer. *Eur J Surg Oncol* 1987;**13**:419–424.

29 Guillou PJ. Tumour escape mechanisms. In: Rees RC. ed. *The Biological and Clinical Applications of Interleukin-2*, edited by Rees RC. IRL Press, Oxford, 1990:164–175.

30 Wright SC, Tam AW, Kumar P. Selection of tumour cell variants for resistance to tumour necrosis factor also induces a form of pleiotropic drug resistance. *Cancer Immunol Immunother* 1992;**34**:399–406.

31 Zaloom Y, Brokks B, Camobell D, Field M, Gallagher G. Localisation of cytokines and cytokine receptors within human tumours. Proc British Society for Immunology, Spring Meeting 1992, Abstract No. 2.35.

32 Dolbaum C, Craesey AA, Dairkee SH *et al*. Specificity of tumour necrosis factor toxicity for human mammary carcinomas relative to normal mammary epithelium and correlation with response to doxorubicin. *Proc Natl Acad Sci USA* 1988;**85**:4740–4744.

33 Naylor MS, Stamp WH, Foulkes WD, Eccles D, Balkwill FR. Tumour necrosis factor and its receptors in human ovarian cancer. Potential role in disease progression. *J Clin Invest* 1993;**91**:2194–2206.

34 Gamble J, Smith WB, Vadas MA. TNF modulation of endothelial and neutrophil adhesion. In: *Tumour Necrosis Factors, The Molecules and their Emerging Role in Medicine*. edited by Beutler B. Raven Press, New York, 1992:65–87.

35 Aderka D, Engelmann H, Hornik V *et al*. Increased serum levels of solubile receptors for tumour necrosis factor in cancer patients. *Cancer Res* 1991;**51**:5602–5607.

36 Porteau F, Brockhaus M, Wallach D, Engelmann H, Nathan CF. Human neutrophil elastase releases a ligand-binding fragment from the 75-kDa tumour necrosis factor receptor *J Biol Chem* 1991;**266**:18846–18856.

37 Danforth DN, Sgagias MK. Tumour necrosis factor-alpha modulates oestradiol responsiveness of MCF-7 breast cancer cells *in vitro*. *J Endocrinol* 1993;**138**:517–528.

38 Sedlak J, Speiser P, Hunakova L, Duaj J, Chorvath B. Modulation of RGF-receptor and CD15 (Lewisx) antigen on the cell surface of breast carcinoma cell lines induced by cytokines, retinoic acid, 12-*O*-tetradecanoylphorbol 13-acetate and 1,25(OH)$_2$-vitamin D$_3$. *Chemotherapy* 1994;**40**:51–56.

39 Leek RD, Lewis CE, Harris AL. The role of macrophages in tumour angiogenesis. In: *Tumour Angiogenesis*, edited by Bicknell R, Lewis CE, Ferarra N. Oxford University Press, Oxford (in press).

40 Scannell G, Waxman K, Kaml GJ *et al*. Hypoxia induces a human macrophage cell line to release tumor necrosis factor-alpha and its soluble receptors *in vitro*. *J Surg Res* 1993;**54**:281–285.

41 Pusztai L, Lewis CE, McGee JO'D. Growth arrest of the breast cancer cell line, T47D, by TNF alpha: cell cycle specificity and signal transduction. *Br J Cancer* 1993;**67**:290–296.

42 Pusztai L. *Regulation of the Growth of Breast Cancer by Tumour Necrosis Factor α*. DPhil thesis. Oxford University, Oxford, 1993.

43 Pusztai L, Lewis CE, McGee JO'D. Epidermal growth factor, insulin-like growth factor-1 and basic growth factor modulate the cytostatic effect of tumour necrosis factor-α on the breast cancer cell line, T47D. *Cytokine* 1993;**5**:169–172.

44 Rosenberg SA. Adoptive immunotherapy for cancer. *Sci Am* 1990;**27**:34–41.

45 Rosenberg SA. Immunotherapy and gene therapy of cancer. *Cancer Res* 1991;**51** (suppl.):5074–5079.

MULTIPLE CHOICE QUESTIONS

1 In solid tumours, TNF-α is produced by

a macrophages
b B cells
c CD4+ and CD8+ T cells
d endothelial cells
e tumour cells

2 Cytokines made within the tumour microenvironment directly regulate

a proliferation and metastasis of tumour cells

   b enzymatic degradation of the extracellular matrix
   c angiogenesis
   d immunocompetence of tumour-infiltrating leukocytes
   e deposition of extracellular matrix proteins

3 In malignant breast tumours, TNF-α-R p55 is expressed by
   a endothelial cells
   b macrophages
   c tumour cells
   d fibroblasts
   e neutrophils

4 Growth factors shown to modulate the cytostatic effect of TNF-α include
   a insulin-like growth factor (IGF-1)
   b platelet-derived growth factor (PDGF)
   c epidermal growth factor (EGF)
   d basic fibroblast growth factor (bFGF)
   e transforming growth factor (TGF-β)

5 The cytostatic effect of TNF-α
   a is mediated by the p55 receptor
   b blocks cell proliferation in the G1/S transition of the cell cycle
   c is abrogated by the protein kinase C inhibitor H7
   d involves an increase in protein kinase activity in T47D cells
   e inhibited by protein phosphorylases

Answers

1 a True	2 a True	3 a True
b False	b False	b True
c True	c True	c True
d False	d True	d True
e True	e True	e False

4 a True	5 a True
b False	b True
c True	c False
d True	d True
e False	e False

The clinical use of
insulin-like growth factors in diabetes

DAVID B. DUNGER

The identification of the insulin-like growth factors, IGF-1 and IGF-2, arose out of the observation of three quite distinct biological effects in serum, namely sulphation factor activity, non-suppressible insulin-like activity and multiplication-stimulating activity. Subsequent investigation has revealed a complex system of interactions between the IGFs, their binding proteins, receptors and insulin. Both IGF-1 and IGF-2 consist of single-chain polypeptides which share remarkable sequence homology with human proinsulin [1]. Although IGF-1 and IGF-2 have their own distinct receptors [2], receptor interactions with insulin do occur and there is overlap in their respective biological functions.

The IGF-1 receptor is structurally very similar to the insulin receptor, comprising two extracellular α subunits which are primarily concerned with hormone binding and two β subunits with transmembrane and tyrosine kinase domains which are involved in intracellular signalling. The IGF-1 receptor has the highest affinity for IGF-1 and a much lower affinity for IGF-2 and insulin. It is thought to mediate most of the biological effects of IGF-1 and IGF-2. Hybrid receptors have also been described consisting of one insulin receptor α and β subunit and one IGF-1 receptor α and β subunit. The hybrid receptors seem to be most abundant in tissues such as muscle and appear to have a higher affinity for IGF-1 than insulin. The regulation of production of these hybrid receptors is still unclear.

IGF-2 also has its own receptor which is structurally unrelated to either the IGF-1 or the insulin receptor. It consists of a single-chain polypeptide with a large extracellular domain containing binding sites for IGF-2 and mannose-6-phosphate. It would appear that most of the biological actions of IGF-2 are mediated through the type 1 receptor and the full role of the type 2 receptor is not clear but it may include removal of excess hormone by internalization of ligand and also the regulation of lysosomal enzymes. Although IGF-2 circulates in very high concentrations in plasma its functions are still unclear and for this article I will concentrate on developments in our understanding of the function of IGF-1.

It has been shown that both IGF-1 and insulin may induce either metabolic or mitogenic effects through their own receptors and there has been considerable interest in how, under normal physiological conditions, insulin largely regulates intermediary metabolism, whereas IGF-1 is involved in the regulation of growth and development [3]. Furthermore, the increasing availability of recombinant human IGF-1 (rhIGF-1) has permitted a re-examination of its role in the regulation of metabolism.

THE INSULIN-LIKE ACTIONS OF IGF-1

In vitro studies have demonstrated that IGF-1 can induce a metabolic signal through its own receptor and in the isolated soleus muscle of the rat it can stimulate glucose transport and intermediary metabolism in ways which are quite distinct from those of insulin [4]. *In vivo* administration of IGF-1 in the rat and humans lowers blood glucose levels, although the hypoglycaemic effect is less potent than that of insulin [5,6]. Insulin and IGF-1 appear to have differential tissue effects which may be explained by differences in receptor distribution. For example, IGF-1 appears to be more effective in stimulating glucose uptake by muscle and has less effect on hepatic glucose production, presumably because of the relative paucity of IGF-1 receptors on the adult liver. Similarly, IGF-1 effects on adipocytes are less marked than those of insulin, whereas IGF-1 appears to be more effective than insulin in stimulating protein synthesis [7]. However, in all of the *in vivo* studies, rhIGF-1 administration has led to a suppression of insulin and glucagon secretion and this may be relevant to the interpretation of hepatic glucose production data [8]. Furthermore, in many of these studies, very high doses of IGF-1 were administered in order to overcome the effects of the IGF-binding proteins.

THE ROLE OF THE IGF-BINDING PROTEINS

The concentrations of IGF-1 and IGF-2 in the serum are 10–100 times higher than those of insulin and, although the glucose-lowering effects may be less than those of insulin, this does represent a formidable amount of insulin-like activity. However, unlike insulin, IGF-1 circulates bound to a series of binding proteins, of which six have been identified [9]. The principal IGF-binding protein, IGFBP-3, when bound to IGF-1 and an acid-labile subunit produced by the hepatocyte, produces a 150 kDa complex which provides a reservoir of IGFs in the circulation. Thus the amount of free IGF-1 in the circulation is relatively small. It has always been argued that the IGFBPs prevent the expression of any insulin-like actions of the IGFs, but this may need to be revised in the light of recent observations concerning the functions of the smaller IGF-binding proteins [10], and in particular IGFBP-1.

IGFBP-1 is also produced by the hepatocyte and it shows a marked diurnal rhythm as its levels in the circulation are inversely regulated by insulin [11]. In most bioassay systems, IGFBP-1 is an inhibitor of IGF bioactivity and, although the amount of IGF bound to IGFBP-1 is relatively small, it may represent a mechanism by which the availability of free IGF-1 in the tissues is regulated by insulin. Lewitt *et al.* recently showed that in the rat an injection of IGFBP-1 led to a prompt rise in glucose levels which could be reversed by the simultaneous injection of rhIGF-1 [12]. This presents the first evidence that the IGFs may play a role in glucose homeostasis. The complex interactions between insulin and the growth hormone (GH)/IGF-1 axis are summarized in Fig. 1. Insulin has a role in the regulation of IGF-1 production by the liver and IGF bioactivity through the actions of IGFBP-1. In the presence of high portal concentrations of insulin, increased availability of free IGF-1 brought about by a fall in IGF/IGFBP-1 concentrations could lead to direct effects of IGF-1 on glucose homeostasis via the type 1 receptor.

Thus, circulating levels of IGF-1 are a potent source of insulin-like activity which could lead to increased glucose uptake through signalling of the IGF-1 receptor quite independent of the effects of insulin. These considerations have led to an exploration of the possible use of rhIGF-1 as a treatment for insulin-resistant states and type 2 diabetes.

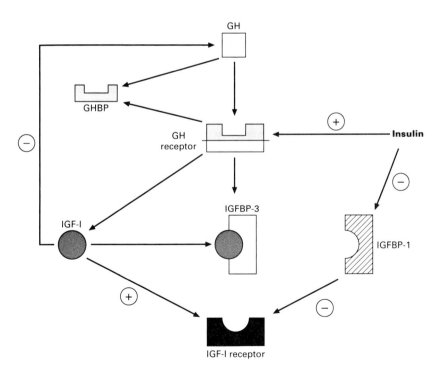

Fig. 1 The relationship between insulin and the growth hormone/insulin-like growth factor I axis.

STUDIES OF rhIGF-1 IN INSULIN-RESISTANT STATES AND TYPE 2 DIABETES

Extreme insulin resistance usually results from either mutations in the insulin receptor gene or from post-receptor defects which are critical to the effects of insulin on glucose metabolism [13]. rhIGF-1 could have a therapeutic role in stimulating glucose uptake in skeletal muscle through the IGF-1 receptor. In a patient with the Mendenhall syndrome who had a mutation in both alleles of the insulin receptor gene, high doses of rhIGF-1 were effective in reversing ketoacidosis but the improvements in glycaemic control were less impressive in the long term [14]. The results of studies in patients with type A insulin resistance have yielded rather variable results [15,16]. One interpretation of these findings might be that, although the metabolic role of IGF-1 is largely mediated through the IGF-1 receptor, its effect may still be limited by failure of activation of pathways common to the insulin receptor.

The rationale for the use of IGF-1 in type 2 diabetes was very similar in that it was thought that this treatment might result in reduced hyper-glycaemia by direct effects on glucose uptake through the IGF-1 receptor. In early studies, rhIGF-1 appeared to improve insulin sensitivity [17] and longer-term studies were undertaken. However, when administered at a dose of 160 μg/kg twice daily, although rhIGF-1 appeared to control blood glucose nearly as well as insulin in obese type 2 patients, adverse experiences led to early termination of these trials [18]. The principal adverse events experienced were jaw pain, myalgia and oedema. Thus, very high-dose rhIGF-1 results in adverse effects which are quite distinct from those of insulin when it is used as a single therapy in type 2 diabetes.

In all of the studies where high doses of rhIGF-1 were used, there was a dramatic suppression of endogenous insulin secretion and C-peptide levels. Thus, the high-dose strategy may not have been the most appropriate, for under normal physiological conditions there is likely to be synergy between the effects of IGF-1 and insulin. Subsequent studies of the use of rhIGF-1 in type 2 diabetes will be directed towards evaluating the role of lower doses or combinations of IGF-1 and insulin in the treatment of these patients.

THE USE OF rhIGF-1 IN THE TREATMENT OF TYPE 1 DIABETES (INSULIN-DEPENDENT DIABETES MELLITUS, IDDM)

The rationale for the use of rhIGF-1 in the treatment of IDDM has differed from that applied to the treatment of type 2 and insulin-resistant states. Abnormalities of the GH/IGF-1 axis are well-documented in IDDM and have been implicated in the pathogenesis of deteriorating glycaemic control during adolescence. It has been argued that correction of these abnormalities using physiological doses of rhIGF-1 might lead to improvements in glycaemic control [19].

Abnormalities of the GH/IGF-1 axis in IDDM

GH hypersecretion has been well-documented, particularly during adolescence in subjects with IDDM [20], yet circulating levels of IGF-1 and IGF bioactivity are reduced [21]. Thus there appears to be partial GH insensitivity at the level of the hepatic GH receptor. Some confirmation of this has come from studies of the circulating GH binding protein (GHBP) which is identical to the extracellular domain of the GH receptor. Low levels of GHBP have been observed in adolescents with IDDM [22] (Fig. 1).

The hepatic GH receptor is, in part, insulin-dependent and the circulating levels of IGF-1, IGFBP-3 and GHBP are related to insulin dose [22]. Intensification of insulin therapy leads to increases in the circulating level of IGF-1 [23]. Arslanian *et al.* have recently demonstrated that, with the introduction of insulin therapy to newly diagnosed patients, GHBP levels increase, although levels remain lower than those seen in normal subjects [24]. Insulin also has a direct role in regulating IGFBP-1 levels and the circulating concentrations of this inhibitor of IGF bioactivity are increased overnight in IDDM [25].

The persisting abnormalities of IGF-1 and IGFBP-1 in patients on standard insulin therapy appear to stem from the peripheral rather than the direct portal vein route of administration of insulin. Brismar *et al.* recently showed that the hepatic secretion of IGFBP-1 and IGF-1 were directly related to the levels of insulin in the hepatic vein [26] and studies of intraportal administration of insulin have shown complete correction of abnormalities of the GH/IGF-1 axis [27].

Metabolic effects of abnormalities of the GH/IGF-1 axis

The low circulating levels of IGF-1 and the reduced IGF-1 bioactivity appear to be the major stimulus of GH hypersecretion in IDDM. GH hypersecretion has been implicated in the insulin resistance which develops during puberty and the pathogenesis of the 'dawn phenomenon' [28]. The extent to which insulin requirements increase overnight are directly related to GH pulsatility and can be reversed by suppression of nocturnal GH release with agents such as pirenzipine. Furthermore, GH hypersecretion results in enhanced ketogenesis overnight [29].

It could also be argued that the reduced circulating levels of IGF-1 and the elevated levels of IGFBP-1 might have direct effects on insulin-sensitivity in adolescents with IDDM. Thus restoration of normal physiological levels of IGF-1 using rhIGF-1 could lead to enhanced insulin sensitivity, either indirectly through the suppression of GH or by the direct effect of enhanced IGF bioactivity.

Short-term studies of rhIGF-1 in IDDM

Some confirmation of this hypothesis has come from short-term studies of rhIGF-1 in IDDM. These studies have employed a much lower dose of rhIGF-1 than that used in type 2 diabetes and the choice of dose (40 µg/kg subcutaneously) reflects the estimated IGF-1 production rate. In double-blind placebo-controlled studies Cheetham et al. were able to show that this dose of rhIGF-1 led to restoration of normal circulating levels of IGF-1, sustained reductions in GH secretion and a corresponding fall in the insulin requirements for euglycaemia overnight [30,31].

These studies have now been extended and in an analysis of the results from 17 subjects who were studied either on a night when rhIGF-1 was administered or on a control night, the authors were able to show that the greatest reductions in GH levels were seen in those patients with the highest baseline GH levels and those with the poorest glycaemic control as judged by glycated haemoglobin (HbA1C) concentrations. The improvements in insulin insensitivity overnight were directly related to the fall in GH secretion following rhIGF-1 administration. Thus, in these short-term studies a possible role for rhIGF-1 therapy has been demonstrated.

Longer-term studies of rhIGF-1 in IDDM

These short-term effects of rhIGF-1 therapy in IDDM appear to be sustained over longer periods. In a small study involving 6 subjects with IDDM, Cheetham et al. showed that sustained increases in IGF-1 levels could be obtained after a month of daily injections and that reductions in GH secretion and basal insulin requirements were sustained [32]. Levels of IGF-1 did not fall during the study despite the reductions in GH secretion, and there was a modest increase in IGFBP-3 levels.

In those studies Cheetham et al. were not able to observe any adverse effects of IGF-1 therapy and the small reduction in HbA1c levels was encouraging [32]. However, this was an unblinded study and the balance between efficacy and possible adverse effects on diabetic microangiopathic complications will need to be assessed by longer-term double-blind placebo-controlled studies.

CONCLUSIONS

Although we have gained considerable knowledge over the last 10 years of the complex interactions between IGF-1 and its binding proteins, we are still unclear as to whether IGF-1 plays a normal physiological role in the regulation of carbohydrate metabolism. Studies with rhIGF-1 indicate that it has metabolic actions which are quite distinct from those of insulin, although it is unclear as to whether levels of free IGF-1 are ever sufficient for this activity to be expressed. Recent studies of the effects of IGFBP-1 *in vivo* do, however, suggest a mechanism whereby IGF-1 may play a role in the regulation of glucose metabolism.

The use of IGF-1 as an alternative to insulin in the treatment of insulin-resistant states has produced variable results which must be, in part, related to the bioavailability of IGF-1 in these conditions and interactions between the IGF-1 and insulin receptors. The use of rhIGF-1 as a replacement for insulin in type 2 diabetes had to be abandoned because of the development of unacceptable side-effects. Further study will probably be directed towards using rhIGF-1 in lower doses or as an adjunct to insulin therapy in these patients.

The use of rhIGF-1 as an adjuvant to standard insulin replacement therapy in IDDM has led to consistent short- and long-term reductions in GH hypersecretion and improvements in insulin sensitivity. No adverse effects have been observed in short-term studies and longer-term placebo-controlled trials are now underway.

Over the next few years we should see further exciting developments in the application of rhIGF-1 or its analogues, in combination with insulin and perhaps recombinant binding proteins to the regulation of metabolism. These studies will undoubtedly improve our understanding of the complex interrelationships between insulin and the GH/IGF-1 axis and they may also lead to promising developments in the treatment of diabetes.

REFERENCES

1 Rinderecht E, Hambil RE. The amino acid sequence of IGF-I and its structural homology with proinsulin. *J Biol Chem* 1978;**253**:2769–2776.
2 Massague J, Czech MP. The subunit structure of two distinct receptors for insulin-like growth factors I and II and their relationships to the insulin receptor. *J Biol Chem* 1982;**257**:5038–5045.
3 Le Roith D, Sampson PC, Roberts CT. How does the mitogenic insulin-like growth factor-I receptor differ from the metabolic insulin receptor? *Horm Res* 1994;**41**(suppl 2):74–79.
4 Dimitriadis G, Parry-Billings M, Piva T *et al*. Effects of insulin like growth factor I on the rates of glucose transport and utilisation in rat skeletal muscle *in vitro*. *Biochem J* 1992;**285**:269–274.
5 Zapf J, Hauri M, Wadvogel M, Froesch ER. Acute metabolic effects and half lives of intravenously administered IGF-I and II in normal and hypophysectiomised rats. *J Clin Invest* 1986;**77**:1768–1775.
6 Guler HP, Zapf J, Froesch ER. Short term metabolic effects of recombinant human insulin-like growth factor I in healthy adults. *N Engl J Med* 1987;**317**:137–140.
7 Boulware SD, Tamborlane WV, Matthews LS, Sherwin RS. Diverse effects of insulin-like growth factor I on glucose lipid and amino acid metabolism. *Am J Physiol* 1992;**262**:E130–E133.

8 Sherwin RS, Borg WP, Boulware SD. Metabolic effects of insulin-like growth factor I in normal humans. *Horm Res* 1994;**41**(suppl 2):97–102.

9 Ballard FJ, Baxter RC, Binoux M *et al.* Report on the nomenclature of the IGF binding proteins. *J Clin Endocrinol Metab* 1992;**74**:1215–1216.

10 Clemmons DR. IGF binding proteins: regulations of cellular actions. *Growth Regul* 1992;**2**:80–87.

11 Holly JMP, Biddlecombe RA, Dunger DB *et al.* Circadian variation of GH-independent IGF-binding protein in diabetes mellitus and its relationship to insulin. A new role for insulin? *Clin Endocrinol* 1988;**29**:667–675.

12 Lewitt MS, Denyer GS, Cooney GJ, Baxter RC. Insulin-like growth factor binding protein-I modulates blood glucose levels. *Endocrinology* 1991;**129**:2254–2256.

13 Moller DE, Flier JS. Insulin-resistance-mechanisms, syndromes and implications. *N Engl J Med* 1991;**325**:938–948.

14 Quin JD, Smith K, Beastall GH, Miell JP, MacCuish AC. The effects of recombinant insulin-like growth factor I on ketone body, lipid and apolipoprotein concentrations and its use to treat ketoacidosis in severe insulin resistance. *Diabetic Med* 1994;**11**:590–592.

15 Ishihama H, Suzuki Y, Muramatsu K *et al.* Long term follow-up in type A insulin resistant syndrome treated by insulin-like growth factor I. *Arch Dis Child* 1994;**71**:144–146.

16 Marrow LA, O'Brian MB, Mollar DE, Flier JS, Moses AC. Recombinant human insulin-like growth factor I therapy improves glycaemic control and insulin action in type A syndrome of severe resistance. *J Clin Endocrinol Metab* 1994;**79**:205–210.

17 Zenobi PD, Jaeggi-Croisman SE, Riesen W, Roder ME, Froesch ER. Insulin like growth factor I improves glucose and lipid metabolism in type 2 diabetes mellitus. *J Clin Invest* 1992;**90**:2234–2241.

18 Jabri N, Schalch DS, Schwartz SL *et al.* Adverse effects of recombinant human insulin-like growth factor I in obese insulin resistant type II diabetic patients. *Diabetes* 1994;**43**:369–374.

19 Dunger DB, Cheetham TD, Holly JMP, Matthews DR. Does recombinant insulin-like growth factor-I have a role in the treatment of insulin-dependent diabetes mellitus during adolescence? *Acta Paediatr* 1993;**388**(suppl):49–52.

20 Edge JA, Dunger DB, Matthews DR, Gilbert JP, Smith CP. Increased overnight growth hormone concentrations in diabetics compared with normal adolescents. *J Clin Endocrinol Metab* 1990;**71**:1356–1362.

21 Taylor AM, Dunger DB, Grant DB, Preece MA. Somatomedin-C IGF-I measured by radioimmunoassay and somatomedin bioactivity in adolescents with insulin dependent diabetes compared with puberty matched controls. *Diabetes Res* 1989;**9**:177–181.

22 Clayton KL, Holly JMP, Carlsson LMS *et al.* Loss of the normal relationship between growth hormone, growth hormone binding protein and insulin like growth factor in adolescents with insulin dependent diabetes mellitus. *Clin Endocrinol* 1994;**41**:517–524.

23 Amiel SA, Sherwin RS, Hintz RL, Gertner JM, Press M, Tamborlane WV. Effects of diabetes and its control on insulin-like growth factors in the young subject with type 1 diabetes. *Diabetes* 1984;**33**:1175–1179.

24 Arslanian SA, Menon RK, Gierl AP, Heil BV, Foley TP Jr. Insulin therapy increases low plasma growth hormone binding protein in children with new onset type 1 diabetes. *Diabetic Med* 1993;**10**:833–838.

25 Taylor AM, Dunger DB, Preece MA *et al.* The growth hormone independent insulin-like growth factor-I binding protein BP-28 is associated with serum insulin-like growth factor-I inhibitory bioactivity in adolescent insulin dependent diabetes. *Clin Endocrinol* 1990;**32**:229–239.

26 Brismar K, Fernqvist-Forbes E, Wahren J, Hall K. Effect of insulin on the hepatic production of insulin-like growth factor-binding protein-1 (IGFBP-1), IGFBP-3, and IGF-I in insulin-dependent diabetes. *J Clin Endocrinol Metab* 1994;**79**:872–878.

27 Shisko PI, Kovaler PA, Goncharov VG, Zajarny IU. Comparison of peripheral and portal (via the umbilical vein) routes of insulin infusion in IDDM patients. *Diabetes* 1992;**41**:1042–1049.

28 Dunger DB. Diabetes in puberty — annotation. *Arch Dis Child* 1992;**67**:569–570.

29 Edge JA, Harris DA, Phillips PE, Pal BR, Dunger DB. Evidence for a role for insulin and growth hormone in the overnight regulation of 3-hydroxybutyrate in normal and diabetic adolescents. *Diabetes Care* 1993;**16**:1011–1019.
30 Cheetham TD, Jones J, Taylor AM, Holly JMP, Matthews DR, Dunger DB. The effects of recombinant insulin-like growth factor-I administration on growth hormone levels and insulin requirements in adolescents with type I (Insulin-dependent) diabetes mellitus. *Diabetologia* 1993;**36**:678–681.
31 Cheetham TD, Clayton KL, Taylor AM, Holly J, Matthews DR, Dunger DB. The effects of recombinant human insulin-like growth factor I (rhIGF-I) on growth hormone secretion in adolescents with insulin dependent diabetes mellitus. *Clin Endocrinol* 1994;**40**:515–522.
32 Cheetham TD, Clayton KL, Holly JM, Taylor AM, Connors M, Dunger DB. *In vivo* use of recombinant human IGF-I: studies in type 1 diabetes. In: *The Insulin-like Growth Factors and their Regulatory Proteins*, edited by Baxter RC, Gluckman PD, Rosenfeld RG. Elsevier Science, The Netherlands, 1994:437–448.

PART 6
RENAL

New aspects of lupus nephritis

J. STEWART CAMERON

Systemic lupus erythematosus remains a perenially fascinating syndrome, even though it is now more than 100 years since Moritz Kaposi in Vienna first described the systemic component of what had been until then a dermatological condition. Amongst the most serious organ manifestations of lupus is, of course, nephritis. In this brief account I wish to concentrate on some recent ideas about the treatment of lupus patients with nephritis.

THE DESCRIPTION OF LUPUS NEPHRITIS

Most patients with lupus will have, on renal biopsy, at least minor changes visible on either immunocytochemical examination or electron microscopy which suggest formation or deposition of immune aggregates within the glomeruli, most prominently in the mesangial areas. This is so even in those whose urine in normal on clinical testing [1], and some of these have microalbuminuria [2].

Between 40 and 80% of patients with systemic lupus will develop clinically evident nephritis. This is usually not present at onset, the commonest initial manifestations being rashes, arthralgia without deformity and pleuropericarditis. However a minority have nephritis from onset, and occasional patients with single-organ disease in the form of nephritis later develop immunological and/or clinical signs of systemic lupus. Usually these patients show membranous or mesangiocapillary patterns of nephritis on renal biopsy.

In overt clinical lupus nephritis a bewildering variety of appearances may be seen in the glomeruli, accompanied in the majority by immune aggregates in the tubular basement membranes and an interstitial celullar infiltrate [3]. Appearances may vary between and even within glomeruli, although a mixture of proliferative/infiltrative patterns predominates, together with membranous changes characterized by diffuse extracapillary immune aggregates. The World Health Organization (WHO) classification is usually employed to describe these various appearances [4], but the limitations of trying to force a polymorphic pattern into a few categories must be kept in mind. Perhaps more useful in approaching the question

295

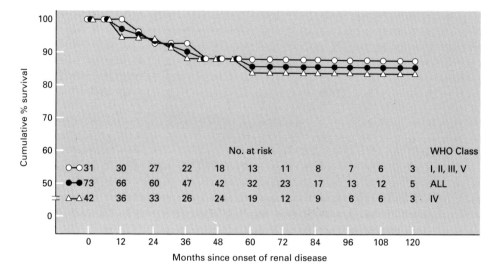

Fig. 1 Renal survival in a cohort of 73 patients with lupus nephritis (58% WHO class IV) followed at Guy's Hospital during 1980–90. There is no difference in outcome between milder forms of nephritis (classes I–III and V) and those with class IV during the first decade. Reproduced with permission from [7].

of what treatment should be given is the concept of activity versus chronicity, i.e inflammation versus scarring. This was suggested during the 1970s and popularized by workers at the National Institutes of Health (NIH) in the 1980s [5]. Not every observer, however, finds this analysis to be of predictive value [6].

Predicting outcome in lupus is complicated by the fortunate fact that the prognosis of the patient can be favourably influenced in the great majority of cases. Thus if more severe nephritis is given more intense treatment, the prognostic value of the biopsy appearances is almost completely lost (Fig. 1). The presence of hypertension, a raised plasma creatinine at onset, and tubulointerstitial scarring and infiltrate are reliable predictors of a poor outcome.

TODAY'S TREATMENTS

Induction phase in acute severe disease

Lupus is a disorder of immune reactivity against self antigens, and immunosuppressive therapy is logical. Unfortunately, today we still have only non-specific agents to depress the immune system. Thus the agents used involve corticosteroids and cytotoxic agents [7,8]. There is general agreement that milder forms of lupus nephritis can be controlled with corticosteroids alone. Corticosteroids remain the mainstay in the treatment of acute severe lupus. Today, most units, including our own, use initial intravenous daily injections of 1 g methylprednisolone followed by maintenance treatment (7.5–15 mg daily according to body weight) rather than high-dose tapering oral doses in the past. The main reason for this is that there are fewer side-effects using the initially high-dose intravenous regime. Induction treatment should include a cytotoxic agent, preferably cyclophosphamide, and there seems no reason not to give this orally in a dose of 100–200 mg daily by mouth according to body weight and renal function. This regime can be continued for 12 weeks, and then converted to the maintenance regime (see next section).

Two trials, one in milder lupus [9] and one in more severe lupus [10], have shown that up to thrice-weekly plasma exchange has no effect on outcome, although it is theoretically attractive. The only reasons for using plasma exchange today are severe lupus resistant to all other forms of treatment, severe cerebral lupus and the rare pulmonary haemorrhage. There are, however, no controlled data to support this policy, even though it is widespread.

Maintenance treatment in initially severe disease

After 12 weeks, when the disease is relatively under control, one can continue the maintenance corticosteroids, but what cytotoxic agent should be used? Oral cyclophosphamide cannot be continued because of bladder toxicity and the risk of oncogenesis, so the alternative is between 1 and 2 years' treatment with monthly or bimonthly intravenous cyclophosphamide boluses, or daily oral azathioprine. As outlined below, there is nothing to choose between these at the moment, although to my mind azathioprine has advantages. How many patients will eventually come off treatment altogether using either regime is a crucial point, but there are as yet no comparative data on this important point.

Stopping treatment

When can treatment be stopped? There is no clear answer to this question. Some patients' disease appears to be immunologically and clinically quiescent after only a year or two, but others can relapse on withdrawal of treatment up to 30 years later. Certainly, before stopping treatment one would like the patient to have normal complement and anti-DNA antibody levels, an inactive biopsy if one is done, clinical inactivity of the disease (perhaps with the exception of proteinuria, which may be a con-sequence of inactive glomerular scarring). At this point one can stop the cytotoxic agent first, then the corticosteroids by gradually transferring the corticosteroids to double the dose on alternate days, to give the hypothalamic–pituitary–adrenal axis a chance to recover. Then the dose can be gradually reduced over several months towards zero, watching for clinical and immunological signs of activity.

EXAMINATION OF THE ROLE OF CYTOTOXIC AGENTS

Thus the prognosis for patients with severe (WHO class IV) lupus nephritis has improved steadily during the past 30 years (Table 1), whilst the better prognosis of those with initially milder appearances has remained much the same. In the former group of patients with severe nephritis, the possibility that this improvement is the result of different diagnostic criteria is not present, and it must be attributed to treatments received. For example, in our unit between 1969 and 1978 [11] the 10-year cumulative *patient* survival for all patients, and for those with WHO class IV lupus nephritis, were 57% and 52% respectively, compared to 87% and 87% in a cohort of 82 patients studied during 1980–89 [7,12]. Corresponding figures for cumulative *renal* survival in the two groups were 65% and 63%

Table 1 Survival of patients with severe diffuse lupus nephritis (WHO class IV) in different periods.

Date of publication	Authors	5-year actuarial survival (%)
1957	Muehrcke *et al.*	10*
1969	Pollak and Pirani	25
1970	Baldwin *et al.*	23
1971	Estes and Christian	25
1973	Striker *et al.*	76
1973	Nanra and Kincaid-Smith	78
1976	Morel-Maroger *et al.*	78
1979	Cameron *et al.*	78
1986	Austin *et al.*	83
1987	Ponticelli *et al.*	93
1987	Leaker *et al.*	74+
1989	Esdaile *et al.*	87
1991	Mc'Ligeyo *et al.*	82
1991	McLaughlin *et al.*	74
1992	GISNEL	85

* two-year survival.
† Class IVb only.
Note: These series are not strictly comparable because different starting points have been taken in some series (onset of lupus/onset of nephritis), and some report patient rather than renal survival. Also the small numbers in all these individual series mean that the confidence limits on all these figures are large. However, the trend is so strong as to overcome all these objections.
Reproduced with permission from [7]; for detailed references see this paper.

for the earlier decade and 86% and 84% in the latter study; the differences are significant at a level of less than 1 : 20. As in 1979, we found that the large differences in survival between milder and more severe forms of lupus nephritis reported by Baldwin et al. [13] and Pollak et al. [14] are no longer evident in our population (Fig. 2).

The data are now overwhelming that one of the major factors in better survival and lower morbidity has been the addition of a cytotoxic agent to the corticosteroids: in the controlled trials done during the 1970s, meta-analysis [15] shows clear clinical benefit for those on cytotoxic drugs, and the careful work of the NIH shows that scarring in repeat renal biopsies does not progress in those taking these agents as it does in those on corticosteroids alone [16].

However, neither of these sets of data gives any clue as to which is the optimum cytotoxic regime; in both sets of data only oral drugs, overwhelmingly azathioprine or cyclophosphamide, were used. Little use

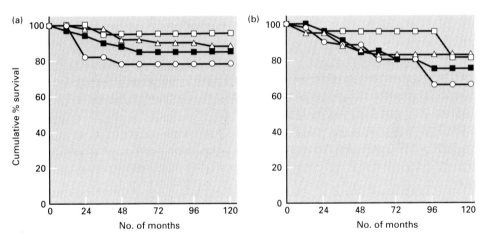

Fig. 2 (a) Renal survival in patients with lupus nephritis of all World Health Organization (WHO) classes in recent series, treated with a variety of maintenance regimes consisting of prednisolone plus a cytotoxic agent. □ = Intravenous cyclophosphamide (20 cases [19]); △ = azathioprine (84 cases [20]); ■ = azathioprine (73 cases [12]); ○ = azathioprine (19 cases [19]). There is no statistical difference (Kaplan–Meier) between the outcomes in the different series, including the two limbs of the NIH trials, which include only very small numbers of cases. The proportion of different WHO classes in the different series is similar in all the series. (b) Renal survival in patients with WHO class IV nephritis only treated with a variety of maintenance regimes of prednisolone plus a cytotoxic agent. △ = Azathioprine (42 cases [12]); □ = azathioprine (43 cases [21]); ■ = various treatments [16]; ○ = azathioprine (41 cases [11]). Again there is no statistical difference between the four sets of results. Reproduced with permission from [7].

has been made of chlorambucil and methotrexate in lupus nephritis to date, although it is beginning to emerge that the latter drug may be a useful adjunct, as it already is in rheumatoid arthritis, given weekly by mouth in a dose of 10–20 mg.

During the 1970s and early 1980s, azathioprine was the usual immuno-suppressant, and has every right to be considered the 'gold standard' treatment [17]. Nevertheless, in the 1980s cyclophosphamide has come to be so regarded, especially when given by the intravenous route [18]. Is this justified, and what do the data show?

LONG-TERM SURVIVAL UNDER VARIOUS TREATMENT REGIMES

A comparison of the renal survival data in our recent study [12] with those from other centres for patients with all forms of lupus nephritis shows that Austin *et al.* [19] described a somewhat poorer overall renal survival than ours in a group of patients treated only with oral pred-nisone and azathioprine, whereas their results were better — although not significantly so — using oral prednisone and intravenous boluses of cyclo-phosphamide every 2 or 3 months (Fig. 2a). On the other hand Esdaile *et al.* [20], using only oral steroids together with either oral cyclophosphamide or azathioprine, showed results almost exactly the same as ours. None of the curves differs from the others at a 1 : 20 level of significance, with 10-year renal survivals averaging 85–90%. It is worth emphasizing that the distribution of the renal lesions in these patients by WHO histological class was similar in all three studies.

As already mentioned, patients with the most severe form of lupus nephritis, WHO class IV, have shown a dramatic improvement in some centres during the past two decades. Our own data for the last decade have been compared with those of Ponticelli *et al.* [21] and with data from the NIH [22] (Fig. 2b). Ponticelli *et al.* used a similar regime to ours, of initial intravenous pulse methylprednisolone (with plasma exchange in a few patients) and prednisolone for follow-up, whilst the NIH group used various regimes of maintenance treatment, including corticosteroids together with oral or intravenous cyclophosphamide or with azathioprine. Again, none of the survival curves differs statistically from the others at a 1 : 20 level (Kaplan–Meier).

The NIH group trials of various combinations of prednisolone and cytotoxic therapy over a period of 16 years showed that only the group of patients treated with intravenous boluses of cyclophosphamide had a statistically improved renal survival over those treated with corticosteroids alone [19,23]. Groups treated with oral prednisolone in combination with azathioprine, oral cyclophosphamide, or oral cyclophosphamide and azathioprine had long-term renal survivals not statistically different from those treated with oral prednisolone only. However, it is important to note also that the renal survivals in the last three groups were also not significantly different from that in the patients who received intravenous boluses of cyclophosphamide. Also, the numbers in these trials are small with wide confidence limits [23], and the prednisolone-treated group was to some extent a group of historical rather than contemporary controls.

There are many problems and pitfalls in retrospective comparisons between different centres in different countries. However, the NIH data seem to us slender grounds for advocating the use of regular intravenous cyclophosphamide as some sort of standard against which other forms of maintenance therapy should be judged, when results as good can be obtained — even in WHO class IV lupus nephritis patients — using intravenous pulse methylprednisolone followed by oral prednisolone and azathioprine, as in the present series and in the series of Esdaile *et al.* [20] and Ponticelli *et al.* [21]. Whether or not oral cyclophosphamide as part of a brief induction regime improves results over azathioprine from the outset has never been tested, and would need a separate trial. It is however attractive to use cyclophosphamide in the initial phases of the treatment of active disease, because of the great capacity of mustard-like drugs to inhibit B cells and thus autoantibody formation.

The more recent NIH trial [24] comparing *induction* treatment with methylprednisolone versus monthly intravenous cyclophosphamide for different periods of time showed a clear advantage of the latter regime over the former; however, the methylprednisolone group received *no* cytotoxic agent. A trial comparing monthly intravenous cyclophosphamide versus oral azathioprine maintenance has never been done but is now underway in Europe.

One important point is that the NIH data apply only to patients receiving the regime originally described: 1 g/m^2 of body surface area, which generally produces nausea, vomiting and a quite profound leukopenia. Because of this many observers have used only 500 mg, or weekly low-dose intravenous regimes. The long-term efficacy of these modified intravenous regimes remains unknown.

SIDE-EFFECTS OF CYTOTOXIC DRUGS

The rationale for the use of intravenous cyclophosphamide was to avoid the bladder toxicity of the drug, which is common in those treated chronically with oral cyclophosphamide, and may eventually lead to bladder cancer [25], as in one of our own patients [26], who developed cancer of the bladder after a latent period of 15 years. The general oncogenic risk of cyclophosphamide is not avoided, however, [27].

Obviously, the best way to avoid the toxicity of long-term cyclophos-phamide is by avoiding the drug altogether for maintenance, using it only during the acute phase of the disease if this is felt to be desirable. An important advantage for the azathioprine maintenance regime over any form of mustard-like drug is that there is abundant evidence, from now more than 1000 pregnancies [28] that fertility is unimpaired on this regime, and that it is safe to conceive and carry a fetus whilst under treatment with this agent; neither of these facts is confirmed for intravenous cyclophos-phamide [29], and ovarian failure and premature menopause are common in patients treated with intravenous cyclophosphamide maintenance in the NIH studies (18 of 34 patients) [30] as well as considerable terartogenicity.

This point is crucial, because lupus is a disease predominantly of young women or adolescent girls, and already 26 of our patients have had 55 pregnancies whilst on treatment [31], with successful pregnancies in 20 out of 30 cases in whom prednisolone and azathioprine were taken before, throughout and following the pregnancy. Full rehabilitation of patients with lupus should include the ability to have a family.

One major advantage of the intravenous regime, however, is in patients who live a long way from the treatment centre, or have poor comprehension of the treatment regime and poor compliance. This is a major problem in poor, city-centre populations with lupus. The knowledge that the treatment has been received is important to both doctor and patient.

REFERENCES

1 Leehey DJ, Katz AI, Azaran AH, Aronson AJ, Spargo BH. Silent diffuse lupus nephritis: long term follow-up. Am J Kidney Dis 1984;2(suppl 1):188–196.
2 Terai C, Nojima Y, Takano K, Yamada A, Takaku F. Determination of urinary albumin excretion by radioimmunoassay in patients with subclinical lupus nephritis. Clin Nephrol 1987;27:79–83.
3 Alexopoulos E, Cameron JS, Hartley BH. Lupus nephritis: correlation of interstitial cells with glomerular function. Kidney Int 1990;37:100–109.
4 Churg J, Sobin LH. Renal Disease: Classification and Atlas of Glomerular Diseases. Igaku Shoin, Tokyo, 1982.
5 Austin HA III, Muenz LR, Joyce KM et al. Prognostic factors in lupus nephritis. Contribution of renal histologic data. Am J Med 1983;75:382–391.
6 Schwartz MM, Bernstein J, Hill GS, Holley K, Phillips EA and the Lupus Nephritis Study Group. Predictive value of renal pathology in diffuse proliferative glomerulo-nephritis. Kidney Int 1989;36:891–896.
7 Cameron JS. What is the role of long-term cytotoxic agents in the treatment of lupus nephritis? J Nephrol 1994;6:172–176.
8 Donadio JV, Glassock RJ. Immunosuppressive drug therapy in lupus nephritis. Am J Kidney Dis 1993;21:239–250.
9 Wei N, Klippel JH, Huston DP et al. Randomized trial of plasma exchange in mild systemic lupus erythematosus. Lancet 1983;i:17–21.
10 Lewis EJ, Hunsicker LG, Lan S-P, Rohde RD, Lachin JM. A controlled trial of plasmapheresis therapy in severe lupus nephritis. N Engl J Med 1992;326:1373–1379.

11 Cameron JS, Turner DR, Ogg CS *et al.* Systemic lupus with nephritis: a long term study. *Q J Med* 1979;**48**:1–24.

12 Mc'Ligeyo SO, Cameron JS, Williams DG *et al.* Improved survival in lupus nephritis in the modern era (1979–1989) using only azathioprine and corticosteroids as maintenance immunosuppression. Unpublished data, 1993.

13 Baldwin DS, Lowenstein J, Rothfield NF, Gallo G, McCluskey RT. The clinical course of the proliferative and membranous forms of lupus nephritis. *Ann Intern Med* 1970;**73**:924–929.

14 Pollak VE, Pirani CL, Schwartz FD. The natural history of the renal manifestations of systemic lupus erythematosus. *J Lab Clin Med* 1964;**63**:537–550.

15 Felson DT, Anderson J. Evidence for the superiority of immunosuppressive drugs and prednisone over prednisone alone in lupus nephritis. *N Engl J Med* 1984;**311**:1528–1533.

16 Balow JE, Austin HA III, Muenz LR *et al.* Effect of treatment on the evolution of renal abnormalities in lupus nephritis. *N Engl J Med* 1984;**311**:491–495.

17 Ginzler E, Sharon E, Diamond H, Kaplan D. Long-term maintenance therapy with azathioprine in systemic lupus erythematosus. *Arthritis Rheum* 1975;**18**:27–34.

18 Balow JE. Treatment and monitoring of patients with lupus nephritis. *Nephrol Dial Transplant* 1990;**5**(suppl 1):58–59.

19 Austin HA III, Klippel JH, Balow JE *et al.* Therapy of lupus nephritis: Controlled trial of prednisolone and cytotoxic drugs. *N Engl J Med* 1986;**314**:614–619.

20 Esdaile JM, Levinton C, Federgreen W, Hayslett JP, Kashgarian M. The clinical and renal biopsy predictors of long term outcome in lupus nephritis: a study of 87 patients and review of the literature. *Q J Med* 1989;**72**:779–833.

21 Ponticelli C, Zucchelli P, Moroni G, Cagnoli L, Banfi G, Pasquali S. Long term prognosis of diffuse lupus nephritis. *Clin Nephrol* 1987;**28**:263–271.

22 Austin KA III, Muenz LR, Joyce KM *et al.* Prognostic factors in lupus nephritis. Contribution of renal histologic data. *Am J Med* 1983;**75**:382–387.

23 Steinberg AD, Steinberg SC. Long-term preservation of renal function in patients with lupus nephritis receiving treatment that includes cyclophosphamide versus those treated with predisolone only. *Arthritis Rheum* 1991;**34**:945–950.

24 Boumpas DT, Austin HA III, Vaughn EM *et al.* Controlled trial of pulse methylprednisolone versus two regimes of pulse cyclophosphamide in severe lupus nephritis. *Lancet* 1992;**340**:741–745.

25 Pedersen-Bjergaard J, Ersboll J, Hansen VL. Carcinoma of the urinary bladder after treatment with cyclophosphamide for non-Hodgkin's lymphoma. *N Engl J Med* 1988;**318**:1028–1032.

26 Cameron JS, Boulton-Jones M, Robinson RJ, Ogg CS. Treatment of lupus nephritis with cyclophosphamide. *Lancet* 1970;**ii**:846–849.

27 Gibbons RB, Westerman E. Acute lymphocytic leukemia following short term intermittent intravenous cyclophosphamide treatment of lupus nephritis. *Arthritis Rheum* 1988;**31**:1552–1554.

28 Davison JM. Pregnancy in renal transplant recipients: clinical perspectives. *Contr Nephrol* 1984;**37**:170–178.

29 Kirshon B, Wasserstrum N, Willis R, Herman GE, McCabe ER. Teratogenic effects of first trimester cyclophosphamide therapy. *Obstet Gynecol* 1988;**72**:462–464.

30 Boumpas DT, Austin HA III, Vaughn EM *et al.* Risk for sustained amenorrhea in patients with systemic lupus erythematosus receiving intermittent pulse cyclophosphamide therapy. *Ann Intern Med* 1993;**119**:366–369.

31 Oviasu E, Hicks J, Cameron JS. The outcome of pregnancy in women with lupus nephritis. *Lupus* 1991;**1**:19–25.

FURTHER READING

Cameron JS. Lupus nephritis in childhood and adolescence. *Pediatr Nephrol* 1994;**8**:230–249.

Cameron JS. Systemic lupus erythematusus. In: *Immunologic Renal Disease*, edited by Causer W & Neilson E. Raven Press, New York, 1996; (in press).

Golbus J, McCune JW. Lupus nephritis: classification, prognosis, immunopathogenesis and treatment. *Rheum Dis Clin North Am* 1994;**20**:213–242.

Mills JA. Systemic lupus erythematosus. *N Engl J Med* 1994;**330**:1871–1879.

Wallace DJ, Hahn BV. *Dubois' Systemic Lupus Erythematosus*. Lea & Febiger, Philadelphia, 1993.

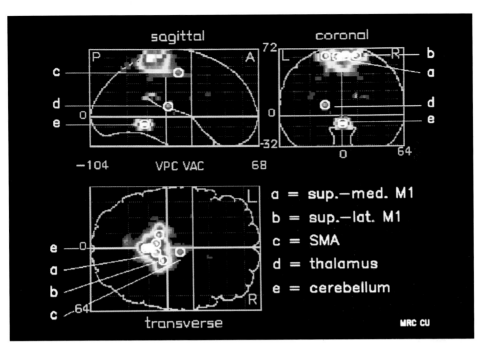

Plate 1 Areas of significant relative regional cerebral blood flow (rCBF) increase during leg exercise, averaged from the group of 6 subjects, are shown as through-projections on to representations of sterotactic space. The upper left (sagittal) image views the brain from the side, the upper right (coronal) image from the back and the lower (transverse) image from the top. L = Left; R = right; A = anterior; P = posterior; VAC = vertical plane through the anterior commissure; VPC = vertical plane through the posterior commissure. Axis numbers refer to atlas coordinates. Areas of activation are shown with increasing significance by an arbitrary colour scale ranging from green, through yellow and red, to white. Foci of maximally significant local relative rCBF increases (indicated by white circles) are seen bilaterally in (a) the superomedial and (b) the superolateral motor cortex. Midline activation is seen in (c) the supplementary motor area and (d) the left thalamus. (e) The cerebellar activation is midline. See text for explanation.

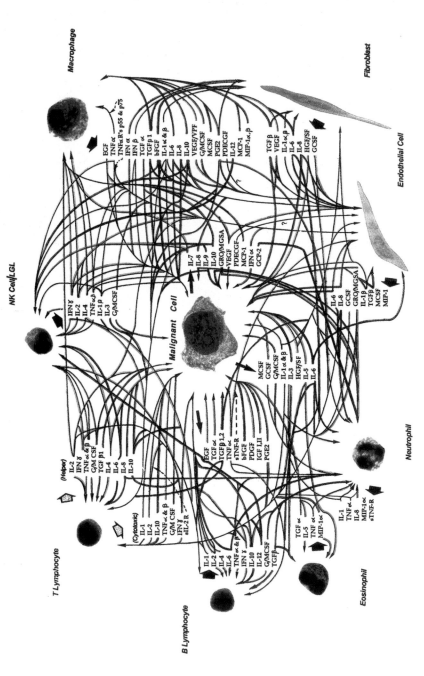

Plate 2 The complex network of cytokines thought to mediate communication between different cell types present within solid human tumours. Note the promiscuity of this network, with different cell types capable of producing and/or responding to the same cytokines. This means that many cytokines have multiple effects within the tumour microenvironment.

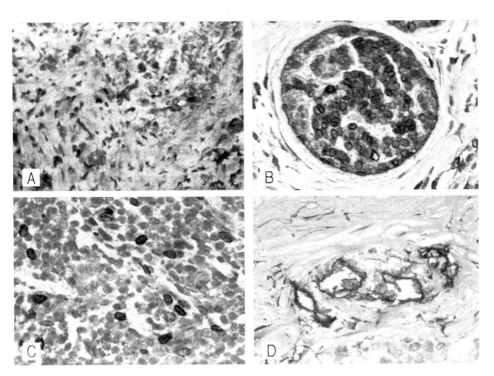

Plate 3 Expression of tumour necrosis factor-α (TNF-α) and its receptors in breast carcinoma. Frozen sections were stained with antibodies 6/35 (A) htr-9 (B,C,D) respectively, and counterstained with haematoxylin. Positive cells are indicated by the red staining in the cytoplasm. (A) Sporadic TNF-α-producing cells displaying macrophage-like morphology in the stroma. (B) Some fibroblast-like cells in the stroma and neoplastic cells of *in situ* lesions express TNF-R p55. (C–D) Some leukocytes and capillary endothelial cells also express this receptor. Tumour-infiltrating leukocytes and some neoplastic cells also express TNF-R p75 (not shown here but illustrated in [27].)

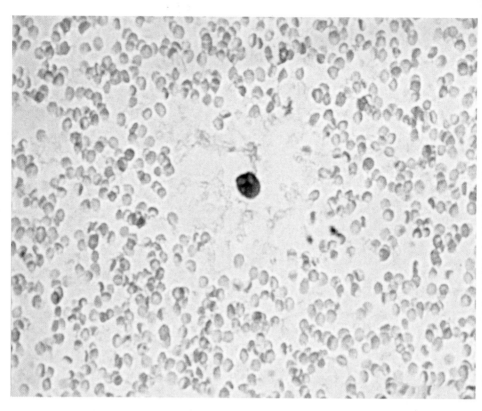

Plate 4 Light micrographs of a haemolytic plaque (areas of lysis) formed around a CD68 positive macrophage secreting tumour necrosis factor-α (TNF-α) in the reverse haemolytic plaque assay (RHPA). Invasive breast carcinomas were enzymatically dispersed within 1 hour of surgical removal, and the whole resultant single-cell suspension washed and used in the RHPA. In this assay, single human cells are mixed with equimolar proportions of protein A-coated sheep erythrocytes and plated onto a glass slide to form a confluent monolayer of cells. The cells are then incubated with a specific anti-cytokine followed by guinea pig complement. During these incubations, the cytokine released by individual human cells is picked up by the antibody which then binds to protein A on erythrocytes neighbouring the producer cell. The addition of complement causes these erythrocytes to lyse, forming an area of lysis around each producer cell. These cells in the monolayer are then identified by immunocytochemistry using monoclonal antibodies (in this case, KP-1 antibody to CD68).

Plate 5 (*opposite*) (a) Section from a 92-year-old kidney, showing a sclerosed glomerulus with related tubular atrophy and interstitial fibrosis. Alongside there is a relatively normal glomerulus with healthy adjacent tubules. (b) Section from an ageing renal arteriole showing intimal thickening and reduplication of the internal elastic lamina. (c) Tubular diverticula in an ageing kidney. (Specimens kindly provided by Dr Angus MacIver.)

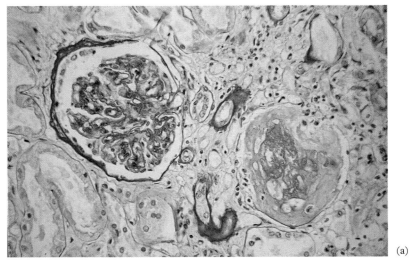

(a)

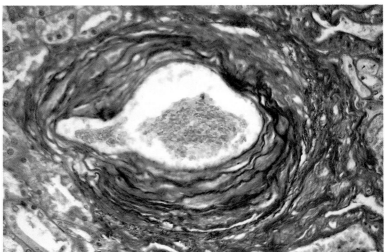

(b)

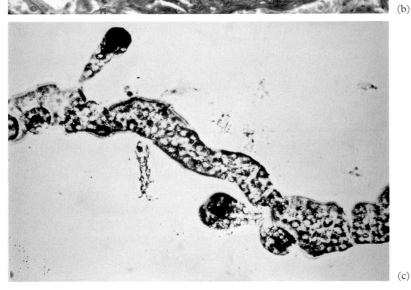

(c)

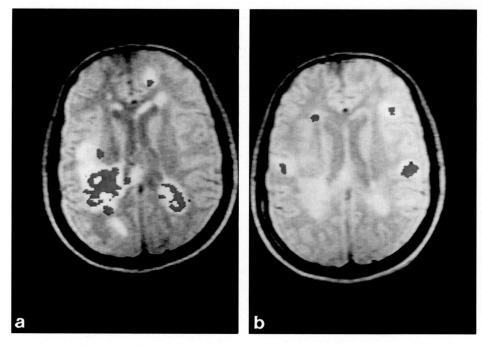

Plate 6 T2-weighted magnetic resonance imaging scans taken 3 months apart, of the brain in a patient with multiple sclerosis. The irregular white areas in the parenchyma correspond with lesions. The red areas represent regions of disruption of the blood–brain barrier shown by enhancement after injection of gadolinium — diethylenetriamine-pentaacetic acid (DTPA), superimposed by computer on the unenhanced images. Note: 1 The regions enhancing in (a) are no longer doing so in (b) 2 There are four new enhancing lesions in b 3 The areas of the old lesions in (b) are smaller than in (a) as a result of resolution of oedema. Reprinted from McDonald WI, Barnes A. *Trends in Neuroscience* 1989;**12**:376–379

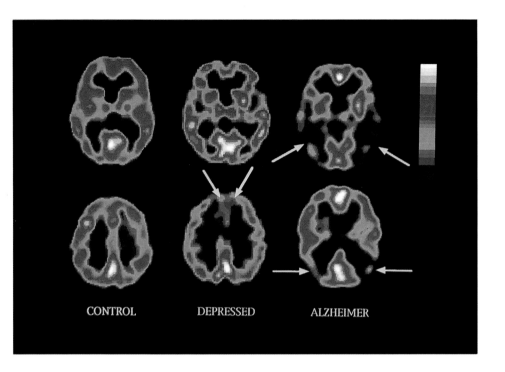

CONTROL   DEPRESSED   ALZHEIMER

Plate 7 99mTc-exametazime single-photon emission tomography (SPET) scans for (left) a control (middle) a case of major depression and (right) a case of Alzheimer-type dementia. Arrows show areas of apparent perfusion deficits in depressed and Alzheimer case. To the right of the figure is the colour scale used to represent tracer uptake: bright is high uptake. The upper slices are at the level of the basal ganglia in the transverse plane; the lower slices are 2 cm higher. These are representative cases of similar age. The decrements in this single case of depression may be compared with the average effect shown in Fig. 1 (p. 421).

Autosomal dominant polycystic kidney disease: molecular analysis

PETER C. HARRIS

Cyst development is one of the commonest abnormalities of the kidney which can occur because of an inherited defect, be acquired during life, or, in animal systems, can be induced by cystogenic chemicals. The similarity of cysts arising by these different ways indicates that a common or related cystic pathway may be involved that can be initiated in various ways. At this stage, however, the initiation step is unknown in any human renal cystic disease and so much effort has been devoted to identifying this primary defect, by genetic means, in inherited polycystic kidney diseases.

INHERITED HUMAN POLYCYSTIC DISEASES

Renal cyst development has been noted in two diseases generally associated with tumorous growths and thought to be due to tumour-suppressor genes, tuberous sclerosis (TSC) and von Hippel–Lindanu disease (reviewed in [1]), and with malformation syndromes, such as some chromosome disorders. However, the vast majority of inherited human polycystic disease is associated with disorders that primarily affect the kidney. These are autosomal dominant polycystic kidney disease (ADPKD), autosomal recessive polycystic kidney disease (ARPKD) and juvenile nephronophthisis (JN). Both ARPKD and JN are recessively inherited, present in infancy and relatively rare conditions; ARPKD has an incidence of ~ 1/25 000 while the incidence of JN is not known, but it probably accounts for 2–10% of childhood renal failure. Some recent progress has been made in the localization of the genes for these two disorders, with JN mapped to chromosome 2 [2] and ARPKD mapped to chromosome 6 [3]. However, most progress has been made in identifying the primary defects in ADPKD, and it is that disorder which will be discussed in detail here.

ADPKD — CLINICAL FEATURES

ADPKD is characterized by progressive cyst formation and enlargement, typically leading to end-stage renal disease (ESRD) by late middle age:

approximately 8% of all renal transplant and dialysis patients have this disease [4]. Considerable variability in disease severity is seen (partly due to genetic heterogeneity; see below) with ~ 25% of patients having adequate renal function at 70 years [5], while a small minority present in childhood; approximately one-third of childhood polycystic kidney disease is due to ADPKD [6,7].

Although the vast majority of morbidity and mortality in ADPKD is due to renal disease, a spectrum of extrarenal manifestations are also seen. These include cysts in many other organs, most notably the liver, and a higher prevalence of abnormalities of connective tissue. These include intracranial aneurysms, which can rupture to cause subarachnoid haemorrhage; heart valve defects; colonic diverticula; inguinal herniae (reviewed in [8]) and an overlap connective tissue disorder (OCTD) [9]. The range of associated abnormalities indicates that ADPKD is a systemic disorder.

ADPKD IS GENETICALLY HETEROGENEOUS

ADPKD is one of the commonest genetic disorders; with a frequency of 1/1000, it is twice as common as cystic fibrosis and 10 times more frequent than Huntington's disease. ADPKD is now known to be genetically heterogeneous, with at least three different genes causing this disorder. The first ADPKD locus to be genomically localized, polycystic kidney disease 1 (PKD1), lies close to the end of the short arm of chromosome 16, in the region 16p13.3 [10] and accounts for approximately 85% of ADPKD [11]. In 1993 a second locus (PKD2) was mapped to the region 4q13–q23 [12,13] and is thought to be responsible for the majority of non-PKD1 ADPKD. PKD2 is a milder condition with an average age of ESRD of ~ 72.5 years compared to ~ 56 years for PKD1 [14]. Recent studies have shown one ADPKD family which is not linked to PKD1 or PKD2 and hence it is likely that there is a third, as yet unmapped, ADPKD locus [15].

POSITIONAL CLONING OF ADPKD LOCI

Despite detailed studies of the biochemistry and cell biology of ADPKD it has not been possible to determine the primary defects which lead to cyst formation. Recent effort has focused on employing genetic means to identify the genes which are defective in this disorder and then using that information to determine the primary protein abnormality. By the method of positional cloning the mutated gene can be identified without determining the biochemical defect. This involves very precisely localizing the gene within the genome by tracing genetic markers through families which segregate the disease. The positional cloning approach seemed likely to succeed with ADPKD because the disease is frequent and usually affects individuals later in life, with the result that many large pedigrees are available for study. Furthermore, individuals inheriting the disease nearly always develop cysts in their kidneys (at least by middle age), which can be assayed by ultrasound, and so the gene can be reliably traced within a family. Nevertheless, the gene search was complicated by genetic heterogeneity and the genomic structure of the region containing the PKD1 gene, so that 9 years elapsed between linkage of the PKD1 locus to chromosome 16 and the final identification of the gene.

CLONING THE PKD1 GENE

The PKD1 locus was mapped to chromosome 16 in 1985 by linkage with α-globin [10]. Subsequently, several years followed in which new markers were identified, and physically and genetically localized relative to each other, and to the PKD1 locus. By 1992 the PKD1 locus had been mapped to an area of 600 kb of DNA [16–18], but because this area is very gene-rich (containing ~ 20 different genes [16]), it proved difficult to identify the gene and some further clue to pinpoint its position was required. This clue finally emerged after the discovery that a locus for another genetic disease, tuberous sclerosis (TSC), termed the TSC2 locus, was also mapped to the PKD1 region [19]. At this stage a Portuguese family with both ADPKD and TSC was recognized and cytogenetic analysis showed that a chromosome translocation between chromosomes 16 and 22 also segregated within this pedigree. Carriers of the balanced exchange had ADPKD, while the son with an unbalanced karyotype, which resulted in monosomy for a region of 16p13.3, had TSC [20]. One explanation for these findings was that the deleted chromosome region found in the son contained the TSC2 locus, while the translocation breakpoint itself disrupted the PKD1 gene. Consequently, this rearrangement was studied in detail and after extensive cloning and mapping the breakpoint in 16p13.3 was precisely localized ([20]; Fig. 1). By this stage the TSC2 gene had also been identified by analysis of a number of large DNA deletions that disrupt this gene in typical TSC patients [21]. The translocation breakpoint lies close to the TSC2 gene (~ 25 kb) and disrupts a gene which is positioned immediately adjacent to it (Fig. 1). This gene encodes a large transcript (~ 14 kb) and was clearly a strong candidate as the PKD1 gene. However, to prove this, other mutations of the gene in typical PKD1 patients were required.

MUTATIONS OF THE PKD1 GENE

Initial analysis of this gene in ~ 300 PKD1 patients revealed two deletions detected by Southern blotting. One deletion of 5.5 kb resulted in a 3 kb

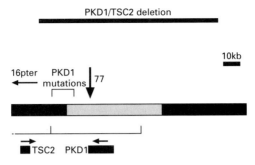

Fig. 1 The polycystic kidney disease 1 (PKD1) gene. The locations of the PKD1 and tuberous sclerosis 2 (TSC2) genes (solid boxes) in 16p13.3 are shown below the line with the direction of transcription (arrow) and genomic extents (brackets) indicated. The duplicated genomic region is hatched. The position of the Portuguese translocation breakpoint (large arrow 77), the region where typical PKD1 mutations have been detected so far and the region deleted in a representative PKD1/TSC2 deletion are shown.

deletion of the transcript, while the second was a genomic deletion of 2 kb which removed 446 bp from the transcript and was therefore a frameshift deletion [20]. The smaller deletion was a *de novo* change which occurred concurrently with the onset of PKD1 within this family, providing further evidence that mutation of this gene results in PKD1.

Three other splicing mutations of this gene have also been described, including a substitution in a splice donor site, resulting in the skipping of a 135 bp exon [20] and two cases of deletion within the same 75 bp intron [22]. These intronic deletions of 18 or 20 bp result in aberrant splicing with three different transcripts produced from the abnormal gene. As the deletions do not disrupt the splice donor or acceptor sites they probably cause aberrant splicing because the deleted intron is too small to be spliced out effectively.

DELETIONS OF THE PKD1 AND THE TSC2 GENES

The PKD1 and TSC2 genes lie within 2 kb of each other in genomic DNA and this raised the possibility that mutations affecting both genes would be found. So far, six large deletions that disrupt the TSC2 gene and the PKD1 gene (often completely deleting it; Fig. 1) have been described [23]. In each case this contiguous gene syndrome is associated with a specific phenotype of TSC and severe polycystic kidney disease that is manifest at birth or within the first few months of life. The polycystic kidney disease in these cases is more severe than is normally seen in PKD1 or TSC alone.

WHAT IS THE MUTATIONAL MECHANISM IN PKD1?

ADPKD is a dominant disease but it is not yet clear if disease occurs because a novel protein is produced (gain of function) or if the mutations are inactivating and disease results from loss of one copy of the gene, haplo-insufficiently, or only after the normal allele is eliminated in renal cells by a second somatic mutation (as occurs in many inherited cancer syndromes). At this stage there is evidence of both inactivating mutations, and changes that produce a novel transcript, which may generate a novel protein. All of the clear inactivating mutations of PKD1 are large deletions that also disrupt the adjacent TSC2 gene. It is not clear whether the inactivation of PKD1 or a combined affect of disrupting both genes results in the severe disease seen in these cases [23]. All mutations in typical adult-onset PKD1 patients so far described generate an abnormal transcript but analysis of further mutations and study at the cellular level for aberrant protein are required to determine if these are gains of function mutations.

THE PKD1 GENE LIES IN A DUPLICATED GENOMIC REGION

A significant complication in studying the PKD1 gene is the unusual structure of the genomic region encoding most of the gene. All but 3.5 kb at the 3′ end of the transcript is encoded by a region of DNA which is reiterated at least four times in a position more proximal on chromosome 16 (Fig. 1). The duplicated area (termed the HG locus) also encodes

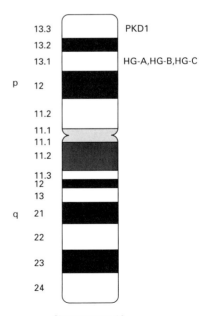

Fig. 2 The chromosome location of the PKD1 and HG genes.

Chromosome 16

three genes: HG-A (21 kb), HG-B (17 kb) and HG-C (8.5 kb) which share substantial homology to the PKD1 transcript (Fig. 2); preliminary analysis indicates that the HG transcripts and the PKD1 transcript show a sequence divergence of less than 3%. Consequently, it has proved difficult to study the PKD1 gene by Southern blotting and polymerase chain reaction (PCR) methods without simultaneously analysing the duplicate area and this has showed progress in detecting mutations and characterizing a full-length transcript. It is not yet known whether the HG genes produce functional proteins.

THE PKD1 TRANSCRIPT

Analysis by Northern blotting shows that the PKD1 transcript is ~ 14 kb and expressed in a wide range of tissue-specific cell lines [20]. A high level of expression was found in an astrocytoma cell line and in primary fibroblasts, with a lower level detected in cell lines derived from kidney and liver cells. Significant expression was also detected in lymphoblast cells and leukocytes so that the PKD1 transcript can be assayed by reverse transcriptase-PCR (RT-PCR) directly from peripheral blood.

The complication caused by duplication has hampered the characterization of a full-length transcript and at present sequence from only 5.7 kb at the 3' of the transcript has been published. Analysis of this has not revealed the likely role of the PKD1 protein. Several groups worldwide are presently attempting to clone a full-length transcript. Initial efforts have focused on sequencing the genomic region containing the gene [24] so that the sequence of the PKD1 gene can be established.

To clone the bona fide PKD1 transcript we are employing a method of exon linking by RT-PCR with RNA from a cell line which contains the PKD1 gene but not the duplicate HG loci. In this way a contig containing the whole PKD1 transcript will be isolated and full analysis of the predicted protein sequence will be possible.

CONCLUSIONS

Over the last 5–10 years the approach of positioned cloning has revolutionized our understanding of some of the most frequent genetic diseases of humans. This method identifies the primary defect in what are often complex disorders so that an insight into the basis of disease and possible therapeutic approaches is provided. For ADPKD that process has now begun with the identification of the major disease gene PKD1. The identification process and now analysis of the PKD1 gene have been complicated by an unusual duplication involving much of the PKD1 gene, that has occurred on chromosome 16 in recent evolutionary time. For this reason it is likely that new methods will be required to characterize the gene and to detect mutations effectively. So far only a few mutations have been detected and the mutational mechanism causing PKD1 is not clear; further studies are required. It is likely that in the next year the full sequence of the PKD1 transcript will be available and so allow analysis of the predicted protein, while studies of immunohistochemistry will reveal its cellular localization and help to define the likely role of the PKD1 protein. An understanding of the early stages of cyst formation in this disease is likely to provide insight into the mechanisms underlying cyst formation in other inherited and acquired forms of cystic disease in humans and may suggest candidate molecules involved in these disorders.

The entire sequence of the PKD1 transcript and the predicted PKD1 protein, polycystin, has now been described [25,26]. Polycystin is an integral membrane protein of ~ 460 KD which may be involved in cell–cell and/or cell–matrix interactions. The protein has been immunolocalized to tubular epithelia in fetal, adult and cystic kidney [27].

REFERENCES

1 Fick GM, Gabow PA. Hereditary and acquired cystic disease of the kidney. *Kidney Int* 1994;**46**:951–964.
2 Antignac C, Arduy CH, Beckmann JS *et al*. A gene for familial juvenile nephronophthisis (recessive medullary cystic kidney disease) maps to chromosome 2p. *Nature Genet* 1993;**3**:342–345.
3 Zerres K, Mücher G, Bachner L *et al*. Mapping of the gene for autosomal recessive polycystic kidney disease (ARPKD) to chromosome 6p21-cen. *Nature Genet* 1994;**7**:429–432.
4 Gabow PA. Autosomal dominant polycystic kidney disease. *N Engl J Med* 1993;**329**:332–342.
5 Gabow PA, Johnson AM, Kaehny WD *et al*. Factors affecting the progression of renal disease in autosomal-dominant polycystic kidney disease. *Kidney Int* 1992;**41**:1311–1319.
6 Zerres K, Rudnik-Schöneborn S, Deget F, German working group on paediatric nephrology. Childhood onset autosomal dominant polycystic kidney disease in sibs: clinical picture and recurrence risk. *J Med Genet* 1993;**30**:583–588.
7 Fick GM, Johnson AM, Strain JD *et al*. Characteristics of very early onset autosomal dominant polycystic kidney disease. *J Am Soc Nephrol* 1993;**3**:1863–1870.
8 Gabow PA. Autosomal dominant polycystic kidney disease — more than a renal disease. *Am J Kidney Dis* 1990;**16**:403–413.
9 Somlo S, Rutecki G, Giuffra LA, Reeders ST, Cugino A, Whittier FC. A kindred exhibiting cosegregation of an overlap connective tissue disorder and the chromosome 16 linked form of autosomal dominant polycystic kidney disease. *J Am Soc Nephrol* 1993;**4**:1371–1378.
10 Reeders ST, Breuning MH, Davies KE *et al*. A highly polymorphic DNA marker linked to adult polycystic kidney disease on chromosome 16. *Nature* 1985;**317**:542–544.
11 Peters DJM, Sandkuijl LA. Genetic heterogeneity of polycystic kidney disease in Europe. In: *Contributions to Nephrology: Polycystic Kidney Disease*, edited by Breuning MH, Devoto M, Romeo G. Karger, Basel, 1992:128–139.
12 Peters DJM, Spruit L, Saris JJ *et al*. Chromosome 4 localization of a second gene for autosomal dominant polycystic kidney disease. *Nature Genet* 1993;**5**:359–362.
13 Kimberling WJ, Kumar S, Gabow PA, Kenyon JB, Connolly CJ, Somlo S. Autosomal dominant polycystic kidney disease: localization of the second gene to chromosome 4q13-q23. *Genomics* 1993;**18**:467–472.

14 Ravine D, Walker RG, Gibson RN *et al*. Phenotype and genotype heterogeneity in autosomal dominant polycystic kidney disease. *Lancet* 1992;**340**:1330–1333.

15 Daoust MC, Reynolds DM, Bichet DG, Somlo S. Evidence for a third genetic locus for autosomal dominant polycystic kidney disease. *Genomics* 1995;**25**:733–736.

16 Germino GG, Weinstat-Saslow D, Himmelbauer H *et al*. The gene for autosomal dominant polycystic kidney disease lies in a 750-kb CpG-rich region. *Genomics* 1992;**13**:144–151.

17 Somlo S, Wirth B, Germino GG *et al*. Fine genetic localization of the gene for autosomal dominant polycystic kidney disease (PKD1) with respect to physically mapped markers. *Genomics* 1992;**13**:152–158.

18 Harris PC, Thomas S, Ratcliffe PJ, Breuning MH, Coto E, Lopez-Larrea C. Rapid genetic analysis of families with polycystic kidney disease by means of a microsatellite marker. *Lancet* 1991;**338**:1484–1487.

19 Kandt RS, Haines JL, Smith M *et al*. Linkage of an important gene locus for tuberous sclerosis to a chromosome 16 marker for polycystic kidney disease. *Nature Genet* 1992;**2**:37–41.

20 European Polycystic Kidney Disease Consortium. The polycystic kidney disease 1 gene encodes a 14 kb transcript and lies within a duplicated region on chromosome 16. *Cell* 1994;**77**:881–894.

21 European Chromosome 16 Tuberous Sclerosis Consortium. Identification and characterization of the tuberous sclerosis gene on chromosome 16. *Cell* 1993;**75**:1305–1315.

22 Peral B, Gamble V, San Millán JL *et al*. Splicing mutations of the polycystic kidney disease 1 (PKD1) gene induced by intronic deletion. *Hum Mol Genet* 1995;**4**:569–574.

23 Brook-Carter PT, Peral B, Ward CJ *et al*. Deletion of the TSC2 and PKD1 genes associated with severe infantile polycystic kidney disease — a contiguous gene syndrome. *Nature Genet* 1994;**8**:328–332.

24 Burn TC, Connors TD, Dackowski WR *et al*. Analysis of the genomic sequence for the autosomal dominant polycystic kidney disease (PKD1) gene predicts the presence of a leucine-rich repeat. *Hum Mol Genet* 1995;**4**:575–582.

25 International Polycystic Kidney Disease Consortium: Polycystic kidney disease: the complete structure of the *PKD1* gene and its protein. *Cell* 1995;**81**:289–298.

26 Hughes J, Ward CJ, Peral B, Aspinwall R, Clark K, San Millán JL, Gamble V, Harris PC. The polycystic kidney disease 1 (*PKD1*) gene encodes a novel protein with multiple cell recognition domains. *Nature Genet* 1995;**10**:151–160.

27 Ward CJ, Turley H, Ong ACM, Comley M, Biddolph S, Chetty R, Ratcliffe PJ, Gatter K, Harris PC. Polycystin, the polycystic kidney disease 1 protein, is expressed by epithelial cells in fetal, adult and polycystic kidney. *Proc Natl Acad Sci* USA 1996;**93**:1524–1528.

MULTIPLE CHOICE QUESTIONS

1 Autosomal dominant polycystic kidney disease

  a affects about 1/10 000 individuals

  b most often causes cysts in the liver (apart from the kidney)

  c is responsible for approximately 8% of patients with end-stage renal disease

  d is usually an infantile disease

  e is associated with various disorders of connective tissue

2 Autosomal recessive polycystic kidney disease

  a is more frequent than ADPKD

  b is a childhood disease

  c has been mapped to chromosome 16

d is more frequent than juvenile nephronophthisis
e usually affects individuals in late middle age

3 Polycystic kidney disease 1
a accounts for approximately 50% of all ADPKD
b is a more severe disease than PKD2
c and PKD2 account for all cases of ADPKD
d usually affects adults
e is located in chromosome region 16q13.3

4 The PKD1 gene
a was localized to chromosome 16 in 1990
b lies close to a tuberous sclerosis gene
c was pinpointed by a chromosome translocation
d is located in a region with many other genes
e lies in a duplicated genomic region

5 Positional cloning
a involves precisely localizing a disease gene within the genome
b requires knowledge of the biochemical defect in a disease
c of the PKD1 gene took 9 years after initial linkage
d of PKD1 was complicated by genetic heterogeneity
e involves genetic linkage analysis

Answers

1 **a** False	2 **a** False	3 **a** False
b True	**b** True	**b** True
c True	**c** False	**c** False
d False	**d** True	**d** True
e True	**e** False	**e** False

4 **a** False	5 **a** True
b True	**b** False
c True	**c** True
d True	**d** True
e True	**e** True

Renal disease in the elderly

TERRY G. FEEST

In a famous editorial in 1982 Berlyne [1] observed that in the UK the combination of uraemia and age over 50 lead to inevitable death. Such people were not offered renal replacement treatment. This contrasted with figures from Europe [2]. In many countries the median age of starting renal replacement therapy was over 60, the European average was around 55, but in the UK the median age was only 45. Unless different patterns of renal disease existed in the rest of Europe it was clear that in the UK the elderly were discriminated against. They were not offered renal replacement therapy, they died and were not perceived to be a problem. This led to a widespread perception that renal diseases were relatively common in young people and relatively uncommon in the elderly. There is a need to focus more on the problems of the elderly with renal disease.

THE INCIDENCE OF RENAL FAILURE IN THE ELDERLY

Community-based surveys conducted in the late 1980s showed that the incidence of severe renal failure increases dramatically with age [3–5] (Fig. 1). An incident of severe renal failure was defined as the first time serum creatinine was known to rise above 500 μmol/l. The condition was defined as acute if the serum creatinine subsequently fell below that level, or the patient died and an acute lesion was confirmed. If the creatinine remained elevated the failure was defined as chronic. Similar results were obtained in Devon, Blackburn and Northern Ireland. After excluding people with terminal disease such as malignancy, the incidence of chronic renal failure per million population per year was around 140. The incidence of acute renal failure follows a similar pattern. The incidence of both conditions rises 10-fold with age (Fig. 1). For chronic renal failure this is a rise from around 60 per million per year for people in their 20s and 30s to over 600 per million per year for those in their 80s. There was an even greater proportional rise in acute renal failure.

The observed patterns of referral of chronic renal failure for a specialist opinion showed that the elderly were referred relatively infrequently

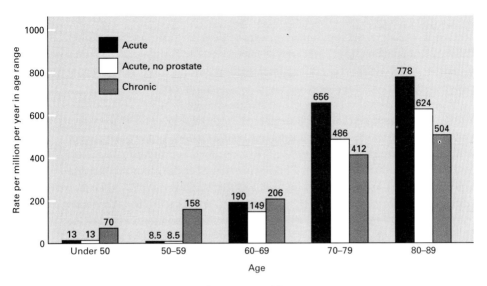

Fig. 1 Age-related incidence of severe renal failure.

(Table 1) [3]. All patients under 60 willing to be referred saw a specialist. In the 60–80-year age group, even in a health district which contained a renal unit, one-third of patients were not referred for specialist opinion. Where there was no renal unit two-thirds of patients were not referred. Those over the age of 80 had very little chance at all of seeing a specialist. When nephrologists assessed the case histories of the 23 patients aged between 65 and 80 who were not referred, they judged that they would have offered renal replacement therapy to 14 of these patients, all of whom died quickly without it. From this information it would appear that low treatment rates in the elderly are less due to the ageism of nephrologists than to the unwillingness of other physicians to refer to a specialist centre.

The overall need for renal replacement therapy, assuming that all patients whom nephrologists considered suitable under the age of 80 are to be treated, was estimated at around 80 per million per year in areas

Table 1 Non-referral of chronic renal failure.

Age of patients (years)	With renal unit	Without	Total (%)
Under 60	3% of 31	4% of 27	3
60–80	33% of 42	64% of 59	51
Over 80	71% of 24	100% of 26	86
All patients			46

Figures are the percentage of patients with advanced chronic renal failure not referred for a specialist opinion by age in districts with and without a local renal unit.

where there are no large ethnic communities. In patients of Asian or Afro-Caribbean descent the incidence appears to be three or four times higher than in Caucasians [6]. This may explain the very high dialysis rates achieved in the USA where it has been estimated that up to 200 patients per million per year may be starting renal replacement therapy.

In recent years the British situation has changed. In 1992 in Europe 37% of those starting renal replacement therapy were over 65. The overall acceptance rate in the UK for adults has risen from 19.1 new patients per million population per year in 1982 [2] to around 66 per million population in 1992 (unpublished figures). The proportion of these patients over the age of 65 is now 36.5%, which is similar to that in Europe (37%) [7]. It is rather higher for men at 38% than women (25%). As the UK acceptance rate has steadily risen (Fig. 2) there has been little change in acceptance rates for the younger age groups who were relatively well-catered-for in the past. The major increase has been in the elderly and diabetic patients. The current acceptance rate for patients between 60 and 84 years is 190 per million per year.

Thus, like most other diseases, renal failure is predominantly a problem of the elderly. The situation for renal replacement therapy in the UK has significantly improved in recent years but there is still a shortfall below the estimated need of 80 new patients per million per year in areas where

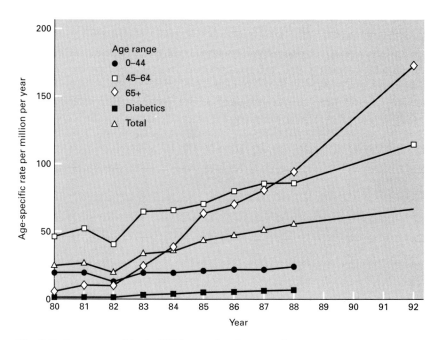

Fig. 2 Patients accepted in the UK for renal replacement therapy.

there are no ethnic communities. The major area of shortfall is in the provision for the elderly.

THE AGEING KIDNEY

Like neurons, nephrons start to die in the third decade of life. Changes occur first in the outer cortex with hyalinization and collapse of glomeruli leading to glomerulosclerosis — changes similar to those observed in hypertension [8,9]. There is subsequent tubular degeneration and interstitial fibrosis related to the affected nephrons. Unlike neurons, the remaining nephrons hypertrophy to compensate for nephron loss. Thus in the ageing kidney one sees sclerosed glomeruli with related nephron atrophy alongside healthy glomeruli with related tubular hypertrophy (Plate 5a).

It is thought that the primary renal lesion is vascular [8–10]. In the third and fourth decade of life renal arterioles begin to develop intimal thickening, sometimes with hyaline subintimal deposits, with thickening and reduplication of the elastic lamina (Plate 5b). The end-result of the vascular damage is that elderly renal vessels become tortuous, irregular and less elastic. This damage probably makes them more susceptible to diminished perfusion and may partly explain the high incidence of acute renal failure observed in elderly people.

The rate of nephron loss tends to be greater in men, but is highly variable. The proportion of sclerosed glomeruli in subjects over 50 may vary from 1% to 30% [9]. The compensatory hypertrophy of surviving nephrons tends to protect from declining creatinine clearance until the sixth or seventh decade. At this point creatinine clearance begins to decline, but the ageing subject is then losing muscle mass and thus producing less creatinine each day. The plasma creatinine may thus remain stable, masking the loss of renal function, until the eighth or ninth decade. By this time, of the 600 000–1.2 million nephrons originally present, up to one-third or one-half will have sclerosed [11]. The end-result of this nephron loss is reduction in renal size, length decreasing by up to 2 cm, with development of small superficial punctate scars over the surface of the kidney (Table 2).

Table 2 Aged kidney.

Small (loss of 20% of weight)
Scarred surface
Tubule change
Dehydration when stressed
Infection
Vascular change
Vulnerable to acute renal failure
Early nephron loss, mid clearance change, late creatinine rise

Creatinine clearance may fall by age 80 to between 40 and 75 ml/min [12] with plasma creatinine rising to 140 μmol/l. Creatinine clearance in millilitres per minute can be approximately calculated from the plasma creatinine with correction for age and body weight using the following formula [13].

$$\text{Creatinine clearance} = \frac{(140 - \text{Age}) \ (\text{kg body weight}) \ (1.23)}{\text{serum creatinine (μmol/l)}}$$

There are also age-related changes within the renal tubule. Multiple diverticula develop (Plate 5c) which are thought to be responsible for the increased incidence of pyelonephritis in old people. There is also peritubular fibrosis and associated loss of urinary concentration, acidification and toxin secretion. Thus, in addition to renovascular vulnerability, the elderly, when stressed metabolically, easily become dehydrated, acidotic and accumulate drugs, on a background of reduced renal function. The high incidence of acute renal failure is not surprising.

DISEASES OF THE AGEING KIDNEY

The spectrum of diseases causing failure of older kidneys is different from that found in younger patients (Fig. 3). In the community, 71% of those developing severe chronic renal failure over the age of 70 received no diagnosis [3], largely because they were not referred for specialist opinion. Only 16% of those under 70 remained undiagnosed (Table 3). With such a large undiagnosed group it is impossible to interpret the relative incidence

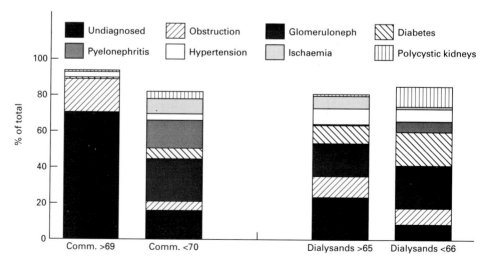

Fig. 3 Causes of severe renal failure in the elderly.

Table 3 Diagnosis of chronic renal failure (%).

	Age	Not diagnosed	Obstruction	GN	Diab	Pyel	Hyp	Isch	PCK
Community	> 69	71	18	0	1	0	3	0	1
	< 70	16	5	24	6	15	4	8	4
Recent	> 65	42	11	19	5/5*	1	8	7	3
dialysands	> 66	9	9	24	10/8*	6	7	1	11

* Insulin dependent/non-insulin dependent.
GN, glomerulonephritis; Diab, diabetes; Pyel, pyelonephritis; Hyp, hypertension; Isch, ishaemia; PCK, polycystic kidneys.

of the other diseases in the few cases where a diagnosis was made. Better information is available from those patients starting dialysis. Studying 200 consecutive patients starting dialysis at the Richard Bright Renal Unit, Bristol in 1993–94 — admittedly a selected group — there is a higher rate of diagnosis. It is disappointing that 42% of those over the age of 65 still remained undiagnosed, compared with 9% of younger patients. This is approximately twice the proportion of undiagnosed older patients reported to the European Dialysis and Transplant Association (EDTA) Registry for the whole of Europe in 1992 [7]. All the Bristol patients who were undiagnosed had bilateral small, non-obstructed kidneys which many clinicians may have classified as 'glomerulonephritis not histologically proven' — a diagnosis made in 11% of the older European patients. The European data were otherwise similar to the Bristol data illustrated. The proportion of patients in Europe with glomerulonephritis has progressively fallen since 1977 and the proportion with undiagnosed disorders, diabetes and renovascular disorders has progressively risen [7]. Analysis of these data indicates that this is not due to a reduction in incidence of glomerulo-nephritis. The proportion with glomerulonephritis has decreased, as increasing numbers of older patients have started treatment. There is a disproportionate contribution of diabetes, vascular disease and undiagnosed patients in this group.

The number of potentially treatable disorders causing end-stage renal failure is disappointing. Of older patients, 11% had renal failure due to obstruction. These were all men with prostatic obstruction, which account-ed for nearly 20% of all older men with chronic renal failure. In the younger age group the obstructive causes of chronic renal failure were congenital lesions, and a few renal stones: there were no cases of prostatic obstruction. Renal failure in 8% of the elderly and 7% of the young was attributed to hypertension — another treatable cause.

Renal ischaemia due to renovascular disease, which accounts for 7% of elderly dialysands, is being diagnosed with increased frequency in the UK and in Europe, where it was the cause of renal failure in 17% of all patients starting renal replacement therapy in 1992 [7]. It is probably still underdiagnosed and may account for a significant proportion of the undiagnosed elderly patients. In any elderly patient with renal failure who does not have heavy proteinuria, renal ischaemia should be considered. This is especially true if there is any other evidence of other peripheral vascular disease, or if there is a discrepancy between the size of the two kidneys of 1 cm or more. Awareness of the possibility of this diagnosis in elderly arteriopaths is especially important as angiotensin-converting enzyme (ACE) inhibitors may lead to disastrous renal decline in such patients, which is not always reversible. As type II diabetics have a high incidence of vascular disease, special care is needed when treating them with ACE inhibition.

Some recent papers have shown encouraging improvements or protection of renal function following revascularization of ischaemic kidneys, even at a very late stage, although this is not a universal experience [14]. In patients with poor renal function non-invasive diagnosis of arterial disease is difficult. Poorly functioning kidneys take up radioisotopes very slowly, and renography is rarely able to give a firm diagnosis. Diagnosis still depends upon renal angiography. This technique is not without risk in arteriopathic patients as it can precipitate showers of cholesterol emboli to the kidneys and elsewhere. This situation often mimics vasculitis with widespread petechiae, eosinophilia and similar histological appearances. The relative merits of treatment of renal arterial stenosis by angioplasty, renal revascularization or renal autotransplantation are still not clear [14].

Diabetes was the cause of renal failure in 18% of younger dialysands, and 10% of older dialysands. These figures are slightly below the European average, although in some Scandinavian countries and in Germany the overall figure approaches 30% of all dialysands. In 50% of the older patients and 40% of the younger ones renal failure was attributed to non-insulin-dependent diabetes mellitus. This is likely to be an underestimate of the contribution of type II diabetes to nephropathy. It is probable that several patients receiving insulin were classified as type I diabetics when, with the use of more stringent criteria, they would have been considered type II diabetics who had subsequently required insulin.

The important contribution of type II diabetes in renal failure has often been underestimated. In 1974 in a study of 6800 deaths in diabetics, renal death was reported as the cause of 48% of deaths of those developing diabetes before the age of 20 and only 6% of those developing diabetes later [15]. What was often overlooked is that the incidence of diabetes in older people is so overwhelmingly greater than that in young people that the number of renal deaths in this series in older diabetics outnumbers younger diabetics by 1.7 to 1 (386 versus 229). There are also studies which suggest that when followed for similar lengths of time, the cumulative incidence of renal failure is similar in both type I and type II diabetics [16]. As more and more older patients are accepted for therapy, the proportion of dialysands with Type II diabetes will progressively grow. In the late 1980s estimates of the proportion of diabetics with renal failure due to type II diabetes from Italy, Germany and the USA ranged from 56% to 66% [16], although one report from New York placed it at over 80% [17]. As much care must be taken with elderly patients with type II diabetes to try to prevent nephropathy as with younger type I patients.

Other common renal diseases of the elderly are important because of their potential reversibility. The importance of prostatic obstruction has already been emphasized. Acute interstitial nephritis is primarily a disease which occurs in people aged over 65. It must be considered in any patient with renal dysfunction and a relatively inactive urine deposit with little proteinuria, especially if the kidneys are of normal size. It is nearly always a drug reaction. It is most commonly seen with the penicillins, analgesics and diuretics, but almost every drug has been associated with this condition. The predominance of this disorder in the elderly probably reflects the fact that they are the group who take most drugs. If the condition is recognized before there is advanced fibrosis and the offending drug is stopped there is then an excellent chance of recovery.

Myelomatosis is another disorder of the elderly which occasionally presents with renal failure. The large majority have renal failure due to myeloma kidney in which the tubules are overloaded with filtered light chains. The common opinion that myeloma patients with severe renal failure have a universally poor prognosis is not borne out by experience. Several patients have lived active lives for over 3 years after starting dialysis. Rapid diagnosis is important, as early institution of fluid repletion, cytotoxic therapy and occasionally plasmapheresis may reverse the renal failure before fibrosis and permanent damage occur.

Wegener's arteritis and microscopic polyarteritis (polyangiitis) are most common in middle-aged and elderly people with a slight male predominance [18]. Both may present with renal manifestations. In microscopic polyangiitis systemic symptoms are mild or absent in many elderly patients, the disease being largely limited to the kidneys. Renal biopsy shows segmental necrotizing glomerulitis, and in the most active cases epithelial crescents are present [19]. Before effective therapy was available mean survival was only 5 months [20]. Rapid diagnosis and therapy are important as the kidneys may be destroyed within a few days. To be effective, treatment must be given in this early phase. These disorders should be suspected in any elderly patient with unexplained advancing renal dysfunction and heavy proteinuria with microscopic haematuria. Immediate renal biopsy is indicated.

Initial therapy is with prednisolone and cyclophosphamide. In rapidly advancing cases induction with pulse intravenous methylprednisolone 500 mg daily for 3 days is carried out, followed by prednisolone 60 mg daily in a slowly tapering dose. Cyclophosphamide is given orally 2 mg/

kg per day in older people, with conversion to azathioprine at 3–6 months. With such therapies overall survivals up to 5 years of around 70% have been obtained in many series, the majority of deaths occurring in the first few months [18]. Plasma exchange has been added to these therapies in severe rapidly progressive cases, especially when dialysis-dependent. There are reports of success in uncontrolled series. No controlled trial of plasma exchange versus intravenous methylprednisolone is available. The prognosis of those surviving 1 year is excellent, with only a slow death rate thereafter.

Most series have not analysed separately the survival of older and younger patients. An early series, before modern therapies were widely used, showed a 1- and 10-year survival of patients over 60 of 42% and 25% respectively, compared with 68% and 48% in younger patients [21]. With modern therapies survival has improved, indicating that even in the elderly, therapy for these conditions is indicated and worthwhile.

The frequency of these common renal disorders in the elderly makes urgent referral for aggressive diagnosis mandatory. Renal ultrasound will identify most cases of obstruction, will identify chronic renal failure with shrunken kidneys, and unequal renal size may point to renal ischaemia. If the kidneys are symmetrical and normal in size, especially when there is heavy proteinuria and an active urinary deposit, immediate renal biopsy is indicated to allow the institution of timely therapy, especially for conditions such as microscopic polyarteritis and acute interstitial nephritis.

In elderly patients presenting with nephrotic syndrome, the most common cause is membranous nephropathy, which is found in about one-third [22]. The next most common condition is minimal-change disease (24%). Most other lesions seen are essentially untreatable and include amyloidosis (10%), proliferative glomerulonephritis and focal sclerosis. Effective treatment in the form of steroid therapy is available for minimal-change disease, but this should not be given without accurate diagnosis. Response in this condition is slower and less predictable in the old than in the young and cannot be used as an indicator of diagnosis. Furthermore, membranous nephropathy often follows a remitting and relapsing course and a spontaneous remission may be falsely interpreted as a response to steroids, leading to an unnecessary prolonged course of a useless and potentially toxic therapy. A definitive diagnosis of membranous glomerulonephritis is also important, as there have been many proposed therapeutic regimes for this condition, although the value of these is uncertain [23]. In addition, in up to 9% of patients membranous nephropathy is associated with underlying malignancy. The most common conditions are lymphomas and leukaemias. The finding of membranous nephropathy should increase clinical awareness of potential underlying malignancy, and should at least stimulate a search to exclude underlying haematological malignancies and a chest X-ray to exclude carcinoma of the lung.

ACUTE RENAL FAILURE

The increasing incidence of advanced acute renal failure with age is illustrated in Fig. 1 [5]. Prostatic obstruction accounts for 25% of cases, only caused advanced renal failure in men over 65, and in over one-third of all men with advanced acute renal failure was the underlying cause. If these prostatic cases are excluded from analysis, the dramatic increase in acute renal failure with age, and the male preponderence, are still present (Fig. 1).

The significant contribution of prostatic obstruction to severe renal failure, whether acute or chronic, as previously described, is not widely appreciated. There does not seem to be a relationship between occurrence of renal failure and severity of prostatic symptoms or apparent prostate size on rectal examination. Many patients undergo tertiary referral before such a simple and treatable diagnosis is made. Although only present in a very small minority of the huge numbers of men who develop prostatic obstruction with advancing age, this small proportion of a large number becomes significant when considering elderly men presenting with renal failure. Prostatic obstruction as a cause of renal failure must be considered in all elderly men presenting with renal dysfunction without heavy proteinuria in whom there is no obvious cause.

The high incidence of acute renal failure in the elderly is not surprising. They have a high incidence of severe predisposing illness and, as has already been discussed, their kidneys will be susceptible to circulatory and metabolic insults. Figure 4 shows the survival of patients following advanced acute renal failure at 3 months and 2 years. The analysis was repeated excluding patients with prostatic disease as this was one condition which was shown to have a particularly good prognosis. Even with this exclusion, and in contrast to some other studies [5], there is no suggestion that with increasing age above 50 there is a decreased prognosis. This information confirms that 70-year-olds just as much as 50-year-olds with acute renal failure should be referred for specialist support and treatment.

Recovery of renal function after acute renal failure in patients over the age of 50 is frequently incomplete. In only 30% of cases did the creatinine return to a level below 110 µmol/l, in 48% it was between 110 and 300 µmol/l, and in 22% it remained above 300 µmol/l. Many of the older patients therefore will need long-term follow-up after recovery from the acute illness.

CHRONIC RENAL FAILURE

Renal replacement therapy in the elderly presents a challenge. Older people are slow to acclimatize to new conditions and techniques and do not learn their treatments easily. They have an increased incidence of comorbidity,

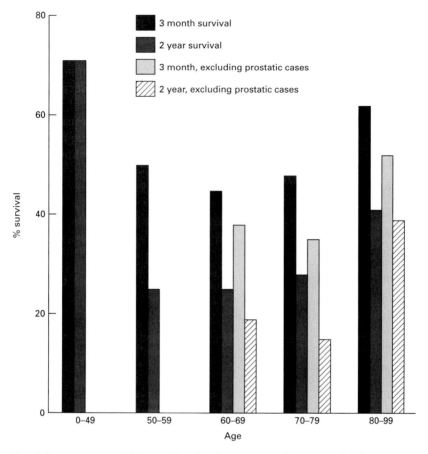

Fig. 4 Severe acute renal failure with and without prostate disease – survival by age.

especially cardiovascular disease. The older, more rigid vascular system is very sensitive to fluid changes seen in haemodialysis, predisposing to hypotension during dialysis and hypertension between dialyses. Old ischaemic hearts lead to pulmonary oedema when fluid-overloaded. The old on dialysis are admitted to hospital more frequently than the young. Many of the elderly are unfit for major surgery and thus renal transplantation, and when the operation is performed there is a relatively high peritransplant mortality. Overall therefore they are more difficult and more expensive to treat than younger patients.

Actuarial survival of older patients may initially seem low. Recent European data give 1-year survival for those aged 65–74 when starting renal replacement therapy of 76%, and 5-year survival of 30% [7]. This compares with 81% and 45% respectively for those aged 55–64. A recent study of 50 patients over the age of 80 starting renal replacement therapy, representing 7.2% of a total programme, found a 1-year survival of 78%

and 2 years of 48% [24]. Any assessment of prognosis in this older age group must be judged against the life expectation of patients of a similar age without renal failure. A review of published data suggested that for the over-65s the mortality was less than three times the expected mortality for the age group, compared with at least 20 times the expected mortality for those starting dialysis at age 45 [25]. In all of these studies there will have been some selection of patients for therapy with rejection of some of the most high-risk patients, but they do indicate that when applied appropriately, renal replacement therapy can be effective for elderly patients, even those above the age of 80.

In the UK it has been traditionally held that continuous ambulatory peritoneal dialysis (CAPD) is the dialysis modality of choice for the elderly. There are many problems in dialysing the elderly which influence the choice of modality (Table 4).

With CAPD old patients are slow to learn, take longer to train, need more home support and have more readmissions [26]. The persistent presence of fluid in the abdomen leads to a high incidence of hernia development. Patients with diverticulitis may experience recurrent peritonitis with bowel organisms and will then have to cease this therapy. In addition a treatment self-administered alone at home often increases the social isolation of a group of people who are already lonely and often relatively immobile. As a result the treatment frequently fails.

With haemodialysis home treatment is not viable for the elderly. In addition, the old are intolerant of fluid change and experience frequent dialytic hypotension. With their fragile vessels there is an increased incidence of subdural and intracranial haemorrhage related to recurrent heparinization. There is frequent myocardial ischaemia and heart failure and many patients experience atrial fibrillation related to dialysis. Dialysis access is difficult to establish, leading to multiple admissions and operations [25]. Fluid accumulation between dialyses may lead to hypertension and pulmonary oedema, and the elderly will need dialysis three times weekly.

Despite these problems, with the recent more widespread use of bicarbonate dialysis, volume-controlled proportionating units and sodium

Table 4 Dialysis problems in the elderly.

HD	CAPD
Intolerant of fluid change	Slow to learn
Subdural/intracranial haematoma	Hernias
Dialysis, atrial fibrillation	Diverticulitis
Poor shunt flows	Social isolation
	Often fails

HD, Haemodialysis; CAPD, continuous ambulatory peritoneal dialysis.

profiling, many of the intradialytic complications have been alleviated and haemodialysis has become a more attractive treatment for older patients.

The dialysis modality used to treat elderly people in many European countries is illustrated in Fig. 5. In Europe as a whole, as illustrated by France and Germany, the huge majority of elderly patients are treated with hospital-based haemodialysis, much more so than younger patients. In the UK there is an unusually large number of elderly patients receiving CAPD, a treatment also favoured in this country for younger patients. The difference from the rest of Europe is much greater in the older age group. Even so, over half the elderly patients receiving dialysis in the UK are on unit-based haemodialysis. It would appear therefore that in practice unit-based haemodialysis is the method of choice for these patients. When CAPD was first introduced in the early 1980s it was inevitably the method of choice for elderly patients, who due to the limited dialysis resources were not being offered haemodialysis treatment at the time. As hospital haemodialysis facilities have increased it appears that the UK is following the European trend, and despite the fact that it is a relatively more expensive form of treatment, is offering unit-based haemodialysis to the majority of its elderly dialysands.

In Europe, with the exception of some Scandinavian countries (Fig. 5), relatively little renal transplantation is undertaken in patients over 65. Cardiovascular and other comorbidity excludes many such patients. There are, however, many reports of excellent 5-year survival in elderly transplantees, especially when compared with the expected life expectancy.

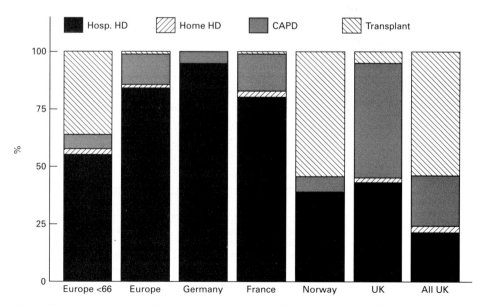

Fig. 5 Modalities of treatment by country and age. Hosp. HD, hospital haemodialysis; CAPD, continuous ambulatory peritoneal dialysis.

For those aged 65–75 the average European 5-year survival is 50% [27] but individual centres have reported better figures, with 5-year survival of up to 80% in the over 60s [28] and in Norway 5-year survival of 55% in those over 70 when transplanted — the same as the 55–70 age group [29]. Raw data from the USA show that transplantation of older patients on renal replacement therapy reduces the death rate compared with continued dialysis by more than threefold from 326 per 1000 to 97 per 1000 [30]. Other similar analyses have been made, but such figures are difficult to interpret as those transplanted are a selected group on the basis of fitness for operation.

Perioperative mortality in those over 65 receiving a kidney is at least five times higher than in young adults, largely due to cardiovascular disease which is also the major cause of later death in this group. There is also an increased incidence of postoperative bronchopneumonia and of later pulmonary embolism [31]. It is essential to undertake a comprehensive screening programme for older patients prior to transplantation in order to avoid this high cardiovascular mortality. Advanced peripheral and cerebrovascular disease are contra-indications to operations. Thorough investigation for myocardial ischaemia is essential. Some physicians recommend exercise testing where appropriate and echocardiography for all elderly patients entering the transplant waiting list. Where identified, significant coronary artery disease should be treated surgically prior to transplantation. Where there is severe myocardial dysfunction, transplantation should not be considered.

Older transplant recipients have a higher rate of infection than younger patients and a lower rate of graft rejection [32], presumably due to a degree of immune incompetence in the elderly. Immunosuppressive regimes must therefore be reduced in this group to avoid fatal infection.

Although transplantation may be successful in the elderly there is evidence that postoperative rehabilitation is very slow during the first postoperative year with relatively little gain in strength [33]. However, as with younger patients, the quality of life of elderly transplantees seems to be better than on dialysis [34].

There is therefore little doubt that when applied with appropriate selection, transplantation can be an effective treatment for older patients with renal failure. However, transplant kidneys are in short supply and the donor rate in most of Europe is slowly falling due to improvements in road traffic accident rates and treatment of cerebrovascular disease. Donor kidneys are thus a very valuable and scarce resource and questions have been raised as to whether giving such kidneys to older patients is justified [28]. Concomitant with the short supply has been an increasing proportion of older donors whose kidneys seem to survive for shorter periods when transplanted. A useful compromise when considering transplantation in the elderly would seem to be to try to age-match donors and recipients, giving the elderly patients the older kidneys.

Good studies of the quality of life of elderly patients receiving renal replacement therapy are difficult to find. A recent British study [34] of 616 adults being treated in 40 renal units showed that when patient selection was corrected for comorbidity and age there was no difference in quality of life between the various modalities of dialysis, but that in all age groups transplantation gave better quality of life. This study showed a good quality of life in elderly patients, perhaps because they are not frustrated by not being able to meet the extreme expectations of youth which dialysis inhibits.

Economic realities may force rationing of care. Despite the fact that older people are rather more difficult to treat with renal replacement therapy, and therefore rather more expensive to treat, the worldwide experience indicates that blanket withholding of such treatments on the grounds of age is not justified.

As more older patients are accepted for renal replacement therapy the issue of withdrawal of treatment, often at the patient's request, becomes more prominent. Treatment withdrawal is the reason for death in 7% of older European patients [7], is estimated at about 10% of all deaths in the USA, is the second commonest cause of death in Canada, and may account for more than 20% of deaths in American patients over 70 [35]. The issue is beset by many cultural and religious problems which may lead to underreporting, and may inhibit appropriate care and counselling. A 'good' death can be achieved with an appropriate multidisciplinary approach [35].

SUMMARY

Renal disease and failure, like everything else, is largely a problem of the elderly. There are many acute diseases of the elderly which are reversible when treated early, especially prostatic obstruction, acute interstitial nephritis and microscopic polyarteritis, rendering early diagnosis and treatment mandatory. The prognosis of older people with acute renal failure compares favourably with that of younger patients, and they deserve referral and renal support. British acceptance rates of old people for renal replacement therapy have risen progressively in the last 10 years, although the estimated need is not yet being met. The prognosis of renal replacement therapy for the elderly and the quality of life obtained are sufficiently good that patients in this age group must be referred for specialist opinion and possible treatment.

REFERENCES

1 Berlyne G. Editorial. *Nephron* 1982;**31**:189–190.

2 Wing AJ, Broyer M, Brunner FP *et al*. Combined report on regular dialysis and transplantation in Europe, XIII, 1982. *Proc EDTA* 1983;**20**:5–78.

3 Feest TG, Mistry CD, Grimes DS, Mallick NP. Incidence of advanced chronic renal failure and the need for end stage renal replacement treatment. *Br Med J* 1990;**301**:897–900.

4 McGeown MG. Prevalence of advanced renal failure in Northern Ireland. *Br Med J* 1990;**301**:900–903.

5 Feest TG, Round A, Hamad S. Incidence of severe acute renal failure in adults: results of a community based study. *Br Med J* 1993;**306**:481–483.

6 Roderick PJ, Jones I, Raleigh VS, McGeown MG, Mallick N. Population need for renal replacement therapy in Thames regions: ethnic dimension. *Br Med J* 1994;**309**:1111–1114.

7 Valderrabano F, Jones EHP, Mallick N. Report on management of renal failure in Europe, XXIV, 1993. *Nephrol Dial Transplant* 1995;**10**(suppl 5):1–25.

8 Oliver JR. Urinary system. In: *Cowdry's Problems of Aging*, edited by Lansing AI, Williams & Wilkins, Baltimore, 1952:631–650.

9 McManus JFA, Lupton CH. Ischemic obsolescence of renal glomeruli. *Lab Invest* 1960;**9**:413–434.

10 McLachlan MSF, Guthrie JC, Anderson CK, Fulker MJ. Vascular and glomerular changes in the ageing kidney. *J Pathol* 1977;**121**:65–77.

11 Moore RA. The total number of glomeruli in the normal human kidney. *Anat Rec* 1931;**48**:153–168.

12 Kampmann J, Siersbaek-Nielsen K, Kristensen M, Molholm Hansen J. Rapid evaluation of creatinine clearance. *Acta Med Scand* 1974;**196**:517–520.

13 Cockroft DW, Gault MH. Prediction of creatinine clearance from serum creatinine. *Nephron* 1976;**16**:31–41.

14 Zuccala A, Zucchelli P. Atherosclerotic renal artery stenosis — when is intervention by PTA or surgery justified? *Nephrol Dial Transplant* 1995;**10**:585–600.

15 Knowles HC Jr. Magnitude of the renal failure problem in diabetic patients. *Kidney Int* 1974;**6**:S2–S7.

16 Catalano C, Marshall SM. Epidemiology of end-stage renal disease in patients with diabetes mellitus: from the dark ages to the middle ages. *Nephrol Dial Transplant* 1992;7:181–190.

17 Friedman EA. Diabetes with kidney failure (letter). *Lancet* 1986;**ii**:1285.

18 Gaskin G, Pusey CD. Systemic vasculitis. In: *Oxford Textbook of Clinical Nephrology*, edited by Cameron JS, Davison A, Grünfeld J, Kerr D, Ritz E, Oxford University Press, Oxford, 1992:612–636.

19 Heptinstall RH. Polyarteritis (periarteritis) nodosa, other forms of vasculitis, and rheumatoid arthritis. In: *The Pathology of the Kidney*, vol. 2, 3rd edn, edited by Heptinstall RH. Little, Brown, Boston, 1983:793–807.

20 Walteon EW. Giant-cell granuloma of the respiratory tract (Wegener's granulomatosis). *Br Med J* 1958;**2**:265–270.

21 Serra-Cardus A, Cameron JS. Renal vasculitis in the aged. In: *Renal Function and Disease in the Elderly*. Butterworths, London, 1987:321–347.

22 Murray BM, Raij L. Glomerular disease in the aged. In: *Renal Function and Disease in the Elderly*, edited by Nuñez J, Cameron JS, Butterworths, London, 1987:288–320.

23 Cameron JS. Membranous nephropathy and its treatment. *Nephrol Dial Transplant* 1992;S1:72–79.

24 Neves PL, Sousa A, Bernardo I *et al*. Chronic haemodialysis for very old patients. *Age Ageing* 1994;**23**:358–359.

25 Mignon F, Michel C, Mentre F, Viron B. Worldwide demographics and future trends of the management of renal failure in the elderly. *Kidney Int* 1993;**43**(suppl 41):S18–S26.

26 Nissenson AR. Chronic peritoneal dialysis in the elderly. *Geriatr Nephrol Urol* 1991;**1**:3–12.

27 Raine AEG, Margreiter R, Brunner FP *et al*. Report on management of renal failure in Europe XXII 1991. *Nephrol Dial Transplant* 1992;7(suppl 2):7–35.

28 Briggs JD. Should older patients receive transplants? *Nephrol Dial Transplant* 1995;**10**:18–19.

29 Albrechsten D, Leivestad T, Bentdal O *et al*. Kidney transplantation in patients older than 70 years of age. *Transplant Proc* 1995;**27**:986–988.

30 US Renal Data System. USRDS 1993 Annual Data Report. The National Institutes of Health, 1993.

31 Nyberg G, Nilsson B, Norden G, Kalrberg I. Outcome of transplantation to patients over the age of 60: a case-control study. *Nephrol Dial Transplant* 1995;**10**:83–86.

32 Cantarovich D, Baatard R, Baranger T *et al*. Cadaveric renal transplantation after 60 years of age: a single center experience. *Transplant Int* 1994;**7**:33–38.

33 Nyberg G, Hallste G, Norden G, Hadimeri H, Wramner L. Physical performance does not improve in elderly patients following successful kidney transplantation. *Nephrol Dial Transplant* 1995;**10**:86–90.

34 Gudex C. Health-related quality of life in endstage renal failure. *Qual Life Res* 1995;**4**:359–366.

35 Cohen LM, McCue JD, Germain M, Kjellstrand CM. Dialysis discontinuation. A 'good' death? *Arch Intern Med* 1995;**155**:42–47.

PART 7
IMMUNOLOGY

HLA and disease

ROBERT I. LECHLER

The observation that certain alleles of human leukocyte antigens (HLAs) were associated with susceptibility to a variety of diseases was made long before any clear understanding of the function of HLA molecules was acquired. The first reported association was between Hodgkin's lymphoma and a cross-reactive group of HLA-B antigens, B5, B15, B18 and B35 [1]. A short time later an association was described between HLA-A2 and acute lymphoblastic leukaemia. These particular associations have not proven to be consistently reproducible, but shortly afterwards the remarkable association between the rheumatological disorder, ankylosing spondylitis, and HLA-B27 was described [2,3]. These observations provided the impetus for further studies of HLA and disease associations; over the ensuing decade a large number of diseases have been shown to be associated with the possession of particular HLA types. Some of the major associations are summarized in Table 1.

STRUCTURE OF HLA MOLECULES

Solution of the three-dimensional structure of HLA-A2 in 1987 was a critical landmark in the modern discipline of immunology in that it shed considerable light on the process of antigen presentation [4,5]. The two membrane-proximal domains, the α_3 domain of the heavy chain, and the β_2-microglobulin light chain, were shown to fold into typical immunoglobulin-like domains. The two membrane-distal domains proved to have a unique structure that is elegantly tailored to their function. Each domain is composed of a floor of antiparallel strands of β-pleated sheet structure, and a section of α-helical sequence lying on top of the β-pleated sheet floor. This arrangement leads to the creation of a groove, flanked on either side by the α-helices, and supported by the floor. This groove represents the peptide-binding site of the major histocompatibility complex (MHC) molecule, and was noted to be entirely occupied, in the molecules in the crystals, with electron-dense material corresponding to bound peptide. One of the striking findings was that almost all the polymorphism between MHC alleles was located in the surfaces comprising

Table 1 Some examples of human leukocyte antigen (HLA)-associated diseases, classified according to their pathogenetic mechanism.

Group	Disease	HLA marker
No autoimmune aetiology	21-hydroxylase deficiency	Deletion of the 21-OH B gene, (Bw47)*
	Idiopathic haemochromatosis	A3
Autoimmune aetiology	Ankylosing spondylitis	B27
	Rheumatoid arthritis	DR4Dw4/14, DR1
	Coeliac disease	B8 DR3 DQw2
	Insulin-dependent diabetes mellitus	DR3,4 DQw7/8
	Multiple sclerosis (in Caucasians)	DRw15 DQw6
	Goodpasture's syndrome	DRw15 DQw6
Unknown aetiology	Narcolepsy	DRw15

* The 21-OH B deletion is in linkage disequilibrium with Bw47.

the peptide-binding and T-cell receptor-contacting regions of the molecule. Furthermore, a series of pockets were observed in the peptide-binding groove, into which the side chains of the amino acids of bound peptide were buried. The amino acids of the MHC molecule that line these pockets show considerable allele-specific variation. As a consequence, individual alleles of MHC molecules bind and display different arrays of peptides. This has subsequently been demonstrated directly by the characterization of bound peptides from a variety of different alleles. Several groups have extracted peptides from purified MHC molecules by acid elution, and subjected these peptides to microsequencing. This has highlighted the existence of allele-specific motifs in bound peptides. It has also been shown that almost all the peptides bound by MHC class I molecules are between eight and 10 amino acids in length [6]. This conservation of size reflects the fact that the peptide-binding groove of class I molecules is closed at both ends.

The three-dimensional structure of MHC class II molecules was solved a few years later, using the same technique [7]. The overall structure of the two classes of MHC molecule are remarkably similar, despite the fact that class two molecules have a different domain organization, in that both chains have two domains. The major difference between the two classes of molecule is that the peptide-binding groove of the class II molecule is more open-ended. Consistent with this finding, the peptides occupying class II molecules have been shown to be longer and more heterogeneous in size, ranging from 14 to 25 amino acids. As for class I molecules, class

II-bound peptides have allele-specific motifs, although these motifs are less conserved than for class I molecules [8].

FUNCTIONS OF MHC MOLECULES

MHC molecules play a central role in immune recognition of antigen, in that T-cells only recognize antigens in the form of peptides bound to self MHC molecules. This phenomenon is referred to as MHC restriction, and reflects the fact that T-cells have dual specificity both for the antigenic peptide, and for the self MHC molecule by which the peptide is displayed. The trimolecular complex involving T-cell receptor, MHC molecule, and bound peptide is illustrated schematically in Fig. 1. Accessory molecular and costimulatory interactions are also shown.

There is functional specialization between the two classes of MHC molecule, which was noted several years ago, before any insights were available to explain how this was achieved. It was first noted that cells pulsed with inactivated virus failed to be recognized by class I-restricted cytotoxic T-cells (CTL), but were effective stimulators of class II-restricted T-cells. CTL recognition by class I-restricted CD8+ T-cells required that the target cells were infected with live virus [9]. Subsequent experiments showed that the critical event was intracellular synthesis of antigen for class I-restricted recognition. It is now clear that the peptides are loaded on to class I molecules in the endoplasmic reticulum (ER) [10]. Peptides that are available at this site arise from cytosolic proteins that are degraded by proteasome complexes, and then actively transported into the ER by

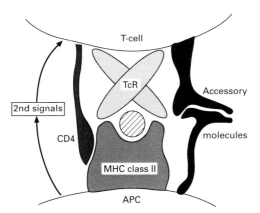

Fig. 1 Molecular interactions in T-cell activation. Signals required for triggering interleukin-2 (IL-2) release by T-cells. The molecular interactions involved in the activation of IL-2-secreting T-cells are shown. In addition to the specific interaction between the T-cell's receptor and its peptide major histocompatibility complex (MHC) ligand, and a variety of accessory molecule interactions, there is a requirement for receipt by the T-cell of second or costimulatory signals.

an adenosine triphosphate (ATP) dependent complex, known as the TAP (transporter associated with antigen processing) complex. MHC class II molecules, in contrast, are loaded with peptide in endosomal/lysosomal

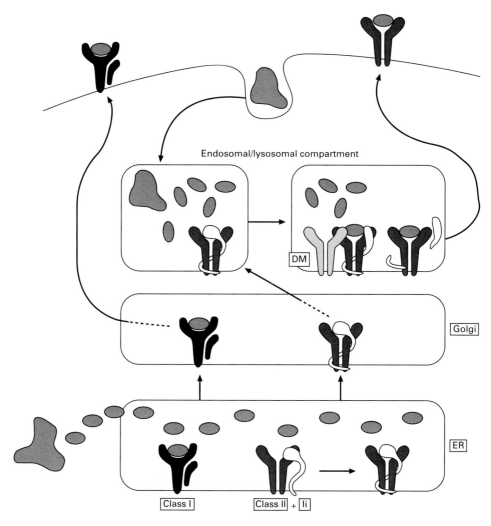

Fig. 2 The pathways of antigen presentation for major histocompatibility complex (MHC) class I and class II molecules are illustrated. Once inserted into the endoplasmic reticulum (ER), the class I heavy chain assembles with the β2-microglobulin light chain, and immediately binds peptide. The assembly of these three components allows the molecule to fold into its mature conformation. The class I molecule then traffics through the Golgi network, undergoes glycosylation and travels to the cell surface.

Class II molecules, once inserted into the ER associate with the invariant (Ii) chain; this inhibits peptide binding, and targets the class II molecule to endosomal/lysosomal compartments of the cell. Here, under low pH conditions, the Ii chain is cleaved from the class II molecule, and peptide binds. The human leukocyte antigen (HLA)-DM molecule is instrumental in facilitating the removal of the Ii chain and the loading of peptide.

compartments of the cell. Peptides that are available in these compartments are mostly derived from proteins that have been endocytosed from the cell surface, or from the extracellular space. The molecule that plays a key role in maintaining the distinction between these two pathways is a conserved protein that is coexpressed with class II molecules, called the invariant (Ii) chain. The dichotomy between the two classes of MHC molecule in antigen presentation and the manner in which this is influenced by the Ii chain are illustrated in Fig. 2. The Ii chain binds to class II molecules in the ER, and inhibits class II molecules from binding peptide at this site. In addition, the Ii chain targets the class II molecule to endosomal compartments, where it is proteolytically cleaved, thus allowing peptide to bind [11]. At least one other molecule is involved in facilitating class II peptide binding, namely the HLA-DM molecule. The mechanism of action of DM is not yet clear; however, in mutant cells that express class II and Ii molecules, the cell-surface class II molecules are almost entirely occupied by a single sequence of the Ii chain, known as the CLIP peptide. This indicates that DM serves in some way to liberate the class II molecule from the Ii chain, and facilitates the binding of peptides derived from endocytosed proteins [12].

The logic of this functional specialization is that the only cells that display viral peptides and act as targets for antiviral CTL are cells that are actually infected with virus. These, of course, are the only cells that need to be killed in order to eradicate a virus infection. MHC class II+ antigen-presenting cells that internalize inert viral proteins or particles will present viral peptides with class II molecules and stimulate CD4+ T-cells. There is no need to kill such cells.

GENETICS OF THE HLA REGION

The HLA complex spans some 4 million base pairs of DNA on the short arm of chromosome 6. It is the most densely populated region of the mammalian genome, containing in excess of 200 genes. Most of these are not genes that encode HLA molecules; the functions of some of these non-HLA genes are known, but many are currently of unknown function. The complex can be divided into class I, class II and class III regions. These are represented schematically in Fig. 3 [13]. The class I region carries the genes encoding the classical class I HLA molecules, HLA-A, -B and -C, together with many non-classical class I genes, whose functions are unknown. The class III region carries the genes encoding several complement components, heat shock proteins and tumour necrosis factor-α (TNF-α). There are numerous other genes in this region whose functions are currently undefined. The class II region includes the genes encoding the three major class II isotypes, and in addition, the genes encoding the TAP transporters, two components of the proteasome complex and the

(a)

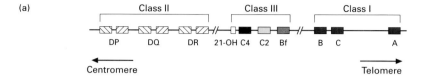

(b)

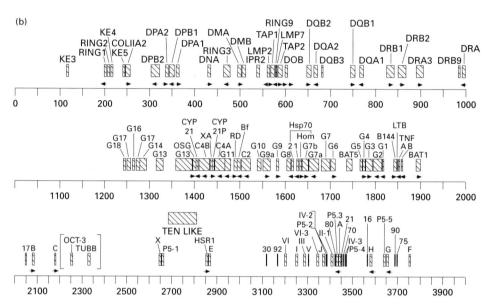

Fig. 3 (a) The arrangement of the three major regions of the human leukocyte antigen (HLA) region are shown; the distances between the loci are not to scale. (b) Map of the human major histocompatibility complex.

DM molecule. It is of interest that these genes, whose functions are so intimately related to the functions of the HLA molecules themselves, are located in the middle of the class II region.

LINKAGE DISEQUILIBRIUM

One of the striking features of the HLA complex is the tendency to inherit extended haplotypes *en bloc*. This is referred to as linkage disequilibrium. This phenomenon was established when it was noted that alleles of separate HLA class I and class II genes occurred together on the same haplotype with a frequency far greater than would have been predicted from the individual gene frequencies within the study population. Furthermore, there is considerable ethnic variation in the haplotypes that are over-represented within populations. For example, in northern European caucasoids, approximately 10% of the population carry the A1 B8 DR17 haplotype, whereas in American Indians this haplotype is only present in 3.7%, but the A2 B35 DR4 haplotype is present in almost 15%. Several explanations can be offered to account for these observations, but the most plausible one is that these combinations of HLA alleles conferred selective advantage on individual ethnic groups in combating particular pathogens at some point in human history.

Linkage disequilibrium is of particular importance in the context of HLA and disease studies, because it means that caution must be exercised in the interpretation of an association between an HLA allele and a disease. It cannot be assumed that the disease-associated allele is necessarily the HLA-encoded susceptibility factor; the possibility must be borne in mind that the true susceptibility gene is in linkage disequilibrium with the HLA allele that has been typed for. This point is well-illustrated by the fact that the early HLA and disease associations were with HLA class I alleles, because they were the only alleles that could be typed for at the time. Once class II typing techniques were established, it became clear, in almost all cases, that stronger associations existed between class II alleles and the disease in question. Given the profusion of genes in the HLA complex, it remains possible that, in some diseases, the susceptibility locus is a non-HLA gene in close linkage with the defined HLA allele.

MECHANISMS OF HLA AND DISEASE ASSOCIATIONS

Before contemplating the question of mechanisms, it is helpful to divide HLA-associated diseases according to their pathogenesis. Some of these diseases have an aetiology that appears to have nothing to do with immune recognition. Two outstanding examples of this category are haemochromatosis and narcolepsy. It is almost certain that the first of these examples, which is closely associated with HLA-A3, reflects linkage with a gene whose product is involved in iron metabolism. Narcolepsy is more of a mystery. Until the pathogenesis of this condition is better understood, the significance of the strong association with HLA DR15 is a matter of speculation. All that can be said at present is that there is no known mechanism whereby MHC class II molecules influence sleep patterns.

A second category of HLA-associated diseases are immune complex-mediated. A major example is provided by systemic lupus erythematosus (SLE). SLE is associated with the HLA A1 B8 DR17 haplotype; it has been argued that this reflects the fact that this haplotype carries null (non-functional) genes for one of the C4 proteins of the classical pathway of the complement cascade [14]. Given the importance of C4 in maintaining the solubility of immune complexes, one explanation for this association is that the susceptibility factor is the null C4 gene. Although this remains a point of debate, it provides another illustration of the possibility that associations between diseases and HLA class I and II alleles may have other explanations.

The third, and major, category of HLA-associated diseases are auto-immune in origin. Typical examples in this category are rheumatoid arthritis, myasthenia gravis, multiple sclerosis and Goodpasture's syndrome. These diseases are almost invariably associated with HLA class II alleles. The pathogenesis of these diseases almost certainly involves autoimmune reactions that are triggered by a breakdown in T-cell tolerance to self, and it is difficult to resist the suggestion that the HLA class II association reflects the function of HLA class II molecules in the presentation of peptide to T-cells. Rheumatoid arthritis (RA) is of particular interest in that it is associated with more than one HLA-DR type. The commonest association is with the broad serologically defined specificity HLA-DR4, but there is also an association with HLA-DR1. It is now known that there are 14 DR4 subtypes which are referred to as DRB1*0401 to DRB1*0414. These subtypes share sequence identity in the floor of the peptide-binding groove, but differ by a small number of amino acids in the α-helical sequence of the β1 domain. Several of the DR4 subtypes are associated with RA; the ones that are not differ at amino acid positions that are known to be highly influential in T-cell recognition, namely positions 67, 70, 71 and 74 [15]. Furthermore, of the DR1 subtypes, only DRB1*0101 is associated with RA [16]. This DR type is almost identical to the RA-associated DR4 subtypes in the α-helical region of the β1 domain. The conservation of sequence in this influential portion of the DR molecule amongst the DR types that are associated with RA argues strongly that it is the DR molecule itself, rather than anything that is in linkage disequilibrium with it, that confers susceptibility for this disease.

Further insights into the precise mechanisms underlying HLA and disease associations will require the identification of the relevant auto-antigens, and the availability of disease-inducing T-cell clones in order to determine whether mechanisms such as the preferential binding of autoantigenic peptide account for these phenomena.

REFERENCES

1 Amiel JL. Study of the leukocyte phenotypes in Hodgkin's Disease. In: *Histocompatibility Testing*, edited by Curtoni ES, Mattiuz PL, Tosi RM. Munksgaard, Copenhagen, 1967:79–81.
2 Brewerton DA, Caffrey M, Hart FD *et al.* Ankylosing spondylitis and HL-A27. *Lancet* 1973;**1**:904–907.
3 Schlosstein L, Terasaki PI, Bluestone J *et al.* High association of a HLA-A antigen, w27, with ankylosing spondylitis. *N Engl J Med* 1973;**288**:704–706.
4 Bjorkman PJ, Saper MA, Samraoui B *et al.* The foreign antigen binding site and T cell recognition regions of class I histocompatibility antigens. *Nature* 1987;**329**:512–518.
5 Bjorkman PJ, Saper MA, Samraoui B *et al.* Structure of the human class I histocompatibility antigen, HLA-A2. *Nature* 1987;**329**:506–512.
6 Rotzke O, Falk K. Naturally occurring peptide antigens derived from the MHC class I-restricted processing pathway. *Immunol Today* 1991;**12**:447–455.

7 Brown JH, Jardetzky T, Gorger JC *et al.* Three-dimensional structure of the human class II histocompatibility antigen. *Nature* 1993;**364**:33–39.

8 Chicz RM, Urban RG, Lane WS *et al.* Predominant naturally processed peptides bound to HLA-DR1 are derived from MHC-related molecules and are heterogenous in size. *Nature* 1992;**358**:764–768.

9 Morrison LA, Lukacher AE, Braciale VL *et al.* Differences in antigen presentation to MHC class I and class II-restricted influenza virus-specific cytolytic T lymphocyte clones. *J Exp Med* 1986;**163**:903–921.

10 Townsend A, Ohlen C, Bastin J *et al.* Association of class I major histocompatibility heavy and light chains induced by viral peptides. *Nature* 1989;**340**:443–448.

11 Teyton L, O'Sullivan D, Dickson PW *et al.* Invariant chain distinguishes between the exogenous and endogenous antigen presentation pathways. *Nature* 1990;**348**:39–45.

12 Sanderson F, Kleijmeer MJ, Kelly A *et al.* Accumulation of HLA-DM, a regulator of antigen presentation, in MHC-class II compartments. *Science* 1994;**266**:1566–1568.

13 Trowsdale J, Campbell RG. Map of the human MHC. *Immunol Today* 1993;**14**:349–352.

14 Fielder AHL, Walport MJ, Batchelor JR *et al.* Family study of the major histocompatibility complex in patients with systemic lupus erythematosus: importance of null alleles of C4A and C4B in determining disease susceptibility. *Br Med J* 1983;**286**:425–428.

15 Nepom GT, Byers P, Seyfried *et al.* HLA genes associated with rheumatoid arthritis. Identification of susceptibility alleles using specific oligonucleotide probes. *Arthritis Rheum* 1989;**32**:15–21.

16 Goronzy J, Weyand CM, Fathman CG. Shared T cell recognition sites on human histocompatibility leukocyte antigen class II molecules of patients with seropositive rheumatoid arthritis. *J Clin Invest* 1986;**77**:1042–1049.

MULTIPLE CHOICE QUESTIONS

1 The following statements concerning major histocompatibility complex (MHC) molecules are correct

a CD8 T cells recognize antigens with MHC class I molecules

b MHC class II molecules predominantly present peptides derived from intracellular proteins

c MHC molecules preferentially bind peptides from foreign, rather than self, proteins

d MHC class I and II molecules have a very similar structure

e cell-surface MHC molecules are almost entirely occupied with self peptides

2 The HLA region

a is located on the short arm of chromosome 16

b occupies almost 1 megabase of DNA

c contains 2–300 genes

d contains many genes encoding for non-HLA molecules

e is characterized by linkage disequilibrium

3 As regards HLA and disease associations

a they mostly involve autoimmune diseases

b most associations are with HLA class II alleles

c identification of the true HLA-linked susceptibility gene may be confounded by linkage disequilibrium
d account for genetic susceptibility in monogenic disorders
e the pattern of HLA and disease associations can vary in different ethnic groups

Answers

1		2		3	
a	True	**a**	False	**a**	True
b	False	**b**	False	**b**	True
c	False	**c**	True	**c**	True
d	True	**d**	True	**d**	False
e	True	**e**	True	**e**	True

Homoeostatic regulatory mechanisms in rheumatoid arthritis synovium: interleukin-10 is the major anti-inflammatory cytokine

MARC FELDMANN, FIONULA M. BRENNAN,
MARITA WALMSLEY, SHARA B. A. COHEN,
PETER KATSIKIS & R. N. MAINI

SUMMARY

In recent years, it has been clearly documented that the rheumatoid synovium synthesizes a number of proinflammatory mediators, including the cytokines tumour necrosis factor-α (TNF-α) interleukin-1 (IL-1), IL-6, IL-8 and granulocyte-macrophage colony-stimulating factor (GM-CSF). These proinflammatory cytokines are linked in a network or cascade, and neutralization of TNF-α also leads to diminished production of the others listed above. Based on these observations, the concept was generated that blocking TNF-α would be sufficient to ameliorate the disease process. This prediction has been successfully tested *in vivo* in animal models and clinical trials, and TNF-α is thus now a recognized therapeutic target. The same experimental approach has been used to explore the expression of anti-inflammatory cytokines, and to evaluate whether these may be useful as therapeutic agents. We found that transforming growth factor-β (TGF-β) and IL-10 were highly expressed; and even after many years into the disease process, neutralizing IL-10 *in vitro*, in rheumatoid joint cultures yielded two to three times more IL-1 and TNF-α within 24 hours. These results established IL-10 as an important endogenous regulator. Adding IL-10 to these rheumatoid joint cell cultures diminished IL-1 and TNF-α production, and injecting mice with collagen induced arthritis, after disease onset ameliorated the inflammation. Thus, our work suggests that IL-10 is a potential therapeutic candidate in rheumatoid arthritis (RA), and clinical trials to test this hypothesis are warranted.

INTRODUCTION

In all biological systems, knowledge of agonists precedes that of antagonists, as understanding or assaying the latter depends on knowledge of the former. This also applies to cytokines and their regulation. Thus, it is not surprising that, while it is now well-accepted that the rheumatoid synovium synthesizes abundant proinflammatory cytokines, including (IL-1), TNF-α, IL-6, IL-8 and GM-CSF, much less is known concerning the

343

production and relative importance of various anti-inflammatory cytokines. The current list of cytokines with mostly inhibitory activity includes TGF-β, IL-4, IL-10 and IL-13. However, it is likely that more will be found, and many cytokines are agonists for some actions, but inhibitory for others, e.g. interferon-γ (IFN-γ).

Many studies of cytokine physiology have been performed *in vitro*, with limitless quantities of recombinant cytokine, and with homogeneous target cells. These studies are useful to reveal the potential properties of cytokines, but it is not clear from such studies which of these properties really matters in the complexities of inflammatory disease lesions, for example the RA joint. In this situation, the cells are heterogeneous, and there are many cytokines competing for attention, as well as serum and cell-derived inhibitors. Thus we have for many years studied the cytokine expression and regulation of the cells dissociated by collagenase from RA synovium. From this work we showed that the proinflammatory cytokines were highly expressed, and organized in a hierarchy. Thus, blocking the pivotal cytokine TNF-α was sufficient significantly to down-regulate IL-1, GM-CSF, IL-6 and IL-8 [1–3]. This provided much of the rationale for the testing of anti-TNF-α monoclonal antibody in long-standing RA patients, as described in detail by Maini *et al.* ([4,5]; see p. 53).

The same experimental approach has been used to study the expression of the chiefly anti-inflammatory cytokines IL-4, TGF-β and IL-10. We and others have not been able to detect IL-4 and, as this is produced in other joint diseases, such as reactive arthritis [6] it is possible that a lack of IL-4 is of importance in the pathogenesis of RA. In contrast, TGF-β and IL-10 were both abundantly produced [7,8].

TGF-β is a family of molecules (TGF-β_{1-3} in humans) widely expressed in the body, which tend to inhibit the function of haemopoietic and blood-borne cells — thus, haemopoiesis, immunity and inflammation can all be down-regulated by TGF-β. However TGF-β augments the function of connective tissue cells. In RA tissue, abundant TGF-β, both β_1 and β_2 isoforms, is produced [7]. The levels of bioactive TGF-β is less in RA than in monoarthritis (Table 1), and it was thus possible that a relative lack of TGF-β may be of importance in the pathogenesis of RA. This was tested by adding exogenous recombinant TGF-β to RA synovial cells, but there was no diminution of TNF-α (Fig. 1) or IL-1 synthesis. Thus, while it is likely that TGF-β is part of the homeostatic regulation, it is not a therapeutic candidate, as adding more *in vitro* was without effect.

Interleukin-10 inhibits macrophage production of IL-1, TNF-α, IL-6, IL-8, GM-CSF, and also inhibits T-cell proliferation [9]. These properties suggested that it may be of importance in RA homeostasis and prompted our studies of its expression in RA joints. The levels produced by RA synovium are clearly in the active range (0.5–5 ng/ml per 24 hours; Fig. 2). Neutralizing monoclonal antibodies to IL-10 up-regulated IL-1

Table 1 Synovial fluid transforming growth factor-β (TGF-β) in arthritis.

Disease	TGF-β (ng/ml)		Acid-activated
	Untreated		
Rheumatoid arthritis	2.6		45
	0.5		26
	0.6	Mean = 1.83 ng/ml	27
	2.2		20
	3.0		46
	2.1		3
Monoarthritis	10.0		13
Monoarthritis	21.0		13
Monoarthritis	2.0		15
Gout	15.0	Mean = 11 ng/ml	30
Psoriatic arthritis	1.5		8
Polyarthritis	9.0		28

Synovial fluid samples from patients with rheumatoid arthritis (RA) and non-RA arthropathies were tested for TGF-β activity using the radioreceptor-binding assay. Active TGF-β was detected in treated samples: latent TGF-β was rendered active by acid activation. Reproduced with permission from [7].

and TNF-α production on the dissociated RA synovial cultures by two- to threefold within 24 hours. Addition of IL-10 halved the IL-1 and TNF production (Fig. 3a [8]). This demonstrates that, while IL-10 is part of the homeostatic regulatory process, and is also a potential candidate therapeutic agent, additional IL-10 was as effective *in vitro*.

Analogous experiments were performed, analysing the effect of IL-10 and anti IL-10 on the production of IL-6 and IL-8 in the RA synovial cultures. The results show that IL-8 production was also regulated by IL-10, but not that of IL-6 (Fig. 3b). This could be because a large part of the IL-6 produced in these cultures is by the fibroblast, which are not inhibited by IL-10. We have thus become interested in the properties of IL-10 which are of possible relevance to the arthritic process. Of interest is the effect of IL-10 on TNF receptor expression — IL-10 inhibits p55 and p75 TNF receptor expression on the membrane of monocytic cells, but it also up-regulates the production of the TNF inhibitor, the soluble TNF receptor (TNF-R) [10]. This is in contrast to IL-4 and TGF-β, both of which also down-regulate membrane TNF-R expression, but unlike IL-10 diminish soluble TNF-R production. As the soluble form of TNF-R is derived from the membrane form by proteolytic cleavage, the results suggest that IL-10 up-regulates the cleavage process. The effects on membrane and soluble TNF-R should, in theory, add to the anti-inflammatory effect of reduced proinflammatory cytokine production.

During our studies of IL-10 expression in RA, we verified that the IL-10 detected in RA synovial cultures was a reflection of synthesis *in vivo*. It

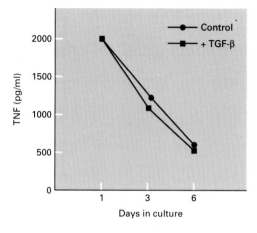

Fig. 1 Dissociated synovial membrane cells were cultured with/without 10 ng/ml transforming growth factor-β$_1$ (TGF-β$_1$). Supernatants were harvested after 24 hours and assayed for tumour necrosis factor-α (TNF-α) by enzyme-linked immunosorbent assay. Reproduced with permission from [7].

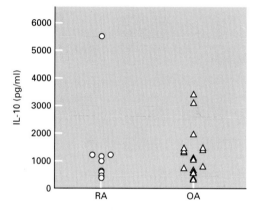

Fig. 2 Interleukin-10 (IL-10) protein is expressed in rheumatoid arthritis (RA) and osteoarthritis (OA) synovial membranes. IL-10 is produced spontaneously by RA ($n = 11$) and OA ($n = 17$) synovial membrane cultures cultured for 24 hours and supernatants assayed for IL-10 by enzyme-linked immunosorbent assay at 24 hours. Reproduced with permission from [8].

is possible that dissociation of cells by collagenase may induce cytokine synthesis, and to exclude this, small pieces of synovium were snap-frozen in liquid nitrogen for immunohistology and other pieces dissolved in guanadinium chloride for analysis of messenger RNA expression by reverse transcription polymerase chain reaction (rt-PCR), using IL-10-specific primers. By rt-PCR, IL-10 messenger RNA was found in all RA synovial preparations. Immunohistology confirmed the IL-10 expression *in vivo* and also yielded interesting results. By distribution and double staining it looked as if most IL-10 was produced by macrophages (CD68-expressing cells), but some IL-10 was also produced in the T-cell-rich perivascular clusters. Double staining with anti-CD3 demonstrated that about 1.5% of the T-cells immunostained for IL-10, indicating that some of the IL-10 produced in synovium was produced by T-cells [8,11].

This led us to investigate the IL-10 production by T-cells extracted from the rheumatoid synovium. Initially we have looked at the *in vivo*-activated (IL-2 receptor-expressing cells) T-cells and have cloned these in the absence of antigen, using IL-2 and anti-CD3. Even 8 or more weeks

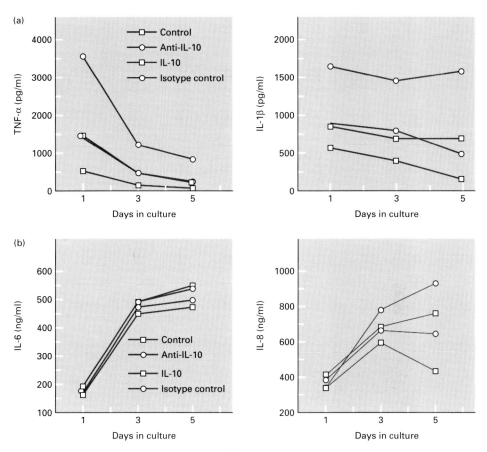

Fig. 3 Rheumatoid arthritis (RA) synovial membrane cultures: effect of neutralizing endogenously produced interleukin-10 (IL-10) and of the addition of exogenous IL-10. Representative experiment showing (a) tumour necrosis factor-α (TNF-α), IL-1β, (b) IL-6 and IL-8 levels produced by RA synovial membrane culture SM1376. Synovial membrane culture was treated with neutralizing rat monoclonal anti-IL-10 antibody 9D7 (2 μg/ml), isotype-matched control rat monoclonal GL113 or 10 ng/ml of recombinant IL-10 for 24, 72 and 120 hours. Reproduced with permission from [8].

after cloning, a large fraction of these cells produced very large amounts of IL-10 (> 7 ng/ml per $24 \, h/10^6$ cells) after restimulation (Fig. 4). In contrast, T-cells cloned from the same patient's blood did not contain the subset producing large amounts of IL-10, suggesting that these cells are specifically recruited, induced or expanded in the RA synovium [11].

ROLE OF IL-10 (AND OTHER IMMUNOREGULATORS) IN THE PATHOGENESIS OF RHEUMATOID ARTHRITIS

RA has a strong genetic association with HLA-DR4 and DR1, the DR4 subtypes expressing the amino acids abbreviated QRR AA at positions

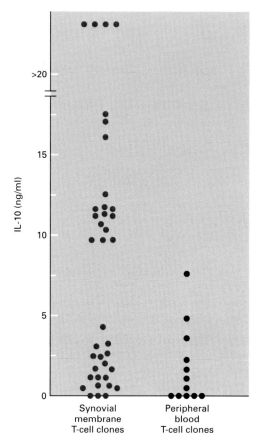

Fig. 4 Cells were stimulated with 10 ng/ml phorbol-12-myristate-13-acetate and 1 μg/ml soluble OKT3. Interleukin-10 (IL-10) was assayed by enzyme-linked immunosorbent assay. Clones derived from the synovium of chronic rheumatoid arthritis were compared with clones derived from the autologous peripheral blood lymphocytes.

70–74 of the DRβ chain. This strongly implies a role of T-cells in the development of the disease, as the only known function of the HLA-DR molecule is peptide presentation to thymocytes and T-cells. However, in long-standing and active RA T-cell responses *in vitro* or on skin test to recall antigens (tet toxoid, purified protein derivative of mycobacterium tuberculosis (PPD), streptokinase streptodornase (SKSD)) are often diminished [12] and in the rheumatoid joint, T-cell activity seems to be down-regulated, as judged by the lack of T-cell blasts and low levels of T-cell-derived cytokine expression. This has led some workers to question the role of lymphocytes in late RA [13].

We think that the down-regulated T-cell activity in late RA is not an indication that these cells are not involved but rather that their activity is depressed by the presence of active quantities of IL-10 and perhaps TGF-β. Evidence to support this was obtained by adding anti-IL-10 to RA synovial cultures: in 2 of 7 samples IFN-γ production reached high levels within 24 hours. This suggests to us that activated T-cells are still present, but inhibited by cytokine and perhaps other inhibitors in the rheumatoid joint.

IS IL-10 A POTENTIAL THERAPY IN RHEUMATOID ARTHRITIS?

Based on the above considerations, it seems that IL-10 may be useful in the therapy of RA. Accordingly, we have investigated its use in the collagen-induced model of arthritis in DBA/1 mice, in which blocking TNF after onset of arthritis is beneficial [14]. Injecting IL-10 after onset of arthritis was beneficial. The degree of benefit depended on dose, with high dosage inhibiting joint inflammation as effectively as anti-TNF [15].

Not all the effects of IL-10 are likely to be beneficial in RA. IL-10 has some chemotactic activity, especially for natural killer and CD8+ T-cells [16]. But the most detrimental effect may be on B lymphocytes. IL-10 is involved in B-cell proliferation and is a strong stimulus for immunoglobulin production [16]. It is thus possible that rheumatoid factor and immune complex levels may be augmented, and this may be deleterious. There are reports that IL-10 may precipitate the onset of systemic lupus in susceptible mouse strains [17] and this may also occur in RA patients, as discussed previously [18].

Thus, depending on toxicology and the safety of injecting recombinant IL-10 in appropriate concentrations, it is a promising therapeutic candidate. In view of it being a major endogenous regulator in diseases such as RA, adding a little more should be safe, and may conceivably tip the balance back to the equilibrium found in health. Figure 5 shows the balance between proinflammatory and anti-inflammatory cytokines.

Since the manuscript was written, clinical trials of IL-10 in rheumatoid arthritis have been initiated. We await the results with interest.

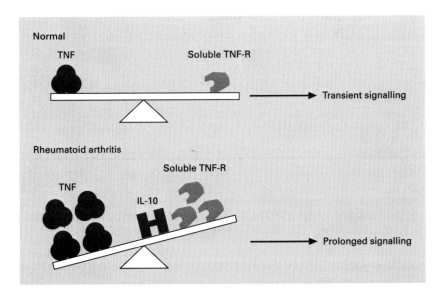

Fig. 5 Tumour necrosis factor (TNF) and its inhibitors in disease.

REFERENCES

1 Brennan FM, Chantry D, Jackson A, Maini R, Feldmann M. Inhibitory effect of TNFα antibodies on synovial cell interleukin-1 production in rheumatoid arthritis. *Lancet* 1989;2:244–247.

2 Haworth C, Brennan FM, Chantry D, Turner M, Maini RN, Feldmann M. Expression of granulocyte-macrophage colony-stimulating factor in rheumatoid arthritis: regulation by tumor necrosis factor-α. *Eur J Immunol* 1991;21:2575–2579.

3 Butler D, Maini RN, Feldmann M, Brennan FM. Modulation of proinflammatory cytokine release in rheumatoid synovial membrane cell cultures with an anti TNFα monoclonal: comparison with blockade of IL-1 using the recombinant IL-1 receptor antagonist. *Eur Cyt Network* 1996;6:225–230.

4 Elliott MJ, Maini RN, Feldmann M *et al.* Treatment of rheumatoid arthritis with chimeric monoclonal antibodies to TNFα. *Arthritis Rheum* 1993;36:1681–1690.

5 Elliott MJ, Maini RN, Feldmann M *et al.* Randomised double blind comparison of a chimaeric monoclonal antibody to tumour necrosis factor α (cA2) versus placebo in rheumatoid arthritis. *Lancet* 1994;344:1105–1110.

6 Simon AK, Seipelt E, Sieper J. Divergent T-cell cytokine patterns in inflammatory arthritis. *Proc Natl Acad Sci USA* 1994;91:8562–8566.

7 Brennan FM, Chantry D, Turner M, Foxwell B, Maini RN, Feldmann M. Transforming growth factor-β in rheumatoid arthritis synovial tissue: lack of effect on spontaneous cytokine production in joint cell cultures. *Clin Exp Immunol* 1990;81:278–285.

8 Katsikis P, Chu CQ, Brennan FM, Maini RN, Feldmann M. Immunoregulatory role of interleukin 10 (IL-10) in rheumatoid arthritis. *J Exp Med* 1994;179:1517–1527.

9 de Waal Malefyt R, Haanen J, Spits H *et al.* Interleukin 10 (IL-10) and viral IL-10 strongly reduce antigen-specific human T cell proliferation by diminishing the antigen-presenting capacity of monocytes via downregulation of class II major histocompatibility complex expression. *J Exp Med* 1991;174:915–924.

10 Joyce DA, Gibbons D, Green P, Feldmann M, Brennan FM. Two inhibitors of pro-inflammatory cytokine release, IL-10 and IL-4, have contrasting effects on release of soluble p75 TNF receptor by cultured monocytes. *Eur J Immunol* 1994;24:2699–2705.

11 Cohen SBA, Katsikis PD, Chu CQ *et al.* High IL-10 production by the activated T cell population within the rheumatoid synovial membrane. *Arthritis Rheum* 1995;38:946–952.

12 Silverman HA, Johnson JS, Vaughan JH, McGlamory JC. Altered lymphocyte reactivity in rheumatoid arthritis. *Arthritis Rheum* 1976;19:509–515.

13 Firestein GS, Zvaifler NJ. How important are T cells in chronic rheumatoid synovitis? *Arthritis Rheum* 1990;33:768–773.

14 Williams RO, Feldmann M, Maini RN. Anti-tumor necrosis factor ameliorates joint disease in murine collagen-induced arthritis. *Proc Natl Acad Sci USA* 1992;89:9784–9788.

15 Walmsley M, Katsikis PD, Abrey E, Parry S, Williams R, Maini RN, Feldmann M. IL-10 inhibits progression of established collagen induced arthritis. *Arthritis Rheum* 1996;39:495–503.

16 Moore KW, O'Garra A, de Waal Malefyt R, Vieira P, Mosmann TR. Interleukin-10. *Annu Rev Immunol* 1993;11:165.

17 Ishida H, Muchamuel T, Sakaguchi S, Andrade S, Menon S, Howard M. Continuous administration of anti-interleukin 10 antibodies delays onset of autoimmunity in NZB/W F$_1$ mice. *J Exp Med* 1994;179:305.

18 Maini RN, Elliott MJ, Charles PJ, Feldmann M. Immunological intervention reveals reciprocal roles for TNFα and IL-10 in rheumatoid arthritis and SLE. *Springer Semin Immunopathol* 1994;16:327–336.

MULTIPLE CHOICE QUESTIONS

1 Rheumatoid arthritis.
  a is more common in women
  b affects joints asymmetrically
  c has a genetic predisposition
  d responds poorly to therapy
  e is associated with increased mortality

2 Interleukin-10
  a stimulates T-cells
  b is produced by T-cells, not by macrophages
  c stimulates B-cells
  d is involved in homeostasis in rheumatoid arthritis
  e is closely related to transforming growth factor-β

3 Cytokines
  a are protein mediators
  b are carried in the blood
  c are locally active
  d are neutralized by soluble receptors found in body fluids
  e are not made by epithelial cells

Answers

1		2		3	
a	True	**a**	False	**a**	True
b	False	**b**	False	**b**	False
c	True	**c**	True	**c**	True
d	True	**d**	True	**d**	True
e	True	**e**	False	**e**	False

Treating allergy — any progress?

ROBYN E. O'HEHIR

In genetically predisposed individuals, exposure to common environmental aeroallergens results in a cascade of physiopathological events that lead to the aberrant production of specific immunoglobulin E (IgE), which is the main specific effector molecule of the allergic immune response ([1]; Fig. 1). Approximately 40% of the population produce IgE in this way — the atopic population — and approximately one-third of these people suffer from one or more of the common allergic diseases, including extrinsic asthma, rhinitis and atopic dermatitis. Despite widespread clinical use of allergen immunotherapy for hyposensitization in pollen, house dust mite (HDM) and insect venom allergy, a systematic approach to the development of immunotherapy has been lacking due to limited understanding of the immunological principles that govern allergic inflammation and the down-regulation of these responses. Different hypotheses are proposed to explain the observed effectiveness of immunotherapy, including increased membrane stability of mediator-releasing cells, decreased IgE antibody levels, increased competitive IgG antibodies, decreased lymphocyte reactivity, the generation of suppressor T-cells and the induction of anti-idiotypic networks [2].

Our knowledge of the allergic immune response has increased greatly over the last decade and it is now clearly recognized that the CD4+ T lymphocyte plays a central role in the initiation and regulation of allergic inflammation [1]. Moreover, effective immunotherapy may be achieved at a practical level by mimicking the mechanisms of T-cell non-responsiveness that occur *in vivo* to prevent autoimmune disease. These mechanisms include clonal deletion (physical elimination) of specific cells from the T-cell repertoire or clonal anergy (antigen-specific non-responsiveness). Anergy is defined immunologically as the inability of antigen-specific T-cells to respond to subsequent specific antigen stimulation following an anergic stimulus.

Clonal deletion normally occurs in the neonatal thymus when the self-reactive thymocytes are physically removed during the maturation of T-cells. In contrast, clonal anergy occurs in the peripheral, mature T-cell compartment. First, in normal development, autoreactive T-cells are

352

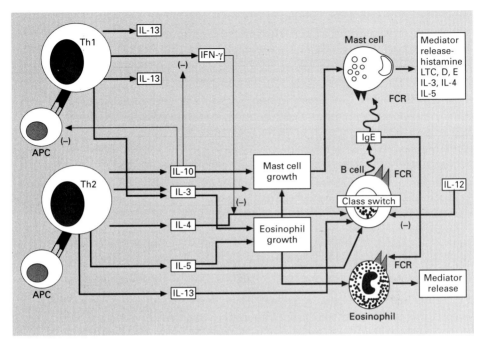

Fig. 1 The cellular interactions of the allergic immune response, with the CD4+ T lymphocyte occupying a pivotal position.

functionally but not physically removed from the repertoire and, second, anergy may be induced in mature T-cells that have already survived thymic deletion. The ability to render selected subsets of peripheral T-cells from atopic individuals anergic to rechallenge with specific allergen may help control allergic disease or, ideally, prevent its development prior to sensitization in predisposed individuals.

T-LYMPHOCYTE SUBSETS: TH1 AND TH2

Two distinct functional subsets of CD4+ T cells, designated Th1 and Th2, have been identified in the peripheral T-cell compartment of the mouse [3]. Although the clear polarity of function described in the mouse is not observed in human T-cells, there is a tendency for their cytokine secretion to favour a Th1-like or Th2-like pattern [4]. Each subset is characterized by the profile of cytokines released; Th1 cells secrete interleukin-2 (IL-2), IL-3, interferon-gamma (IFN-γ), tumour necrosis factor-α (TNF-α), TNF-β and granulocyte-macrophage colony-stimulating factor (GM-CSF), whilst Th2 cells secrete predominantly IL-3, IL-4, IL-5, IL-6 and IL-10 [5]. In addition to the varied effects of Th2-derived cytokines on the non-specific effector cells of the allergic immune response, IL-4 is primarily responsible for regulating the IgG to IgE isotype switch [6]. Cytokines derived from Th1 cells also influence eosinophils and indirectly modulate B-cell function but of major importance is the ability of IFN-γ to antagonize IL-4 and so prevent IgE production [7,8]. The response to allergens, in atopic individuals, is dominated by CD4+ T-cells that produce IL-4 and IL-5 [9–11] whereas, in non-atopic individuals, the cytokines IFN-γ and IL-2 are predominantly secreted, therefore the Th2 functional subset is an obvious target for manipulation. However, the lack of a distinct dichotomy of cytokine production by human CD4+ T-cells offers the opportunity for preferential induction of a particular cytokine and redirection of the immune response. The preferential secretion of IFN-γ rather than IL-4 favours redirection of the immune response towards IgG production and away from IgE production.

MODULATION OF IMMUNE RESPONSIVENESS

Activation of CD4+ T-cells requires the interactions of allergen in peptide form presented in association with major histocompatibility complex (MHC) class II molecules on the surface of an antigen-presenting cell (APC) to the specific T-cell antigen–receptor complex (TcR/CD3; Fig. 2; [12]). In addition, costimulatory signals are required, including engagement of the

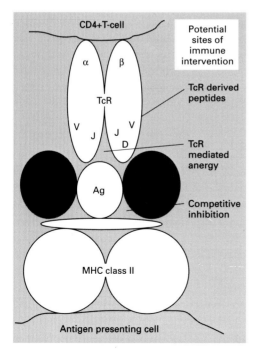

Fig. 2 Schematic interactions of TcR with peptide bound to major histocompatibility complex (MHC) class II.

CD28 molecule on the T-cell by the ligand B7 on the APC [13]. Disruption of the molecular interactions resulting in T-cell activation may lead to the down-regulation of allergen-specific responses [14]. Theoretically, this may be achieved in several ways. One approach depends on the binding of allergenic peptides to those human leukocyte antigen (HLA) class II molecules associated with responsiveness in atopic individuals by immunization with non-stimulatory, non-allergen-derived peptides [15,16]. These competitive inhibitors bind with greater affinity and so displace or prevent the potentially pathogenic allergen epitopes from occupying the antigen-combining site of the HLA class II molecules. An alternative approach for down-regulating T-cell-dependent IgE responses to allergen is to present peptide fragments of the allergen or their structural analogues under conditions that induce antigen-specific anergy of the specific T-cells [17,18]. The result may be to disrupt the physiological function of the T-cells such that they fail to provide B-cell help and undergo clonal expansion on re-exposure to allergen. In addition, there is evidence to suggest that peptide-mediated inhibition may operate by selectively altering patterns of cytokine secretion and so reprogramme the functional activity of the T-cells from the Th2 to Th1 pathway [17]. The advantage of using allergen-derived peptides to regulate the response is the unique specificity in the inhibitory effects that it allows due to the clonal distribution of TcRs. With this in mind, the efficacy of allergen-derived peptides as immunotherapeutics is being assessed.

Before the potential of peptide-mediated immunotherapy in the regulation of immune responses to allergens can be determined it is necessary to characterize both the antigen and restriction specificity of the T-cell repertoire reactive with these allergens. We have chosen initially to investigate anergy induction using peptides from HDMs as they are the most common source of perennial allergens and have been well-characterized at the molecular level.

MAPPING HUMAN T-CELL EPITOPES

The selective stimulation of distinct profiles of cytokine production may be dictated in part by the physical characteristics of antigen encountered and influence the nature of the immune response generated. Now that the genes encoding many of the major environmental allergens have been cloned and sequenced [19–21], it has been possible to use truncated recombinant proteins and overlapping sets of synthetic peptides to identify the important antigen recognition sites (epitopes). Information on the specificity of human T-cell responses to mite allergens at the population level at present remains incomplete, and analysis of antigen specificity has been directed predominantly to the group I (*Der p* I) and group II (*Der p* II) allergens of *Dermatophagoides pteronyssinus* [18,22–26]. The

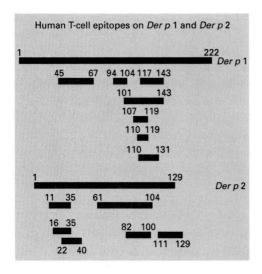

Fig. 3 Human T-cell epitopes recognized on *Der p* I and *Der p* II. Epitopes were identified by lymphocyte proliferation *in vitro* using overlapping synthetic peptides derived from the primary sequence of each allergen. Adapted from [22] with permission.

investigation of polyclonal T-cell responses suggests that in both *Der p* I and *Der p* II there are regions of dominant immune recognition ([22], Fig. 3). However, despite this there is considerable variation in T-cell responses between individuals [23,26,27]. Furthermore, over time in the same individual the array of T-cell epitopes recognized remains relatively constant, which may be the result of chronic exposure to HDM. This pattern is also reflected by a bias of TcR-Vα and β gene usage and the presence of long-lived HDM-specific T-cell clones *in vivo* [28]. In contrast there is a great deal of heterogeneity in the MHC class II restriction specificity of T-cell recognition of HDM responses involving HLA-DR, -DP and -DQ molecules of different specificities ([18,24–26,28,29]; Table 1) and within a single individual a single T-cell epitope may bind to more than one HLA class II molecule.

Table 1 Major histocompatibility complex (MHC) class II restriction of house dust mite (HDM) allergens: heterogeneity of the MHC class II restriction specificity of T-cell recognition of HDM responses involving HLA-DR, -DP and -DQ molecules of different specificities.

HLA-D region genes	Antigen specificity
DRB1 (DR1;DR2;DR5;DR8)	*D. pter.*, *D. far.*, *Der p* I
DRB3 (DR52b)	*D. far.*, *Der f* II
DRB4 (DR53)	*D. far*
DRB5 (DR2Dw2; -Dw12; -Dw21)	*D. pter.*, *D. far.*, *Der p* I, *Der f* I
DPB1 (*0401; *0402)	*D. pter.*, *Der p* I
DQB1 (*0301)	*D. pter.*, *Der p* II

FUNCTIONAL INACTIVATION OF ALLERGEN-REACTIVE T-CELLS

These findings prompted us to develop an *in vitro* model of peptide anergy using human T-cells with which to investigate the cellular and molecular basis of HDM peptide-mediated T-cell desensitization. T-cells, irrespective of the HLA class II restriction specificity, when exposed to supraoptimal concentrations of HDM peptides in either the presence or absence of APCs, become refractory to a subsequent immunogenic challenge, although their responsiveness to IL-2 is enhanced due to up-regulation of the CD25 receptor (Fig. 4). The loss of antigen-dependent proliferation is accompanied by complex changes in the T-cell phenotype, including down-regulation of the TcR and CD28. The molecule CD4 is comodulated with the TcR on some but not all of the T-cells ([30,31]; Table 2). Within 3–4 days

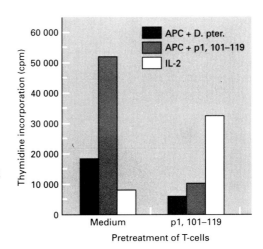

Fig. 4 Allergen peptide-mediated clonal anergy induced following overnight incubation with the dominant peptide from *Der p* I. Adapted from [18] with permission.

Table 2 Effect of allergen peptide-mediated anergy on the T-cell phenotype.

Membrane proteins		
Elevated	Diminished	No change
CD2	TcR	CD71
CD11a/18	CD3	MHC class II
CD25	CD4 +/−	
CD44	CD5 +/−	
CD54	CD28	
MHC class I +/−	CD29	
	CD43	

MHC, Major histocompatibility complex.

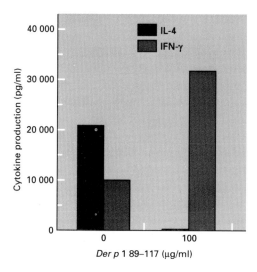

Fig. 5 Cytokine dysregulation in allergen-reactive cloned T-cells *in vitro* following the induction of anergy using a dominant peptide from *Der p* I with subsequent rechallenge using an immunogenic stimulus of peptide and antigen-presenting cells (APCs). A switch of cytokine secretion from a Th2-like pattern to a Th1-like pattern is observed. Adapted from [17] with permission.

the phenotype of the anergic T-cells is similar to that of resting T-cells but they remain unable to respond to further immunogenic challenge, suggesting that mechanisms other than receptor modulation are involved.

During the induction phase of non-responsiveness, cytokine-specific messenger RNA levels are enhanced and for the majority of the cytokines there is also increased production of the soluble product [32]. However, when the anergic T-cells are restimulated with an immunogenic challenge, selective regulation of the cytokine production is observed. The anergic HDM reactive T-cells fail to secrete both IL-4 and IL-5, whereas IFN-γ production remains unaltered (Fig. 5). The synthesis of HDM-specific IgE is regulated in part by the balance between IL-4 and IFN-γ production, with the latter having negative effects [7,8]. Therefore, the overall effect of down-regulating IL-4 while maintaining IFN-γ production would be to reduce the synthesis of IgE.

MODULATION OF ALLERGEN IMMUNE RESPONSIVENESS IN A MOUSE MODEL

In parallel, in order to determine if peptides were able to modulate the function of HDM-specific T-cells *in vivo*, a murine model of T-cell recognition of *Der p* I was investigated. The results of our experiments demonstrate that inhalation of low concentrations of peptide containing the major T-cell epitope of *Der p* I (residues 111–139) induces marked non-responsiveness to both the specific peptide and the intact protein in naive H-2^b mice ([33]; Fig. 6). Lymph node-derived T-cells from the tolerant mice, when restimulated *in vitro*, proliferated poorly and produced only low levels of IL-2. Additionally, these anergic T-cells are unable to

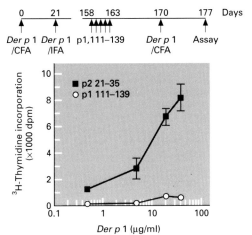

Fig. 6 Inhalation of low concentrations of the dominant peptide from *Der p* I induces marked anergy to both the specific peptide and the intact protein in naive H-2^b mice. Adapted from [33] with permission.

provide cognate help for the production of *Der p* I-specific antibodies. HDM allergy is a chronic disease, so these studies were extended to investigate the effects of immunotherapy on established immune responses. We observed that peptide administered intranasally was able to inhibit both ongoing and long-term responses to HDM in mice [33]. In similar *in vivo* studies addressing peptide-mediated allergen immunotherapy in a murine model, it was demonstrated that dominant peptides from the major cat allergen, *Fel d* I, administered subcutaneously, were able to decrease the T-cell response to subsequent challenge with the peptide in naive and primed animals. Furthermore, pretreatment with two dominant peptides was able to induce tolerance to a challenge with whole recombinant *Fel d* I, thereby down-regulating responses to other epitopes within *Fel d* I [34]. Taken together, these *in vitro* and *in vivo* models allow the efficacy and immunological basis of peptide-mediated immunotherapy to be investigated.

REFERENCES

1 O'Hehir RE, Garman R, Greenstein J, Lamb JR. The specificity and regulation of T cell responsiveness to allergen. *Annu Rev Immunol* 1991;9:67–95.

2 Rocklin RE. Clinical and immunologic aspects of allergen-specific immunotherapy in patients with seasonal allergic rhinitis and/or allergic asthma. *J Allergy Clin Immunol* 1983;72:323–328.

3 Mosmann TR, Coffman RL. Two types of mouse helper T-cell clone. *Immunol Today* 1987;8:223–227.

4 Romagnani S. Th1 and Th2 subsets: doubt no more. *Immunol Today* 1991;12:256–257.

5 Maggi E, Del Prete GF, Macchia D *et al.* Profiles of lymphokine activities and helper function for IgE in human T cell clones. *Eur J Immunol* 1988;18:1045–1050.

6 Esser C, Radbruch A. Immunoglobulin class switching: molecular and cellular analysis. *Annu Rev Immunol* 1990;8:717–735.

7 Finkelman FD, Holmes J, Katona IM *et al.* Lymphokine control of *in vivo* immunoglobulin isotype selection. *Annu Rev Immunol* 1990;**8**:303–333.

8 Vercelli D, Jabara HH, Aria K, Geha RS. Induction of human IgE synthesis requires IL-4 and T/B cell interactions involving the T cell receptor/CD3 complex and MHC class II antigens. *J Exp Med* 1989;**169**:1295–1308.

9 O'Hehir RE, Bal V, Quint DE *et al.* An *in vitro* model of allergen-dependent IgE synthesis by human B lymphocytes: comparison of the responses of an atopic and a nonatopic individual to *Dermatophagoides* spp. (house dust mite). *Immunology* 1989;**66**:499–504.

10 Wierenga EA, Snoek M, de Groot C *et al.* Evidence for compartmentalisation of functional subsets of CD4+ T lymphocytes in atopic patients. *J Immunol* 1990;**144**:4651–4657.

11 Wierenga EA, Snoek M, Bos JD *et al.* Comparison of diversity and function of house dust mite-specific T lymphocyte clones from atopic and nonatopic donors. *Eur J Immunol* 1990;**20**:1519–1526.

12 Schwartz RH. T lymphocyte recognition of antigen in association with gene products of the major histocompatibility complex. *Annu Rev Immunol* 1985;**3**:237–261.

13 Linsley PS, Ledbetter JA. The role of the CD28 receptor during T cell responses to antigen. *Annu Rev Immunol* 1993;**11**:191–212.

14 Lanzavecchia A. Identifying strategies for immune intervention. *Science* 1993;**260**:937–944.

15 Adorini L, Nagy ZA. Peptide competition for antigen presentation. *Immunol Today* 1990;**11**:21–24.

16 O'Hehir RE, Busch R, Rothbard JB, Lamb JR. An *in vitro* model of peptide-mediated immunomodulation of the human T cell response to *Dermatophagoides* spp. (house dust mite). *J Allergy Clin Immunol* 1991;**87**:1120–1127.

17 O'Hehir RE, Yssel H, Verma S *et al.* Clonal analysis of differential lymphokine production in peptide and superantigen induced T cell energy. *Int Immunol* 1991;**3**:819–826.

18 Higgins JA, Lamb JR, Marsh SGE *et al.* Peptide-induced non-responsiveness of HLA-DP restricted human T cells reactive with *Dermatophagoides* spp. (house dust mite). *J Allergy Clin Immunol* 1992;**90**:749–756.

19 Chua KY, Stewart GA, Thomas WR *et al.* Sequence analysis of cDNA encoding for a major house dust mite allergen, *Der p* I. Homology with cysteine proteases. *J Exp Med* 1988;**167**:175–182.

20 Chua KY, Dilworth RJ, Thomas WR. Expression of *Dermatophagoides* pteronyssinus allergen, *Der p* II, in *Escherichia coli* and the binding studies with human IgE. *Int Arch Allergy Appl Immunol* 1990;**91**:124–129.

21 Thomas WR. Mite allergens group I-VII. A catalogue of enzymes. *Clin Exp Allergy* 1993;**23**:350–353.

22 O'Hehir RE, Hoyne GF, Thomas WR, Lamb JR. House dust mite allergy: from T cell epitopes to immunotherapy. *Eur J Clin Invest* 1993;**23**:763–772.

23 O'Hehir RE, Verhoef A, Panagiotopoulou E *et al.* Analysis of human T cell responses to the group II allergen of *Dermatophagoides* spp. (house dust mite): localisation of major antigenic sites. *J Allergy Clin Immunol* 1993;**92**:105–113.

24 Yssel H, Johnson KE, Schneider PV *et al.* T cell activation inducing epitopes of the house dust mite allergen *Der p* I. Proliferation and lymphokine production patterns by *Der p* I-specific CD4+ T cell clones. *J Immunol* 1992;**148**:738–745.

25 Verhoef A, Higgins JA, Thorpe CJ *et al.* Clonal analysis of the atopic immune response to the group 2 allergen of *Dermatophagoides* spp.: identification of HLA-DR and -DQ restricted T cell epitopes. *Int Immunol* 1993;**12**:1589–1597.

26 Joost van Neerven R, van t'Hof W, Ringrose JH *et al.* T cell epitopes of house dust mite major allergen *Der p* II. *J Immunol* 1993;**151**:2326–2335.

27 O'Brien RM, Thomas WR, Wootton AM. T cell responses to the purified major allergens for the house dust mite *Dermatophagoides pteronyssinus*. *J Allergy Clin Immunol* 1992;**89**:1021–1031.

28 Wedderburn LR, O'Hehir RE, Hewitt CRA, Lamb JR, Owen MJ. *In vivo* clonal dominance and limited T cell receptor usage in human CD4+ T cell recognition of house dust mite allergens. *Proc Natl Acad Sci USA* 1993;**90**:8214–8218.

29 O'Hehir RE, Mach B, Berte C *et al.* Direct evidence for a functional role of HLA-DRB3

gene products in the recognition of *Dermatophagoides* spp. by helper T cell clones. *Int Immunol* 1990;**2**:885–892.

30 O'Hehir RE, Aguilar BA, Schmidt TJ, Gollnick SO, Lamb JR. Functional inactivation of *Dermatophagoides* spp. (house dust mite) reactive T cell clones. *Clin Exp Allergy* 1991;**21**:209–214.

31 O'Hehir RE, Lamb JR. Induction of specific clonal anergy in human T lymphocytes by *Staphylococcus aureus* enterotoxins. *Proc Natl Acad Sci USA* 1990;**87**:8884–8888.

32 Schall TJ, O'Hehir RE, Goeddel DV, Lamb JR. Uncoupling of cytokine mRNA expression and protein secretion during the induction of T cell anergy. *J Immunol* 1992;**148**:381–387.

33 Hoyne GJ, O'Hehir RE, Wraith DC, Thomas WR, Lamb JR. Inhibition of T-cell and antibody responses to house dust mite allergen by inhalation of the dominant T-cell epitope in naive and sensitised mice. *J Exp Med* 1993;**178**:1783–1788.

34 Briner TJ, Kuo M-C, Keating KM, Rogers BL, Greenstein JL. Peripheral T-cell tolerance induced in naive and primed mice by subcutaneous injection of peptides from the major cat allergen *Fel d* I. *Proc Natl Acad Sci USA* 1993;**90**:7608–7612.

MULTIPLE CHOICE QUESTIONS

1 The atopic state is associated with

  a the production of serum-specific immunoglobulin E (IgE) to common aeroallergens

  b increased incidence of allergic disease, e.g. asthma, rhinitis, eczema

  c use of allergen immunotherapy for hyposensitization in some patients

  d increased risk of occult malignancy

  e a Th2-like cytokine response by allergen-reactive T-cells

2 Human CD4+ T-cells

  a play a pivotal role in the allergic immune response

  b may be functionally defined as Th1-like or Th2-like

  c differentiate into plasma cells and secrete IgE

  d do not secrete cytokines

  e cooperate with B cells to induce immunoglobulin synthesis

3 Immunoglobulin E

  a is the main specific effector molecule in allergic inflammation

  b synthesis is favoured by Th1-like cytokines

  c production is induced by a high interleukin-4/interferon-γ ratio

  d may be induced in all individuals with parasite infection

  e is usually elevated in non-atopic subjects

4 Human T-cell allergen epitopes

  a can be identified using truncated recombinant proteins and peptide sets

  b are important T-cell antigen recognition sites

  c are always carbohydrate

d can be identified in the major aeroallergens, e.g. *Der p* I and *Der p* II

e are subject to antigenic drift and shift, as observed in influenza

5 Induction of allergen-specific anergy using dominant T-cell epitopes

a can be achieved with *in vitro* and *in vivo* experimental models

b is associated with decreased expression of the T-cell receptor

c prevents all cytokine secretion on rechallenge

d may be associated with Th2 to Th1 cytokine shift

e can be achieved via the intranasal or subcutaneous routes

Answers

1 a True		**2 a** True		**3 a** True				
b True		**b** True		**b** False				
c True		**c** False		**c** True				
d False		**d** False		**d** True				
e True		**e** True		**e** False				

4 a True   **5 a** True
  b True   **b** True
  c False   **c** False
  d True   **d** True
  e False   **e** True

Complement deficiency

MARK J. WALPORT

There are three phenotypes associated with the presence of inherited complement deficiency — robust good health, systemic lupus erythematosus (SLE) and recurrent pyogenic infections, including particularly neisserial infections. These phenotypes tell us a great deal about the normal physiological activities of the complement system in human beings. The exact phenotype varies according to the position of the missing complement protein in the complement activation and effector pathways, which demonstrates that different parts of the complement system subserve particular functions. The role of complement as part of the innate immune system is demonstrated by the markedly increased prevalence of pyogenic bacterial infections in patients with impaired complement function. The activation pathways of the complement system and the major effector functions are shown in Figs 1 and 2.

Even the nature of the pyogenic bacteria to which complement-deficient subjects are susceptible varies according to the deficient portion of the complement pathway. Deficiency of the pathways leading to the activation of C3 is associated with susceptibility to a wide range of pyogenic organisms, with a similar spectrum to that seen in immunoglobulin or phagocyte dysfunction. This illustrates the role of complement as bacterial opsonin, enhancing phagocytosis and killing of bacteria. In contrast, deficiency of the lytic pathway of complement is solely associated with an increased susceptibility to neisserial infection. These organisms are capable of intracellular survival and this association demonstrates the important role of complement as bacteriolysin for this group of bacteria.

The humoral adaptive immune system engages complement as an effector pathway through a linking molecule, C1q, which binds to antibody which has engaged antigen. The binding of C1q to antibody–antigen immune complexes triggers the classical pathway of complement, leading to the cleavage of C3 and the covalent attachment of this molecule to the antibody–antigen complex, promoting immune complex clearance by phagocytic cells.

Of great interest are the observations that absence or deficiency of classical pathway of complement normally protects humans from the

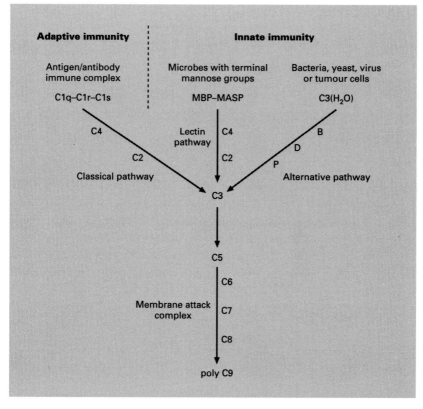

Fig. 1 An overview of the complement system showing: (a) the three activation pathways; (b) the central role of C3 cleavage in the activation of complement; and (c) the formation of the membrane attack complex.

development of SLE. One hypothesis that links classical pathway complement deficiency with predisposition to SLE is that the normal physiological role of complement in clearing immune complexes is impaired. This may allow immune complexes to deposit in tissues, stimulating inflammation, with the release of autoantigens and the subsequent development of an autoantibody response.

In this review, each of these associations will be considered in more detail. Deficiencies of cell-surface regulatory molecules of the complement system and of complement receptors will not be considered and for recent reviews on these topics the interested reader is referred to [1–5].

COMPLEMENT DEFICIENCY AND AUTOIMMUNITY

Complement deficiency in SLE — inherited or acquired?

The association of complement deficiency with SLE is paradoxical. On

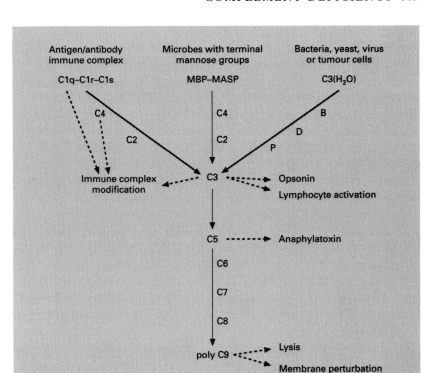

Fig. 2 The major effector activities of the complement system.

the one hand, active SLE is associated with activation of the complement pathway and hypocomplementaemia and there is evidence that complement plays a causal role in causing inflammatory injury to tissues. On the other hand, inherited deficiency of classical pathway complement proteins, reviewed below, plays a causal role in the induction of SLE.

Faced with a patient with SLE with low complement levels, how does one decide whether the complement deficiency is inherited or acquired? In the case of homozygous complement deficiency, this is a fairly straightforward problem, as long as the routine laboratory undertakes a functional haemolytic complement assay, such as the CH_{50} (essentially a measure of the quantity of serum that causes 50% haemolysis of target erythrocytes sensitized with antibody). The main pathway of complement activation in active SLE is the classical pathway, mediated by antigen–antibody immune complexes. This causes activation and increased turnover of C1, C4, C2 and, to a lesser extent, of C3. Most laboratories measure the levels of C3 and C4 using antigenic assays, and a typical patient with active SLE will show reductions in C4 levels, CH_{50} and, to some degree, C3 levels. These will vary with disease activity.

Results that should trigger suspicion that there may be homozygous complement deficiency are: (i) an absence of CH_{50} activity with persistently normal C3 and C4 levels; (ii) absent C4 levels and CH_{50} with persistently normal C3 levels, which would imply C4 deficiency; or (iii) absent or severely reduced C3 levels and CH_{50} with normal C4 levels, implying deficiency of C3 or of one of the regulatory molecules of the alternative pathway. From this point on, specialized assays are needed to identify the precise nature of the deficient protein. If the routine laboratory does not measure CH_{50}, it becomes much harder to identify complement-deficient patients and factors that should increase the index of suspicion and trigger further investigation are: (i) persistently normal C3 and C4 levels in a patient with very active disease; (ii) two or more siblings with disease; (iii) early-onset disease; and (iv) parental consanguinity.

Measurement of C3, C4 and CH_{50} levels does not allow the identification of deficiencies of alternative pathway complement proteins such as factors B, D or properdin. The easiest screen for deficiency of one of these proteins is a functional assay such as an AP_{50}, which is a haemolytic assay of lysis of rabbit erythrocytes by the alternative pathway in a buffer that inhibits classical pathway activation by the selective chelation of calcium. It is important to perform such assays in patients with recurrent pyogenic infections, particularly those caused by *Neisseria*, but less relevant in patients with SLE, where there appears to be no strong association with inherited deficiencies of alternative pathway proteins.

Mechanisms of acquired deficiency in SLE

There is abundant evidence that complement is activated in patients with SLE. Tissue biopsies show deposits of C4, C3 and associated complement proteins. However, the presence of complement does not necessarily coincide with the presence of tissue injury, for example the presence of fixed C3 at the dermoepidermal junction in clinically and histologically normal skin in SLE (the lupus band test). Some effort has been devoted to identifying markers of complement deposition in tissue which may act as markers of tissue inflammation. For example, the presence of proteins of the membrane attack complex of complement shows a better correlation with inflammatory lesions in the skin and the kidneys than the presence of C3 and C4 [6,7].

There are a number of diseases where there is good evidence that complement activation causes local tissue injury but where there is very little that can be measured in the circulation to show for this. Examples include rheumatoid arthritis, Goodpasture's disease, membranous nephritis and myasthenia gravis. In each of these diseases, the scale of complement activation in tissues is too small to have measurable large-scale consequences in the circulation, though more subtle tests of complement activation, which measure fragments of complement proteins split by the process of complement activation, may be positive in serum from patients with rheumatoid arthritis, reflecting the large amounts of complement activation within joints [8]. In contrast, autoimmune haemolytic anaemia such as cold agglutinin disease, in which activation of the complement system in the circulation is induced by antierythocyte antibodies, is associated with a pattern of classical pathway complement activation similar to that measured in SLE. What is the explanation of the difference between autoimmune haemolytic anaemia and rheumatoid arthritis? It may be a question of the scale of complement activation, but the site may also be very important, i.e. complement activation occurring within the circulation may be more likely to be reflected by changes in serum C4 and C3 concentrations.

There have been a number of factors correlated with the degree of reduction in C4 and C3 levels in sera from patients with SLE. These include disease activity *per se* [9–11], the presence of haemolytic anaemia and the levels of particular autoantibodies, including anti-dsDNA [11,12], anticardiolipin [13,14] and anti-C1q antibodies [15]. Other autoantibodies do not seem to be associated with much in the way of systemic complement activation, e.g. anti-Ro and anti-La antibodies, which are characteristically found in patients with subacute cutaneous lupus erythematosus or with primary Sjögren's syndrome.

In the case of anti-dsDNA antibodies, it seems likely that their association with complement activation in serum does reflect large-scale activation of the complement occurring in tissues. This may also be the case for anti-C1q antibodies, which may act to amplify C1q activation in tissues, though definite evidence for this is lacking. In the case of anticardiolipin antibodies, it is not known if, how or where they act to cause complement activation *in vivo*.

The association of inherited complement deficiency with SLE

Homozygous complement protein deficiencies are extremely rare. In recent years a clear picture has emerged of rather precise disease associations which show subtle but important variations according to the position of the missing protein in the complement-triggered enzyme cascade. Only specific complement deficiencies have been associated with SLE, particularly of the classical pathway proteins, C1q, C1r and C1s, C4, C2 and C3. Amongst these proteins there appears to be a hierarchy of association of both disease prevalence and severity with SLE, according to the position of the protein in the activation pathway of complement. C1q, C1r, C1s (reviewed in [16,17]), and C4 deficiency (reviewed in [18]) are each associated with a very high apparent prevalence of disease (> 75%), which tends to be severe. Deficiency of C2, the next protein in the pathway, is associated with a lower prevalence of disease, about 33%, and disease tends to be of a similar severity to that seen amongst cohorts of patients with SLE in the absence of complement deficiency [19]. C3 deficiency, reported in 24 subjects [20], has only been associated with lupus-like disease in 3 patients in two families, one with autoantibodies [21] and the other two without [22]. These findings would suggest that a physiological activity of the early part of the classical pathway of complement serves to prevent the development of SLE. Two candidate activities of complement in this respect would be the processing of immune complexes and host defence against an unknown infecting agent. Discussion of these falls outside the scope of this review and the interested reader is referred to [23].

Could these associations of SLE with complement deficiency be due to ascertainment artefact? The first two complement-deficient humans to be identified were immunologists, a group who have a propensity to use their own serum as an experimental reagent. It could follow in a similar fashion that the finding of complement deficiency in patients with SLE is an artefactual consequence of the selective measurement of complement in that particular cohort of patients.

There are data that refute this trivial explanation for the association between complement deficiency and SLE. There have been some very large population surveys of healthy individuals, of blood donors in Osaka [24] and recruits into the Swiss army [25]. Amongst these individuals no examples were found of patients with inherited deficiencies of classical pathway proteins, though, amongst the Japanese blood donors, subtotal C9 deficiency was relatively common and small numbers of patients with homozygous deficiencies of other membrane attack complex proteins were identified [24]. This evidence effectively excludes ascertainment artefact as accounting for the association between SLE and classical pathway complement protein deficiencies. However, there have been some isolated cases of SLE reported in association with deficiency of a membrane attack complex protein (references given in [23]) and it is possible that these cases may represent ascertainment artefact.

A second important question when establishing whether a gene is causally related to a disease is to ask whether the association is with the identified gene or a linked unknown gene. This is easily answered in the case of the complement deficiency and SLE. The relevant classical pathway complement proteins are encoded on different chromosomes: C1q on chromosome 1, C4 and C2 on chromosome 6 in the MHC, and C3 on chromosome 19. It would be pushing coincidence too far to argue that each of these associations was due to linked genes on three different chromosomes.

Finally there is an association between acquired complement deficiency and the development of SLE. Inherited deficiency of C1 inhibitor, the cause of hereditary angioedema, is associated with unregulated consumption of C4 and C2. About 1% of patients with this condition develop SLE [26].

Complement deficiency in SLE — does it matter?

The association of complement deficiency with SLE is important for two reasons, one academic, the other practical. The academic reason is that insight into the aetiology of at least a subset of patients with SLE may follow from studying the mechanisms of the association of inherited complement deficiency with disease.

The practical reason is that complement deficiency impairs host defence against pyogenic infections, reviewed below. Patients with acquired hypocomplementaemia secondary to SLE and other diseases feature in several of the series characterizing abnormalities of the complement system amongst patients presenting with meningococcal infections. We have found (unpublished data) a strong association between acquired hypocomplementaemia and overwhelming pneumococcal and menin-gococcal infections amongst our patients with SLE. A practical implication of these observations is that we probably should be treating patients with SLE and hypocomplementaemia with prophylactic penicillin and immunization against pneumococcal and meningococcal infection. There are no prospective data to support this approach but the anecdotal data provide a strong argument for setting up an appropriate study.

COMPLEMENT DEFICIENCY AND INFECTION

Complement deficiency and pyogenic infection

Important mechanisms of host defence against infectious disease have been illuminated by analysis of patients with specific immunodeficien-cies. There is an increased susceptibility to pyogenic bacteria such as *Staphylococcus aureus* in patients who have defects of antibody production, classical pathway complement proteins or phagocyte function. This dem-onstrates that the normal pathway of host defence against these bacteria is opsonization with antibody, followed by complement, followed by uptake by phagocytosis and intracellular killing.

The most notable association between inherited deficiency of com-plement and pyogenic bacterial infection is that between Neisserial disease, particularly *N. meningitidis*, and inherited deficiencies of membrane attack complex proteins [27]. This appears to be the only significant disease association of inherited deficiencies of these proteins and illustrates an important point. It may be necessary to stress an organism in a particular way to identify the biological role *in vivo* of a pathway or protein. *Neisseria* are capable of intracellular survival. The association between an inability to form the lytic plug of the complement system with infection by these organisms implies that extracellular lysis is of major physiological importance as a mechanism of killing these organisms.

There are several intriguing features of the association of meningococcal disease with complement deficiency. Infections appear to be milder than in complement-sufficient subjects [27]. The explanation for this may be that formation of the membrane attack complex in large amounts in patients with meningococcal disease is injurious to the host. This might be by releasing large amounts of endotoxin from the bacteria and by direct effects on autologous cell membranes causing cellular activation and promoting inflammation [28]. An alternative explanation for the observation that meningococcal disease is milder in complement-deficient compared with complement-sufficient subjects is that the observation is artefactual. It may be that complement deficiency is less likely to be diagnosed in a subject who presents with rapidly fatal disease in whom measurement of complement levels takes a low priority in the assessment and management of a critically ill patient.

Epidemiology of membrane attack complex deficiency

In several parts of the world where meningococcal infections are highly endemic, such as around the Mediterranean basin [29] and in South Africa [30], there appears to be a high prevalence of membrane attack complex protein deficiencies. It has been argued that the heterozygous deficiency state may offer some selective advantage, possibly by protecting against the deleterious effects of complement activation by endotoxin [30]. However, C9 deficiency is also remarkably common in Japan [31], where meningococcal disease is rare, and there is no obvious hypothesis to explain a selective advantage of C9 deficiency in this population.

The strength of the association of membrane attack complex (MAC) protein deficiency with neisserial disease has in the past been overestimated due to ascertainment artefact. Based on a survey of the families of patients presenting with meningococcal sepsis, it was suggested that the prevalence of meningococcal infection in subjects with MAC deficiency may be as high as 44% [27]. However, a survey of nearly 150 000 consecutive blood donors in Japan [24] revealed 154 with complete deficiency of one of the MAC proteins (138 with C9 deficiency, 16 with deficiency of C5, C6, C7 or C8), none of whom had suffered from neisserial infection. As has been noted above, the prevalence of meningococcal infection is low in Japan — of the order of 1 in 10^6 [32]. An interesting result emerged when the strength of the association of complement deficiency with meningococcal disease in Japan was studied in a different way, by asking what the prevalence was of complement deficiency in patients presenting with meningococcal disease. Amongst 17 patients with meningococcal disease ascertained from a register in Fukuoka, 8 had inherited complement deficiency, 4 of C7 and 4 of C9, and a ninth patient had SLE with acquired complement deficiency [32]. Combining the incidence data for meningococcal disease, the prevalence of complement deficiency amongst sporadic cases of meningococcal disease and the frequency of inherited complement deficiency amongst Japanese blood donors [24,32], the estimated risk to a complement-deficient subject in Japan of developing meningococcal disease is approximately 0.5% per annum. This estimate suggests that the strength of the association of isolated inherited deficiencies of membrane attack complement proteins with the development of meningococcal sepsis has been grossly overestimated in the past by only including families in which one member had presented with meningococcal infection.

Mannose-binding protein deficiency

In 1976 [33] a group of young children aged mainly between 6 months and 2 years was described from Great Ormond Street Hospital suffering from recurrent pyogenic infections and failure to thrive. It was subsequently found that serum from these children failed to opsonize the yeast *Saccharomyces cerevisiae* normally with C3 [34]. A similar opsonic defect was present in approximately 5% of the adult population and was not associated with any obvious immunodeficiency. The pathophysiological basis for these findings remained a mystery until it was discovered that the opsonic defect correlated with reduced serum levels of mannose-binding protein (MBP) [35]. MBP is a member of a family of calcium-dependent lectins, the collectins (collagenous lectins), which includes C1q. MBP binds to arrays of terminal mannose groups, present on a variety of bacteria, and activates complement by interaction with a serine proteinase called MASP (mannose-binding protein-associated serine proteinase), which cleaves and activates C4 and C2 [36].

Three point mutations have now been identified in the MBP gene which are associated with reduced levels of expression of MBP (reviewed in [37]). Allele B, with a gene frequency of 0.11–0.17, is found in Caucasoid, Asian and Eskimo populations, and varies from the normal A allele by a glycine to aspartic acid substitution at codon 54. Alleles C, gene frequency 0.23–0.29, and D, gene frequency 0.05, are found in black African populations and vary by a glycine to glutamic acid substitution at codon 57 and by an arginine to cysteine substitution at codon 52, respectively. Each of these polymorphic variants is associated with markedly reduced levels of MBP when present as heterozygous with the normal A alleles, and very low levels when present in homozygous form. Present evidence suggests that MBP containing the B, C or D allotype may be unstable in plasma compared with MBP comprised solely of the A allotype.

Activation of complement through the binding of MBP is a further part of the innate immune system and provides a carbohydrate-dependent route for triggering complement. The association of low levels of MBP with recurrent infections in young children suggests that this mechanism of host defence may be of particular importance during the window of time between loss of passively acquired maternal antibody and the acquisition of a mature adaptive immunological repertoire. The surprising observation is that there is a high frequency of dominantly expressed alleles of MBP which result in low levels of expression of MBP protein in several different human races. This suggests that the immunodeficiency of early childhood must be counterbalanced by some selective advantage at some other time in life. A recent study [38] showed that Ethiopians with lepromatous leprosy had higher levels of serum MBP than their counterparts without disease. The hypothesis that follows from this observation is that the opsonization of organisms with complement by binding of MBP might enhance the uptake into cells of pathogens with an intracellular lifestyle, such as mycobacteria. Expression of reduced levels of MBP might confer host resistance against such infections. This interesting hypothesis awaits further experimental evaluation.

CONCLUSION

Study of patients with inherited and acquired deficiencies of complement proteins has provided a powerful analysis of the physiological activities of the complement system *in vivo*. The paradoxical observation that complement deficiency causes SLE, yet SLE causes complement deficiency, has been partially resolved. There is an intricate but changing balance between the host and pathogenic agents. The host uses the complement system as a weapon against microorganisms and in turn, microbial pathogenicity may depend on microorganisms using host complement as a mechanism for enhancing their own pathogenesis. The observation that some individuals with complement deficiency are healthy emphasizes that host defence mechanisms against infectious disease show a considerable degree of redundancy, a reassuring observation given the rapidity with which potential infectious agents can evolve!

REFERENCES

1 Walport MJ, Lachmann PJ. Erythrocyte complement receptor type 1, immune complexes and the rheumatic diseases. *Arthritis Rheum* 1988;**31**:153–158.
2 Lachmann PJ. The control of homologous lysis. *Immunol Today* 1991;**12**:312–315.
3 Harlan JM. Leukocyte adhesion deficiency syndrome: insights into the molecular basis of leukocyte emigration. *Clin Immunol Immunopathol* 1993;**67**:S16–S24.
4 Arnaout MA. Leukocyte adhesion molecules deficiency: its structural basis, pathophysiology and implications for modulating the inflammatory response. *Immunol Rev* 1990;**114**:145–180.

5 Schieren G, Hansch GM. Membrane-associated proteins regulating the complement system: functions and deficiencies. *Int Rev Immunol* 1993;**10**:87–101.

6 Biesecker G, Katz S, Koffler D. Renal localisation of the membrane attack complex in systemic lupus erythematosus. *J Exp Med* 1981;**154**:1779–1794.

7 Biesecker G, Lavin L, Ziskind M, Koffler D. Cutaneous localization of the membrane attack complex in discoid and systemic lupus erythematosus. *N Engl J Med* 1982;**306**:264–270.

8 Mallya RK, Vergani D, Tee DE *et al*. Correlation in rheumatoid arthritis of concentrations of plasma C3d, serum rheumatoid factor, immune complexes and C-reactive protein with each other and with clinical features of disease activity. *Clin Exp Immunol* 1982;**48**:747–753.

9 Valentijn RM, van Overhagen H, Hazevoet HM *et al*. The value of complement and immune complex determinations in monitoring disease activity in patients with systemic lupus erythematosus. *Arthritis Rheum* 1985;**28**:904–913.

10 Lloyd W, Schur PH. Immune complexes, complement, and anti-DNA in exacerbations of systemic lupus erythematosus (SLE). *Medicine* 1981;**1**:208–217.

11 Koffler D, Schur P, Kunkel HG. Immunological studies concerning the nephritis of systemic lupus erythematosus. *J Exp Med* 1967;**126**:607.

12 Cameron JS, Lessof MH, Ogg CS, Williams BD, Williams DG. Disease activity in the nephritis of systemic lupus erythematosus in relation to serum complement concentrations. DNA-binding capacity and precipitating anti-DNA antibody. *Clin Exp Immunol* 1976;**25**:418–427.

13 Norberg R, Nived O, Sturfelt G, Unander M, Arfors L. Anticardiolipin and complement activation: relation to clinical symptoms. *J Rheumatol* 1987;**14**:149–153.

14 Hammond A, Rudge AC, Loizou S, Bowcock SJ, Walport MJ. Reduced numbers of complement receptor type 1 on erythrocytes are associated with increased levels of anticardiolipin antibodies: findings in patients with systemic lupus erythematosus and the antiphospholipid syndrome. *Arthritis Rheum* 1989;**32**:259–264.

15 Siegert C, Daha M, Westedt ML, van der Voort E, Breedveld F. IgG autoantibodies against C1q are correlated with nephritis, hypocomplementemia, and dsDNA antibodies in systemic lupus erythematosus. *J Rheumatol* 1991;**18**:230–234.

16 Loos M, Heinz H-P. Component deficiencies. 1. The first component: C1q, C1r, C1s. *Prog Allergy* 1986;**39**:212–231.

17 Reid KBM. Deficiency of the first component of human complement. *Immunodefic Rev* 1989;**1**:247–260.

18 Hauptmann G, Goetz J, Uring-Lambert B, Grosshans E. Component deficiencies. 2. The fourth component. *Prog Allergy* 1986;**39**:232–249.

19 Ruddy S. Component deficiencies 3. The second component. *Prog Allergy* 1986;**39**:250–266.

20 Botto M, Walport MJ. Hereditary deficiency of C3 in animals and humans. *Intern Rev Immunol* 1993;**10**:37–50.

21 Nilsson UR, Nilsson B, Storm KE, Sjolin Forsberg G, Hallgren R. Hereditary dysfunction of the third component of complement associated with a systemic lupus erythematosus-like syndrome and meningococcal meningitis. *Arthritis Rheum* 1992;**35**:580–586.

22 Sano Y, Nishimukai H, Kitamura H *et al*. Hereditary deficiency of the third component of complement in two sisters with systemic lupus erythematosus-like symptoms. *Arthritis Rheum* 1981;**24**:1255–1260.

23 Morgan BP, Walport MJ. Complement deficiency and disease. *Immunol Today* 1991;**12**:301–306.

24 Inai S, Akagaki Y, Moriyama T *et al*. Inherited deficiencies of the late-acting complement components other than C9 found among healthy blood donors. *Int Arch Allergy Appl Immunol* 1989;**90**:274–279.

25 Hassig A, Borel JF, Ammann P. Essentielle hypocomplementemia. *Pathol Microbiol* 1964;**27**:542–547.

26 Donaldson VH, Hess EV, McAdams AJ. Lupus-erythematosus-like disease in three unrelated women with hereditary angioneurotic edema *Ann Intern Med* 1977;**86**:312–313.

27 Ross SC, Densen P. Complement deficiency states and infection: epidemiology,

pathogenesis and consequences of neisserial and other infections in an immune deficiency. *Medicine* 1984;**63**:243–273.

28 Lehner PJ, Davies KA, Cope AP *et al.* Meningococcal septicaemia in a C6-deficient patient, the effects of plasma infusion on LPS release. *Lancet* 1992;**340**:1379–1381.

29 Schlesinger M, Nave Z, Levy Y, Slater PE, Fishelson Z. Prevalence of hereditary properdin, C7 and C8 deficiencies in patients with meningococcal infections. *Clin Exp Immunol* 1990;**81**:423–427.

30 Orren A, Potter PC, Cooper RC, Toit Edu. Deficiency of the sixth component of complement and susceptibility to *Neisseria meningitidis* infections: studies in 10 families and five isolated cases. *Immunology* 1987;**62**:249–253.

31 Fukumori Y, Yoshimura K, Ohnoki S, Yamaguchi H, Akagaki Y, Inai S. A high incidence of C9 deficiency among healthy blood donors in Osaka, Japan. *Int Immunol* 1989;**1**:85–89.

32 Nagata M, Hara T, Aoki T *et al.* Inherited deficiency of ninth component of complement: an increased risk of meningococcal meningitis. *J Pediatr* 1989;**114**:260–264.

33 Soothill JF, Harvey BAM. Defective opsonisation: a common immunity deficiency. *Arch Dis Child* 1976;**51**:91–99.

34 Soothill JF, Harvey BA. A defect of the alternative pathway of complement. *Clin Exp Immunol* 1977;**27**:30–33.

35 Super M, Lu J, Thiel S, Levinsky RJ, Turner MW. Association of low levels of mannan-binding protein with a common defect of opsonisation. *Lancet* 1989;**2**:1236–1239.

36 Matsushita M, Fujita T. Activation of the classical complement pathway by mannose-binding protein in association with a novel C1s-like serine protease. *J Exp Med* 1992;**176**:1497–1502.

37 Madsen HO, Garred P, Kurtzhals JA *et al.* A new frequent allele is the missing link in the structural polymorphism of the human mannan-binding protein. *Immunogenetics* 1994;**40**:37–44.

38 Garred P, Harboe M, Oettinger T, Koch C, Svejgaard A. Dual role of mannan-binding protein in infectious disease: another case of heterosis. *Eur J Immunogen* 1994;**21**:125–131.

MULTIPLE CHOICE QUESTIONS

1 Complement deficiency is associated with

a recurrent viral infections
b scleroderma
c pyogenic bacterial infections
d meningococcal meningitis
e systemic candidiasis

2 Hypocomplementaemia may be found in association with

a subacute bacterial endocarditis
b partial lipodystrophy
c polyarteritis nodosa
d post-streptococcal glomerulonephritis
e cold agglutinin disease

3 Hereditary angioedema

a shows autosomal recessive inheritance
b may be associated with reduced or normal levels of C1 inhibitor
c acute attacks respond to adrenaline

d may present with abdominal pain
e stanozolol is effective prophylaxis

Answers

1			2			3		
	a	False		**a**	True		**a**	False
	b	False		**b**	True		**b**	True
	c	True		**c**	False		**c**	False
	d	True		**d**	True		**d**	True
	e	False		**e**	True		**e**	True

Cytokines in the regulation of metabolic and immune responses to infection

GEORGE E. GRIFFIN

Clinical syndromes relating to infectious diseases and inflammatory processes have been recognized for many centuries and many still remain as important diagnostic pointers. For example, fever and weight loss, whilst not being specific, have classically been associated with clinical infection and inflammation. Until recently we have been ignorant of the definitive agents responsible for the mediation of such basic patho-physiological features of disease and many of the previously postulated chemical mediators which have been measured in serum are now regarded as either secondary or trigger agents. The discovery of cytokines has had immense importance in the understanding of pathophysiology of infection and inflammation. Since the discovery of the first cytokine, cachectin or tumour necrosis factor (TNF), many other agents in this group have been discovered and these have principally been called interleukins (IL) with a numerical designation currently from IL-1 to IL-17. The action of these polypeptide hormones in the inflammatory response is turn-ing out to be exceedingly complex; however, the integrated effect of the cascade of cytokines released by various infectious stimuli orchestrates the immune and metabolic adaptation to infection. An immense amount of information has amassed concerning these agents and it is now apparent that cytokines are autocrine and paracrine signal molecules crucial in the integration of the generation of appropriate immune and metabolic responses to infectious agents and antigens. However, in the setting of sepsis the massive release of cytokines with dissemination throughout the body in blood causes physiological and metabolic chaos with devastating effects.

CYTOKINES, SEPTIC SHOCK AND LIPOPOLYSACCHARIDE

Animal models

Cytokines have been strongly implicated in the pathogenesis of septic shock [1]. A consensus view now appears that septic shock situation represents massive and overwhelming cytokine release with the appearance of these agents in the circulation.

Animal models provided initial detailed knowledge of the cytokine cascade in septic shock. The defined nature of the stimulus used in these models, namely either administration of lipopolysaccharide (LPS) or live organisms, or surgical procedures such as caecal ligation, have enabled detail of the cytokine network to be evaluated *in vivo*, both in the circulation and at tissue level.

The uniformity of the cytokines involved in the response and the very similar pattern of the cytokine cascade observed in the plasma of diverse animal models indicates that this response and its control are conserved across species (Table 1). The principal characteristic feature in the model systems is that peak proinflammatory cytokine plasma concentration appears very early. For example, TNF peak levels are detected at about 1 hour and those of IL-6 and IL-8 at between 6 and 8 hours following stimulus [2–9]. It might be expected that plasma levels of cytokines, such as TNF, which appear to be central in mediating septic shock, would be accurate predictors of outcome given the defined nature of the animal models and stimulus. However, the situation appears to be considerably more complex *in vivo* [1], for example, in a pig model of sepsis, high TNF levels are markers of survival rather than mortality. In addition, in the rat caecal ligation model, protection is afforded by TNF administered 24 hours before the insult (Remick, personal communication).

The brisk up-regulation of TNF production and its rapid appearance in plasma are characteristic features across all species. Tissue sites of TNF

Table 1 Synthesis of cytokines after endotoxin or live bacterial challenge. There is remarkable uniformity of the cytokine response to a bacterial challenge; regardless of the bacterial species, or the experimental animal, cytokines are quickly induced within a few hours.

Animal	Stimulus	Peak cytokine production (h)	Cytokines
Mice	LPS	1	TNF, IL-1
Pigs	LPS	0.5–1	TNF
		1–2	IL-6
Mice	*Salmonella*	1.5	TNF
Baboons	*Escherichia coli*	1	TNF
		2	IL-1
		2	IL-6
Rats LPS		1	TNF
Baboons	*Escherichia coli*	2	TNF
		6	IL-1β, IL-6
Baboons	*Escherichia coli*	1	TNF
		8	IL-1, IL-6, IL-8

LPS, Lipopolysaccharide; IL, interleukin; TNF, tumour necrosis factor.

production have been defined in the rat [7]. Studies of cytokine release from isolated macrophages in tissue culture exposed to LPS indicate a brisk increase in messenger RNA for TNF, which peaks at approximately 45 minutes after exposure and rapidly declines. It is therefore surprising that *in vivo* the level of TNF messenger RNA in tissues increases very little in the face of massive elevation of the concentration of this cytokine in plasma. Further studies [10] using chloramphenicol acetyl transferase linked to the TNF promoter suggest that the principal regulation of this cytokine *in vivo* occurs at post transcriptional level. In addition, since information on control of TNF synthesis has accumulated, the phenomenon of tolerance to repeated LPS injection has been understood in that there is a failure both of macrophages in culture and *in vivo* to produce TNF for several days after the last exposure to LPS [11]. Such a phenomenon of tolerance indicates a crucial very well-regulated control for TNF production which attempts to restrict massive release of this potentially lethal cytokine.

Human studies

Studies of the cytokine cascade in human sepsis have been somewhat confusing in that variable levels of proinflammatory cytokines have been detected in the plasma of patients admitted with Gram-negative septi-caemia. Meningococcal septicaemia provides one of the best human situations in which to study the cascade of plasma cytokines, since in classical cases the rash allows an accurate clinical diagnosis at presentation, unlike most other forms of sepsis [12]. In meningococcal sepsis plasma TNF may be undetectable, presumably since clinical presentation is several hours, if not longer, after the initial stimulus, resulting in tolerance, described above.

However, when this cytokine is detected in plasma the absolute level (> 140 pg/ml) bears a strong relationship to bad prognosis [13]. Since other cytokines are released into the circulation during sepsis, longitudinal studies have attempted to measure the pattern of release of TNF and IL-6 during the clinical course of meningococcal sepsis. A highly complex pattern of these cytokines is present in the circulation as this disease progresses [12]. Such a complex pattern is not surprising given the variability of the duration of stimulus before presentation to hospital and probable genetic differences in host response in terms of the generation of cytokine release [13,14].

Measurement of plasma TNF, IL-6 and IL-8 in another form of human Gram-negative sepsis, namely that due to *Pseudomonas pseudomallei*, revealed no relationship between survival and TNF or IL-6 levels but IL-8 plasma concentration was a better prognostic index [15]. Interestingly, in the latter study plasma IL-6 and IL-8 levels were found to be elevated up to 30 days after admission to hospital and presumably are a measure of the continuing stimulus for the acute-phase response.

Since an exceedingly complex pattern of plasma cytokines has been detected in the course of human sepsis [1], attempts have been made to define the plasma cytokine cascade in more defined conditions. These have principally involved studies in human volunteers infused with endo-toxin and blood sampled at short time intervals. Similar to the animal models, the cytokines peak within a few hours and then decline rapidly to undetectable plasma levels [1,16]. Both TNF and IL-1 have been infused into patients as trials of cancer therapy. Such treatment has not been efficacious in terms of malignant disease but have given insights into toxicity. Not surprisingly, fever, rigors and malaise developed; however, the dose-limiting toxicity was hypotension [17]. The only wild-type infection in which a defined cytokine cascade has been detected in human plasma relates to the Jarisch–Herxheimer reaction (J-HR) of relapsing fever [18]. This infection is caused by the organism *Borrelia recurrentis* which can be detected by microscopy of blood smears taken from infected subjects. Following treatment with penicillin there is a very clearly defined clinical syndrome, J-HR, consisting of fever with rigors, hypotension and a sudden drop in peripheral blood white cell count. Measurement of plasma cytokines during the evolution of this syndrome showed that plasma TNF rose soon after the injection of penicillin and preceded coincidental peaks of IL-6 and IL-8 (Fig. 1). Interestingly, the rise in plasma TNF concentration preceded the elevation of body temperature and rigors, whereas elevation of IL-6 and IL-8 concentrations coincided with the development of symptoms.

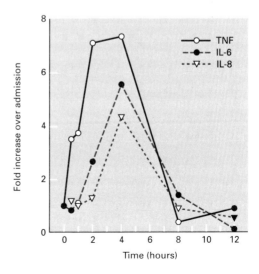

Fig. 1 Kinetics of cytokine release in the Jarisch–Herxheimer of louse-borne relapsing fever. Data are expressed as fold increase over admission levels of tumour necrosis factor (TNF) and interleukins-6 and 8 (IL-6 and IL-8) measured in plasma. Compared with baseline levels. TNF showed the most rapid induction, and attained the greatest relative increase. The TNF level was significantly increased over baseline by 1 hour, IL-6 by 2 hours and IL-8 by 4 hours. Reproduced with permission of *J Exp Med*.

ANTICYTOKINE THERAPIES

Several studies have revealed protective effects of monoclonal antibodies directed against TNF (see review [1]). These studies have involved mouse, pig and baboon models. From these studies it is apparent, however, that at the same time as TNF bioactivity may be completely removed from plasma of these animals, plasma levels of other cytokines, such as IL-6, are attenuated, suggesting that TNF has an important paracrine effect of inducing the release of other cytokines [19]. Polyclonal ovine antiserum directed against human TNF given to patients experiencing the J-HR of relapsing fever ablates many of the adverse symptoms (Warrell, personal communication). However, in general, many of the human studies involving anti-TNF in the intensive care sepsis situation have been very disappointing and the early hope of such a definitive mode of therapy has greatly diminished. In addition, it has been shown that the receptors for TNF and IL-1 leave the cell membrane and exist in soluble form in the circulation. Such molecules are endogenous inhibitors of their specific cytokine ligand. IL-1 receptor antagonist is one such molecule on which early experiments demonstrated protective efficacy in animal models of septic shock but which were very disappointing in the human clinical situation.

The role of cytokines in appropriate and protective immune responses evoked in animal models of infection is now becoming clearer. In non-lethal *Listeria monocytogenes* infection of mice, treatment with anti-TNF monoclonal antibodies results in mortality [20]. In addition, humoral responses to oral *Salmonella typhimurium* in a mouse model of infection are greatly diminished by pretreatment with monoclonal antibody directed against TNF (Dougan, personal communication). Thus the benefit of any strategy directed against cytokines in a specific clinical situation must be weighed against deleterious side-effects, the most serious of which appears to be the ability to mount an appropriate immune response.

CYTOKINES AND INTRACELLULAR PARASITES

Macrophages are the principal cells of the immune system which encounter and phagocytose infecting organisms and cell debris. Since macrophages is potent cytokine producers it is hardly surprising that these cells respond to phagocytosis of microbial organisms they ingest with the production of cytokines. It is very likely that the particular pattern of cytokines which is evolved is then responsible for discrete tissue reactions, for example, granuloma formation [21]. Granulomas consist of cells of the monocyte lineage, including epithelial cells, multinucleate giant cells and antigen-specific T-cells. Following phagocytosis of *mycobactèria*, for example, such granulomas are the hallmark of the tissue response. Their formation and maintenance are brought about by specific cell–cell contact under the paracrine influence of cytokines. This is likely to be mediated by the specific interaction of cytokine-induced adhesion molecules on the surface of the cells. The purpose of such granuloma formation is to contain the microorganism and another principal role of cytokines in this respect is to activate the macrophage to restrict mycobacterial replication within the cell. In the latter respect interferon-γ (IFN-γ) appears to be the key up-regulatory molecule acting in synergy with TNF. The production of TNF by macrophage cell lines is a transient phenomenon resulting in a burst peak of TNF production with very similar kinetics to that induced by LPS [22]. IL-6, a potent stimulus of the acute-phase protein response and T-cell activation, is thought to be of particular significance in terms of the mediation of the whole-body and cellular response to mycobacterial infection. For example, IL-6 enhances the antimycobacterial activity of murine macrophages and some *Mycobacterium avium-intracellulare* are capable of down-regulating IL-6 release [23], suggesting that IL-6 might be a crucial part of host defence [24]. Components of mycobacteria responsible for activating macrophages are currently being investigated. The major cell-wall component with such activity is lipoarabinomannan (LAM), a molecule similar to LPS. Interestingly, LAM has been shown to bind to CD14, the LPS receptor, and it may well be that after binding to this ligand, common intracellular signalling pathways are involved, resulting in the generation of cytokines.

In order for granulomata to form, one of the major driving factors is the production of chemotactic cytokines which attract mononuclear cells to the site of phagocytosis. In this respect the principal chemotactic cytokines involved have been shown to be monocyte chemotactic protein-1 (MCP-1) and IL-8. Macrophages have evolved mechanisms whereby the simple act of phagocytosis does not simply result in an identical pattern of evolution of cytokine production and release but is specific for different particles. Thus, whilst phagocytosis of latex particles, zymosan and mycobacteria all induce similar MCP-1 production, these agents vary greatly in their ability to induce IL-8 secretion [25]. Phagocytosis of *M. tuberculosis* was demonstrated to be a very potent stimulus for IL-8 secretion, with 8–15 times more IL-8 being secreted by THP-1 cells after this mode of stimulation than by LPS. Inert particles such as latex or, to some extent, zymosan caused much less release of IL-8 following phagocytosis being undetectable for latex. Interestingly, monoclonal antibodies directed against murine TNF-α inhibit the formation of hepatic granulomata in tail vein-infected mice, suggesting a pivotal role of this proinflammatory cytokine in this model [26].

THERAPY OF INFECTIOUS DISEASES USING CYTOKINES

Since some cytokines exert powerful effects in inducing specific appropriate protective immune cell activation, it is not surprising that their use has been employed in animal models of infection and more recently in chronic human infections. The principal example of a cytokine investigated and used in this way is IFN-γ. This cytokine induces activation in macrophages and increases their ability to kill intracellular pathogens such as *Mycobacterium* and *Leishmania* species. IFN-γ has been injected via the subcutaneous route into lesions of lepromatous leprosy. Biopsy of these infected lesions has revealed a brisk infiltration of CD4-positive lymphocytes and monocytes, followed by a reduction in mycobacterial load but no inhibition of granuloma formation [27]. Trials are currently underway using systemic IFN-γ in disease caused by *Mycobacterium* tuberculosis, particularly that induced by human immunodeficiency virus (HIV). The use of IFN-γ has potentially very great significance in the management of patients infected with multidrug-resistant mycobacterial infection, for which there are currently few therapeutic options.

The rationale for using IFN-γ for therapy of *Leishmania* ingestion is very strong and based on *in vitro* animal and clinical data [28]. Clinical trials with IFN-γ have shown great promise in the field in which this agent has been used as an adjunct to chemotherapy. This is likely to be particularly important in patients with T-cell deficiency, for example, HIV-infected patients who are subject to leishmanial infection. In addition, two other cytokines have been suggested to be of use in conjunction with IFN-γ, namely IL-2 and granulocyte-macrophage colony-stimulating factor (GM-CSF). These agents may induce anti-leishmanial activity by cytotoxic T-cell stimulation, diminishing leukopenia and enhancing human macrophage anti-leishmanial activity. Delivery mechanisms for IFN-γ are currently being investigated to optimize activity. The clinical use of IFN has already received product licence and is in clinical use in the management of chronic carriage of hepatitis B [29]. In this condition subcutaneous pulsed administration of IFN-α has demonstrated clinical efficacy in many trials. Approximately 40% of patients benefit from such treatment in that their carriage of hepatitis B e antigen can be permanently reversed. Under these conditions replication of hepatitis B is inhibited in the first stage and subsequently the presentation of viral proteins by hepatocytes is thought to induce a cytotoxic T-cell response which eliminates infected hepatocytes.

ACKNOWLEDGEMENTS

George E. Griffin acknowledges support from the Medical Research

Council, the Wellcome Trust and the Association of Physicians. Acknowledgements are extended to Dr Robin Shattock, Dr Jon Friedland and Dr Derek Macallan for helpful discussion and support.

REFERENCES

1 Remick DG. Cytokines and septic shock. In: *Clinical Infectious Diseases: Cytokines in Infection*, vol. 1, edited by Griffin GE. Baillière Tindall, London, 1994:37–50.

2 Remick DG, Strieter RM, Eskandari MK *et al*. Role of tumor necrosis factor-alpha in lipopolysaccharide-induced pathologic alterations. *Am J Pathol* 1990;**136**:49–60.

3 Mozes T, Ben-Efraim S, Tak CJ *et al*. Serum levels of tumor necrosis factor determine the fatal or non-fatal course of endotoxic shock. *Immunol Lett* 1991;**27**:157–162.

4 Klosterhalfen B, Hortmann-Jungemann K, Vogel P *et al*. Time course of various inflammatory mediators during recurrent endotoxaemia. *Biochem Pharmacol* 1992;**43**:2103–2109.

5 Mayoral JL, Schweich CJ, Dunn DL. Decreased tumor necrosis factor production during the initial stages of infection correlates with survival during murine Gram-negative sepsis. *Arch Surg* 1990;**125**:24–27.

6 Fong Y, Tracey KJ, Moldawer LL *et al*. Antibodies to cachectin/tumor necrosis factor reduce interleukin 1 beta and interleukin 6 appearance during lethal bacteremia. *J Exp Med* 1989;**170**:1627–1633.

7 Ulich TR, Guo KZ, Irwin B *et al*. Endotoxin-induced cytokine gene expression *in vivo*. II. Regulation of tumor necrosis factor ad interleukin-a alpha/beta expression and suppression. *Am J Pathol* 1990;**137**:1173–1185.

8 Creasey AA, Stevens P, Kenney J *et al*. Endotoxin and cytokine profile in plasma of baboons challenged with lethal and sublethal *Escherichia coli*. *Circul Shock* 1991;**33**:84–91.

9 Redl H, Schlag G, Bahrami S *et al*. Plasma neutrophil-activating peptide-1/interleukin-8 and neutrophil elastase in a primate bacteremia model. *J Infect Dis* 1991;**164**:383–388.

10 Giroir BP, Johnson JH, Brown T *et al*. The tissue distribution of tumour necrosis factor biosynthesis during endotoxaemia. *J Clin Invest* 1991;**90**:693–698.

11 Mathison JC, Virca GD, Wolfson E *et al*. Adaptation to bacterial lipopolysaccharide controls lipopolysaccharide induced tumour necrosis factor production in rabbit macrophages. *J Clin Invest* 1990;**85**:1108–1118.

12 Waage A, Halstenen A, Espevik T, Brandtzaeg P. Cytokines in meningococcal disease. In: *Clinical Infectious Diseases*, vol. 1, edited by Griffin GE. Baillière Tindall, London 1994:97–108.

13 Waage A, Halsensen A, Espevik T. Association between tumour necrosis factor in serum and fatal outcome in patients with meningococcal disease. *Lancet* 1987;**1**(8529):355–357.

14 McGuire W, Hill AVS, Allsopp EM, Greenwood BM, Kwjatkowski D. Variation in the TNF-α promoter region associated with susceptibility to cerebral malaria. *Nature* 1994;**371**:508–511.

15 Friedland JS, Suputtamongkol Y, Remick DG *et al*. Prolonged elevation of interleukin-8 and interleukin-6 concentrations in plasma and of leukocyte interleukin-8 mRNA levels during septicaemic and localised *Pseudomonas pseudomallei* infection. *Infect Immun* 1992;**60**:2402–2408.

16 Michie HR, Manogue KR, Spriggs DR *et al*. Detection of circulating tumour necrosis factor after endotoxin administration. *N Engl J Med* 1988;**318**:1481–1486.

17 Saks S, Rosenblum M. Recombinant human TNF-alpha; preclinical studies and results from early clinical trials. In: *Tumour Necrosis Factor: Structure, Function and Mechanisms of Action*, edited by Aggarwal BB, Vilcek J. Marcel Dekker, New York, 1993:567–587.

18 Negussie Y, Remick DG, De Forge LE *et al*. Detection of plasma tumour necrosis factor, interleukin-6 and interleukin-8 during the Jarisch–Herxheimer reaction of relapsing fever. *J Exp Med* 1992;**175**:1207–1212.

19 Sharma RJ, Macallan DC, Sedgewick P *et al*. Kinetics of endotoxin induced acute phase

protein gene expression and its modulation by TNF-α monoclonal antibody. *Am J Physiol* 1992;**262**:R786–R793.

20 Havell EA. Evidence that tumour necrosis factor has an important role in antibacterial resistance. *J Immunol* 1989;**143**:2894–2899.

21 Friedland JS. Mycobacteria, chronic inflammation and granuloma formation In: *Clinical Infectious Diseases, Cytokines in Infection*, vol. 1, edited by Griffin GE. Baillière Tindall, London, 1994:51–64.

22 Friedland JS, Shattock RR, Johnson J *et al*. Differential cytokine gene expression and secretion after phagocytosis by a human monocyte cell line of *Toxoplasma gondii* and *Mycobacterium tuberculosis*. *Clin Exp Immunol* 1993;**91**:282–286.

23 Shiratsuchi H, Johnson JL, Ellner JJ. Bidirectional effects of cytokines on the growth of *Mycobacterium avium* within human monocytes. *J Immunol* 1991;**140**:3971–3977.

24 Denis M. Growth of *Mycobacterium avium* in human monocytes: identification of cytokines which reduce and enhance intracellular microbial growth. *Eur J Immunol* 1991;**21**:391–395.

25 Friedland JS, Shattock R, Griffin GE. Phagocytosis of *M. tuberculosis* or particulate stimuli by human monocytic cells induced equivalent MCP-1 gene expression. *Cytokine* 1993;**5**:150–156.

26 Kindler V, Sappino A, Grau GE *et al*. The inducing role of tumour necrosis factor in development of bactericidal granulomas during BCG infection. *Cell* 1989;**56**:731–740.

27 Kaplan G, Mathur NK, Kob CK *et al*. Effect of multiple interferon α injections on the disposal of *Mycobacterium leprae*. *Proc Natl Acad Sci USA* 1989;**86**:8073–8077.

28 Murray HW. Cytokines in the treatment of leishmaniasis. In: *Clinical Infectious Diseases: Cytokines in Infection*, vol. 1, edited by Griffin GE. Baillière Tindall, 1994:127–143.

29 Foster GR, Jacyna MR, Thomas HC. Interferon treatment of hepatitis. In: *Clinical Infectious Diseases: Cytokines in Infection*, vol. 1, edited by Griffin GE. Baillière Tindall, London, 1994:145–149.

MULTIPLE CHOICE QUESTIONS

1 Tumour necrosis factor
a is an effective anticancer agent
b causes hypotension in humans
c reduces human immunodeficiency virus (HIV) transcription in macrophages
d may act in an autocrine fashion
e is produced by endothelial cells

2 Tumour necrosis factor
a is detected in plasma of normal individuals
b is often absent in plasma of patients admitted with septic shock
c has a long plasma half-life
d can be blocked by monoclonal antibodies with therapeutic efficacy in rheumatoid arthritis
e has been associated with weight loss

Answers

	1		2	
a	False		a	False
b	True		b	True
c	False		c	False
d	True		d	True
e	True		e	True

Immunoendocrine interactions in chronic infection — a clue to the pathogenesis of tuberculosis?

GRAHAM A. W. ROOK &
ROGELIO HERNANDEZ-PANDO

SUMMARY

There are numerous ways in which the endocrine system interacts with the immune response. The balance of hormones within lymphoid tissue, some derived locally from circulating prohormones, regulates the type of response that is first generated. Then cytokines released as a consequence of immunological activity cause systemic feedback from the hypothalamo–pituitary–adrenal axis (HPA). It is likely that this feedback can influence the balance of type 1 to type 2 T-cell-derived cytokines, partly via changes in relative levels of glucocorticoid and antiglucocorticoid steroids. Long-term changes in the HPA axis may play an important role in the tendency for type 1 to type 2 shift in chronic infections. The HPA axis also regulates the toxicity of cytokines, and failure of rapid feedback exacerbates such toxicity. Recent findings in human and murine tuberculosis using gas chromatography and mass spectrometry have demonstrated profound alterations in adrenal function that have been missed by studies that have been confined to serum cortisol levels. This disease is therefore used to illustrate the role of these immunoendocrine interactions.

THE CYTOKINE–HYPOTHALAMO–PITUITARY–ADRENAL AXIS

The pioneering observations of Besedovsky and Sorkin in the 1970s proved that there is a two-way flow of information between the immune system and the HPA axis, though this has tended to be ignored until recently [1]. Rats were immunized with sheep erythrocytes, and a peak of antibody-forming cells in the spleen was observed 5–8 days later. However, there was simultaneously a peak in serum cortisol, a trough in thyroxine and a threefold increase in the firing rate of neurons in the ventromedial hypothalamic nuclei. Equally striking was the poor response to a second immunogen given at the time of the cortisol peak. This antigenic competition was eliminated by adrenalectomy. The cytokines tumour necrosis factor-α (TNF-α), interleukin-1 (IL-1) and IL-6 have been identified as important mediators of the HPA axis in response to activation of the immune system *in vivo* [2]. In general, these cytokines act by causing release of corticotrophin-releasing hormone (CRH) from the parvocellular cells of the paraventricular nucleus (PVN). This in turn leads to adrenocorticotrophic hormone (ACTH) production by the corticotrophs in the anterior pituitary. However, recent studies reveal that there is another pathway which can activate the pituitary adrenal axis, because in the chronic phase of adjuvant arthritis, levels of messenger RNA for CRH, and the levels of CRH peptide in hypophyseal portal blood, are in fact below normal, but increased production of ACTH and glucocorticoids persists [3]. It is probable that arginine vasopressin (AVP), also derived from the parvocellular cells in the PVN, takes over some of the role of CRH during chronic inflammatory states.

THE CYTOKINE–HPA AXIS AND MANIFESTATIONS OF AUTOIMMUNITY

The fundamental importance of the cytokine–HPA axis has been obvious in models of autoimmunity for several years. Table 1 lists some experimental systems in which this can be demonstrated. The most striking is the susceptibility of the Lewis rat to experimental autoimmune encephalitis (EAE) and to a form of adjuvant arthritis [4,5]. Susceptibility correlates

Table 1 Defects in the hypothalamo–pituitary–adrenal (HPA) axis associated with autoimmune manifestations.

	Disease	Defect in cytokine–HPA axis
Animal		
Lewis rats	EAE and arthritis	Low IL-1α-induced ACTH release due to defect in CRH release
Obese chicken	Thyroiditis	IL-1 production OK. Block in hypothalamo–pituitary axis
NOD mice	Diabetes	Low TNF-α and IL-1α from macrophages Giving either cytokine inhibits insulitis
BB rat	Diabetes and thyroiditis	Low IL-1α from macrophages. Steroid response to recombinant IL-1 is OK
Human		
Rheumatoid arthritis	Autoantibody and arthritis, etc.	Hypothalamic defect. Pituitary–adrenal OK
Tuberculosis	Autoantibody and arthritis	Flat cortisol rhythm, variable ACTH response. Low DHEA. Liable to tuberculin shock. Striking adrenal atrophy

EAE, Experimental autoimmune encephalitis; IL-1α, interleukin-1α; ACTH, adrenocorticotrophic hormone; CRH, corticotrophin-releasing hormone; TNF-α, tumour necrosis factor-α; DHEA, dehydroepiandrosterone.

with inadequate feedback via the HPA axis. In susceptible rats IL-1 evokes less corticosterone production than it does in resistant rats. Susceptible rats can be rendered resistant by boosting the glucocorticoid levels at the early stage of disease induction. Similarly, resistant rats can be made susceptible by reducing corticosterone production. Recently evidence has accumulated that suggests a similar defect in human rheumatoid arthritis [6].

These findings are widely accepted, yet few workers have extended this thinking to chronic infectious disease. This is odd because infections such as tuberculosis and leprosy are accompanied by precisely the same manifestations of autoimmunity as are seen in rheumatoid arthritis, and there is even overlap with features of systemic lupus erythematosus [7]. If endocrine factors regulate autoimmunity in models of autoimmune disease, may they not also be relevant to the same types of autoimmunity occurring in tuberculosis and leprosy?

THE CYTOKINE–HPA AXIS AND CYTOKINE-MEDIATED IMMUNOPATHOLOGY

Another crucial role of the cytokine–HPA axis is in the limitation of acute tissue damage mediated by cytokines. The toxicity or lethality of cytokines such as TNF-α, or of cytokine triggers such as endotoxin, is enormously enhanced if feedback via the cytokine–HPA axis is compromised. Inhibition of cytokine-mediated tissue damage requires rapid peaks of cortisol in response to the cytokine release [8,9]. Toxicity and lethality are enhanced if adrenal function is subnormal. However, this feedback is regulated at many other levels. For instance, IL-1 is a major mediator of the feedback from inflammatory sites to the hypothalamus, and induction of gluco-corticoid production by endotoxin can be blocked by administration of the IL-1 receptor antagonist (IL-1ra), which is a physiological competitive inhibitor of IL-1 [10–12]. The potential relevance of this mechanism becomes clear when one remembers that production of IL-1ra is a type 2 phenomenon. It is increased by IL-10 [13], soluble CD23 [14], IL-13 [15] and IL-4 [16,17]. Therefore activation of inappropriate Th2 cells, leading to increased production of these type 2 cytokines, will tend to block the feedback from the cytokine network via the hypothalamus, and cytokine-mediated tissue damage would be expected to be more severe when the immune response has undergone a type 1 to type 2 shift. Evidence that this is indeed the case is outlined later.

THE ROLE OF THE ENDOCRINE SYSTEM IN THE REGULATION OF THE TH1/TH2 BALANCE

Under some circumstances, CD4+ T lymphocytes differentiate into cells

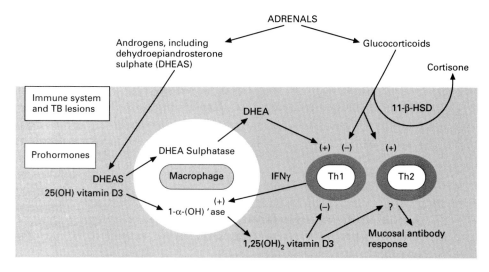

Fig. 1 The complex interaction of hormones and locally activated prohormones within antigen-stimulated lymphoid tissue. The complexity of the modifications of steroids that take place in the periphery is greatly simplified. As mentioned in the main text, 7-hydroxylated derivatives of dehydroepiandrosterone (DHEA) may be crucial. Enzymes that can inactivate glucocorticoids such as 11β-hydroxysteroid dehydrogenase (11β-HSD) may also be present in lymphoid tissue.

releasing predominantly IL-2 and interferon-γ (IFN–γ) or IL-4 and IL-5. The former (Th1) tend to drive correlates of cell-mediated immunity (CMI) such as macrophage activation and induction of cytotoxic T-cells (CD8+ CTL), whereas the latter (Th2) tend to drive antibody production, and in extreme cases, immunoglobulin E (IgE) and eosinophilia. In reality CD8+ cells can also be Th1-like or Th2-like in terms of cytokine release patterns, and cytokines such as IL-10 can be released from cells that are not T-cells, although tending to drive a Th2 pattern. Similarly, IL-12 is not a T-cell product, yet it tends to drive a Th1 pattern. Therefore the preferred terminology is type 1 and type 2, where type 1 refers to a pattern of cytokine release leading to CMI, and including IFN-γ, IL-2 and IL-12, from whatever source, and type 2 includes IL-10, IL-4 and IL-5, from whatever source. The endocrine system plays a key role in predetermining the Th1/Th2 balance that develops following immunization, and can also be shown to play a role in causing shifts from type 1 towards type 2 in established immune responses. Some of this regulation of the type of immune response involves conversion of circulating prohormones into active metabolites in the periphery (Fig. 1).

Peripheral conversion of prohormones and Th1/Th2 regulation

Dehydroepiandrosterone sulphate (DHEAS) is the major adrenal steroid in the serum of both men and women. Specific receptors for the free hormone (DHEA) are found in T-cells [18]. A single injection of DHEA before a large dose of dexamethasone can almost completely block the ability of the dexamethasone to cause apoptosis of thymocytes and unresponsiveness of peripheral T-cells [19]. This antiglucocorticoid effect is indirectly Th1-enhancing because glucocorticoids preferentially suppress Th1 activity, and can synergize with Th2 cytokines such as IL-4. Moreover, DHEA also directly enhances Th1 T-cell activity. It was found that the balance of Th1 to Th2 cytokines released from normal mouse lymphoid tissue in response to anti-CD3 is related to the DHEA sulphatase activity in each lymphoid compartment [20]. DHEA levels fall to very low levels in old age, and DHEA supplements can correct many of the immunological defects and excessive cytokine release seen in old mice [21,22], and cause clear immunological changes in postmenopausal women [23].

Not only may changes in DHEAS sulphatase affect Th1 T-cell activity, but also loss of circulating DHEAS, if sufficiently gross, may deprive the enzyme of substrate (reviewed in [24]). A fall in serum DHEAS heralds the down-grading from human immunodeficiency virus (HIV)-positive to acquired immunodeficiency syndrome (AIDS) [25], regarded by many as at least partly attributable to loss of Th1 activity.

Not all of the effects of DHEA are directly attributable to DHEA itself, and some are demonstrable *in vivo* but not *in vitro*. This implies that further downstream metabolites are involved. Particular attention is being paid to certain 7-hydroxylated derivatives [26,27] that are generated in the skin and in the stromal cells of adipose tissue [28].

25-hydroxy cholecalciferol as immunoregulatory prohormone

Another major prohormone, 25-hydroxy cholecalciferol ($25(OH)D_3$) may have the reverse effect on Th1/Th2 balance (Fig. 2). There is intense conversion of $25(OH)D_3$ to $1,25(OH)_2D_3$ (calcitriol) in the lesions of chronic T-cell-dependent inflammatory disorders such as tuberculosis or sarcoidosis [29]. Calcitriol is best known for its systemic effects on calcium balance, but hypercalcaemia, although it can occur, is uncommon in tuberculosis and sarcoidosis [29]. Therefore calcitriol can act independently in the systemic and lymphoid compartments in which it exerts entirely unrelated functions, with little cross-talk between the two. This is an important fundamental principle which may be relevant to our thinking about the roles of several other hormones. In the lymphoid compartments calcitriol is an important regulator of T-cell function. It decreases output of IL-2 and IFN-γ [30]. Calcitriol cannot be used systemically to obtain this down-regulation of Th1 activity because at immunologically relevant doses it causes severe hypercalcaemia. However, new calcitriol analogues such as KH1060 from Leo Pharmaceuticals have increased effects on

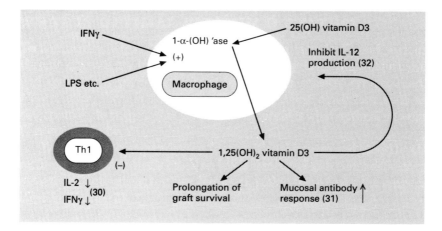

Fig. 2 The multiple immunological roles of calcitriol. It is not yet clear how many of the effects are secondary to its ability to decrease production of interleukin-12 from monocytes and B-cells. Numbers in parentheses refer to references.

T-cells relative to their effects on calcium balance, so they can be given systemically (Touraine, personal communication). They prove to rival cyclosporin A in their ability to prolong skin graft survival by inhibiting Th1 activity, while sparing antibody production, and their effects are additive, perhaps synergistic with those of cyclosporin.

One striking new finding may be interpreted as an effect of calcitriol on lymphocyte homing. When calcitriol is administered peripherally with or shortly after antigen, it evokes a response which tends to localize to mucosal surfaces [31], resulting in high IgA titres and mucosal immunity. Thus, mucosal immunity can be evoked by merely painting calcitriol on to skin sharing lymphatic drainage with the immunization site. Following exposure to calcitriol, the draining node behaves temporarily like gut-associated lymphoid tissue [31].

It is probable that some of the immunoregulatory effects of calcitriol are attributable to its ability to switch off production of the Th1-promoting cytokine IL-12 [32].

Regulation of the prohormone-converting enzymes

We know remarkably little about the regulation of 1α-hydroxylase in lymph node macrophages. It is up-regulated in human macrophages exposed to IFN-γ or to bacterial components such as lipopolysaccharides, and the enzyme is also present in murine lymphoid tissues (Rook *et al.*, unpublished observations).

We know still less about the regulation of DHEA sulphatase. This is a microsomal enzyme, and it is not clear how the DHEAS, which cannot cross membranes, gains access to it. Does the enzyme shuttle backwards and forwards to the cell surface? Investigating the regulation of the enzyme is proving remarkably difficult. Levels are high in triton X-100 lysates of the human macrophage lines U937 and MonoMac 6, but absent from murine J774 macrophages, in which we have been unable to induce it. When present, the activity of intact cultured cells is less than 1% of that of triton X-100 lysates. Thus, trivial changes in cell viability and permeability cause huge problems for *in vitro* studies of stimuli that might increase or decrease the activity of intact cells (Setloboko and Rook, unpublished observations). The recent discovery of potent inhibitors of the enzyme [33] will facilitate rapid dissection of its immunological role *in vivo*. Meanwhile there is one claim that certain cytokines will down-regulate the enzyme in macrophages [34].

SWITCHING ESTABLISHED CELL-MEDIATED RESPONSES FROM TYPE 1 TO TYPE 2

Immunity to most chronic infections requires the Th1 pattern of cytokine release. Under some circumstances the type 1 response is stable, but at other times it is readily suppressed and replaced by type 2. This type 1 to type 2 shift is a crucial step in the pathogenesis of many chronic infections such as syphilis, schistosomiasis, leishmaniasis and the mycobacterioses (referenced in [24]). For instance, in tuberculosis a type 1 response is protective, but patients, in whom immunity has evidently failed, can have an IgE response to *Mycobacterium tuberculosis*, eosinophilia and circulating T-cells that release IL-4 in response to a specific antigen of *M. tuberculosis*, and circulating T-cells expressing the IL-4 gene (discussed in [35]). Similarly, there has been speculation that the appearance of HIV sero-positivity in individuals exposed to HIV represents a detrimental shift from Th1 to Th2, since loss of Th1 cytokine release by peripheral blood lymphocytes (PBL) precedes loss of Th2 cytokine release, and individuals (homosexuals, haemophiliacs, needlestick health care workers and babies born to HIV-positive mothers) who remain healthy after many years of exposure to HIV tend to have T-cells that secrete IL-2 in response to HIV-derived peptides, but no antibody response [36,37]. If this — currently controversial — view proves correct, the mechanisms leading to such switching will be of crucial contemporary importance.

Defective cytokine–HPA axis during chronic infection

Since disruption of the cytokine-HPA axis is one obvious way to distort immunoregulation and the type 1/type 2 cytokine balance, it is not surprising that a number of infectious agents appear to have evolved ways of doing this, and no doubt more will be found as we start to look. Figure 3

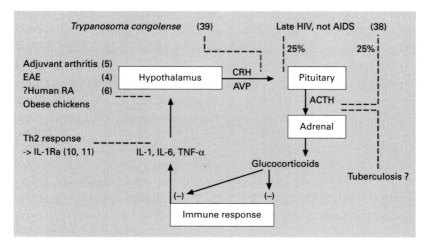

Fig. 3 Tentative map of sites where there is a block in the cytokine–hypothalamo–pituitary–adrenal (HPA) axis in chronic infection. Numbers in parentheses refer to references.

illustrates some points in the cytokine–HPA axis where the block appears to occur. For instance, attempts to unravel the site of the defects in the HPA axis in HIV infection without AIDS suggest that 25% have reduced pituitary reserve, while 25% have reduced adrenal reserve [38]. Cattle infected with *Trypanosoma congolense* show reduced cortisol response to CRH, but normal response to ACTH, suggesting changes at the pituitary level [39].

The cytokine–HPA in tuberculosis

It has long been suspected that there is abnormal adrenal function in tuberculosis, mainly because of the occurrence of sudden death during treatment, resembling acute adrenal insufficiency [40]. Attempts to prove it have been limited to measuring early-morning serum cortisol, and testing changes in serum cortisol following administration of synthetic ACTH. Such studies have given equivocal results [41]. However, using gas chromatography and mass spectrometry to quantify and identify the steroid output in 24-hour urine collections, we have established that there is a profound deficit in adrenal function in human tuberculosis, except in very early disease [42]. Output of glucocorticoid derivatives and androgen derivatives is reduced by approximately 50%. Nevertheless, cortisol levels are maintained, while DHEAS levels are not. As explained above, this constitutes a stimulus for type 1-to-type 2 shift. The findings in humans are reinforced by the observation that, when mice are infected with tuberculosis by the intratracheal route, the adrenals increase in size for 2 weeks and then decrease to 50% of their normal weight [43]. This is an early stage of the lung infection, and the adrenals themselves are not directly infected. The mechanism leading to the atrophy is uncertain, but we have found that mycobacteria contain factors that disturb adrenal cell function *in vitro*. Other possible mechanisms are discussed later.

It is now apparent why the earlier investigations missed the striking abnormalities of the adrenals in tuberculosis. First, the patients' serum cortisol is usually relatively normal, and the same is true of tetra-hydrocortisol levels we have detected in the urine. However, this is because cortisol is not being catabolized normally. In patients there is little dehydrogenation of the 11β-hydroxyl group, or reduction of the ketone on carbon 20. Thus there is little conversion to cortisone derivatives or cortols. The *total* output of glucocorticoids and of adrenal androgens is in fact down by ~ 50%. Secondly, the standard short Synacthen test uses 250 μg of synthetic ACTH. This is a vast dose, since physiological ACTH levels are in the picogram range. A response that is 70% maximal can be evoked in normal people with as little as 150 ng [44] and 500 ng evokes maximal cortisol output. The short Synacthen test is therefore a poor measure of the adrenal response to physiological levels of ACTH. We now suggest, therefore, that there is a profound and early change in adrenal function in tuberculosis that can contribute to a Th1-to-Th2 switch and, as explained later, to enhanced immunopathology.

Stress, the adrenals and the type 1 to type 2 switch

Endocrine effects on the immune response can also be triggered by stress. As little as 5 minutes of restraint stress cause readily apparent increased expression of messenger RNA for c-*fos* and CRH in the rat hypothalamus [45]. Students stressed by their exams show increased titres of antibody to Epstein–Barr virus, implying transient reactivation of the latent infection which is normally controlled by CTL (reviewed in [46]). This could imply that stress drives a Th1-to-Th2 switch. A study of the consequences of an intensely stressful training course to which the US Rangers are exposed (E. W. Bernton, personal communication) showed that thyroid hormone levels fell so dramatically (as in Besedovsky's early studies, where antigen rather than stress was the stimulus) that the subjects became clinically hypothyroid. Testosterone levels fell to castrate levels. From an immuno-logical point of view it is particularly important to note that the ratio of DHEAS to cortisol fell, and that there was loss of delayed hypersensitivity (DTH) responses with relative sparing of humoral immunity. This also suggested that stress drives a shift in the Th1/Th2 balance towards Th2. The stress of chronic infections is therefore one more factor tending to distort the Th1 response.

Cytokines and adrenal function

There is a second set of endocrine changes in chronic infectious disease which may contribute to the shift from type 1 to the type 2 cytokine pattern that is often seen in these situations. The changes may be attributable to TNF-α, and to other cytokines released with it, because *in vitro* at least, TNF-α acts directly on the adrenal to reduce steroid output [47]. In particular, TNF-α causes a dose-related reduction of DHEAS production by human fetal adrenal *in vitro* [47]. Transforming growth factor-β (TGF-β) has a similar effect and, like TNF-α, it inhibits DHEAS more than cortisol [48]. This may be important because TGF-β is also abundant in tuberculous lesions and has been implicated in the suppressive effects of patients' monocytes *in vitro*. Thus, these cytokine-mediated effects could partly explain the adrenal changes seen in tuberculosis.

On the other hand, as outlined earlier, once a switch towards a Th2 pattern of response has occurred, there may be an excess of cytokine inhibitors (such as IL-1ra and soluble TNF-α receptors) over free cytokine, so feedback to the hypothalamus could be compromised. These two mutually exclusive possibilities can clearly be distinguished, but available data using immunoassays do not tell us whether there is net functional cytokine, or net excess of inhibitor in the sera of tuberculosis patients.

THE CONSEQUENCES OF TH1-TO-TH2 SWITCHING

One consequence of an inappropriate Th1-to-Th2 switch is persistent infection and disease progression. This is seen in *Leishmania* infection in Balb/c mice, in the mycobacterioses and in secondary syphilis. Even when the Th1 cytokines continue to be produced, their efficacy is reduced if Th2 cytokines are also present. This may be due in part to the ability of IL-4 and IL-10 to oppose macrophage-activating effects of IFN-γ and TNF-α. It may also result from the inability of the immune system to develop CD8+ cytotoxic T-cell activity when the underlying Th1 response is undergoing suppression from a superimposed Th2 response. For instance, mice in this phase of schistosomiasis cannot develop a CTL response to a virus infection [49]. An obvious example in human disease is the hepatitis B carrier state, where a Th1-to-Th2 shift has resulted in massive antibody production, eosinophil infiltration and a lack of protective CTL.

Th1-to-Th2 switching and immunopathology

A second consequence is less obvious, but clinically important. There is evidence that inflammatory lesions mediated by mixed Th1 + Th2 (or Th0?) T-cell activity are susceptible to necrosis. For instance, in murine schistosomiasis there is initially a relatively pure Th1 pattern of response, with priming for release of IFN-γ. Subsequently (when the ova are produced at about day 42), a Th2 response becomes superimposed on this Th1 pattern and release of IL-4 and IL-5 can be demonstrated [50]. At this point tissue damage begins to occur in the granulomata, and further tissue damage can be evoked if systemic cytokine (TNF-α) release is triggered by endotoxin [51]. Then from day 84 the Th2 component starts to decline, the Th1 component returns and the granulomata promptly become less tissue-damaging.

Subsequent studies have confirmed this pathway in a model that uses mycobacterial antigen [35]. Direct injection of TNF-α into T-cell-mediated DTH responses to mycobacterial antigen often causes necrosis. The effect is dependent on CD4+ T cells. However, the sensitivity of a DTH skin-test site to a subsequent injection of TNF-α into the same site, depended not on the size of the DTH response but on the immunization schedule. DTH reaction sites elicited in mice with apparently pure Th1 response (and suppressed IL-4 release) are not affected by a subsequent injection of TNF-α, whereas when such DTH sites are elicited in mice with a mixed Th1/Th2 (or perhaps Th0) response, the site is exquisitely sensitive to TNF-α [35].

In tuberculous mice this effect may be exacerbated, because by day 60 not only is there a mixed type 1 + type 2 pattern of cytokine response, but there is also profound adrenal atrophy, as explained earlier. Therefore DTH sites elicited in these animals are not only inherently TNF-α-sensitive, but also unable to benefit from the protective effect of efficient corticosterone feedback.

CONCLUSIONS

This paper is an attempt to use tuberculosis to illustrate the potential importance of immunoendocrine interactions in chronic infection. There is a tendency for immunologists to confine their thinking to elements that are traditionally regarded as part of the immune system. Physiology, in the sense of the study of emergent properties of interacting complex systems *in vivo*, has become unpopular, and difficult to fund. Nevertheless, these systems do interact, and always have done. They evolved interactively and it is absurd to ignore this interaction. Indeed, it is entirely logical, even if unproven, to suggest that the immunoregulatory disturbance in tuberculosis, leading to tissue damage rather than to microbial functions, is not attributable to a problem within the immune system itself, but rather to inappropriate regulation of the immune system by the endocrine system.

REFERENCES

1 Besedovsky H, Sorkin E. Network of immune–neuroendocrine interactions. *Clin Exp Immunol* 1977;**27**:1–12.

2 Besedovsky HO, del-Rey A, Klusman I *et al.* Cytokines as modulators of the hypothalamus–pituitary–adrenal axis. *J Steroid Biochem Mol Biol* 1991;**40**:613–618.

3 Harbuz MS, Rees RG, Eckland D, Jessop DS, Brewerton D, Lightman SL. Paradoxical responses of hypothalamic CRF mRNA and CRF-41 peptide and adenohypophyseal POMC mRNA during chronic inflammatory stress. *Endocrinology* 1992;**130**:1394–1400.

4 Mason D, MacPhee I, Antoni F. The role of the neuroendocrine system in determining genetic susceptibility to experimental allergic encephalomyelitis in the rat. *Immunology* 1990;**70**:1–5.

5 Calogero AE, Sternberg EM, Bagdy G *et al.* Neurotransmitter-induced hypothalamic–pituitary–adrenal axis responsiveness is defective in inflammatory disease-susceptible Lewis rats: *in vivo* and *in vitro* studies suggesting globally defective hypothalamic secretion of corticotropin-releasing hormone. *Neuroendocrinology* 1992;**55**:600–608.

6 Chikanza IC, Petrou P, Kingsley G, Chrousos G, Panayi GS. Defective hypothalamic response to immune and inflammatory stimuli in patients with rheumatoid arthritis. *Arthritis Rheum* 1992;**35**:1281–1288.

7 Rook GAW, Lydyard PM, Stanford JL. A reappraisal of the evidence that rheumatoid arthritis, and several other idiopathic diseases, are slow bacterial infections. *Ann Rheum Dis* 1993;**52**(suppl):S30–S38.

8 Zuckerman SH, Shellhaas J, Butler JD. Differential regulation of lipopolysaccharide-induced interleukin 1 and tumour necrosis factor synthesis; effects of endogenous and exogenous glucocorticoids and the role of the pituitary–adrenal axis. *Eur J Immunol* 1989;**19**:301–305.

9 Bertini R, Bianchi M, Ghezzi P. Adrenalectomy sensitizes mice to the lethal effects of interleukin 1 and tumor necrosis factor. *J Exp Med* 1988;**167**:1708–1712.

10 Schotanus K, Tilders FJ, Berkenbosch F. Human recombinant interleukin-1 receptor antagonist prevents adrenocorticotropin, but not interleukin-6 responses to bacterial endotoxin in rats. *Endocrinology* 1993;**133**:2461–2468.

11 Ebisui O, Fukata J, Murakami N *et al.* Effect of IL-1 receptor antagonist and antiserum to TNF-alpha on LPS-induced plasma ACTH and corticosterone rise in rats. *Am J Physiol* 1994;**266**:E986–E992.

12 Kakucska I, Qi Y, Clark BD, Lechan RM. Endotoxin-induced corticotropin-releasing hormone gene expression in the hypothalamic paraventricular nucleus is mediated centrally by interleukin-1. *Endocrinology* 1993;**133**:815–821.

13 Jenkins JK, Malyak M, Arend WP. The effects of interleukin-10 on interleukin-1 receptor antagonist and interleukin-1 beta production in human monocytes and neutrophils. *Lymphokine Cytokine Res* 1994;**13**:47–54.

14 Herbelin A, Elhadad S, Ouaaz F, de-Groote D, Descamps-Latscha B. Soluble CD23 potentiates interleukin-1-induced secretion of interleukin-6 and interleukin-1 receptor antagonist by human monocytes. *Eur J Immunol* 1994;**24**:1869–1873.

15 Muzio M, Re F, Sironi M *et al.* Interleukin-13 induces the production of interleukin-1 receptor antagonist (IL-1ra) and the expression of the mRNA for the intracellular (keratinocyte) form of IL-1ra in human myelomonocytic cells. *Blood* 1994;**83**:1738–1743.

16 Sone S, Orino E, Mizuno K *et al.* Production of IL-1 and its receptor antagonist is regulated differently by IFN-gamma and IL-4 in human monocytes and alveolar macrophages. *Eur Respir J* 1994;**7**:657–663.

17 Jenkins JK, Arend WP. Interleukin 1 receptor antagonist production in human monocytes is induced by IL-1 alpha, IL-3, IL-4 and GM-CSF. *Cytokine* 1993;**5**:407–415.

18 Meikle AW, Dorchuck RW, Araneo BA *et al.* The presence of a dehydroepiandrosterone-specific receptor-binding complex in murine T cells. *J Steroid Biochem Mol Biol* 1992;**42**:293–304.

19 Blauer KL, Poth M, Rogers WM, Bernton EW. Dehydroepiandrosterone antagonises

the suppressive effects of dexamethasone on lymphocyte proliferation. *Endocrinology* 1991;**129**:3174–3179.

20 Daynes RA, Araneo BA, Dowell TA, Huang K, Dudley D. Regulation of murine lymphokine production *in vivo*. III. The lymphoid tissue microenvironment exerts regulatory influences over T helper cell function. *J Exp Med* 1990;**171**:979–996.

21 Araneo BA, Woods ML, Daynes RA. Reversal of the immunosenescent phenotype by dehydroepiandrosterone: hormone treatment provides an adjuvant effect on the immunization of aged mice with recombinant hepatitis B surface antigen. *J Infect Dis* 1993;**167**:830–846.

22 Daynes RA, Araneo BA, Ershler WB, Maloney C, Li G-Z, Ryu S-Y. Altered regulation of IL-6 production with normal aging; possible linkage to the age-associated decline in dehydroepiandrosterone and its sulphated derivative. *J Immunol* 1993;**150**:5219–5230.

23 Casson PR, Andersen RN, Herrod HG *et al*. Oral dehydroepiandrosterone in physiologic doses modulates immune function in postmenopausal women. *Am J Obstet Gynecol* 1993;**169**:1536–1539.

24 Rook GAW, Onyebujoh P, Stanford JL. TH1→TH2 switch and loss of CD4 cells in chronic infections; an immuno-endocrinological hypothesis not exclusive to HIV. *Immunol Today* 1993;**14**:568–569.

25 Wisniewski TL, Hilton CW, Morse EV, Svec F. The relationship of serum DHEA-S and cortisol levels to measures of immune function in human immunodeficiency virus-related illness. *Am J Med Sci* 1993;**305**:79–83.

26 Morfin R, Courchay G. Pregnenolone and dehydroepiandrosterone as precursors of native 7-hydroxylated metabolites which increase the immune response in mice. *J Steroid Biochem Mol Biol* 1994;**50**:91–100.

27 Padgett DA, Loria RM. *In vitro* potentiation of lymphocyte activation by dehydroepiandrosterone, androstenediol and androstenetriol. *J Immunol* 1994;**153**:1544–1552.

28 Khalil MW, Strutt B, Vachon D, Killinger DW. Effect of dexamethasone and cytochrome P450 inhibitors on the formation of 7 alpha-hydroxydehydroepiandrosterone by human adipose stromal cells. *J Steroid Biochem Mol Biol* 1994;**48**:545–552.

29 Rook GAW. The role of vitamin D in tuberculosis. *Am Rev Respir Dis* 1988;**138**:768–770.

30 Rigby WF, Denome S, Fanger MW. Regulation of lymphokine production and human T lymphocyte activation by 1,25-dihydroxyvitamin D_3. Specific inhibition at the level of messenger RNA. *J Clin Invest* 1987;**79**:1659–1664.

31 Daynes RA, Araneo BA. The development of effective vaccine adjuvants employing natural regulators of T cell lymphokine production *in vivo*. *Ann NY Acad Sci* 1994;**730**:144–161.

32 Lemire JM. Immunomodulatory actions of 1,25-dihydroxyvitamin D3. *J. Steroid Biochem Mol Biol* 1995;**53**:599–602.

33 Howarth NM, Purohit A, Reed MJ, Potter BVL. Estrone sulphamates: potent inhibitors of estrone sulphatase with therapeutic potential. *J Med Chem* 1994;**37**:219–221.

34 Hennebold JD, Daynes RA. Regulation of macrophage dehydroepiandrosterone sulfate metabolism by inflammatory cytokines. *Endocrinology* 1994;**135**:67–75.

35 Hernandez-Pando R, Rook GAW. The role of TNF-α in T cell-mediated inflammation depends on the Th1/Th2 cytokine balance. *Immunology* 1994;**82**:591–595.

36 Meyaard L, Otto SA, Meyaard L, Otto SA, Keet IP, Van LRA, Miedema F. Changes in cytokine secretion patterns of CD4+ T-cell clones in human immunodeficiency virus infection. *Blood* 1994;**84**:4262–4268.

37 Clerici M, Shearer GM. A TH1 to TH2 switch is a critical step in the etiology of HIV infection. *Immunol Today* 1993;**14**:107–111.

38 Azar ST, Melby JC. Hypothalamic–pituitary–adrenal function in non-AIDS patients with advanced HIV infection. *Am J Med Sci* 1993;**305**:321–325.

39 Abebe G, Eley RM, Ole-MoiYoi OK. Reduced responsiveness of the hypothalamic–pituitary–adrenal axis in Boran (*Bos inducus*) cattle infected with *Trypanosoma congolense*. *Acta Endocrinol (Copenh)* 1993;**129**:75–80.

40 Scott GM, Murphy PG, Gemidjioglu ME. Predicting deterioration of treated tuberculosis by corticosteroid reserve and C-reactive protein. *J Infect* 1990;**21**:61–69.

41 Post FA, Soule SG, Willcox PA, Levitt NS. The spectrum of endocrine dysfunction in active pulmonary tuberculosis. *Clin Endocrinol* 1994;**40**:367–371.

42 Rook GAW, Honour J, Kon OM, Wilkinson RJ, Davidson R, Shaw RJ. Urinary steroid metabolites in tuberculosis; a new clue to pathogenesis. *Q J Med* 1996; (in press).

43 Hernandez-Pando R, Orozco H, Honour JP, Silva J, Leyva R, Rook GAW. Adrenal changes in murine pulmonary tuberculosis; a clue to pathogenesis? *FEMS Immunol Med Microbiol* 1995;**12**:63–72.

44 Roberts NA, Barton RN, Horan MA. Ageing and sensitivity of the adrenal gland to physiological doses of ACTH in man. *J Endocrinol* 1990;**126**:507–513.

45 Harbuz MS, Chalmers J, De Sousa L, Lightman SL. Stress-induced activation of CRF and c-fos mRNAs in the paraventricular nucleus are not affected by serotonin depletion. *Brain Res* 1993;**609**:169–173.

46 Zwilling BS. Stress affects disease outcomes. *ASM News* 1992;**58**:23–25.

47 Jaattela M, Ilvesmaki V, Voutilainen R, Stenman UH, Saksela E. Tumor necrosis factor as a potent inhibitor of adrenocorticotropin-induced cortisol production and steroidogenic P450 enzyme gene expression in cultured human fetal adrenal cells. *Endocrinology* 1991;**128**:623–629.

48 Stankovic AK, Dion LD, Parker CR. Effects of TGFβ on human fetal adrenal steroid production. *Mol Cell Endocrinol* 1994;**99**:145–151.

49 Actor JK, Shirai M, Kullberg MC, Buller RM, Sher A, Berzofsky JA. Helminth infection results in decreased virus-specific CD8+ cytotoxic T-cell and Th1 cytokine responses as well as delayed virus clearance. *Proc Natl. Acad Sci USA* 1993;**90**:948–952.

50 Grzych JM, Pearce E, Cheever A *et al.* Egg deposition is the stimulus for the production of Th2 cytokines in murine *Schistosomiasis mansoni. J Immunol* 1991;**146**:1322–1340.

51 Carswell EA, Old LJ, Kassel RL, Green S, Fiore W, Williamson B. An endotoxin-induced serum factor that causes necrosis of tumours. *Proc Natl Acad Sci USA* 1975;**72**:3666–3670.

PART 8
CENTRAL NERVOUS SYSTEM

What nuclear magnetic resonance has revealed about the natural history of multiple sclerosis

W. IAN McDONALD

The introduction of magnetic resonance imaging (MRI) and spectroscopy (MRS) to clinical investigation has greatly increased our understanding of the pathogenesis of new lesions in multiple sclerosis (MS) and has shed light on the natural history of the disease as a whole.

In 98% of patients with clinically definite multiple sclerosis, areas of abnormally high signal on T_2-weighted images are seen in a distribution corresponding to the distribution of lesions found at postmortem (Plate 6). That these lesions represent plaques has been established by scanning formalin-fixed postmortem brains [1,2]. It soon became clear, however, that there was more to the story than this. First, lesions were seen to wax and wane in size over a matter of weeks [3,4]. Second, the use of gadolinium-diethylenetriaminepentaacetic acid (DTPA) as an enhancing agent revealed that some lesions enhanced, while others did not [5,6].

Quantitative MR techniques showed that the disappearing elements of new lesions represented, as expected, oedema [7,8]. Pathological studies established that pathological enhancement was due to an increase in permeability of the blood–brain barrier in lesions showing histological evidence of active inflammation [9]. Serial studies have shown that the earliest detectable event in the development of a new lesion is such a focal increase in permeability [10]. Oedema develops and reaches a peak at about a month. Thereafter enhancement ceases, presumably indicating subsidence of inflammation. The oedema is absorbed over the next few weeks to leave a smaller residual lesion. Both *in vivo* quantitative MR studies and postmortem studies show that the residual lesions are of two extreme types: one is made up of demyelinated axons embedded in a mass of astrocytic processes with little expansion of the extracellular space, while the other is characterized by a great expansion of the extracellular space due to axonal loss [11].

When does demyelination, the characteristic feature of MS, occur? Serial proton MRS has shown that myelin breakdown occurs during the inflammatory phase of the lesion [12], and electrophysiological evidence suggests that it probably occurs very early (within 24 hours) in it (Kapoor *et al.*, unpublished observations).

FUNCTIONAL EVOLUTION

It has long been known that demyelination of sufficient severity results in conduction block [13,14]. Observations on evoked potentials have provided confirmation that this occurs early in the development of the new lesion [15]. The latter studies also provided evidence that the inflammatory process itself probably contributes. The mechanism is not yet clear, though it is known that certain cytokines modify the function of ion channels in excitable membranes and it is possible that they play a part. Compensatory mechanisms permit the restoration of conduction in persistently demyelinated axons, and involve the extension of sodium channels into the demyelinated axon, thus permitting continuous or microsaltatory conduction [16]. These processes can account for the rapid development of functional loss and its resolution in the new lesion.

Later in the course of MS, however, the great majority of patients develop irrecoverable neurological deficit. In principle, two mechanisms might be operating. First, it is possible that the local axonal compensatory mechanisms fail, leading to persistent conduction block. This phenomenon is known to occur in the peripheral nervous system [17], but has not yet been demonstrated in the central nervous system.

Several lines of evidence suggest that another mechanism is important — axonal loss [18]. The most convincing evidence is derived from MRS where a strong correlation has been demonstrated between the presence of severe ataxia, cerebellar atrophy and a reduction in the concentration of *N*-acetyl aspartate (an amino acid virtually confined to neurons, including axons, in the adult brain) [19]).

LATER COURSE AND PATTERNS OF DISEASE ACTIVITY

The use of serial MRI in different clinical subgroups (relapsing/remitting, primary progressive, secondary progressive) has helped to elucidate the natural history of the disease process as a whole. Evidence of new disease activity is 5–10 times more frequent than clinical relapse, though the frequency of new lesions is lower in patients with the primary progressive form of the disease than in other types [20]. As time goes by there is an increase in the extent of abnormality in the brain: Paty *et al.* [21] observed an 18% increase over 2 years in patients with relapsing/remitting disease. There was, however, a poor correlation with disability. An important factor contributing to this discrepancy is the development of many of the lesions in the periventricular white matter where they produce neither neurological symptoms nor signs, though cognitive impairment does correlate with the extent of lesions in these regions [22].

These observations have important implications for the assessment of effectiveness of putative therapies. It is now possible to detect an effect on the acute elements of the pathological process by using serial gadolinium-DTPA-enhanced MRI at monthly intervals for 7 months: a 50% reduction in active lesions can be detected with a 90% power with just 30 patients each in placebo- and actively treated groups [23]. But, as expected, and as Paty *et al.* [21] found, the changes on standard MRI are poorly predictive of clinical outcome and cannot properly be used as a surrogate endpoint for therapeutic effectiveness. The complex issues involved have been reviewed elsewhere [18]. The present role of MRI in this context is as a relatively quick screening method; if a favourable effect on disease activity is observed, it may then be worth mounting a full-scale double-blind placebo-controlled trial with disability as the primary endpoint.

REFERENCES

1 Stewart WA, Hall LD, Berry K, Paty DW. Correlation between NMR scan and brain slice data in multiple sclerosis. *Lancet* 1984;**ii**:412.

2 Ormerod IEC, Miller DH, McDonald WI *et al.* The role of NMR imaging in the assessment of multiple sclerosis and isolated neurological lesions. A quantitative study. *Brain* 1987;**110**:1579–1616.

3 Isaac C, Li DK, Genton M *et al.* Multiple sclerosis: a serial study using MRI in relapsing patients. *Neurology* 1988;**38**:1511–1515.

4 Willoughby EW, Grochowski E, Li DKB, Oger J, Kastrukoff LF, Paty DW. Serial magnetic resonance scanning in multiple sclerosis: a second prospective study in relapsing patients. *Ann Neurol* 1989;**25**:43–49.

5 Grossman RI, Gonzalez-Scarano F, Atlas SW, Galetta S, Silberberg DH. Multiple sclerosis: gadolinium enhancement in MR imaging. *Radiology* 1986;**161**:721–725.

6 Miller DH, Kendall BE, Barter S *et al.* Magnetic resonance imaging in central nervous system sarcoidosis. *Neurology* 1988;**38**:378–383.

7 Barnes D, McDonald WI, Johnson G, Tofts PS, Landon DN. Quantitative nuclear magnetic resonance imaging: characterisation of experimental cerebral oedema. *J Neurol Neurosurg Psychiatry* 1987;**50**:125–133.

8 Larsson HBW, Frederiksen J, Kjaer L, Henriksen O, Olesen J. (1988) *In vivo* determination of T_1 and T_2 in the brain of patients with severe but stable multiple sclerosis. *Magn Res Med* 1988;**7**:43–55.

9 Katz D, Taubenberger JK, Cannella B, McFarlin DE, Raine CS, McFarland H. Correlation between MRI findings and lesion development in chronic active multiple sclerosis. *Ann Neurol* 1993;**34**:661–669.

10 Kermode AG, Thompson AJ, Tofts P *et al.* Breakdown of the blood–brain barrier precedes symptoms and other MRI signs of new lesions in multiple sclerosis: pathogenetic and clinical implications. *Brain* 1990;**113**:1477–1489.

11 Barnes D, Munro PMG, Youl BD, Prineas JW, McDonald WI. The longstanding MS lesion. A quantitative MRI and electron microscopic study. *Brain* 1991;**114**:1271–1280.

12 Davie CA, Hawkins CP, Barker GJ *et al.* Serial proton magnetic resonance spectroscopy in acute multiple sclerosis lesion. *Brain* 1994;**117**:49–58.

13 Denny-Brown D, Brenner C. Lesion in peripheral nerve resulting from compression by spring clip. *Arch Neurol Psychiatry* 1944;**52**:1–19.

14 McDonald WI. The effects of experimental demyelination on conduction in peripheral nerve: a histological and electrophysiological study. II. Electrophysiological observations. *Brain* 1963;**86**:501–524.

15 Youl BD, Turano G, Miller DH *et al.* The pathophysiology of acute optic neuritis: an association of gadolinium leakage with clinical and electrophysiological deficits. *Brain* 1991;**114**:2437–2450.

16 Black JA, Felts P, Smith KJ, Kocsis JD, Waxman SG. Distribution of sodium channels in chronically demyelinated spinal cord axons: immuno-ultrastructural localization and electrophysiological observations. *Brain Res* 1991;**544**:59–70.

17 Lewis RA, Sumner AJ, Brown MJ, Asbury AK. Multifocal demyelinating neuropathy with persistent conduction block. *Neurology* 1982;**32**:958–964.

18 McDonald WI, Miller DH, Thompson AJ. Are MRI resonance findings predictive of clinical outcome in therapeutic trials in multiple sclerosis? The dilemma of beta-interferon. *Ann Neurol* 1994;**36**:14–18.

19 Davie CA, Barker GJ, Webb S *et al.* Persistent deficit in multiple sclerosis and autosomal dominant cerebellar ataxia is associated with axon loss. *Brain* 1995;**118**:1583–1592.

20 Thompson AJ, Kermode AG, Wicks D *et al.* Major differences in the dynamics of primary and secondary progressive multiple sclerosis. *Ann Neurol* 1991;**29**:53–62.

21 Paty DW, Li DKB, the UBC MS/MRI study group and the IFNß multiple sclerosis study group. Interferon beta-1b is effective in relapsing-remitting multiple sclerosis. II. MRI analysis results of a multicentre, randomised, double-blind, placebo-controlled trial. *Neurology* 1993;**43**:662–667.

22 Ron MA, Feinstein A. Multiple sclerosis and the mind. *J Neurol Neurosurg Psychiatry* 1992;**55**:1–3.

23 Nauta JJP, Thompson AJ, Barkhof F, Miller DH. Magnetic resonance imaging in monitoring the treatment of multiple sclerosis patients: statistical power of parallel-groups and crossover designs. *J Neurol Sci* 1994;**122**:6–14.

MULTIPLE CHOICE QUESTIONS

1 The following are recognized as increasing the likelihood of clinical relapse in MS
a pregnancy
b the puerpurium
c a major surgical procedure
d hot weather
e trauma

2 The following are pathological features in a chronic MS lesion
a gliosis
b inclusion bodies
c amyloid deposition
d axon loss
e microglial nodules

3 The following conditions may produce changes visible on magnetic resonance imaging similar to those observed in MS
a systemic lupus erythematosis
b acute disseminated encephalomyelitis
c Creutzfeldt–Jakob disease
d benign intracranial hypertension
e tuberous sclerosis

4 The following are common presenting manifestations of MS

a aphasia
b transverse myelitis
c seizures
d faecal incontinence
e cognitive impairment

5 Interferon-ß

a is a cytokine
b is produced exclusively by lymphocytes
c antagonizes the effects of interferon-γ
d inhibits viral replication
e reduces the rate of relapse in early relapsing/remitting multiple
sclerosis

Answers

1 a	False	2 a	True	3 a	True
b	True	b	False	b	True
c	False	c	False	c	False
d	False	d	True	d	False
e	False	e	False	e	False
4 a	False	5 a	True		
b	True	b	False		
c	False	c	True		
d	False	d	True		
e	False	e	True		

The potential use of viral vectors for gene therapy in neurological diseases

PETER G. E. KENNEDY & ISRAEL STEINER

SUMMARY

Gene therapy for a variety of neurological diseases is now feasible using viral vectors such as herpes simplex virus type 1 (HSV-1), retroviruses and adenoviruses. HSV-1 vectors have been developed and enable the efficient delivery of foreign genes under the control of appropriate promoter elements into non-dividing neurons *in vitro* and *in vivo*. Their use is based on the natural ability of HSV-1 to spread throughout the nervous system and to establish a lifelong latent infection in neurons. HSV is present in an episomal form in the neuronal nucleus, and normal neuronal functions remain unaltered. A wide variety of foreign genes can theoretically be packaged into the large HSV genome. A number of technical problems will need to be overcome to ensure the stable expression of the foreign gene products, adequate control of the levels of their expression, the safety of the vectors and the correct targeting of the vectors to the appropriate neuronal cell populations. Such vectors have the potential to replace missing gene products in neurons in patients with a variety of metabolic and neurodegenerative diseases, and also to insert growth factors or enzymes into the local vicinity of neurological lesions to promote neuronal repair. HSV-1 vectors also have the potential to define the genetic basis of various neurophysiological functions which may prove to be useful in evaluating altered neuronal function encountered in disease. Viral vectors may also be used to insert foreign genes into brain tumour cells which may render the tumour susceptible to particular drugs.

INTRODUCTION

The possibility of gene delivery to neurons using viral vectors for treating neurological diseases has now emerged from the realm of science fiction to that of foreseeable reality. This potential 'coming of age' of gene therapy has emerged as a result of major advances in three main areas: (i) the increasing knowledge of virus biochemical genetics; (ii) the rapidly increasing sophistication of molecular genetic engineering techniques; and

Table 1 Strategies for gene therapy in the central nervous system.

Replace missing or defective gene

Replace or enhance local growth factors or enzyme production

Virus-directed enzyme prodrug therapy

Delivery of antisense sequences to particular genes

Use of inserted DNA to increase cellular antigen expression to boost immune response

(iii) the increasing understanding of the genetic basis of both rare and common neurological diseases. Moreover, viral vectors now provide a powerful tool to study neuronal function under normal conditions. Recent advances in the understanding of the molecular biology of HSV-1 latency in the human nervous system have made this virus a particularly promising agent in this area. Our aim here is to summarize the salient principles and issues underlying this therapeutic and scientific approach concentrating on HSV-1-derived vectors (Table 1). We shall consider: (i) the general principles of HSV-1 vector neuronal delivery; (ii) the types of neurological disorder which may benefit from this approach; (iii) ideal properties of, and practical difficulties with, such vectors; and (iv) some examples of *in vitro* and *in vivo* studies of gene delivery to neurons.

GENERAL PRINCIPLES AND PRACTICAL APPROACHES

Viruses which have been used as vectors include HSV-1, retroviruses, Simian Virus 40 (SV40) and adenoviruses [1]. There are a variety of potential ways in which such viral vectors could be used for gene delivery to neurons. The most obvious application is to replace a missing or defective gene where this is known — the rare single-gene disorders, based on the assumption that the gene delivered will be expressed and the appropriate gene product, e.g. enzyme or other protein, will be produced *in situ*. Vulnerability of particular cell types to drugs could be produced by inserting into them genes which render them susceptible to the action of, for example, antiviral agents. Another example of such 'gene knockout' is the delivery of antisense message to particular cells, e.g. virally infected cells, which may abolish the activity of selected viral genes which have been incorporated into the host genome or which are present episomally.

We will concentrate here on HSV-1 which, like other viruses, has the ability to cross cell membranes — a property which is not shared by many gene products such as certain key enzymes. HSV-1 has a number of additional properties which make it particularly suitable for delivering foreign genes into post mitotic, non-dividing cells such as neurons [1,2].

HSV-1 is a large double-stranded DNA virus with a length of 152 kilobases (kb). It has the ability to spread within the nervous system, e.g. from the periphery to the dorsal root ganglia (DRG) and to the central nervous system (CNS, namely the spinal cord and brain) via axonal transport and transsynaptically [3,4]. Indeed, HSV-1 has been used as a neuronal tracer [4]. Having entered the nervous system, HSV-1 has the remarkable property of producing a latent infection in neurons [5,6], primarily in human and animal DRG and trigeminal ganglia [2,7,8], but also elsewhere in the CNS [2]. Under various conditions such as sunlight, trauma, X-ray irradiation and fever, the virus can periodically reactivate from latency, leading to the appearance of cold sores in the area of the skin inner-vated by the appropriate sensory nerve. Rarely, HSV encephalitis may develop [9].

The latent HSV-1 infection is lifelong. During latency the virus is present in an episomal form in the neuronal nucleus, i.e. it is not integrated into the host DNA [10]. Neuronal functions, including electrophysiological activity, remain unaltered, and HSV-induced mutations in neuronal DNA are very unlikely [2]. Understanding of the mechanisms of HSV-1 latency in the nervous system has facilitated the use of this virus as a vector. Prior viral DNA replication is not required for the establishment of latency [11]. During latency, the entire HSV-1 genome is present [12], but only restricted transcriptional activity can be detected in neurons and include the latency-associated transcripts (LATs) [13–15]. The LATs have been the focus of intense interest, and they appear to be important in viral reactivation from latency [16,17] and also possibly in the establishment of latency [18]. LAT genes have both coding and regulatory elements, which can be experimentally manipulated [2]. In contrast to latent infection *in vivo*, HSV-1 produces a lytic infection of cells during primary infection and in tissue culture in which neurons and other cell types such as Schwann cells, fibroblasts and astrocytes are killed following a full cycle of viral replication [2,19,20]. A successful HSV-1 vector must therefore maintain the viral ability to spread through the nervous system and to enter and remain latent in neurons, but be altered so as to eliminate its ability to replicate and reactivate in host tissues [1,2].

In practice, most viral vectors for gene delivery are derived from plasmids rather than recombinant viruses [1]. The genetic engineering techniques which have been used to produce defective HSV-1 vectors will not be described here in any detail (for review see [1]). A prime objective is to 'package' an additional foreign gene, e.g. one which is miss-ing or defective in neurons, into the HSV-1 virion. It has been possible to incorporate at least 30 foreign kb after removing viral sequences not essential for viral replication [21,22]. A prototype defective HSV-1 vector known as pHSVlac contains a number of elements, including a transcrip-tion unit that places the *Escherichia coli lacZ* gene under the control of an

HSV-1 promoter [23]. Since *lacZ* encodes the β-galactosidase enzyme, it is possible, using appropriate staining techniques, to identify cells which contain this enzyme, i.e. those into which *lacZ* has been successfully inserted [1,23]. The blue compound resulting from the enzymic reaction can be easily identified in infected cells and tissues. The promoter is required to allow the inserted gene to be transcribed and expressed in particular cells and tissues, and therefore determines the cell specificity of the expression of the inserted gene. For example, insertion of the neuronal neurofilament gene promoter into a vector should theoretically allow the gene to be expressed only in neurons [23,24]. The pHSVlac vector also contains HSV-1 segments that allow the packaging of plasmid DNA into HSV particles which are combined with a helper virus that is temperature-sensitive, being unable to replicate at the non-permissive temperature of 37–39°C encountered *in vivo* [23]. Such a vector can therefore propagate in the nervous system and infect cells without replicating and causing cell death. Likewise, a wide range of foreign genes can theoretically be delivered to neuronal cells.

ASPECTS OF NEUROLOGICAL DISEASES WHICH MAY RENDER THEM AMENABLE TO HSV-1-TARGETED GENE THERAPY

Inherited metabolic brain diseases

On theoretical grounds, some neurological disorders are more likely than others to be treatable using the viral vector approach. Diseases known to be caused by a specific defect such as enzyme deficiency may prove to be the most amenable. An example is the Lesch–Nyhan syndrome resulting from a deficiency of the enzyme hypoxanthine phosphoribosyltransferase (HPRT) leading to a severe disorder, including behavioural and CNS deficits [25]. Requirements for gene therapy in this group of disorders include knowledge of the complete DNA sequence of the responsible gene coding for the gene product, and the ability to package relevant sequences into the HSV-1 genome [1].

Neurodegenerative disorders

In view of the affinity of HSV-1 for neurons, HSV-1-mediated gene delivery is likely to be particularly appropriate for diseases causing neuronal degeneration, many of which are untreatable at present. However, since many neurodegenerative diseases may have multifactorial causes, the single-gene replacement approach may not be feasible here. Several exceptions have already been identified. Gene therapy may offer a realistic prospect for treatment of Huntington's chorea, now that the genetic defect responsible for this condition has been identified [26]. The recent report of mutations in the gene coding for superoxide dismutase in some patients with familial amyotrophic lateral sclerosis [27] is another example. HSV-1 vectors would have the practical advantage of transporting the gene for this enzyme across cell membranes, since superoxide dismutase itself has very limited ability to traverse cell membranes [28]. In other conditions, with more complex aetiology and pathogenesis, gene therapy may still be feasible, e.g. levels of dopamine in the basal ganglia of patients with Parkinson's disease may be elevated by HSV-1 delivery of the enzyme tyrosine hydroxylase [29]. Whether or not some patients with Alzheimer's disease may benefit from local delivery of enzymes or growth factors is unclear, but the identification of the possible genetic basis of at least some cases with this condition may eventually render it amenable to some form of gene replacement therapy [30].

Brain injury repair

Gene therapy may also be used to deliver the gene coding for an enzyme or growth factor which might be effective in treating the consequences and enhance tissue healing of a particular defect, although the lack of such factors is not the primary underlying abnormality. Neurological diseases such as head trauma, stroke or multiple sclerosis may benefit from treatment with growth factors such as nerve growth factor (NGF, see below) that may be provided by an HSV-1 vector to the site of damage.

Brain tumour therapy

Viral vectors also have considerable potential for the treatment of brain tumours, and there is some promising preliminary evidence to suggest

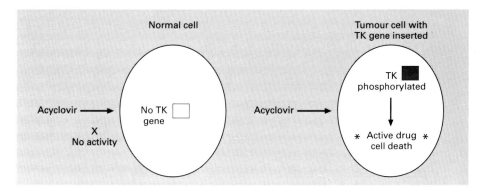

Fig. 1 Virus-mediated delivery of acyclovir for prodrug therapy.

that this may well be feasible. One approach is to use the vector to insert a gene into the tumour which is thereby rendered susceptible to the action of a particular drug. For example, using a rat C6 glioma mouse brain tumour model, Chen *et al.* [31] introduced the HSV thymidine kinase (tk) gene into the tumour *in vivo* using an adenovirus vector. The mice were then treated with the anti-HSV drug ganciclovir, which requires the tk enzyme for its activity. This was followed by a reduction in the size of the tumours in the treated mice compared to controls. This approach offers the real possibility of viral vector-mediated gene therapy in humans to cause regression in brain tumour growth (Fig. 1). This principle is clearly applicable to tumours in other organs.

IDEAL PROPERTIES AND POTENTIAL DIFFICULTIES OF HSV-1 VECTORS

Ideally, viral vector therapy should fulfill the following requirements (Table 2):

1 It must have enough capacity for the foreign gene to be packaged into it. As mentioned, the HSV-1 genome can harbour at least 30 kb of foreign DNA.

2 The vector must be easily delivered to the targeted tissue. HSV spreads easily within the nervous system and thus intracranial inoculation with vectors into, for example, the basal ganglia in Parkinson's disease, which clearly involves significant surgical risks, can be prevented. However, it will be essential for the vector to remain intact and not to be broken down during transit and at the site of action.

3 The vector must reach the *appropriate* population of neurons. In discussing viral vector therapy, there exists the danger of adopting too simplistic a view of target cells and we may still have only limited knowledge of exactly which types of neurons are the ones with genetic defects and/or which are most likely to benefit from foreign gene insertion in particular diseases. With accumulating knowledge about neuronal function and markers, this difficulty may be largely surmounted by judicious choice of promoter elements within the viral construct.

4 The virus must not replicate or reactivate in target neurons. In cases where temperature-sensitive mutant viruses are used, there is a theoretical danger of the virus reverting to a wild-type phenotype capable of producing a lytic infection, possibly through acquiring a missing protein *in vivo*. This could have grave consequences, including the development of herpes simplex encephalitis. Deleting the coding sequence of the LATs may at least render the HSV-1 vector unable to reactivate.

5 The foreign gene must be *stably* expressed in target neurons into which it has been episomally incorporated. Even if the foreign gene is shown to be expressed and its product identified in target tissues, there will be little

Table 2 Ideal properties of viral vectors for gene therapy.

Enough capacity for packaging of foreign gene
Vector must be easily delivered to target cells
Vector must be delivered to *appropriate* target cells, e.g. neuronal population
Viral vector must not replicate in target cells
Foreign gene must be stably expressed in target cells
Must have ability to control the level of expression of the gene products
Vector should not elicit host immune responses

likelihood of therapeutic benefit if its expression is only transient. This failure to be continuously expressed may be a consequence of a variety of factors related to the promoter elements in the vector and/or local adverse metabolic conditions. The regulatory elements of the LATs have the potential to enable stable expression of any gene whose expression they control.

6 Even if expression of the delivered gene is achieved, the ability to control the level of expression of the gene products will be crucial. Underexpression of the gene will render the procedure ineffective, while overexpression may have severe consequences, such as toxicity and the appearance of new cellular malfunctions. Difficulty in controlling the level of production of the required gene product has already been experienced in the case of HSV-1 vectors containing the HPRT gene under the regulatory control of the HSV thymidine kinase gene [25].

A variety of ethical issues must be carefully considered prior to gene therapy. Those are beyond the scope of this discussion, but one example may highlight the extent of the problems involved. Genes may be delivered in order to prevent programmed cell death in certain tissues [32]. While such therapy in localized regions may be highly appropriate for a particular neurological disease, a therapy ultimately designed to slow down or prevent a more general neuronal degeneration would have significant ethical implications.

EXAMPLES OF *IN VITRO* AND *IN VIVO* HSV-1 DELIVERY TO NEURONS

Gene delivery to neuronal cells could be used to study normal function as one of the essential steps eventually to correct a malfunction. Thus, the genetic basis of specific neurophysiological activity in neurons can be studied using HSV-1 vectors such as pHSVlac, into which particular genes critical for various functions have been inserted [33]. Successful results in this field might allow therapeutic approaches *in vivo* by delivering a gene coding for a protein essential for restoring a localized but specific electrophysiological abnormality.

It is interesting that early experiments using pHSVlac demonstrated that the inserted *lacZ* gene was expressed without deleterious effects on cultured neurons from rat superior cervical ganglion and DRG [23] as well as a whole spectrum of other CNS sites (rat neurons in primary cultures derived from the spinal cord, cerebellum, thalamus, basal ganglia, hippocampus and occipital, temporal and frontal cortex) [29,34] using a viral and not a specific neuronal promoter. Stable expression of the gene product β-galactosidase was observed for at least 2 weeks. Moreover, neuronal expression of this gene could be enhanced by replacing the viral promoter with the neurofilament promoter [1]. The identification and characterization of this and other neuron-specific genes should allow the use of various neuronal promoters to control the fine neuronal specificity of the inserted genes.

There have been a limited number of *in vivo* reports of gene delivery by HSV-1 defective vectors, which indicate the latter's therapeutic potential. A particularly elegant example was recently described in which delivery of NGF by a defective HSV-1 vector (pHSVngf) into living rat superior cervical ganglion could prevent the biochemical defects associated with ganglion axotomy [35]. The neuronal cells expressed the NGF gene product, which they do not usually produce, with resultant prevention of the expected axotomy-induced decline in ganglion tyrosine hydroxylase levels. Significant advances in this field have also been made by other groups, including Dobson *et al.* [36] and Ho and Mocarski [37], who achieved stable expression of exogenous β-globin and *E. coli lacZ* genes, respectively, in trigeminal neurons *in vivo* for extended time periods under the control of the LAT promoter.

As explained by Breakefield and DeLuca [1], several additional problems need to be addressed to evaluate the potential of HSV-1 vector gene delivery *in vivo*. These include the questions of whether neurons are the only cells in which the vector may establish latency, the nature of host as well as HSV-1-incorporated non-herpetic promoters active or activated during latency and, crucially, whether a neuron already latently infected with a wild-type HSV strain can also allow a superinfecting HSV to become latent within it. How, under these circumstances, may the two viruses interact?

CONCLUSIONS

The development of viral vectors for delivering foreign genes into neurons *in vitro* and *in vivo* has the potential significantly to enhance both the understanding of the genetic basis of neuronal function and our ability to treat a range of neurological disorders which hitherto have been considered incurable (Table 3). The latter could include neurodegenerative disorders such as Alzheimer's disease, Parkinson's disease and amyotrophic lateral sclerosis, as well as metabolic conditions such as the Lesch–Nyhan

Table 3 The potential use of gene therapy in neurological disorders.

Disorder	Example	Potential gene
Inherited/metabolic	GM2 gangliosidosis	Hexoseaminidase
Degenerative	Familial ALS	Superoxide dismutase
Demyelinating	Multiple sclerosis	β-Interferon
Acute damage	Spinal trauma	NGF
Brain tumours	Glioma	Suicide genes
Infections	SSPE	α- and β-Interferon

ALS, Amyotrophic lateral sclerosis; NGF, nerve growth factor; SSPE, subacute sclerosing panencephalitis.
In each group of nervous system disorders an example of the specific disorder is provided, followed by a gene that can be used for gene transfer and therapy.

syndrome, in which a specific enzyme deficiency has been identified. Although a climate of optimism is reasonable, the practical problems inherent in this genetic approach are likely to be formidable, and need to be rigorously addressed in experimental animal systems before their use in humans can be envisaged. Prominent among the difficulties will be targeting of vectors to specific groups of neurons, probably by skilful use of appropriate promoters for neuronal genes, and the control of the level of expression of the required gene products. The success of HSV-1 vectors will also be critically dependent on increasing knowledge of the LATs promoter in the latency process. Probably the most worrying aspect is the potential risk of the viral vector reverting to wild-type and replicating at and beyond the site intended, leading to encephalitis. Even if these techniques are sufficiently refined to allow trials in patients, various ethical issues regarding their use will almost certainly need to be addressed [38].

ACKNOWLEDGEMENTS

This work was supported in part by grant no. 88-00184 from the United States–Israel Binational Science Foundation (BSF), Jerusalem, Israel and grants by the Chief Scientist, Ministry of Health and the Israel Cancer Association. This article is a very slight modification of a paper which was previously published [39]. The main text is reprinted here by permission of Oxford University Press.

REFERENCES

1 Breakefield XO, DeLuca NA. Herpes simplex virus for gene delivery to neurons. *New Biol* 1991;3:203–218.
2 Steiner I, Kennedy PGE. Molecular biology of herpes simplex virus type 1 latency in the nervous system. *Mol Neurobiol* 1993;**137**:137–159.
3 Kristensson K, Lycke E, Roytta M, Svennerholm B, Vahlne A. Neuritic transport of herpes simplex in rat sensory neurons *in vitro*. Effects of substances interacting with

microtubular function and axonal flow [nocodazole, taxol, and erythro-9-3(2-hydroxynonyl)-adenine]. *J Gen Virol* 1986;**67**:2023–2028.

4 Kuypers HGJM, Ugolini G. Viruses as transneuronal tracers. *TINS* 1990;**13**:71–75.

5 Kennedy PGE, Al-Saadi SA, Clements GB. Reactivation of latent herpes simplex virus from dissociated identified dorsal root ganglion cells in culture. *J Gen Virol* 1983;**64**:1629–1635.

6 McLennan JL, Darby G. Herpes simplex virus latency; the cellular location of virus in dorsal root ganglia and the fate of the infected cell following virus activation. *J Gen Virol* 1980;**51**:233–243.

7 Stevens JG, Cook ML. Latent herpes simplex virus in spinal ganglia of mice. *Science* 1971;**173**:843–845.

8 Steiner I, Kennedy PGE. Herpes simplex virus latency in the nervous system — a new model. *Neuropathol Appl Neurobiol* 1991;**17**:433–440.

9 Whitley RJ. Epidemiology of herpes simplex viruses. In: *The Herpes Viruses*, vol. 3, edited by Roizman B. Plenun Publishing, New York, 1985:1–44.

10 Mellerick DM, Fraser NW. Physical state of the latent herpes simplex virus genome in mouse model system. Evidence suggesting an episomal state. *Virology* 1987;**158**:265–275.

11 Steiner I, Spivack JG, Deshmane SL, Ace CI, Preston CM, Fraser NW. A herpes simplex virus type 1 mutant containing a non-transinducing Vmw65 protein establishes latent infection *in vivo* in the absence of viral replication and reactivates efficiently from explanted trigeminal ganglia. *J Virol* 1990;**64**:1630–1638.

12 Rock DL, Fraser NW. Detection of HSV-1 genome in the central nervous system of latently infected mice. *Nature* 1983;**302**:523–525.

13 Stevens JG, Wagner EK, Devi-Rao GB, Cook ML, Feldman LT. RNA complementary to a herpes virus alpha gene mRNA is prominent in latently infected neurons. *Science* 1987;**235**:1056–1059.

14 Spivack JG, Fraser NW. Detection of herpes simplex type 1 transcripts during latent infection in mice. *J Virol* 1987;**61**:3841–3847.

15 Steiner I, Spivack JG, O'Boyle DR, Lavi E, Fraser NW. Latent herpes virus type 1 transcription in human trigeminal ganglia. *J Virol* 1988;**62**:3493–3496.

16 Steiner I, Spivack JG, Lirette RP *et al*. Herpes simplex virus type 1 latency-associated transcripts are evidently not essential for latent infection. *EMBO* 1989;**8**:505–511.

17 Trousdale MD, Steiner I, Spivack JG *et al*. *In vivo* and *in vitro* reactivation impairment of a herpes simplex virus type 1 latency-associated transcript variant in a rabbit eye model. *J Virol* 1991;**65**:6989–6993.

18 Sawtell NM, Thompson RL. Herpes simplex virus type 1 latency-associated transcription unit promotes anatomical site-dependent establishment and reactivation from latency. *J Virol* 1992;**66**:2157–2169.

19 Read GS, Frankel N. Herpes simplex virus mutants defective in the virion-associated shut-off of host polypeptide synthesis and exhibiting abnormal synthesis of alpha (immediate early) viral polypeptides. *J Virol* 1983;**46**:498–512.

20 Kennedy PGE, Clements GB, Brown SM. Differential susceptibility of human neural cell types in culture to infection with herpes simplex virus. *Brain* 1983;**166**:101–119.

21 Roizman B, Sears AE. Herpes simplex viruses and their replication. In: Virology, edited by Fields BN, Knipe DM, *et al*. 2nd edn. Raven Press, New York, 1990:1795–1841.

22 Longnecker R, Roizman B, Meignier B. Herpes simplex viruses as vectors: properties of a prototype vaccine strain suitable for use as a vector. In: *Viral Vectors*, edited by Gluzman Y, Hughes SH. Cold Spring Harbor Laboratory Press, Cold Spring Harbor, NY, 1988.

23 Geller AI, Breakefield O. A defective HSV-1 vector expresses *Escherichia coli* β-galactosidase in cultured peripheral neurons. *Science* 1988;**241**:1667–1679.

24 Federoff HJ, Geller A, Lu B. Neuronal specific expression of the human neurofilament L promoter in a HSV-1 vector. *Soc Neurosci Abstr* 1990;**16**:154.2.

25 Palella TD, Hidaka Y, Silverman LJ, Levine M, Glorioso J, Kelley WN. Expression of human mRNA in brains of mice infected with a recombinant herpes simplex virus vector. *Gene* 1989;**80**:137–144.

26 Morell V. Huntington's gene finally found. *Science* 1993;**260**:28–30.
27 Rosen DR, Siddique T, Patterson D *et al.* Mutations in Cu/Zn superoxide dismutase gene are associated with familial amyotrophic lateral sclerosis. *Nature* 1993;**362**:59–62.
28 McNamara JO, Fridovich I. Did radicals strike Lou Gehrig? *Nature* 1993;**362**:20–21.
29 Freese A, Geller A. Infection of cultured striatal neurons with a defective HSV-1 vector: implications for gene therapy. *Nucleic Acids Res* 1991;**19**:7219–7223.
30 Friedman T. Progress toward human gene therapy. *Science* 1989;**244**:1275–1281.
31 Chen S-H, Shine HD, Goodman JC, Grossman RG, Woo SLC. Gene therapy for brain tumors: regression of experimental gliomas by adenovirus-mediated gene transfer *in vivo*. *Proc Natl Acad Sci USA* 1994;**91**:3054–3057.
32 Raff MC. Social controls on cell survival and cell death. *Nature* 1992;**356**:397–400.
33 Geller AI, During MJ, Neve RL. Molecular analysis of neuronal physiology by gene transfer into neurons with herpes simplex virus vectors. *TINS* 1991;**14**:428–432.
34 Geller AI, Freese A. Infection of cultured central nervous system neurons with a defective herpes simplex virus 1 vector results in stable expression of *Escherichia coli* beta-galactosidase. *Proc Natl Acad Sci USA* 1990;**87**:149–153.
35 Federoff HJ, Geschwind MD, Geller AI, Kessler JA. Expression of nerve growth factor *in vivo* from a defective herpes simplex virus 1 vector prevents effects of axotomy on sympathetic ganglia. *Proc Natl Acad Sci USA* 1992;**89**:1636–1640.
36 Dobson AT, Sedarati F, Devi-Rao G *et al.* Identification of the latency-associated transcript promoter by expression of rabbit beta-globin mRNA in mouse sensory nerve ganglia latently infected with a recombinant herpes simplex virus. *J Virol* 1989;**63**:3844–3851.
37 Ho DY, Mocarski ES. Herpes simplex virus latent RNA (LAT) is not required for latent infection in the mouse. *Proc Natl Acad Sci USA* 1989;**86**:7596–7600.
38 Anonymous. Gene therapy. *Lancet* 1989;**1**:193–194.
39 Kennedy PGE, Steiner I. The use of herpes simplex virus vectors for gene therapy in neurological diseases. *Quarterly Journal of Medicine* 1993;**86**:697–702.

MULTIPLE CHOICE QUESTIONS

1 The following viruses have been used as viral vectors for gene therapy
a retroviruses
b poliovirus
c measles virus
d adenovirus
e herpes simplex virus-1 (HSV-1)

2 The following are characteristics of HSV-1
a its DNA has a length of 30 kb
b virus is present in episomal form in the neuronal nucelus during latency
c during latency the latency-associated transcripts (LATs) are the only detectable viral transcripts
d prior DNA replication is probably not required for the establishment of latency
e virus does not produce a lytic infection *in vitro*

3 The following features of HSV-1 make it particularly suitable for use as a viral vector for gene therapy
a it is able to infect neurons which are post mitotic cells
b it has the capacity to establish a latent infection in neurons *in vivo*
c it is non-cytopathic for non-neuronal cells *in vitro*
d it has a large genome which is readily amenable to genetic engineering techniques
e it does not easily spread within the nervous system

4 The following statements are true of any potential viral vector for gene therapy
a it must have enough capacity for the foreign gene to be packaged into it
b the viral vector must be able to replicate in target neuronal cells
c the foreign gene must be stably expressed in target neural cells
d overexpression of the foreign gene in target cells is unlikely to be a theoretical or a practical problem
e promoter elements in the vector construct are important in determining the cell specificity of the expressed gene

5 Gene therapy using viral vectors are likely to be applicable for replacing missing or defective genes in the following conditions
a Lesch–Nyhan syndrome
b cerebral haemorrhage
c Huntington's chorea
d migraine
e herpes simplex virus encephalitis

Answers

1		2		3	
a	True	a	False	a	True
b	False	b	True	b	True
c	False	c	True	c	False
d	True	d	True	d	True
e	True	e	False	e	False

4		5	
a	True	a	True
b	False	b	False
c	True	c	True
d	False	d	False
e	True	e	False

What can imaging tell us about brain function in psychiatric disease?

GUY M. GOODWIN

Neuroscience has consistently identified localization of function as a cardinal principle of brain organization. The idea is not a new one and lends itself to parody as a new phrenology. However, the methods of brain imaging that establish localization of function within the brain either *in* or *ex vivo* are now so convincing that no credible model of brain function could ignore its detailed functional anatomy. For example, it is now established that visual information is represented repeatedly in the brains of higher animals as functional maps, each of which deals with a different aspect of visual information processing. The maps provide only a partial answer to how the brain works. We also depend upon the full deployment of anatomical, physiological, neuropharmacological and neuropsychological disciplines which contribute to the evolving status of neuroscience.

Validation of the status of psychiatric syndromes is likely to be a major clinical role for functional brain imaging in humans. The abnormal mental states of dementia, depressive illness and schizophrenia are defined in an arbitrary way. Functional imaging can establish the topography of brain function related to the observed mental state abnormalities. In Alzheimer-type dementia, it proved relatively simple to relate global cognitive impairment to reduced function in temporal and parietal cortex with ^{18}F-deoxyglucose or ^{15}O positron emission tomography (PET) [1–3] and ^{99m}Tc-exametazime single-photon emission (computed) tomography (SPET or SPECT) [4–7]. In schizophrenia, stable chronic symptoms cluster into three subsyndromes which have been mapped on to the baseline pattern of brain activity with ^{15}O-PET [8]. These findings, together with the evidence from structural computed tomography (CT) and magnetic resonance imaging (MRI) promise to underpin the shift to viewing schizophrenia as a disease of disordered neurodevelopment. In the case of both dementia and schizophrenia, the race is on to identify the cellular or molecular basis of the disorders.

Depressive illness poses particular problems and is of particular interest. It is the common cold of psychiatry. The lifetime risk for the syndrome of major depression is of the order of 20% for women. Perhaps optimistically, it is generally regarded as a fully reversible clinical condition. Unfortunately, in its most malignant form it also accounts for the majority of suicides, and in patients who are referred for psychiatric care, the severity and chronicity of the illness consistently predict a poor outcome and difficulty in selecting successful drug treatment and psychosocial management. To understand this gradient of possible outcomes in a common illness is a major challenge for applied neuroscience. Imaging, both structural and functional, has a central role in defining the localization and eventually the nature of abnormal brain function in depressive illness.

STRUCTURAL IMAGING

The evidence for structural abnormality in depressive illness is largely confined to subjects over 40 years of age [9]. In the first studies employing CT, Jacoby et al. [10,11] showed that 9 of 41 elderly depressives had enlarged ventricles on CT scan and a reduced brain substance as determined by the attenuation of CT measures. Indeed, they proposed that simply on the basis of such measures the depressed group more closely resembled a demented group than normal controls of the same age. Subsequent CT studies of elderly depressed patients have confirmed that they tend to show indices of structural brain involvement like Alzheimer patients, especially if onset of illness is late [12], the most severely cognitively impaired patients clustering close to those of the Alzheimer group on the basis of CT radioattenuation estimates [13]. The link between degree of structural change and impairment of cognition was examined by Abas et al. [14], who showed that there was a correlation between ventricular brain ratio on CT and impairment on cognitive tests performed both when depressed and after recovery. These reported similarities between Alzheimer dementia and depression are too non-specific to imply that neuropathologically they are related. It has been possible to improve the topographical focus in cerebral cortex with MRI, suggesting a small reduction in total frontal lobe volume in depressive illness [15]. Reports of subcortical structural abnormalities in depression are proliferating from the improved resolution of MRI, where both ill-defined lesions and gross atrophy are described in basal nuclei, the cerebellum and even the brainstem [15–18]. There is therefore a wealth of evidence that elderly patients with major depression are more likely to show evidence of structural abnormality in the brain than are controls. We do not know whether the same is true in younger patients. The working hypothesis must be that individuals with such changes are actually more at risk of depressive illness. The challenge is to determine whether such illnesses are more severe, refractory or recurrent and how the changes are related to the mechanisms involved in normal ageing. Finally we do not yet understand the relationship between the structural abnormalities and the regional disturbances of function shown by perfusion imaging, described below.

FUNCTIONAL IMAGING: REGIONAL PERFUSION

Methods

Perfusion imaging is based on the detection in the brain of any tracer uptake related to regional brain blood flow. Under conditions of normal physiology it is assumed that regional perfusion is closely yoked to substrate demand or regional brain metabolism. The best method employed is PET with ^{15}O (where the isotope allows the calculation of regional perfusion, not oxygen consumption). PET's unusual cost currently restricts its use to two centres in the UK. Our own work has primarily sought to relate defined mental states to brain activity with the SPET perfusion tracer ^{99m}Tc-exametazime, which is injected intravenously, taken up into brain tissue in proportion to regional perfusion, and trapped. Its distribution within the brain can be measured with an appropriate SPET camera system. The critical difference between PET and SPET is the improved sensitivity of PET, with which it is possible to study whole brain perfusion for 12–18 conditions (30-seconds sampling windows) on the same subject for a radiation exposure comparable to that of a single ^{99m}Tc-exametazime SPET scan. ^{99m}Tc-exametazime SPET is best employed experimentally for simple comparisons within or between patient groups. However, it is feasible to employ SPET in large and fully representative clinical studies and it is likely to be the only isotope-based technique widely available for clinical use.

Finally, there are now methods based on MRI which promise to allow a similar measure of regional perfusion without exposure to ionizing radiation [19,20]. It is too early to say whether this method will replace isotope-based techniques for perfusion imaging.

Image analysis

Functional imaging studies have the capacity to produce immense numbers of measurements. The alternative methods for the assessment of regional brain function are broadly polarized as follows:
1 define anatomical regions of interest from a standard brain atlas and, by combining data from large numbers of picture elements or pixels, reduce the comparisons to a reasonable number;
2 use a pixel-by-pixel approach which allows such functional regions of interest to be defined *post hoc*.

The weakness of the first approach is that predetermined regions of interest impose anatomical boundaries not defined by functional criteria and may miss highly localized effects. The relative disadvantage depends upon the resolution of the method and the variance of intersubject brain anatomy. The use of pixel-by-pixel analysis for comparisons of groups of subjects requires individual brain shapes to be transformed into standard coordinates and the higher spatial frequency signals of the image to be heavily filtered. The resulting spatial localization of any effect is limited (10–20 mm) but the approach is more satisfactory because it includes more of the total available data set. The application of pixel-by-pixel analysis to SPET is a recent innovation. It has depended upon the modification of statistical parametric mapping (SPM) software developed for analysis of PET data at the Medical Research Council Cyclotron Unit [21].

FINDINGS IN MAJOR DEPRESSION

Reductions of anterior brain function have been consistently identified by a variety of techniques when depressed patients are compared with controls [22–24]. In our own experience this effect is most striking in elderly males [25], where the reduced perfusion is correlated with increased psychomotor impairment. A region of interest analysis of the findings is shown in Fig. 1. It appears possible that this effect is related to reports of frontal atrophy in elderly depressed subjects [15]. It is not established that such decrements simply reverse on recovery. Thus, it is our hypothesis that reduced frontal perfusion may be a consequence of age-associated changes in frontal cortex, which predispose to the development of depressive illness. The perfusion of posterior and parietal–temporal regions is preserved in the elderly depressed, but not in Alzheimer patients [25]. This suggests that depression is distinguishable from Alzheimer's disease in the elderly using SPET (see Plate 7). This represents a major clinical application of the method, since impairment of cognitive function in depressive illness may be severe (pseudodementia) and the degree of memory impairment overlaps with that seen in early Alzheimer-type dementia.

Fig. 1 The light areas show the decrements in brain perfusion estimated by ^{99m}Tc-exametazime in depressed elderly male patients compared with controls. The brain is represented as a standard template fitted to the single-photon emission tomography (SPET) images at the level of the basal ganglia and to a site 2 cm higher (4 and 6 cm above the orbitomeatal line). Full details are given in [25].

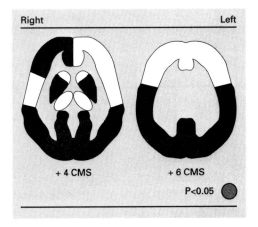

THE FUNCTIONAL ANATOMY OF
DEPRESSIVE SYMPTOMS

The detection of frontal decrements in patients compared with controls is not simply explained by patients being in a depressed state. This would require a negative association between brain perfusion and symptom severity. Instead we found, in younger patients especially, a positive association between uptake and scores on the Newcastle scale — an arbitrary estimate of endogenicity, especially in frontal cortex [26]. This appeared to have been due to the inclusion of patients with mood-congruent delusions and implied that correlations with state variables would be highly influenced by patient selection as well as being confounded in part by global severity. State effects would be better determined by comparing brain topography before and after recovery. We have now used the natural phenomenon of diurnal symptom variation to define further the pattern or patterns of brain function which change in association with amelioration of specific symptoms (Klaus P et al., submitted for publication). The explicit inclusion of a within-subject diurnal improvement in symptom severity has important advantages for the analysis of the depressed state and has been used together with SPM analysis. The limbric and paralimbric cortex where critical correlations are detected are the areas that appear most affected by atrophy in structural studies. Understanding their connectivity will be essential to progress in the neurobiological investigation of mood.

There are considerable difficulties in trying to study patients with severe depressive illness before and after full recovery. However, our own work with SPET, controlling for drug treatment, suggested that the recovery effects are confined to anterior cingulate and basal ganglia regions bilaterally [27]. This finding is important in that it implicates the basal ganglia in the expression of depressive illness; this would have been expected from the neuropsychiatric literature which has associated depressive states with diseases of the basal ganglia such as Parkinson's disease and Huntington's chorea. It further suggests that dopamine pathways may be implicated in core depressive symptoms such as retardation.

SPECIFIC BINDING OF RADIOLIGANDS
WITH SPET

It is a remarkable fact that drug treatment of depression is now possible with highly selective compounds which inhibit only the uptake of serotonin (5-hydroxytryptamine or 5-HT) in the brain (selective serotonin reuptake inhibitors (SSRIs)). Psychopharmacological investigation of the depressed state remains of considerable potential importance in identifying the pathways underlying depressive illness and, indeed, the pathways for regulation of stress responses and anxiety. There is great potential for the extension of *in vivo* psychopharmacology with PET and SPET. It is likely that the long-term application of isotope-based techniques will focus increasingly upon specific ligands for receptors or pathological proteins. The current limitations are in part practical. There are only two commercially available ^{123}I-based ligands for SPET. ^{123}I-iomazenil binds to benzodiazepine receptors and ^{123}I-IBZM binds to dopamine D_2 receptors. A study of ^{123}I-IBZM binding in major depression is underway in our unit. There are a larger number of promising SPET ligands available in precursor form [28]. The problem is efficient local synthesis of the ^{123}I-substituted ligand. The ligand in which we would initially be most interested, given the site of action of the SSRIs, would be selective for the 5-HT reuptake site. 5-Iodo-6-nitroquipazine appears to be an excellent candidate, having high affinity, high specificity and an apparently simple synthesis for ^{123}I substitution [29,30].

There are, broadly, two potential uses for such ligands. High-affinity compounds will indicate the density of receptors and will be highly resistant to displacement by agonists of lower affinity. For example, ^{123}I-iomazenil binding may provide an assay of γ-aminobutyric acid$_A$ (GABA$_A$) receptor numbers. It is highly specific for the benzodiazepine site and has an affinity 10-fold higher than that of the corresponding PET ligand ^{11}C-flumazenil [31,32]. It will, therefore, provide a good measure of receptor density in neocortical areas. This is of interest in several contexts. For example, loss of GABAergic interneurons would be expected to produce increases in postsynaptic GABA receptors, as described in cingulate cortex postmortem in schizophrenia by Benes *et al.* [33]. Alternatively, the loss of pyramidal cells which normally express the receptor should produce decrements, and would be expected in Alzheimer-type dementia and perhaps also in elderly depressed patients. Lower-affinity compounds can be used to indicate displacement from a specific receptor by competing agonists or antagonists. They offer the promise of a pharmacological dissection of drug or hormone action which still appears particularly likely to be of interest in affective disorder. At present, the application is limited to an available ligand such as ^{123}I-IBZM.

CONCLUSIONS

Brain-imaging techniques provide a common focus for neuroscience at both a basic and clinical level. At present functional imaging appears to have the potential to define the critical brain areas involved in the expression of psychiatric symptoms. Whether this localization will lead further to an understanding of disordered anatomy, as may be the case in schizophrenia, or disordered neurotransmitter function, as appears more likely in depressive illness, remains to be seen. At stake is an improved understanding of aetiology, and a better insight into the biological factors that may predispose to refractoriness and poor outcome. The challenge, as for neuroscience in general, is to harness a variety of techniques to answering the central clinical questions.

ACKNOWLEDGEMENTS

I thank the Wellcome Trust and the Gordon Small Trust for support and Norma Brearley for preparation of the manuscript.

REFERENCES

1 Frackowiack RSJ, Pozzilli C, Legg NJ *et al.* Regional cerebral oxygen supply and utilization in dementia: a clinical and physiological study with oxygen-15 and positron tomography. *Brain* 1981;**104**:753–778.

2 Haxby JV, Duara R, Grady CL, Cutler NR, Rapoport SI. Relations between neuro-psychological and cerebral metabolic asymmetries in early Alzheimer's disease. *J Cereb Blood Flow Metab* 1985;**5**:193–200.

3 Foster NL, Chase TN, Patronas NJ, Gillespie MM, Fedio P. Cerebral mapping of apraxia in Alzheimer's disease by positron emission tomography. *Ann Neurol* 1986;**19**:139–143.

4 Neary D, Snowden JS, Shields RA *et al.* Single photon emission tomography using ^{99m}Tc-HM-PAO in the investigation of dementia. *J Neurol Neurosurg Psychiatry* 1987;**50**:1101–1109.

5 Hunter R, McLuskie R, Wyper D *et al.* The pattern of function-related regional cerebral blood flow investigated by single photon emission tomography with ^{99m}Tc-HMPAO in patients with presenile Alzheimer's disease and Korsakoff's psychosis. *Psychol Med* 1989;**19**:847–855.

6 Burns A, Philpot MP, Costa DC, Ell PJ, Levy R. The investigation of Alzheimer's disease with single photon emission tomography. *J Neurol Neurosurg Psychiatry* 1989;**52**:248–253.

7 Montaldi D, Brooks DN, McColl JH *et al.* Measurements of regional cerebral blood flow and cognitive performance in Alzheimer's disease. *J Neurol Neurosurg Psychiatry* 1990;**53**:33–38.

8 Liddle PF, Friston KJ, Frith CD *et al.* Patterns of cerebral blood flow in schizophrenia. *Br J Psychiatry* 1992;**160**:179–186.

9 Dolan RJ, Calloway SP, Mann AH. Cerebral ventricular size in depressed subjects. *Psychol Med* 1985;**15**:873–878.

10 Jacoby RJ, Dolan RJ, Levy R, Baldy R. Quantitative computed tomography in elderly depressed patients. *Br J Psychiatry* 1983;**143**:124–127.

11 Jacoby RJ, Levy R. Computed tomography in the elderly. 3. Affective disorder. *Br J Psychiatry* 1980;**136**:270–275.

12 Alexopoulos GS, Young RC, Shindledecker RD. Brain computed tomography findings in geriatric depression and primary degenerative dementia. *Biol Psychiatry* 1992;**31**:591–599.

13 Pearlson GD, Rabins PV, Kim WS *et al.* Structural brain CT changes and cognitive deficits in elderly depressives with and without reversible dementia ('pseudodementia'). *Psychol Med* 1989;**19**:573–584.

14 Abas MA, Sahakian BJ, Levy R. Neuropsychological deficits and CT scan changes in elderly depressives. *Psychol Med* 1990;**20**:507–520.

15 Coffey CE, Wilkinson WE, Weiner RD *et al.* Quantitative cerebral anatomy in depression. *Arch Gen Psychiatry* 1993;**50**:7–16.

16 Coffey CE, Figiel GS, Djang WT *et al.* Leukoencephalopathy in elderly depressed patients referred for ECT. *Biol Psychiatry* 1988;**24**:143–161.

17 Dupont RM, Jernigan TL, Butters N *et al.* Subcortical abnormalities detected in bipolar affective disorder using magnetic resonance imaging. Clinical and neuropsychological significance. *Arch Gen Psychiatry* 1990;**47**:55–59.

18 Shah SA, Doraiswamy PM, Husain MM *et al*. Posterior fossa abnormalities in major depression: a controlled magnetic resonance imaging study. *Acta Psychiatr Scand* 1992;**85**:474–479.

19 Belliveau JW, Kennedy DN, McKinstry RC *et al*. Functional mapping of the human visual cortex using magnetic resonance imaging. *Science* 1991;**254**:716–719.

20 Kwong KK, Belliveau JW, Chesler DA *et al*. Dynamic magnetic resonance imaging of human brain activity during primary sensory stimulation. *Proc Natl Acad Sci USA* 1992;**89**:5675–5679.

21 Friston KJ, Frith CD, Liddle PF, Frackowiak RSJ. Comparing functional (PET) images: the assessment of significant change. *J Cereb Blood Flow Metab* 1991;**11**:690–699.

22 Baxter LR, Schwartz JM, Phelps ME *et al*. Reduction of prefrontal cortex glucose metabolism common to three types of depression. *Arch Gen Psychiatry* 1989;**46**:243–250.

23 Sackeim HA, Prohovnik I, Moeller JR *et al*. Regional cerebral blood flow in mood disorders. I. Comparison of major depressives and normal controls at rest. *Arch Gen Psychiatry* 1990;**47**:60–70.

24 Bench CJ, Friston KJ, Brown RG *et al*. The anatomy of melancholia — focal abnormalities of cerebral blood flow in major depression. *Psychol Med* 1992;**22**:607–615.

25 Curran SM, Murray CM, Van Beck M *et al*. A single photon emission computerised tomography study of regional brain function in elderly patients with major depression and with Alzheimer-type dementia. *Br J Psychiatry* 1993;**163**:155–165.

26 Austin M-P, Dougall N, Ross M *et al*. Single photon emission tomography with [99mTc]-Exametazime in major depression and the pattern of brain activity underlying the psychotic/neurotic continuum. *J Affect Dis* 1992;**26**:31–44.

27 Goodwin GM, Austin M-P, Dougall N *et al*. State changes in brain activity shown by the uptake of [99mTc]-Exametazime with single photon emission tomography in major depression before and after treatment. *J Affect Dis* 1993;**29**:243–253.

28 Kung HF. SPECT and PET ligands for CNS imaging. *Neurotransmissions* 1993;**IX**:1–4.

29 Mathis CA, Taylor SE, Biegon A, Enas JD. [125I]5-iodo-6-nitroquipazine: a potent and selective ligand for the 5-hydroxytryptamine uptake complex. I. *In vitro* studies. *Brain Res* 1993;**619**:229–235.

30 Biegon A, Mathis CA, Hanrahan SM, Jagust WJ. [125I]5-iodo-6-nitroquipazine: a potent and selective ligand for the 5-hydroxytryptamine uptake complex. II. *In vivo* studies in rats. *Brain Res* 1993;**619**:236–246.

31 Innis R, Zoghbi S, Johnston E *et al*. SPECT imaging of the benzodiazepine receptor in non-human primate brain with [I-123] RO 16-0154. *Eur J Pharmacol* 1991;**193**:249–252.

32 Woods SW, Seibyl JP, Goddart AW *et al*. Dynamic SPECT imaging after injection of the benzodiazepine receptor ligand [123I]-Iomazenil in healthy human subjects. *Psychiatry Res: Neuroimaging* 1992;**45**:67–77.

33 Benes FM, Vincent SL, Alsterberg G, Bird ED, SanGiovanni JP. Increased $GABA_A$ receptor binding in superficial layers of cingulate cortex in schizophrenics. *J Neurosci* 1992;**12**:924–929.

PART 9
ENDOCRINOLOGY AND
METABOLISM

Is intensive control of
diabetes mellitus worthwhile?

DAVID R. HADDEN

There are four important words in the title of this review which require to be considered separately before the overall question can be addressed.

Diabetes is easily recognized from the classical symptoms of thirst, polyuria and weight loss which gave it the Greek name for a siphon: but the definition of a disease by symptoms at its clinical recognition may not be very appropriate when the question is one of long-term survival for 40 or 50 years — often longer than the life expectancy of the doctor who made the original diagnosis. The present division into insulin-dependent and non-insulin-dependent diabetes was a convenient compromise 20 years ago, but recent developments in identifying diabetes-susceptibility genes, and better understanding of the immunological processes which affect the β cells of the pancreatic islets, make this simple split into two types less acceptable. And division by whether or not insulin was used for treatment has always been unacceptable.

The concept and measurement of *control* seeks to emulate both the pattern and the level of blood glucose in the non-diabetic individual, but requires assessment of two factors which do not necessarily go hand in hand. Overall or average blood glucose control can be measured by an average of many blood glucose values, or by the use of a biological integrator such as the glycation of haemoglobin which reflects the average blood glucose over a period approximating to the half-life of a red blood cell — about 8 weeks. But this gives no measure of the lability of blood glucose which is an inevitable consequence of eating and fasting, and of insulin injection — this may be of much more importance to the person with diabetes, but can only be measured by derived indices such as the mean amplitude of glucose excursion (MAGE).

Intensive control is both an old and a new concept in diabetes management by insulin injections. Seventy years ago, when insulin was an exciting new drug, it was quickly realized that one injection of short-acting soluble insulin a day was not sufficient even to relieve the symptoms, let alone reverse the body catabolism: early treatment regimens required short-acting insulin several times a day, before regular meals. The early diabetologists therefore spent much time trying to perfect a long-acting insulin which would theoretically allow only one injection a day — but this never worked satisfactorily, largely because we eat several times a day and then spend a long time fasting when asleep. This fruitless search for a once-a-day panacea may well have been one reason why blood glucose control in those very early days, when diets were strict and the patient did what the doctor said, was probably better on average than it was 30 years later when a *laissez-faire* approach had developed with a concept of simply preventing symptoms, with a free diet and avoidance of hypoglycaemia as the goal. Intensive control returned with the development of insulin infusion pumps which tried to reproduce the physiological response of the β cell to each meal and also the slow continuous release of insulin in the fasting overnight state. But the pumps have been largely overtaken by pen injectors, and self-monitoring of capillary fingerprick blood glucose has had a more profound effect than either on making tight control both possible and acceptable.

Worthwhile is a more difficult word. Does it mean cost-effective, or a longer life expectancy, or a better quality of life, however that is measured, or simply fewer complications of the long-term diabetic state? In this era, it will doubtless have to include a financial cost, and be measured either against the norms for the non-diabetic members of the same population, or even against some future idealized projection of what comprises an ageing society. The costs and benefits of long-term management of a chronic condition which can be remarkably benign and consistent with normal life expectancy or, on the other hand, produce disastrous and crippling complications and morbidity in young people — these concepts require a detailed and sophisticated clinical audit process which is not yet generally available.

The overall question has been addressed in several ways in the past 20 years. A number of well-designed prospective randomized studies of intensive control have now been completed, over sufficient time periods to yield significant results. And these have now been further subjected to meta-analysis with more powerful conclusions. At the same time a much larger and more extensive study has been completed in the USA which has now been reported, and with a more vigorous public presentation has become a 'shot heard round the world'. The Diabetes Control and Complications Trial (DCCT) [1] will now be the standard by which others are judged. During the same period there have been a number of large long-term natural history epidemiological studies on well-defined populations which, although they do not have the methodological correctness of a randomized controlled trial, nevertheless have produced considerable evidence of a strong relationship between blood glucose control and both morbidity and mortality from diabetic complications. Only the prospective randomized trials will be able to answer the basic question of whether the association of good metabolic control with fewer complications is due only to the effectiveness of the treatment, or to a confounding effect of a milder and more easily controlled type of diabetes, perhaps genetically determined.

THE STUDIES: RANDOMIZED CONTROL TRIALS

Over 30 reports of studies of this type have been published, but the design and analysis of these have been different and it is difficult to draw general conclusions. The great majority have compared conventional insulin treatment of insulin-dependent diabetes, using one or two injections of short- or medium-acting insulin daily with conventional attendance at a diabetes clinic for regular review but without intensive medical, nursing or dietetic supervision. This randomly assigned group has been compared with a 'tight control' group where insulin has been given by more frequent subcutaneous injections or by a continuous insulin infusion pump: intensive control has usually meant more frequent medical, nursing and dietetic contact, with increased interest in the results of capillary glucose self-monitoring and a definite aim to achieve as normal a blood glucose profile as possible. Smaller studies of short duration have not had the statistical power required [2]. Almost all of the intervention studies have been of secondary prevention of late complications, and only the DCCT has effectively addressed primary prevention from the date of initial diagnosis of the disease. Three early Scandinavian studies of insulin-dependent diabetes have been extensively analysed.

In Denmark, at the Steno Memorial Hospital, two smaller independent studies (total 70 patients) reviewed for 5-8 years showed a definite improvement in blood glucose control (mean glycosylated haemoglobin) for the intensively treated patients [3]. This group has concentrated on the progression of early nephropathy and showed that among 19 patients with initial microalbuminuria the progression of renal complications was more frequent during conventional treatment — 10 of the 10 conventionally treated patients progressed to clinical nephropathy and 7 developed hypertension, whereas only 2 of 9 intensively treated patients progressed to clinical nephropathy and only 1 developed hypertension.

In Stockholm, 102 patients were randomized to intensive or conventional therapy [4]. After 7 years there was less progression of all measures of microangiopathy in the intensive group — only one developed clinical nephropathy compared to nine on conventional therapy, and laser photocoagulation for retinopathy was needed by only 27% of those intensively treated who developed severe retinopathy, compared to 52% in the conventional group. Nerve conduction velocity in the legs deteriorated less in the intensively treated group.

In Oslo, 45 patients aged 18–42 have been followed up since 1984 [5]. For the first 4 years they were randomized to multiple insulin injections, continuous subcutaneous insulin infusion using a pump, or to two daily injections. After 2 years there was less progression of retinopathy or neuropathy for the continuous subcutaneous infusion group, and the less tight groups were offered the option of more intensive therapy. After 7 years those patients from the whole group who had the best glycosylated haemoglobin had less retinopathy, less urinary albumin excretion and less deterioration in nerve conduction.

Only one meta-analysis has been attempted in this field [6]. The numbers of patients in these long-term randomized trials have been relatively small, and intensive blood glucose control requires considerable effort from both staff and patients, to say nothing of financial support. By pooling results from these smaller trials it is possible to demonstrate significant effects of intensive therapy on retinopathy and nephropathy that may not have achieved statistical significance in the individual studies. In six selected studies after more than 2 years of intensive therapy the risk of retinopathy progression was lower (odds ratio 0.49; 95% confidence interval 0.28–0.85; $P = 0.011$), as was the risk of nephropathy progression (odds ratio 0.34; 95% confidence interval 0.20–0.58; $P < 0.001$; Fig. 1).

The major study in this field is the DCCT which was recently concluded [1]. The study was conceived in 1975, with the aim of assessing the glucose hypothesis using a strict risk/benefit evaluation. After starting to plan in 1980, the first patient was enrolled in 1983 and the study ended in 1993. The conclusion is simple — intensive therapy effectively delays the onset and slows the progression of diabetic retinopathy, nephropathy and neuropathy in patients with insulin-dependent diabetes mellitus. The study followed 1441 patients for 3–9 years (mean 6.5): 99% completed the

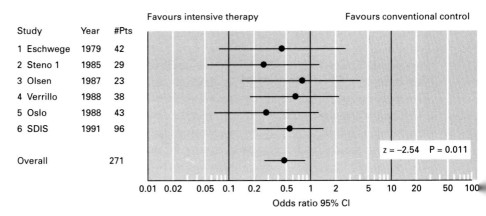

Fig. 1 Meta-analysis of the effects of long-term intensive blood glucose control (more than 2 years) on progression of retinopathy. Overall, for 271 randomized patients, after 2–5 years of intensive therapy the risk of retinopathy was significantly reduced (odds ratio 0.49; 95% confidence interval 0.28–0.85; $P = 0.011$). Reproduced with permission [6].

study and more than 95% of all scheduled examinations were completed. The intensive-therapy regimen (basal/bolus insulin by pump infusor or multiple injections) with frequent self-monitoring, dose adjustment and medical or nursing advice achieved a mean long-term capillary blood glucose of 8.6 (±s.d. 1.7) mmol/l. The conventional regimen consisted of one or two daily injections of insulin on a fixed-dose system, with some education on diet and exercise, and an aim of preventing symptoms of either hyperglycaemia or hypoglycaemia — these patients achieved a mean long-term capillary blood glucose of 12.8 (±s.d. 3.1) mmol/l.

There were two arms of the study — a primary prevention cohort of newly diagnosed (1–5 years' duration) diabetic patients, and a secondary intervention cohort with diabetes for 1–15 years who may already have had mild retinopathy, nephropathy or neuropathy. Considerable trouble was taken to measure glycosylated haemoglobin by an accurate and repro-ducible method; if this is taken as the 'gold standard' for blood glucose control the conventional cohort achieved an average Hb/A_{1c} of 9% compared to the intensive cohort result of 7% — these maintained a highly significant difference ($P < 0.001$) from 3 months to the end of the study. However, it should be stated that the normal non-diabetic range for this assay would be 3.5–5.0%, so that even the intensive cohort were not all that good, and the conventional cohort were really rather bad [7].

The study reached a significant endpoint and closed 1 year earlier than expected. Intensive therapy reduced the risk of development of retinopathy by 76% in newly diagnosed patients, and slowed its progression by 54% in the secondary intervention cohort. For the two cohorts combined, intensive therapy reduced the occurrence of microalbuminuria (≥ 40 mg/ 24 hours) by 39%, of albuminuria (≥ 300 mg/24 hours) by 54%, and of clinical neuropathy by 60%. The treatment effects continued with time, and the differences actually increased with longer duration of intensive therapy (Fig. 2).

The conception and completion of this megastudy is a credit to the vision of Dr Oscar B. Crofford of Vanderbilt University, and to the deter-mination of Dr David Nathan and nearly 700 health care professionals from 29 different North American centres. It cost a great deal, but even at an estimated £10 000 per patient per year, the importance of the clearly stated and easily understood result cannot be overemphasized.

Randomized prospective studies of the treatment of non-insulin-dependent diabetes are even fewer, although epidemiological evidence suggests that the same risks for microvascular disease exist. More important in this older age group is the greater prevalence of macrovascular disease, and the first study to investigate this problem, the University Group Diabetes Programme (UGDP) came to an uncertain conclusion because of a suggested increase in major cardiovascular events in one of the treated groups [8]. The United Kingdom Prospective Diabetes Study (UKPDS)

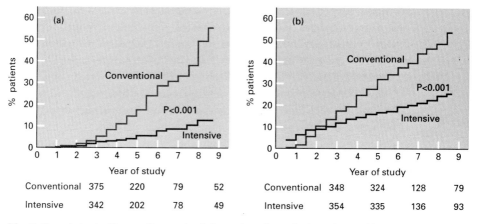

Fig. 2 Cumulative incidence of a sustained change in retinopathy in patients with insulin-dependent diabetes mellitus receiving intensive or conventional therapy, in (a) the primary prevention and (b) the secondary intervention cohort. A sustained change in the severity of retinopathy was defined as a change observed by fundus photography of at least three steps from baseline sustained for at least 6 months. Reproduced with permission from [1].

is now well-advanced, with over 5000 newly diagnosed patients in 23 centres, treated by diet only, or with additional sulphonylurea or diguanide drugs, or with insulin: an interlinked but separate study will assess the effect of antihypertensive therapy in the same population [9]. The randomization has not yet been unmasked: at present the diet-only group has a mean HbA_{1c} of 7.6%, which is significantly higher than any of the other groups (chlorpropamide 6.9%; glibenclamide 7.0%; insulin 7.0%; $P < 0.001$). It should be noted that *all* of these groups are close to the level of HbA_{1c} achieved in the intensively treated cohort of the DCCT, and the conventional cohort in that study was very much worse.

If glycosylated haemoglobin is to be the gold standard for blood glucose control, what at present is the level at which we should aim [10]? It has

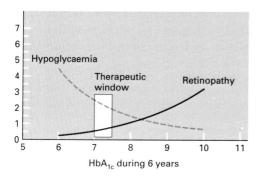

Fig. 3 Graphic presentation of the relative risk of retinopathy and hypoglycaemia based on data from various studies. A therapeutic window is indicated. Reproduced with permission from [11].

been suggested that a long-term HbA_{1c} level of about +4 s.d. above the mean for non-diabetic subjects may be sufficient to avoid serious complications in most patients, but that a level of only +2 s.d. above the normal mean may be necessary completely to avoid their development. Dahl-Jørgensen et al. have [11] indicated that an HbA_{1c} of 7–8% may represent the crossing of the curves of relationship between HbA_{1c} and progression of retinopathy, and HbA_{1c} and the risk of iatrogenic hypoglycaemia — this postulates a 'therapeutic window' of HbA_{1c} as a recommended target (Fig. 3).

NATURAL HISTORY STUDIES

Natural history or epidemiological review studies are less powerful in deciding the best method of treatment but have none the less been important in framing the glucose hypothesis. The major personal analysis by Pirart [12] in Belgium, who followed 2795 diabetic patients for up to 25 years, concluded that poor long-term control of blood glucose was clearly related to a higher prevalence and incidence of all complications, particularly of severe retinopathy. This relationship has also been established in a large population-based study in Wisconsin, where the risk of developing proliferative retinopathy was 22 times higher in those patients with HbA_1 in the highest quartile compared to the lowest quartile during the previous 4 years [13]. 'A prospective study in the past' of insulin-dependent diabetic patients attending the diabetes clinic at the Royal Victoria Hospital, Belfast [14] has also shown a highly significant relationship between increasing mean HbA_1 levels from serial measurements over 6 years with background and proliferative retinopathy, and proliferative changes had not developed in any patient with a mean HbA_1 below 10%.

Natural history studies of non-insulin-dependent diabetes have concentrated more on macrovascular disease, and the incidence of early death from ischaemic heart disease in these patients confounds long-term analysis of microvascular disease. For a cohort of 432 newly diagnosed diabetic patients aged 40–69 at onset followed for 10 years, those who were maintained on diet only showed a steady rise in fasting plasma glucose of about 0.3 mmol/l per year, which is evidence for gradual β-cell failure with time: the overall rate of ischaemic heart disease, both fatal and non-fatal, exceeded that expected in an age/sex-matched population cohort, but there is still no conclusive evidence that macrovascular disease can be prevented by more intensive blood glucose control [15].

PROBLEMS

There are three main problems encountered during all the studies of intensive plasma glucose control. Hypoglycaemia is the most important.

This is well-recognized to need special care in long-standing insulin-dependent patients with hypoglycaemic unawareness who start intensive therapy, and a higher goal of HbA_{1c} may need to be set for them. It should be emphasized that good glycaemic control should mean normoglycaemia, and that hypoglycaemia itself can induce defective counterregulation and thus perpetuate the problem [16].

The chief adverse event associated with intensive insulin therapy in the DCCT was a two- to threefold increase in severe hypoglycaemia. There was no death attributable to hypoglycaemia, and no differences between the treatment groups in major automobile accidents requiring hospital admission (20 in the intensive treatment and 22 in the conventional treatment group). There were two fatal motor vehicle accidents, one in each group, in which hypoglycaemia may have had a causative role, and a non-trial passenger in a car driven by an intensive therapy patient was killed in a motor accident which was probably due to the driver's hypoglycaemia. The authors of the report on this study, although mindful of the potential for severe injury, believe that the risk of severe hypoglycaemia with intensive therapy is greatly outweighed by the reduction in micro-vascular and neurological complications [1,17]. The meta-analysis of the preceding smaller randomized studies of intensive control also showed a trend towards more frequent severe hypoglycaemic reactions among intensively treated patients, but this difference was not significant: they also found a significant increase in diabetic ketoacidosis in patients treated by continuous subcutaneous insulin infusion pumps in three studies [6], but there were insufficient data on patients using multiple injection techniques.

Transient worsening of pre-existing retinopathy with intensive insulin therapy was first noticed in the multicentre Kroc study [18] and was confirmed by the DCCT. This early worsening, which only became apparent because of the extensive photographic records of the retina, consisted of the development of soft exudates or intraretinal microvascular abnormalities, and occurred mainly in the secondary intervention group during the first year of therapy. The abnormalities generally disappeared by 18 months, and those patients with early worsening who were intensively treated ultimately showed a 74% reduction in the risk of progression of retinopathy compared to similar patients with early worsening in the conventional therapy group ($P < 0.001$). The authors considered that evidence of early worsening of retinopathy should not deter clinicians from using intensive therapy.

Quality of life in insulin-treated diabetic patients depends on a number of factors, not all of which are associated with recognized complications of the disease or its treatment. Weight gain was 10 lb (4.5 kg) greater on average in the intensive treatment group in the DCCT, but the patients indicated a better sense of well-being. Whether the intensive medical and nursing contacts that were possible in these specially funded trials would be judged to interfere with a normal lifestyle and thus be an adverse effect on quality of life is difficult to judge. In the Oslo study, after 4 years the patients on conventional therapy were offered the chance to join the intensive treatment protocol and many of them elected to do so, which indicates at least patient enthusiasm for the concept. In Scandinavia, there has been an improvement in the quality of insulin-dependent diabetes treatment in the past 5 years, and nearly all patients may choose intensive treatment if they wish: at present in most clinics 50–80% use multiple injections.

COST-EFFECTIVENESS

This is the question which is left unanswered by all of the studies on intensive control. The DCCT team acknowledged that they employed an expert team of diabetologists, nurses, dieticians and behavioural specialists, and the time, effort and cost required were considerable. They concluded that the health care system should provide the support necessary to make intensive therapy available to those patients who will benefit. The real cost of diabetes in any population is unknown, and very difficult to quantify. An estimate for England and Wales 1986–87 gave a total health care cost for diabetes and its complications of £484 million, which was 3.8% of the total all-cause cost of £12 696 million [19]. This included the inpatient hospital costs where diabetes was the primary or secondary diagnosis, the outpatient costs of diabetic clinics, general practitioner consultations and prescriptions and long-term residential and nursing home care.

In the absence of a register of diabetes any of these figures can only be a rough estimate, and the influence of intensive management can only be guessed. Loss of productivity due to premature mortality in the USA is thought to account for 29% of the total cost of diabetes in that country, with short-term (9%) and long-term morbidity (12%) bringing the total of indirect costs to half of the total estimated cost of $91 848 million [20].

Some speculative figures have been suggested following the DCCT (Crofford, unpublished data). For a typical patient in that study, a 27-year-old insulin-dependent diabetic of 9 years' duration with a background retinopathy of microaneurysms only and 20 mg/24 hours microalbuminuria, the time to develop clinically significant eye complications would be 15 years on conventional treatment and 48 years on intensive therapy. For significant kidney complications the times are 17 and 44 years respectively. On these estimates the typical patient would develop the complications in his or her early 40s on conventional therapy, but not until aged over 70 years on intensive therapy.

The direct costs per patient of the study for physician, nurse and dietician came to about $2000 per year for conventional therapy and $4000 per year for intensive therapy, based on estimates of 85 minutes per year of physician time for conventional care and 307 minutes per year for intensive care. The point at which a cost saving to the US health care system would arise would be after 18 years' treatment.

The aims of the St Vincent Declaration [21] made by the European branch of the World Health Organization and of the International Diabetes Federation include the implementation of effective measures for the prevention of costly complications: whether intensive therapy on the lines proposed by these recent studies will achieve those aims remains uncertain, but the UK Task Force is charged with the responsibility of finding out.

REFERENCES

1 The effect of intensive treatment of diabetes on the development and progression of long-term complications in insulin-dependent diabetes mellitus. The Diabetes Control and Complications Trial Research Group. *N Engl J Med* 1993;**329**:977–986.

2 Bell PM, Sawhney B, Hayes JR, Hadden DR. Effect of plasma glucose control by continuous subcutaneous insulin infusion on nerve conduction. *Ir J Med Sci* 1985;**154**:378–384.

3 Feldt-Rasmussen B, Mathiesen ER, Jensen T, Lauritzen T, Deckert T. Effect of improved metabolic control on loss of kidney function in type 1 (insulin-dependent) diabetic patients: an update of the Steno studies. *Diabetologia* 1991;**34**:164–170.

4 Reichard P, Nilsson B-Y, Rosenqvist U. The effect of long-term intensified insulin treatment on the development of microvascular complications of diabetes mellitus. *N Engl J Med* 1993;**329**:403–409.

5 Brinchmann-Hansen O, Dahl-Jørgensen K, Sandvik L, Hanssen KF. Blood glucose concentrations and progression of diabetic retinopathy: the seven year results of the Oslo study. *Br Med J* 1992;**304**:19–22.

6 Wang PH, Lau J, Chalmers TC. Meta-analysis of effects of intensive blood-glucose control on late complications of type 1 diabetes. *Lancet* 1993;**341**:1306–1309.

7 Hadden DR. The Diabetes Control and Complications Trial (DCCT): what every endocrinologist needs to know. *Clin Endocrinol* 1994;**40**:293–294.

8 Knattrud G, Klimt C, Levin M, Jaccobson M, Goldner M. Effects of hypoglycaemic agents on vascular complications in patients with adult-onset diabetes. VII. Mortality and selected non-fatal events with insulin treatment. *JAMA* 1978;**240**:37–42.

9 United Kingdom prospective diabetes study (UKPDS) 13: relative efficacy of randomly allocated diet, sulphonylurea, insulin or metformin in patients with newly-diagnosed non-insulin dependent diabetes followed for three years. United Kingdom Prospective Diabetes Study Group. *Br Med J* 1995;**310**:83–88.

10 McCance DR, Kennedy L. The concept and measurement of 'control'. In: *Textbook of Diabetes*, edited by Pickup JC, Williams G. Blackwell Science, Oxford, 1991:325–334.

11 Dahl-Jørgensen K, Brinchmann-Hansen O, Bangstad H-J, Hanssen KF. Blood glucose control and microvascular complications — what do we do now? *Diabetologia* 1994;**37**:1172–1177.

12 Pirart J. Diabetes mellitus and its degenerative complications: a prospective study of 4400 patients observed between 1947 and 1973. *Diabetes Care* 1978;**1**:168–188.

13 Klein R, Klein BE, Scott E, Moss MA, Davis MD, Demets DL. Glycosylated hemoglobin predicts the incidence and progression of diabetic retinopathy. *JAMA* 1988;**260**:2864–2871.

14 McCance DR, Hadden DR, Atkinson AB, Archer DB, Kennedy L. Long term glycaemic control and diabetic retinopathy. *Lancet* 1989;**299**:824–828.

15 Hadden DR, Blair ALT, Wilson EA *et al.* Natural history of diabetes presenting age 40–69 years: a prospective study of the influence of intensive dietary therapy. *Q J Med* 1986;**59**:579–598.

16 Cranston I, Lomas J, Maran A, Macdonald I, Amiel S. Restoration of hypoglycae-mia unawareness in patients with long-duration insulin dependent diabetes. *Lancet* 1994;**344**:283–287.
17 The DCCT Research Group. Epidemiology of severe hypoglycaemia in the Diabetes Control and Complications Trial. *Am J Med* 1991;**90**:450–459.
18 The Kroc Collaborative Study Group. Diabetic retinopathy after two years of intensified insulin treatment: follow up of the Kroc Collaborative Study. *JAMA* 1988;**260**:37–41.
19 Diabetes. A Model for Health Care Management. Office of Health Economics, London, 1989:32–42.
20 Diabetes 1993: Vital Statistics. American Diabetes Association, Alexandria, 1993:43–44.
21 Krans HMJ, Porta M, Keen H (eds) Diabetes Care and Research in Europe: the St Vincent Declaration Action Programme. WHO, Copenhagen, 1992:7–8.

Glucokinase mutations and type 2 diabetes

ANDREW T. HATTERSLEY

Clinical and scientific observations as well as molecular biological studies have been important in establishing the role of glucokinase gene mutations in type 2 diabetes. Glucokinase was first recognized as a key enzyme in glucose metabolism in the pancreatic islet in 1968 [1]. The finding in 1992 that mutations in the glucokinase gene could result in type 2 diabetes [2,3] was based on the clinical recognition of maturity-onset diabetes of the young (MODY) as a discrete inherited subgroup of type 2 diabetes.

EARLY DESCRIPTIONS OF MATURITY-ONSET DIABETES OF THE YOUNG

MODY is a discrete subgroup of type 2 diabetes, characterized by an autosomal dominant inheritance of young-onset diabetes (frequently diagnosed before 25 years) [4,5]. This type of non-insulin-dependent diabetes was first recognized in the pre-insulin era. At this time diabetes in childhood was usually fatal within a year of diagnosis, but occasional children had a mild course and were alive many years after diagnosis. Cammidge noted that there was frequently a strong family history in these individuals, writing in 1928 [6] that:

> The dominant variety is almost invariably mild, even in young people, and may persist for many years without causing serious symptoms or materially affecting the general health.

In 1974 it was formally recognized that young patients with type 2 diabetes could have a discrete inherited syndrome. Tattersall described three families in which diabetes was inherited as an autosomal dominant trait and had distinctive clinical features [7]. Although diabetes in these families was frequently diagnosed before age 30, it could be treated without insulin and was not ketoacidosis-prone. Microvascular complications were rare in the families; only 2 of 13 diabetic subjects with a mean duration of 20 years had any retinopathy. This clinical description has been central to the subsequent description and study of MODY.

MODY — A MODEL FOR GENETIC ANALYSIS

The development in the 1980s of the 'new genetics' resulted in techniques becoming available to define the underlying molecular biology of genetic disorders. This resulted in considerable interest in the study of the molecular genetics of type 2 diabetes and MODY.

The importance of genetic factors in type 2 diabetes is clearly illustrated by the near 100% concordance in identical twins [8]. Although type 2 diabetes is a common disorder with a large inherited component, the application of molecular biological methods to type 2 diabetes has been complex. The inheritance of type 2 diabetes is both polygenic and heterogeneous, and the late age of onset and disease-related mortality make the collection of large, multigeneration pedigrees very difficult [9]. Neel in 1965 described diabetes as the 'geneticists' nightmare' and this is still a most apt description for the molecular biological analysis of type 2 diabetes [9].

Genetic analysis in monogenic MODY had many advantages over typical type 2 diabetes, as shown in Table 1. In the late 1980s large MODY families were collected in the UK, France and the USA for molecular biological studies. The homogeneous, multigeneration pedigrees where diabetes resulted from a single gene were ideal for linkage studies. In addition, physiological studies in large Caucasian pedigrees established that diabetes in these pedigrees results from reduced insulin secretion rather than reduced insulin action [5,10]. This reduced the search for causative genes to those genes expressed in the β-cell.

GLUCOKINASE — AN EXCELLENT CANDIDATE GENE

A large body of basic science work principally by Magnuson [11] and Matschinsky [12] suggested that glucokinase was an excellent candidate gene for type 2 diabetes and MODY. Glucokinase is one of the family of

Table 1 Comparison of type 2 diabetes with maturity-onset diabetes of the young (MODY), showing why molecular genetic analysis is easier in MODY.

	Type 2 diabetes	MODY
Age at onset	Middle/old age	Adolescent/young adult
Aetiology	50% genetic 50% environments	100% genetic
Inheritance	Heterogeneous Polygenic	Homogeneous Autosomal dominant
Pathophysiology	β-cell/liver/muscle	β-cell

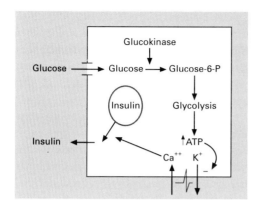

Fig. 1 The pancreatic β-cell, showing the important position of glucokinase, which has been termed the pancreatic glucose sensor. Modified from [29].

hexokinases that catalyses the phosphorylation of glucose to glucose-6-phosphate. This first step in glucose metabolism is the rate-limiting step in glucose metabolism in the β-cell and hepatocyte. Glucokinase is only expressed in the pancreas and liver and its expression is tightly controlled by two tissue-specific promoters [11]. Unlike other hexokinases, it has a low affinity for glucose (high K_m) and is not inhibited by its product, glucose-6-phosphate. These unique kinetic properties result in the rate of glucose phosphorylation being proportional to the physiological glucose concentration, allowing the β-cell and hepatocyte to respond appropriately to the degree of glycaemia [12]. The different regulatory role of glucokinase in these cell types reflects the different roles of glucose metabolism in the two tissues.

In the pancreatic β-cell, glucokinase acts as the 'glucose sensor' [12], ensuring that insulin release is appropriate to the glucose concentration. Figure 1 shows the pathway linking glucose phosphorylation with insulin release. The principal regulator of the expression of β-cell glucokinase is glucose concentration. Increased expression of the pancreatic enzyme will increase glucokinase activity and so further increase insulin secretion.

In the liver the principal response to hyperglycaemia is increased glucose uptake and synthesis of glycogen, in part regulated by glucokinase [12]. Phosphorylation of glucose maintains a concentration gradient for glucose transport across the cell membrane, which facilitates hepatic glucose uptake and metabolism to glycogen. In the liver, expression of glucokinase is increased in response to elevated insulin levels, resulting in an appropriate increase in hepatic glucose uptake after meals.

MUTATIONS OF THE GLUCOKINASE GENE IN MODY

The characteristic of glucokinase strongly suggested that this might be an important candidate gene in type 2 diabetes. Professor Alan Permutt's laboratory in Washington University, St Louis, USA, cloned the human gene and showed that it had a similar structure to rat gene, with 12 exons and discrete pancreatic and hepatic promoters [13].

The identification of two microsatellite polymorphisms flanking the glucokinase gene [13] by Permutt and colleagues led to the description of linkage in French and English MODY pedigrees in early 1992 [2,3]. These were rapidly followed by descriptions of a large number of mutations in the coding region or intron/exon boundaries of the 12 exons of the glucokinase gene. Over 30 different mutations have been described in French, English, Japanese, Swedish, and Afro-Caribbean families [14–19]. Expression studies show that the missense mutations in MODY families alter the enzyme's maximal activity for glucose phosphorylation or alter the affinity for glucose [18]. No common mutation has been described but most mutations are found in exons 7 and 8, which are thought to encode the glucose-binding cleft of the enzyme [18].

CLINICAL PHENOTYPE OF GLUCOKINASE MUTATIONS

The initial descriptions of linkage to the glucokinase gene were in large French [2] and English [3] MODY families characterized by an early onset of hyperglycaemia. In these initial descriptions it was noted that early diagnosis was usually the result of screening and that some patients did not present until middle or old age [3]. Subsequent screening studies have shown that glucokinase mutations have been detected in 10–56% of MODY patients, 0.5–2% of type 2 diabetes patients and 1–5% of subjects with gestational diabetes. There is no evidence to suggest that patients with different clinical diagnoses have a different phenotype. In Oxford we found the same missense mutation, resulting in the substitution of glycine for arginine at position 299 in families diagnosed as having MODY [15], type 2 diabetes [15] and gestational diabetes [20]. All these patients had a very similar phenotype and fasting blood glucose. This shows the limitations of conventional classification, which is based on when a diagnosis is made. In patients with glucokinase mutations it is now possible to propose a classification based on the underlying molecular biology. 'Glucokinase deficiency' or 'glucokinase-deficient type 2 diabetes' has been proposed.

If a diagnostic label based on the underlying molecular biology is to be useful there must be a discrete clinical syndrome [16]. The idea of a distinct clinical phenotype associated with glucokinase mutations is supported by Froguel's series of 18 families [16] (see Table 2 for summary). Hyperglycaemia is mild, with only 46% having diabetes by World Health Organization criteria but almost all subjects with glucokinase deficiency

Table 2 Clinical characteristics of glucokinase deficiency.

Mild fasting hyperglycaemia from childhood
Detected on routine screening, e.g. gestational diabetes
Diet treatment is adequate in most patients outside pregnancy
Most patients require insulin during pregnancy to achieve good glycaemic control
Microvascular complications are rare
Physiological testing shows an abnormality of β-cell function (50% normal)
Obesity and other causes of insulin resistance are not required for hyperglycaemia

have fasting hyperglycaemia (> 6.0 mmol/l). This fasting hyperglycaemia is present very early and has been detected in a 16-month-old child. This means that the age of diagnosis is the age at which the patient is first tested.

There is striking similarity in the level of hyperglycaemia seen with a large variety of mutations (Fig. 2). In contrast, expression studies have shown that the *in vitro* activity of glucokinase mutations that cause hyperglycaemia varies greatly [18]. The minor variation in phenotype between severe and mild mutations suggests that in the severe mutations there must be compensation either by the glucokinase-regulatory protein or by overexpression of the normal allele [21].

The mild hyperglycaemia of glucokinase deficiency rarely needs treatment other than diet until old age when oral agents are usually adequate

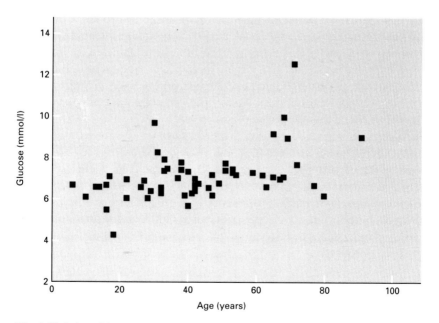

Fig. 2 Variation of fasting plasma glucose of patients with age in patients with nine different mutations in the glucokinase gene (squares). Data taken from [3,19,22,23,24,30].

[3,16]. One exception is during pregnancy when most patients need, or are given, insulin to obtain strict glycaemic control. In keeping with the mild hyperglycaemia found in these patients, diabetic complications, particularly microvascular ones, are rare.

PHYSIOLOGICAL STUDIES IN GLUCOKINASE DEFICIENCY — A GLUCOSE-SENSING DEFECT OF THE β-CELL

The study of patients with mutations of the glucokinase gene is a unique opportunity to observe the action of glucokinase in the β-cell and the hepatocyte. β-cell dysfunction has been seen in glucokinase-deficient subjects using a wide variety of methods of physiological testing. Fasting insulin measurement shows similar values to those found in normal controls [2] and this is inappropriately low for the hyperglycaemia found in these subjects. Modelling of these values suggests that β-cell function is approximately 50% of that found in control patients [3]. The inadequacy of β-cell function is clearly shown during hyperglycaemic clamping; in glucokinase-deficient subjects insulin levels are less than 50% of the matched control subjects [22].

Glucokinase has been described as the 'pancreatic glucose sensor' [11]. It was therefore expected that the defect in insulin secretion seen in patients with glucokinase deficiency would result from an abnormality of glucose sensing. This was elegantly demonstrated by Byrne et al. who measured insulin secretion during a slow stepped glucose infusion [23]. It was shown that in glucokinase-deficient subjects the maximum rate of change of insulin secretion was at a glucose value of 7 mmol/l rather than the 5.5 mmol/l seen in controls. This is consistent with the idea of a resetting of the pancreatic glucose sensor as a result of glucokinase mutations.

As glucokinase plays a major role in hepatic glucose metabolism, some resistance to the action of insulin might be expected. However, physiological studies have not shown a significant difference in the insulin resistance between subjects and controls in a large glucokinase-deficient family [3,24]. This may reflect the insensitivity of such tests to detect a reduction in glucose uptake by the liver. Using nuclear magnetic resonance and labelled glucose isotopes Velho et al. have shown a significant reduction in hepatic glycogen synthesis in 5 glucokinase-deficient individuals [25]. This preliminary result supports the idea that hepatic glucose uptake is reduced.

HOW DOES A HETEROZYGOUS MUTATION CAUSE A CLINICAL SYNDROME?

It is unusual for a *heterozygous* mutation of an *enzyme* to result in a clinical phenotype, even when the mutation has no activity. Inherited diseases resulting from enzyme defects are usually recessive traits, as homozygous or double heterozygous mutations are required for the disease phenotype. The clinical expression of heterozygous mutations of the glucokinase gene as glucose intolerance and diabetes emphasizes the vital role of glucokinase. The tight regulation of enzyme levels [11,12] and possible substrate cycling between glucokinase and glucose-6-phosphatase [1] may make the pancreas very sensitive to changes in enzyme activity. Meglasson and Matschinsky [26] estimated that a 15% reduction in the activity of glucokinase would increase fasting glucose from 5 to 6 mmol/l. This is similar to the change in fasting glucose seen in subjects with glucokinase mutations. It is interesting that increased enzyme expression does not compensate for the reduced enzyme activity. An alternative explanation is that the mutant enzyme may interfere with the wild-type enzyme. Such a 'dominant negative' effect is seen in receptor mutations in cases of thyroxine resistance (page 466) and testosterone resistance (page 479). This is unlikely as glucokinase is a monomer [1] and missense and nonsense mutations have a similar clinical phenotype. Interaction with a nonsense mutation which would stop enzyme synthesis at an early exon is unlikely.

NON-GLUCOKINASE MODY

In France 56% of MODY results from mutations of the glucokinase gene [16] but this is not the case elsewhere. Studies from the UK [27], Germany and Japan [19] all suggest that glucokinase mutations result in under 10% of MODY. In the UK most of the non-glucokinase MODY families have a more marked β-cell defect than glucokinase-deficiency MODY. This results in symptomatic diabetes at an early age, frequently requiring treatment with oral agents or insulin, and microvascular complications are frequent (Hattersley, personal communication).

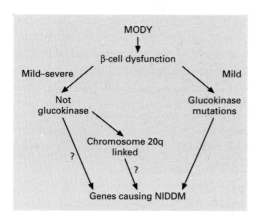

Fig. 3 Summary diagram showing how the clinical recognition of maturity-onset diabetes of the young (MODY) has helped identify genes causing non-insulin-dependent diabetes mellitus.

The underlying molecular biology of non-glucokinase MODY is still unknown. In one large North American pedigree linkage to markers on chromosome 20 (MODY 1) has been found but the gene has not been identified [28]. The genetic defect on chromosome 20 is an unusual cause of MODY, as linkage to these markers is uncommon in both English (Dronsfield and Hattersley, personal communication) and French pedigrees [2]. To define new genes causing MODY, pedigrees that are unlinked to both glucokinase and MODY 1 on chromosome 20 are being studied by linkage using candidate genes and exclusion mapping. It is likely that these will give us more information about β-cell physiology and genetics (Fig. 3).

SUMMARY

MODY is an early onset of type 2 diabetes which is inherited in a dominant fashion. In large Caucasian MODY pedigrees the inherited defect results in β-cell dysfunction. Clinical recognition of patients with MODY was central to the description of the role of glucokinase mutations in a minority of patients with type 2 diabetes. Glucokinase deficiency has a discrete phenotype which is characterized by early-onset mild hyperglycaemia, which results from a glucose-sensing defect in the β-cell.

REFERENCES

1 Randle P. Glucokinase and candidate genes for type 2 (non-insulin dependent) diabetes. *Diabetologia* 1993;**36**:269–275.
2 Froguel Ph, Vaxilaire M, Sun F *et al*. Close linkage of chromosome 7p to early-onset non-insulin-dependent diabetes mellitus. *Nature* 1992;**356**:162–164.
3 Hattersley AT, Turner RC, Permutt MA *et al*. Linkage of type 2 diabetes to the glucokinase gene. *Lancet* 1992;**339**:1307–1310.
4 Tattersall RB, Mansell PJ. Maturity onset-type diabetes of the young (MODY): one condition or many? *Diabet Med* 1991;**8**:402–410.
5 Fajans SS. Maturity-onset diabetes of the young (MODY). *Diabetes Metab Rev* 1989;**5**:579–606.
6 Cammidge PJ. Diabetes mellitus and heredity. *Br Med J* 1928;**ii**:738–741.
7 Tattersall RB. Mild familial diabetes with dominant inheritance. *Q J Med* 1974;**170**:339–357.
8 Barnett AH, Eff C, Leslie RDG, Pyke DA. Diabetes in identical twins. *Diabetologia* 1981;**20**:87–93.
9 O'Rahilly S, Wainscoat JS, Turner RC. Type 2 (non-insulin-dependent) diabetes mellitus. New genetics for old nightmares. *Diabetologia* 1988;**31**:407–414.
10 Hattersley AT, Cook JTE, Scamalan P *et al*. MODY is a dominantly inherited disorder of beta-cell function. *Diabetic Med* 1992;**9**(suppl 1):A25.
11 Magnuson MA. Glucokinase gene structure: functional implications of molecular genetic studies. *Diabetes* 1990;**39**:523–527.
12 Matschinsky FM. Glucokinase as glucose sensor and metabolic signal generator in pancreatic β-cells and hepatocytes. *Diabetes* 1990;**30**:647–752.
13 Permutt MA, Chiu KC, Tanizawa Y. Glucokinase and NIDDM: a candidate gene that paid off. *Diabetes* 1992;**41**:1367–1372.
14 Vionnet N, Stoffel M, Takeda J *et al*. Nonsense mutation in the glucokinase gene

causes early-onset non-insulin dependent diabetes mellitus. *Nature* 1992;**356**:721–722.

15 Stoffel M, Patel P, Lo Y-MD *et al.* Missense mutation in maturity-onset diabetes of the young and mutation screening in late-onset diabetes. *Nature Genet* 1992;**2**:153–156.

16 Froguel P, Zouali H, Vionnet N *et al.* Familial hyperglycemia due to mutations in glucokinase, definition of a subtype of diabetes mellitus. *N Engl J Med* 1993;**328**:697–702.

17 Stoffel M, Froguel Ph,Takede J *et al.* Human glucokinase gene: isolation characterization and identification of two missense mutations linked to early-onset non-insulin-dependent (type 2) diabetes mellitus. *Proc Natl Acad Sci USA* 1992;**89**:7698–7702.

18 Gidh-Jain M,Takeda J, Xu IZ *et al.* Glucokinse mutations associated with non-insulin-dependent (type 2) diabetes mellitus have decreased enzymatic activity implications for structure/function relationships. *Proc Natl Acad Sci USA* 1993;**90**:1932–1936.

19 Sakura H, Eto K, Kadowaki H *et al.* Structure of the human glucokinase gene and identification of a missense mutation in a Japanese patient with early onset non-insulin-dependent diabetes mellitus. *J Clin Endocrinol Metab* 1992;**75**:1571–1573.

20 Hattersley AT, Saker PJ, Barrow B *et al.* A missense mutation in the glucokinase gene in gestational diabetic subjects. *Diabetic Med* 1993;**10**(suppl 2):A15.

21 Sturis J, Kurland IJ, Byrne MM *et al.* Compensation in pancreatic B-cell function in subjects with glucokinase mutations. *Diabetes* 1994;**43**:718–723.

22 Velho G, Froguel P, Clement K. Primary pancreatic beta-cell secretory defect caused by mutations in glucokinase gene in kindreds of maturity onset diabetes of the young. *Lancet* 1992;**22**:444–448.

23 Byrne MM, Sturis J, Clement K *et al.* Insulin secretory abnormalities in subjects with hyperglycaemia due to glucokinase mutations. *J Clin Invest* 1994;**93**:1120–1130.

24 Page RCL, Hattersley AT, Levy JC *et al.* Clinical characteristics of type 2 diabetes associated with a missense mutation in the glucokinase gene. *Diabetic Med* 1995;**12**:209–217.

25 Velho G, Hwang J-H, Petersen K *et al.* Altered hepatic glycogen synthesis in glucokinase deficient subjects. *Diabetologia* 1994;**37**(suppl 1):A131.

26 Meglasson MD, Matschinsky FM. Pancreatic islet glucose metabolism and regulation of insulin secretion. *Diabetes Metab Rev* 1986;**2**:163–214.

27 Hattersley AT, Saker PJ, Patel P *et al.* Linkage of maturity-onset diabetes of the young to the glucokinase gene-evidence of genetic heterogeneity. *Biochem Soc Trans* 1993;**21**:24S.

28 Bell G, Xiang K-S, Newman MV *et al.* The gene for non-insulin dependent diabetes mellitus (maturity onset diabetes of the young subtype) is linked to DNA polymorphism on human chromosome 20q. *Proc Natl Acad Sci USA* 1991;**88**:1484–1488.

29 Hattersley AT,Turner RC. Mutations of the glucokinase gene and type 2 diabetes. *Q J Med* 1993;**86**:227–232.

30 O'Rahilly S, Hattersley AT, Vaag A, Grey H. Impaired glucose tolerance as a state of insulin resistance: a self fulfilling prophecy. *Lancet* 1994;**344**:585–589.

MULTIPLE CHOICE QUESTIONS

1 Analysis of the molecular genetics of classical late-onset type 2 diabetes has been difficult as a result of

a the disease-related mortality in type 2 diabetes
b difficulty collecting multigeneration pedigrees
c type 2 diabetes is a single-gene disorder
d type 2 diabetes is a collection of diseases characterized by hyperglycaemia rather than a single disease
e type 2 diabetes is dominantly inherited

2 Maturity-onset diabetes of the young (MODY) is
  a fatal in the absence of insulin treatment
  b an autosomal recessive disease
  c a subgroup of type 2 diabetes
  d always treated by diet
  e always characterized by β-cell dysfunction

3 Glucokinase
  a is the only enzyme that phosphorylates glucose to glucose-6-phosphate
  b is only expressed in the pancreatic β-cell and the hepatocyte
  c has a high affinity for glucose
  d expression in the pancreatic β-cell is regulated by blood glucose levels
  e is inhibited by glucose-6-phosphate

4 Mutations of the glucokinase gene causing hyperglycaemia
  a frequently affect exons 7 and 8 that encode for the glucose-binding cleft of the enzyme
  b always result in symptomatic diabetes
  c may result in hyperglycaemia in early childhood
  d greatly reduce the action of insulin on skeletal muscle
  e are homozygous or compound heterozygotes

5 Diabetes resulting from glucokinase mutations
  a is not associated with obesity
  b is more severe than MODY not resulting from glucokinase mutations
  c shows a similar phenotype with different mutations
  d may require treatment with insulin during pregnancy
  e frequently results in proliferative retinopathy

Answers

1			2			3		
	a	True		**a**	False		**a**	False
	b	True		**b**	False		**b**	True
	c	False		**c**	True		**c**	False
	d	True		**d**	False		**d**	True
	e	False		**e**	True		**e**	False

4			5		
	a	True		**a**	True
	b	False		**b**	False
	c	True		**c**	True
	d	False		**d**	True
	e	False		**e**	False

Vitamin D: how much do we need?

KAY-TEE KHAW

Vitamin D deficiency is a well-established cause of rickets and osteomalacia. At the turn of this century, rickets was widespread in the northern industrialized cities such as London. The demonstration that rickets could be prevented or cured with ultraviolet light exposure or cod liver oil [1] and consequent public health measures such as vitamin D supplementation of foods led to a dramatic decline in this disease. The introduction of oral vitamin D supplements, however, also led to recognition that excessive supplementation could result in vitamin D toxicity, leading to hyper-calcaemia, soft-tissue calcification and renal damage.

Between the two extremes of deficiency and toxicity, it is less clear what optimal vitamin D status is in terms of health; low circulating levels of vitamin D, though not at levels considered clinically deficient, have been associated with increased risk of several chronic diseases, including coronary heart disease, breast and colon cancer, and osteoporosis and osteoporotic fractures. The association of vitamin D with these chronic diseases and the implications will be discussed here.

SOURCES OF VITAMIN D

Cholecalciferol (vitamin D_3) is made in the skin from 7-dehydrocholesterol in the presence of ultraviolet light (300–320 nm) [2]. It is metabolized in the liver to 25-hydroxyvitamin D, the main form in which vitamin D circulates in the body. 25-Hydroxyvitamin D is converted in the kidney to 1,25-dihydroxyvitamin D, which is the most biologically active form. While much attention has focused on the actions of 1,25-dihydroxyvitamin D [3,4], there is considerable laboratory, clinical and epidemiological evidence indicating a physiological role of circulating 25-hydroxyvitamin D levels, which is the main focus of this review. There are natural food sources of vitamin D (fatty fish, eggs, liver and milk) but these are relatively limited and several studies have indicated that the predominant determinant of circulating vitamin D levels is exposure to sunlight, specifically ultraviolet (UV) light [5]. In winter at latitudes above 50° vitamin D is not formed in the skin and a marked seasonal variation in circulating 25-hydroxyvitamin

D levels has been reported in populations living at increased latitudes [5,6]. Additionally, the ability of skin to synthesize vitamin D at any given UV light exposure declines with increasing age, and older persons have lower levels than younger persons [7].

VITAMIN D AND OSTEOPOROTIC FRACTURES

Conventional teaching is that osteomalacia and osteoporosis are two distinct conditions but there is increasing evidence that they may be part of a continuous spectrum of metabolic bone disease and that vitamin D also has an important aetiological role in osteoporosis and related fractures [8]. A trial of vitamin D_3 (800 IU daily) and calcium (1.2 g) supplementation in elderly women reduced fractures by a third after 18 months compared to placebo [9]. The mean 25-dihydroxyvitamin D level at baseline in this group was about 35 nmol/l, which was raised to about 100 nmol/l after supplementation with no adverse effects. While in this trial it was not possible to distinguish the effects of calcium and vitamin D, other work suggests that vitamin D has an effect independent of calcium. Several studies in both men and younger women have reported an inverse relationship between serum vitamin D levels and bone mass [10,11], which is an important risk factor for fractures. Low levels of vitamin D may result in a rise in parathyroid hormone which increases bone resorption. It is possible that at least some of the decline in bone mass and hence increase in fracture risk with increasing age is associated with the decline in 25-hydroxyvitamin D concentrations and rise in serum parathyroid hormone concentrations. Vitamin D supplementation suppresses parathyroid hormone levels even in apparently healthy older men and women [12].

Osteoporotic fracture rates are generally highest in countries at greatest latitude [13]. There is a strong seasonal variation in fracture rates (higher in winter), bone mass and vitamin D levels (lower in winter) and parathyroid hormone levels (higher in winter) [7,14–17]. Several case-control studies have found lower serum vitamin D levels in cases compared to controls [18,19]. Low vitamin D status is also associated with muscle weakness which may increase predisposition to falls. One estimate of the potential magnitude of impact is that raising serum 25-hydroxyvitamin levels by 40 nmol/l (e.g. from 30 to 70 nmol/l) might be associated with a 20% reduction in fracture risk [10].

VITAMIN D AND CARDIOVASCULAR DISEASE

Concern that vitamin D is adverse for cardiovascular disease arose from early work in which high doses of vitamin D (prolonged consumption of 1000–3000 µg or 40 000–120 000 IU daily) was associated with hypercholesterolaemia and cardiovascular and renal damage; comparable doses in animals produce atherosclerotic-like lesions. However, these are doses which are well-recognized to produce vitamin D toxicity with hypercalcaemia and the lowest daily intake that would contribute to cardiovascular damage among normal people is not known. Certainly, lower doses (e.g. 25 µg or 1000 IU vitamin D daily) or a single dose of 2500 µg/100 000 IU does not appear to raise cholesterol levels [20].

There is now evidence that the relationship of vitamin D with cardio-vascular disease may be U-shaped in nature and that low circulating levels may also predispose to increased cardiovascular risk. Scragg et al. hypo-thesized that the marked winter rise (20–50%) in coronary heart disease mortality observed in most countries at increased latitude was due to summer UV radiation protecting against coronary heart disease by increasing body levels of vitamin D [21].

Several studies have compared levels of 25-hydroxyvitamin D in cases with ischaemic heart disease compared to controls. These studies were often very small in size and with limited statistical power, and most have found no significant differences, though it is notable that mean levels of 25-hydroxyvitamin D were about 4 nmol/l lower in cases (mean level 59 nmol/l) compared to controls in a Norwegian study [22] which analysed 23 cases and about 12 nmol lower in a Danish study [23] with 128 cases (mean levels about 60 nmol/l). In a New Zealand study with 179 cases, Scragg et al. [24] reported a mean difference of about 3.5 nmol/l, significant in this analysis, between cases with myocardial infarction (MI) (mean level 32 nmol/l) and controls. He also reported a dose-related association between vitamin D and estimated risk of MI, persons in the top two quartiles for 25-hydroxyvitamin D plasma level (more than or equal to 33 nmol/l) had one-third the risk of MI compared to those in the bottom quartile (less than 25 nmol/l).

A biological mechanism for this association is not known. However, in experimental animals, vitamin D_3 deficiency produces an increase in sensitivity of the contractile response of cardiac ventricular muscle to noradrenaline and may cause ventricular hypertrophy. In patients with renal failure, elevated parathyroid hormone levels, associated with vitamin D_3 deficiency, may depress cardiac contractile function, and administration of vitamin D will improve left ventricular contractile functions [25]. It is notable that vitamin D supplementation will lower the pulse rate in healthy older persons [20].

VITAMIN D AND CANCER

Garland and Garland have been notable proponents of the hypothesis that both colorectal cancer and breast cancer are linked to low levels of vitamin D [26–28].

Garland and Garland first proposed that calcium and vitamin D might reduce the risk of colon cancer, based on the observation that mortality rates of colon cancer tended to increase with increasing latitude and decreasing sunlight intensity [26]. Several prospective epidemiological studies have reported on an inverse association between dietary intake of vitamin D and/or calcium and subsequent colon cancer incidence [27,28]. For example, the US nurses study [29] reported that there was a weak inverse relationship between vitamin D intake from foods and colorectal cancer: women in the highest vitamin D intake quintile had a relative risk of 0.38 for rectal cancer compared to women in the lowest category. However, not all studies have found a protective effect of dietary intake of vitamin D [30]. It is difficult to separate independent effects of vitamin D and calcium in epidemiological studies of diet, since both are strongly correlated. Additionally, there is considerable measurement error and hence, lack of statistical power, in using dietary intake as a measure of vitamin D status since the substantial contribution from skin exposure to UV light is not accounted for. Nevertheless, there is evidence to suggest an independent effect of vitamin D where studies have used biological measures of vitamin D status.

A cohort study in Maryland [31] found that risk of colon cancer in persons with a serum 25-hydroxyvitamin D concentration of 50 nmol/l or less (the bottom quintile) was threefold that of persons with a 25-hydroxyvitamin D concentration above 50 nmol/ml; mean levels of 25-hydroxyvitamin D in cases (about 76 nmol/l) was 7 nmol/l lower than in controls. Animal and laboratory experiments provide some support for a protective effect of vitamin D: vitamin D metabolites suppress *in vitro* growth and increase differentiation of human colon cancer cell, and vitamin D reduced the incidence of carcinogen-induced tumours in rats [32,33].

Breast cancer has also been linked to vitamin D levels. As with colon cancer, Gorham *et al.* have also observed that mortality and incidence rates in general tend to increase with increasing latitudes. In the USA, breast cancer mortality rates in the south are one-and-a-half to two times higher compared to rates in the north, and Gorham *et al.* reported an inverse correlation between breast cancer incidence in the 15 states of the former USSR and average annual sunlight levels [28]. There was a two-fold variation between states with highest and lowest rates. Although confounding factors such as reproductive patterns, diet and physical activities cannot be excluded in ecological studies, there are plausible biological mechanisms. Vitamin D receptors have been described for breast cancer cells and *in vitro* inhibition of growth of human breast cancer cell lines, and increased cell differentiation by vitamin D has been reported [34,35].

WHAT IS OPTIMAL VITAMIN D STATUS?

To summarize, while the associations between vitamin D and various chronic diseases are intriguing, the evidence is still far from conclusive and more data, particularly from intervention studies, are required. Nevertheless, there is sufficient evidence for some conditions such as osteoporosis, to suggest that we need to reconsider what optimal vitamin D status might be.

Traditional recommendations for nutritional intakes and blood levels set limits which are usually based on levels associated with either deficiency diseases or, conversely, toxicity. However, within these limits the range is large for vitamin D.

BLOOD LEVELS

Rickets or osteomalacia is observed at serum levels of 25-hydroxyvitamin D below 20 μmol/l, and toxicity (hypercalcaemia) at serum levels of above 400 μmol/l [36–38]. Sunlight exposure alone can raise levels to nearly 200 nmol/l; there are no documented cases of vitamin D toxicity from excessive sunlight exposure. Mean levels reported from various studies of chronic diseases such as osteoporosis, colon cancer and cardiovascular disease, examples of which are given above, indicate that increasing blood levels within the range from 30 to 90 nmol/l of 25-hydroxyvitamin D — well below toxicity — may be associated with decreasing risks of these conditions. It is notable that a recent population-based study in healthy men and women aged 65–74 years in the UK found surprisingly low year-round levels, with a mean peak level in the summer of only 35 nmol/l and mean winter levels of 23 nmol/l vitamin D — well below what might be considered optimal [7].

DIETARY INTAKE

Increasing exposure to UV light is feasible but there are concerns about possible risks such as skin cancer and cataracts. If sunlight exposure is limited, then an alternative way to increase circulating vitamin D is by dietary intake. There are three ways to increase dietary vitamin D: (i) by increasing consumption of foods containing vitamin D; (ii) by fortification of staple foods such as fats, milk and flour; and (iii) by dietary supplementation. The main natural food source of vitamin D is from fatty fish such as herring, sardines and mackerel. Regular (daily) fatty fish consumption may not be feasible or palatable for many. Some foods are fortified with vitamin D but policy varies in different countries. Some countries, such as the USA, fortify milk with vitamin D; others, such as the UK, do not. However, in the UK, margarine is required to be fortified with 80–100 IU per ounce (28 g) of vitamin D. A British working party for the Committee on Medical Aspects of Food Policy in 1980 [36] unanimously decided not to recommend mandatory fortification of any sort of flour, milk or butter with vitamin D or any increased fortification of margarine and in 1991 a new working party [37], while recommending continued mandatory fortification of margarine, also recommended that the levels of vitamin D currently added to foods should not be increased and the range of foods to which it is added should not be extended. The third option, dietary supplementation, can be daily, in small doses, e.g. 400–1000 IU as used in some trials, or periodically — a single 100 000 IU (2.5 mg) oral dose of cholecalciferol has been shown to be effective in raising vitamin D levels over a period of 3 months or so without toxicity [12,20].

CLINICAL AND PUBLIC HEALTH IMPLICATIONS

Rickets and osteomalacia and the issues of supplementation in infancy and childhood have been thoroughly examined elsewhere [36]. The main issue considered here is what optimal vitamin D status might be in adult and later life.

It is evident that most adults, in the UK at least, have generally low levels of circulating 25-hydroxyvitamin D throughout the year (25–50 nmol/l) with levels in winter that are close to those considered deficient; this probably reflects low sunlight exposure. Average intakes in the adult population in the UK are around 2–4 μg (80–160 IU) per day [37]; about a third of this comes from fat spreads (particularly fortified margarine), a quarter from cereal products and a quarter from fish [37]. It does not seem, based on the documented circulating 25-hydroxyvitamin levels found in various surveys, that current average dietary intakes of vitamin D in the UK are adequate to maintain average circulating 25-hydroxyvitamin levels in older adults much beyond the marginal levels associated with rickets or osteomalacia.

There are concerns about vitamin D fortification of foods because of the risk of toxicity; reports of vitamin D toxicity from supplemented milk in the USA arose from cases in which poor quality control during production led to massive oversupplementation (e.g. one instance of milk containing about 230 000 IU rather than 400 IU per quart (1.1l)) [38]. Daily vitamin D supplementation (e.g. 400–800 IU daily) has been suggested but compliance is likely to be questionable, particularly in the elderly. An annual single high-dose winter supplement of 100 000 IU in high-risk groups such as the elderly, which has been shown to be safe, might be an appropriate approach. To demonstrate conclusively the effectiveness of such interventions on primary prevention of chronic disease such as fractures, heart disease or cancer will require very large long-term randomized trials; a central issue for debate is whether such trials are required before action is considered justified.

CONVERSIONS

Oral cholecalciferol

IU   = µg × 40
400 IU   = 10 µg cholecalciferol
100 000 IU = 2.5 mg or 2500 µg cholecalciferol

Serum 25-hydroxyvitamin D

nmol/l   = ng/ml × 2.496
50 nmol/l = 20 ng/ml

REFERENCES

1 Chick H, Dalyell EJ, Hume M, Mackay HMM, Henderson-Smith H. The aetiology of rickets in infants. *Lancet* 1922;2:7–11.
2 Holick MF. The photobiology of vitamin D and its consequences for humans. *Ann NY Acad Sci* 1985;**453**:1–13.
3 Richel H, Koeffler HP, Norman AW. The role of the vitamin D endocrine system in health and disease. *N Engl J Med* 1989;**329**:980–991.
4 Fraser DR. Vitamin D. *Lancet* 1995;**345**:104–107.
5 Lawson DEM, Paul AA, Black AE, Cole TJ, Mandal AR, Davie M. Relative cont-ributions of diet and sunlight to vitamin D status in the elderly. *Br Med J* 1979;**ii**:303–305.
6 Hegarty V, Woodhouse P, Khaw KT. Seasonal variation in 25-hydroxyvitamin D and parathyroid hormone concentrations in healthy elderly people. *Age Ageing* 1994;**23**:478–482.
7 MacLaughlin J, Holick MF. Aging decreases the capacity of human skin to produce vitamin D_3. *J Clin Invest* 1985;**76**:1536–1538.
8 Khaw KT, May H. Vitamin D and osteoporosis. *Osteoporosis Rev* (in press).
9 Chapuy MC, Arlot ME, Duboeuf F *et al.* Vitamin D_3 and calcium to prevent hip fractures in elderly women. *N Engl J Med* 1992;**327**:1637–1642.
10 Khaw KT, Sneyd MJ, Compston J. Bone density, parathyroid hormone and 25-hydroxyvitamin D concentrations in middle aged women. *Br Med J* 1992;**305**:263–267.
11 Murphy S, Khaw KT, Prentice A, Compston JE. Relationships between parathyroid hormone, 25-hydroxyvitamin D and bone mineral density in elderly men. *Age Ageing* 1993;**33**:198–204.
12 Khaw KT, Scragg R, Murphy S. Single dose cholecalciferol suppresses the winter increase in parathyroid hormone concentrations in normal older men and women: a randomized trial. *Am J Clin Nutr* 1994;**59**:1040–1044.
13 Cummings SR, Kelsey JL, Nevitt MC, O'Dowd KJ. Epidemiology of osteoporosis and osteoporotic fractures. *Epidemiol Rev* 1985;**7**:178–207.
14 Jacobsen SJ, Goldberg J, Miles TP, Brody JA, Stiers W, Rimm AA. Seasonal variation in the incidence of hip fracture among white persons aged 65 years and older in the United States. *Am J Epidemiol* 1991;**133**:996–1004.
15 Aiken JM, Anderson JB. Seasonal variations in bone mineral content after the menopause. *Nature* 1973;**241**:59–60.

16 Dawson-Hughes B, Dallal GE, Krall EA, Harris S, Sokoll LJ, Falconer G. Effect of vitamin D supplementation on wintertime and overall bone loss in health postmenopausal women. *Ann Intern Med* 1991;**115**:505–512.

17 Krall EA, Sahyoun N, Tannenbaum S, Dallal GE, Dawson-Hughes B. Effect of vitamin D intake on seasonal variations in parathyroid hormone secretion in postmenopausal women. *N Engl J Med* 1989;**321**:1777–1783.

18 Lund B, Sorensen OH, Christensen AB. 25-hydroxycholecalciferol and fractures of the proximal femur. *Lancet* 1975;**ii**:300–302.

19 Lips P, Van Ginkel FC, Jongen MJM, Rubertus F, van der Vijgh WJF, Netelenbos JC. Determinants of vitamin D status in patients with hip fracture and in elderly control subjects. *Am J Clin Nutr* 1987;**46**:1005–1010.

20 Scragg R, Khaw KT, Murphy S. Effect of winter oral vitamin D_3 supplementation on cardiovascular risk factors in elderly adults. *Eur J Clin Nutr* 1995;**49**:640–646.

21 Scragg R. Seasonality of cardiovascular disease mortality and the possible protective effect of ultraviolet radiation. *Int J Epidemiol* 1981;**10**:337–341.

22 Vik T, Try K, Thelle DS, Forde OH. Tromso Heart Study: vitamin D metabolism and myocardial infarction. *Br Med J* 1979;**2**:176.

23 Lund B, Badskjaer J, Lund BJ, Soerensen OH. Vitamin D and ischaemic heart disease. *Horm Metab Res* 1978;**10**:553–556.

24 Scragg R, Jackson R, Holdaway IM, Lim T, Beaglehole R. Myocardial infarction is inversely associated with plasma 25-hydroxyvitamin D_3 levels: a community based study. *Int J Epidemiol* 1990;**19**:559–563.

25 Coratelli P, Petratrulo F, Guongiorno E, Giannattasio M, Antonelli G, Amerio A. Improvement in left ventricular function during treatment of hemodialysis patients with 25 hydroxyvitamin D_3. *Contrib Nephrol* 1984;**41**:433–437.

26 Garland CF, Garland FC. Do sunlight and vitamin D reduce the risk of colon cancer? *Int J Epidemiol* 1980;**9**:227–231.

27 Garland CF, Garland FC, Gorham ED. Can colon cancer incidence and death rates be reduced with calcium and vitamin D? *Am J Clin Nutr* 1991;**54**:193S–201S.

28 Gorham ED, Garland FC, Garland CF. Sunlight and breast cancer incidence in the USSR. *Int J Epidemiol* 1990;**19**:820–824.

29 Martinez ME, Giovannucci E, Colditz G, Stampfer M, Willett W, Speizer F. Relation of calcium, vitamin D and milk consumption to the risk of colorectal cancer in a prospective study among women. *Am J Epidemiol* 1995;**141**:S70.

30 Marcus PM, Newcomb PA, Storer BE. The association of calcium, vitamin D, and dairy products and colon and rectal cancer in Wisconsin women. *Am J Epidemiol* 1995;**141**:S70.

31 Garland CF, Garland FC, Shaw EK, Comstock GW, Helsing KJ, Gorham ED. Serum 25-hydroxyvitamin D and colon cancer: eight year prospective study. *Lancet* 1989;**2**:1176–1178.

32 Pence BC, Buddingh F. Inhibition of dietary fat-promoted colon carcinogenesis in rats by supplemental calcium or vitamin D_3. *Carcinogenesis* 1988;**9**:187–190.

33 De Luca HF, Ostrem V. The relationship between the vitamin D system and cancer. *Adv Exp Med Biol* 1987;**206**:413–429.

34 Eisman JA, Martin TJ, MacIntyre I, Moseley JM. 1,25-dihydroxyvitamin D receptor in breast cancer cells. *Lancet* 1979;**2**:1335–1336.

35 Frampton RJ, Omond SA, Eisman JA. Inhibitions of human cancer cell growth by 1,25-dihydroxy vitamin D_3 metabolites. *Cancer Res* 1983;**40**:4440–4447.

36 Committee on Medical Aspects of Food Policy. *Rickets and Osteomalacia*. Department of Health Report on Health and Social subjects no. 19. HMSO, London, 1980.

37 Committee on Medical Aspects of Food Policy. *The Fortification of Yellow Fats with Vitamins A and D*. Department of Health Report on Health and Social subjects no. 40. HMSO, London, 1991.

38 Jacobus CH, Holick MF, Shao Q *et al*. Hypervitaminosis D associated with drinking milk. *N Engl J Med* 1992;**326**:1173–1177.

39 Gregory J, Foster K, Tyler H, Wiseman M. *The Dietary and Nutritional Survey of British Adults*. OPCS HMSO, London, 1990.

MULTIPLE CHOICE QUESTIONS

1 As regards vitamin D₃ (cholecalciferol)

   a it is converted in the kidney to 25-hydroxyvitamin D

   b low levels of 25-hydroxyvitamin D are predictive of colon cancer in prospective studies

   c toxicity occurs at serum 25-hydroxyvitamin D levels of 100 μmol/l or so

   d toxicity is associated with hypocalcaemia

   e toxicity can occur with excessive sunlight exposure

2 As regards vitamin D₃ (cholecalciferol)

   a average dietary intake in the UK is about 1000 IU (25 μg) daily

   b for a given sunlight exposure, young persons make less vitamin D in their skin compared to older persons

   c doses of 100 000 IU daily (2500 μg) have been associated with hypercholesterolaemia

   d dietary supplementation will suppress parathyroid hormone levels

   e vitamin D₃ and calcium supplementation have been shown to reduce osteoporotic hip fractures

Answers

1		2	
a	False	**a**	False
b	True	**b**	False
c	False	**c**	True
d	False	**d**	True
e	False	**e**	True

Polycystic ovary syndrome
and the risk of coronary heart disease

HOWARD S. JACOBS

In the years since high-resolution diagnostic pelvic ultrasound became available we have become increasingly aware of the prevalence of polycystic ovaries in women with and without reproductive symptoms. Several studies have now confirmed that about one-fifth of asymptomatic women who volunteer for ultrasound examinations have polycystic ovaries [1] (Fig. 1). When these ultrasound findings are associated with a menstrual disturbance (most commonly oligomenorrhoea) or symptoms arising from systemic hyperandrogenization, such as seborrhoea, acne, hirsutism or male-pattern baldness, we speak of *polycystic ovary syndrome* [2]. This is the label now widely used to replace the eponymous Stein–Leventhal syndrome.

The distinction made between morphological identification of polycystic ovaries, a phenotype which runs in families [3] and which can be detected in prepubertal children [4] and patients with hypogonadotrophic hypogonadism [5], and the polycystic ovary syndrome immediately raises the question of what factors operate in women with polycystic ovaries to cause clinical expression of the syndrome [2]. It has been known for years that many women with polycystic ovary syndrome are obese and that it is putting on weight that often leads to the development of symptoms; in women who are already overweight a further increase usually leads to worsening of the clinical condition. These observations have suggested that some endocrine component of obesity links nutritional status with expression of the polycystic ovary syndrome. It was, however, the association in slim women of acanthosis nigricans with polycystic ovary syndrome [6] that made it clear that hypersecretion of insulin occupies a central role in the expression of the polycystic ovary syndrome.

We now recognize that many women with polycystic ovary syndrome have considerable resistance to the extrasplanchnic actions of insulin on glucose transport (reviewed in [7]). Thus we and others have described fasting hyperinsulinaemia in women with oligomenorrhoea caused by the polycystic ovary syndrome. In fact in these women we have found a direct correlation of the patient's fasting serum insulin concentration with the interval between her menstrual periods [8] (Fig. 2). This observation is of considerable importance in relation to the effect that polycystic ovary

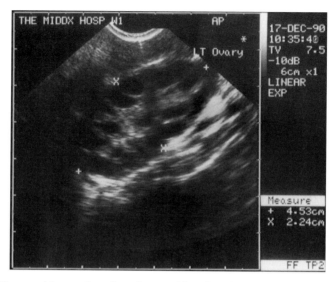

Fig. 1 Ultrasound image of a polycystic ovary. Note the echodense central stroma and the peripherally arranged cysts.

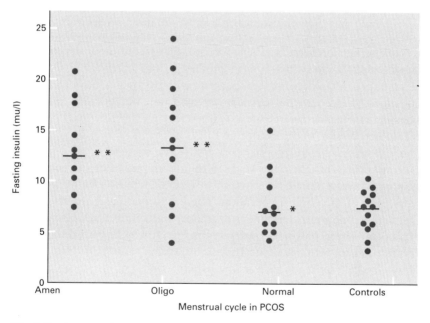

Fig. 2 Fasting serum insulin concentrations in relation to the character of the menstrual cycle in slim women with polycystic ovary syndrome. The asterisks refer to statistically significant differences from the results in women with normal ovaries.

syndrome has on a woman's fertility, since the chance of a woman conceiving is obviously directly related to the frequency with which she ovulates. Other studies have shown a positive correlation of insulin release (as measured by the sum of the serum insulin concentrations in the 2 hours that follow oral glucose loading) with ovarian androgen secretion, as indexed by peripheral serum androstenedione concentrations (Fig. 3). This observation is of importance in understanding the origin of hirsutism in women with polycystic ovary syndrome, particularly since the development of obesity provokes further hyperinsulinaemia. Exposure of the liver to large amounts of insulin depresses secretion of sex hormone-binding globulin (SHBG), to which more than 90% of circulating testosterone is bound. Obesity-provoked insulin release therefore not only enhances ovarian androgen secretion but also amplifies its effect by altering the transport of testosterone. Parenthetically, it is of note that the depression of SHBG that occurs so frequently in obese women with polycystic ovary syndrome conceals a substantial increase in the testosterone production rate and in the free, non-SHBG-bound, testosterone concentration. Thus, in an obese patient, a total serum testosterone concentration that is within the normal range is quite consistent with hormonally mediated hirsutism and, most importantly, does not imply that the patient will not respond to treatment with antiandrogens.

The data reviewed thus far indicate a central role for hypersecretion of insulin in determining clinical expression of the two major reproductive disturbances (anovulation and hyperandrogenization) that characterize women with the polycystic ovary syndrome. The primary cause of the insulin resistance thought to underlie the excessive secretion of insulin is not known with certainty and the prediction that mutations in the gene encoding the insulin receptor would provide an explanation has not been realized [9]. On the other hand, the role of obesity as an amplifier of

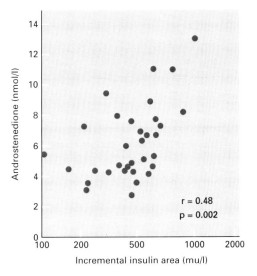

Fig. 3 Serum androstenedione concentrations in slim women with polycystic ovary syndrome in relation to the insulin secreted in response to a standard oral glucose test. The insulin results are presented as the area under the insulin curve less the fasting serum insulin concentration.

insulin resistance and therefore of insulin secretion is not in doubt. The mechanism is thought to involve a perturbation in some postreceptor feature of transduction of the insulin signal [10].Whatever the mechanism proves to be, the clinical implication of these observations is that control of hyperinsulinism forms the centre piece of any strategy of management of patients with polycystic ovary syndrome.Thus, drug therapy with anti-androgens, or ovulation induction with antioestrogens, stands its greatest chance of success if combined with measures to reduce excessive insulin drive to the ovary.Weight loss, through a programme of diet and exercise, which often requires the support of a counsellor or psychologist, is therefore complementary to any drug regimen. Conversely, medications that worsen insulin resistance, such as treatment with glucocorticoids, should be eschewed except in patients in whom a specific adrenal lesion (such as late-onset 21-hydroxylase, or 3β-steroid dehydrogenase deficiency) can be demonstrated [11].

At about the time we were undertaking our studies of the role of hypersecretion of insulin in relation to the reproductive symptoms of patients with polycystic ovary syndrome, Gerald Reaven was developing his concept of a metabolic syndrome X [12]. He and others had noted that insulin resistance was an underlying and unifying metabolic abnormality in many men who demonstrated several of the risk factors for coronary heart disease. For example, he had found strong associations of the risk of coronary events in men with hyperinsulinism, with increased circulating very-low-density lipoprotein cholesterol concentrations and with high blood pressure (Fig. 4). We therefore began to seek these risk factors in our patients with hyperinsulinism and polycystic ovary syndrome. Figure 5 shows the significant reduction of the circulating concentrations of the cardioprotective high-density lipoprotein cholesterol we found in slim women with polycystic ovary syndrome [13]. The concentrations were even lower in the patients who were obese.The lipid abnormalities were associated with a deterioration of carbohydrate tolerance and significant increase of the postglucose serum insulin concentrations. Similar sets of data have been published from Sweden [14] and from the USA (reviewed in [15]). In more recent studies we have found an increase in the concen-trations of circulating plasminogen activator inhibitor 1 — an inhibitor of intravascular fibrinolysis whose production is stimulated by insulin and which is another surrogate marker of the risk of coronary disease.

The results of measuring these surrogate markers of the risk of coronary heart disease has led to the notion that hyperinsulinaemic women with polycystic ovary syndrome may represent the female component of Reaven's syndrome X. Indeed, based on their findings of a 40% prevalence of hyper-tension and a 15% prevalence of diabetes mellitus detected on long-term follow-up of women with surgically proven polycystic ovary syndrome, Dahlgren et al. developed a model that predicted a greater than sevenfold

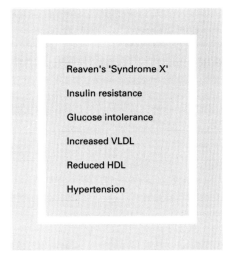

Reaven's 'Syndrome X'

Insulin resistance

Glucose intolerance

Increased VLDL

Reduced HDL

Hypertension

Fig. 4 Features of Reavan's syndrome X (for details see text).

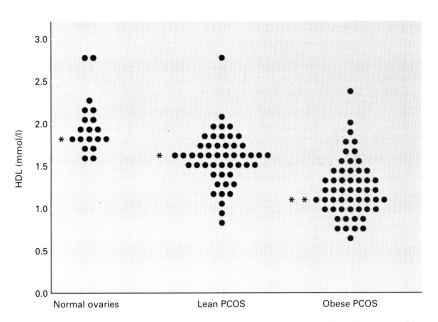

Fig. 5 Serum high-density lipoprotein (HDL) cholesterol concentrations in women with polycystic ovary syndrome, in relation to body weight, compared with the results in age- and weight-matched controls. PCOS, polycystic ovary syndrome.

increase of the lifetime risk of a coronary thrombosis [16]. Our own prediction of a threefold increased risk was more conservative but led my colleagues in the Department of Epidemiology and Population Sciences at the London School of Hygiene and Tropical Medicine to undertake a long-term follow-up study of coronary *mortality* in a group of women whose polycystic ovary syndrome had been confirmed surgically and by histopathology (Pierpoint *et al.*, manuscript in preparation). We managed to trace the records of 842 women in whom the ovarian diagnosis had been made an average of 28 years previously. The mean age of this cohort, which represented an 82% trace rate, was 53.8 years. There were 10 deaths from coronary heart disease, yielding a standardized mortality ratio (SMR) of 1.35 (95% confidence interval (CI) 0.65–2.48). There were only 2 deaths from other circulatory disease (SMR 0.27; 95% CI 0.03–0.96; $P = 0.04$). There were, however, 5 deaths in which diabetes mellitus was cited as an underlying or contributory cause, compared with 1.4 deaths expected from national mortality data (odds ratio 3.9; 95% CI 1.34–9.2; $P = 0.03$).

This study has, therefore, produced the surprising result that, despite the increase we found in the prevalence of fatal diabetes, and the follow-up studies of Dahlgren *et al.* [16] that had shown the increased rate of hypertension and diabetes, the cohort of patients we studied showed no increase in coronary mortality and indeed a statistically significant protection from stroke. The cohort of patients we studied is substantially larger than any other in the literature and of a size whose power had been calculated to be sufficient to detect a threefold increase in the risk of a fatal myocardial infarct. At present, my interpretation of the results is that the resistance of these women to the development of cardiac disease and their protection from stroke is most likely due to some other endocrine feature of the polycystic ovary syndrome. The most probable reason is the marked degree of oestrogenization and it will be recalled that, in women after the menopause, the increased risk of osteoporosis and coronary disease can largely be avoided by oestrogen replacement therapy. We had already shown that patients with polycystic ovary syndrome and amenor-rhoea are protected from developing osteoporosis [17] and it was therefore interesting to read that Dahlgren's group has reported that haemostatic variables were not disturbed in the cohort of patients which on long-term follow-up had exhibited the high rate of diabetes and hypertension [18]. It may therefore be argued that women with polycystic ovary syndrome escape realization of their adverse coronary risk factors because of their coexistent overproduction of oestrogen. It seems likely that follow-up studies of women with this common condition, as they pass through the menopause, may yield important information on the clinical expression of the most common cause of death of postmenopausal women.

REFERENCES

1 Jacobs HS. Prevalence and significance of polycystic ovaries. *Ultrasound Obstet Gynaecol* 1994;4:3–4.
2 Jacobs HS. Polycystic ovaries and polycystic ovary syndrome. *Gynecol Endocrinol* 1987;1:113–131.

3 Hague WM, Adams J, Reeders ST, Peto TEA, Jacobs HS. Familial polycystic ovaries: a genetic disease? *Clin Endocrinol* 1988;**29**:593–606.

4 Bridges NA, Hindmarsh PC, Cooke A, Brook CGD, Healy MJR. Standards for ovarian volume in childhood and puberty. *Fertil Steril* 1993;**60**:456–460.

5 Shoham Z, Conway GS, Patel A, Jacobs HS. Polycystic ovaries in patients with hypo-gonadotropic hypogonadism: similarity of ovarian response to gonadotropin stimulation in patients with polycystic ovarian syndrome. *Fertil Steril* 1992;**58**:37–47.

6 Conway GS, Jacobs HS. Acanthosis nigricans in obese women with polycystic ovary syndrome: disease spectrum not distinct entity. *Postgrad Med J* 1990;**66**:536–538.

7 Conway GS, Jacobs HS. Clinical implications of hyperinsulinaemia in women. *Clin Endocrinol* 1993;**39**:623–632.

8 Conway GS, Jacobs HS, Holly JMP, Wass JAS. Effects of luteinizing hormone, insulin, insulin-like growth factor 1 and insulin-like growth factor small binding protein in the polycystic ovary syndrome. *Clin Endocrinol* 1990;**33**:593–603.

9 Krook A, Kumar S, Laing I, Boulton AJM, Wass JAH, O'Rahilly S. Molecular scanning of the insulin receptor gene in syndromes of insulin resistance. *Diabetes* 1994;**43**:357–368.

10 Marsden PJ, Murdoch A, Taylor R. Severe impairment of insulin action in adipocytes from amenorrheic subjects with polycystic ovary syndrome. *Metabolism* 1994;**43**:1536–1542.

11 Hague WM, Honour JW, Adams J, Vecsei P, Jacobs HS. Steroid responses to ACTH in women with polycystic ovaries. *Clin Endocrinol* 1989;**30**:355–366.

12 Reaven GM. Role of insulin resistance in human disease. *Diabetes* 1988;**37**:1595–1607.

13 Conway GS, Agrawal R, Betteridge DJ, Jacobs HS. Risk factors for coronary artery disease in lean and obese women with the polycystic ovary syndrome. *Clin Endocrinol* 1992;**37**:119–126.

14 Dahlgren E, Johansson S, Linstedt G *et al.* Women with polycystic ovary syndrome wedge resected in 1956 to 1965: a long term follow up focusing on natural history and circulating hormones. *Fertil Steril* 1992;**57**:505–513.

15 Wild RA. Obesity, lipids, cardiovascular risk, and androgen excess. *Am J Med* 1995;**98**:27S-32S.

16 Dahlgren E, Jansen PO, Johansson S, Lapidus L, Oden A. Polycystic ovary syndrome and the risk for myocardial infarction: evaluated from a risk factor model based on a prospective population study of women. *Acta Obstet Gynecol Scand* 1992;**71**:599–604.

17 Di Carlo C, Shoham Z, MacDougal J, Patel A, Hall M, Jacobs HS. Polycystic ovaries as a relative protective factor for bone mineral loss in young women with amenorrhea. *Fertil Steril* 1992;**57**:314–319.

18 Dahlgren E, Janson P-O, Johansson T, Lapidus L, Linstedt G, Tengborn L. Haemostatic and metabolic variables in women with polycystic ovary syndrome. *Fertil Steril* 1994;**61**:455–460.

Response and resistance to thyroid hormone

V. KRISHNA K. CHATTERJEE

Thyroid hormones regulate diverse processes such as growth, the basal metabolic rate and myocardial contractility and are also critical for developmental processes such as differentiation of the central nervous system. The synthesis of thyroid hormones (thyroxine (T_4), triiodothyronine (T_3)) is controlled by thyroid-stimulating hormone (TSH) from the pituitary and in turn, T_4 and T_3 regulate TSH production as part of a classic negative-feedback loop [1]. The physiological actions of thyroid hormones are mediated by its effect on key target genes in different tissues (Table 1). Thus, negative-feedback regulation of TSH secretion is mediated by inhibition of TSH-α and β subunit gene expression and, conversely, many peripheral responses involve thyroid hormone-dependent induction of target gene expression. The transcriptional regulation of target genes by thyroid hormone is now known to be mediated by a nuclear receptor protein which is a member of the steroid receptor superfamily [2]. The receptor contains a highly conserved central 'zinc finger' domain which interacts with specific regulatory DNA sequences or thyroid response elements (TREs), usually located in the promoter regions of target genes. For many target genes, the receptor binds to TREs as a heterodimer with the retinoid X receptor (RXR), but homodimeric interactions have also been demonstrated in some cases. In the absence of hormone, these homo- and heterodimeric receptor complexes exert an inhibitory effect via intermediary corepressor proteins, to repress basal gene transcription [3] (Fig. 1a). Binding of thyroid hormone to the carboxy-terminal region of the receptor induces a marked conformational change in the protein, leading to homodimer dissociation and relief of repression. The TR-RXR heterodimer which remains stable following ligand binding is now able to activate target gene transcription by recruitment of other intermediary proteins or coactivators [4] (Fig. 1b).

In humans, thyroid hormone receptors are encoded by separate α and β genes on chromosomes 17 and 3 respectively. Each gene undergoes alternative splicing to generate distinct proteins with differing properties and tissue distributions [5]. The β gene generates two receptor isoforms: $hTR\beta_1$ is expressed ubiquitously; $hTR\beta_2$ has a divergent amino-terminal

466

Table 1 The effects of thyroid hormones on key target genes in different tissues.

Tissue	Effect of thyroid hormone	Target genes
Central nervous system	Neuronal maturation	Myelin basic protein
Liver	Increased SHBG	SHBG
Heart	Enhanced rate and contractility	Myosin heavy chain and Ca^{2+} ATPase
Pituitary	Inhibits TSH secretion	TSH-α and β subunit
Several	Raised basal metabolic rate	Multiple, e.g. Na-K-ATPase

SHBG, Sex hormone-binding globulin; ATPase, adenosine triphosphatase; TSH, thyroid-stimulating hormone.

region and is selectively expressed in the pituitary and hypothalamus. The major products of the α gene are a receptor isoform designated hTRα_1, together with a splice variant c-*erb*Aα_2 which does not bind thyroid hormone. The role of c-*erb*Aα_2 is unclear, but it can inhibit the action of hTRα_1 and hTRβ_1, suggesting that it may be a naturally occurring negative modulator of receptor action.

DIFFERENTIAL DIAGNOSIS

The syndromes of resistance to thyroid hormone (RTH) are rare disorders characterized by reduced target tissue responsiveness to circulating free thyroid hormones (FT$_4$, FT$_3$). The hallmark of RTH is resistance to thyroid hormone action in the pituitary–thyroid axis, such that continued TSH production drives hypersecretion of T$_4$ and T$_3$ to establish a new equilibrium with high serum levels of free thyroid hormones, together with a non-suppressed TSH. The advent of sensitive immunometric TSH assays has enabled a clear distinction to be made between patients with suppressed versus non-suppressed TSH levels, allowing a diagnosis of inappropriate TSH secretion to be made more easily.

A variety of different conditions may be associated with hyperthyroxinaemia and detectable serum TSH concentrations (Table 2). Familial dysalbuminaemic hyperthyroxinaemia (FDH) is a disorder associated with a qualitatively abnormal serum-binding protein, leading to abnormal T$_4$ but normal T$_3$ levels. Approximately 8% of patients with autoimmune thyroid disease have circulating anti-iodothyronine antibodies which interfere with the measurement of thyroid hormones to produce a biochemical picture which mimics RTH. The use of direct two-step or one-step labelled monoclonal antibody techniques or an equilibrium dialysis assay to measure FT$_4$ overcomes the interference of abnormal forms of albumin or antibodies

(a)

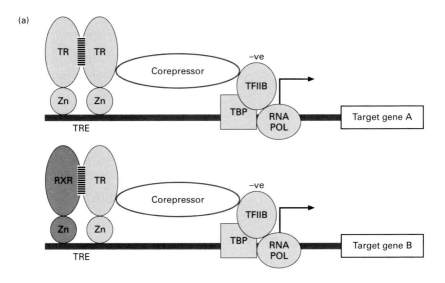

(b) Dissociation

Activation of transcription

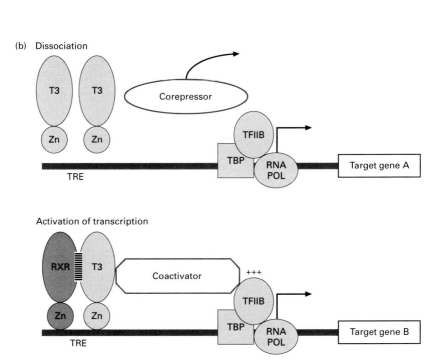

Fig. 1 (a) In the absence of ligand, the thyroid hormone receptor binds to response elements as a homo- or heterodimer and represses basal gene transcription via an intermediary corepressor(s). (b) Thyroid response (TR) homodimers and the corepressor dissociate following hormone binding. The thyroid-retinoid X receptor (TR-RXR) heterodimer remains stable and recruits coactivator(s) to enhance target gene transcription.

Table 2 Causes of elevated thyroxine and non-suppressed thyroid-stimulating hormone (TSH) levels.

Raised serum-binding proteins
Familial dysalbuminaemic hyperthyroxinaemia (FDH)
Anti-iodothyronine antibodies
Anti-TSH antibodies (heterophilic; endogenous)
Non-thyroidal illness
Acute psychiatric disorders
Neonatal period
Drugs (e.g. amiodarone)
Thyroxine replacement therapy
TSH-secreting pituitary tumour
Resistance to thyroid hormone

---

with analogue assay methods. Other causes of hyperthyroxinaemia include the neonatal period, systemic illness, acute psychiatric disorders, various drugs and T_4 replacement. Here, the diagnosis rests on recognition of the abnormal clinical context as well as documenting subsequent normalization of thyroid function tests at a later date.

Hyperthyroxinaemia, non-suppressed TSH levels and thyrotoxic symptoms are also features associated with a TSH-secreting pituitary tumour, which is the major entity that needs to be distinguished from RTH. Table 3 indicates that there are no significant differences in FT_4, FT_3 or TSH levels and the presence of a goitre or thyrotoxic symptoms has often led to inappropriate surgical or ^{131}I thyroid ablation in either group. However, the following investigations can be helpful in differentiating the two conditions: abnormal thyroid function tests in other family members suggests a familial disorder such as RTH; dynamic tests indicate that the majority of patients with autonomous TSH-secreting tumours show no response to thyrotrophin-releasing hormone (TRH), whereas physiological TSH responses are preserved in RTH; the administration of T_3 leads to a suppression (albeit incomplete) of basal or TRH-stimulated TSH secretion in RTH, whereas TSH secretion from a tumour remains unaffected; imaging of the pituitary fossa by computed tomographic (CT) scan or magnetic resonance imaging (MRI) usually confirms the presence of a tumour but abnormal appearances have rarely been documented in RTH as well; elevated serum glycoprotein hormone α-subunit (α-SU) levels and a raised α-SU/TSH ratio are indicative of a TSH-secreting tumour. Lastly, we have observed that serum sex hormone-binding globulin (SHBG) levels can be a useful discriminant, being almost invariably normal in RTH cases, but frequently elevated into the thyrotoxic range in patients with TSH-secreting tumours [6].

Table 3 Comparison of features in resistance to thyroid hormone and TSH-secreting pituitary tumours.

	RTH*	TSHoma
Familial cases (%)	78	0
Mean FT$_4$ (pmol/l)†	31	35
Mean FT$_3$ (pmol/l)†	11	13
TSH (mU/l)†	1.8	3.0
TSH response to TRH (%)	96	9.6
TSH suppression by T$_3$ (%)	100	4.6
CT or MRI lesions (%)	2.3	97
Normal α-SU/TSH ratio (%)	98	8.6
Elevated SHBG (%)	1	95

* Includes generalized and pituitary resistance to thyroid hormone.
† Normal ranges: FT$_4$ 9–20; FT$_3$ 3–7.5; TSH 0.4–4.
RTH, Resistance to thyroid hormone; TSHoma, TSH-secreting pituitary tumour; FT$_4$, free thyroxine; FT$_3$, free triiodothyronine; TSH, thyroid-stimulating hormone; TRH, thyrotrophin-releasing hormone; T$_3$, triiodothyronine; CT, computed tomographic; MRI, magnetic resonance imaging; α-SU, α-subunit; SHBG, sex hormone-binding globulin.

CLINICAL FEATURES

Resistance to thyroid hormone was first described in 1967 in two siblings who were euthyroid despite high circulating thyroid hormone levels and exhibited a number of other abnormalities, including deaf-mutism, stippled femoral epiphyses with delayed bone maturation and short stature as well as dysmorphic facies, winging of the scapulae and pectus carinatum [7]. It is now clear that some of these features are unique to this kindred in which the disorder was recessively inherited.

The majority of RTH cases that have been described since then are dominantly inherited with highly variable clinical features. Many patients with RTH are either asymptomatic or have non-specific symptoms in conjunction with a goitre, prompting thyroid function tests which make the diagnosis. In this context, we have recently shown that the biological activity of circulating TSH is elevated in RTH, which may account for both thyroid hormone hypersecretion and goitre in individuals with normal immunoreactive TSH levels [8]. In these individuals, the high thyroid hormone levels are thought to compensate for generalized resistance (GRTH) in most tissues, resulting in a euthyroid state. In contrast, a number of individuals with the same biochemical abnormalities exhibit signs and symptoms associated with thyrotoxicosis; in adults these can include weight loss, tremor, palpitations, insomnia and heat intolerance or, rarely, cardiac dysrhythmias and failure; in children, failure to thrive, accelerated growth and behavioural abnormalities have also been noted. This clinical entity was first described in 1975, and patients were thought to have selective pituitary resistance to thyroid hormone action (PRTH) with preservation of normal hormonal responses in peripheral tissues [9].

However, we have compared the clinical and biochemical characteristics of individuals classified as GRTH or PRTH on clinical criteria and find that there is a wide overlap between these entities. There are no differences in age, sex ratio, frequency of goitre or levels of FT_4, FT_3 or TSH in patients with the two types of disorder. Significantly, features such as tachycardia, weight loss, anxiety and tremor have also been documented in individuals with GRTH. Conversely, serum SHBG levels are almost invariably normal in patients with PRTH, indicating hepatic resistance to thyroid hormone action [10]. Overall, these observations indicate that, whilst all patients with RTH have abnormal thyroid function tests, the clinical manifestations vary widely both between and within individuals. Nevertheless, the absence or presence of overt thyrotoxic features allows patients to be classified as either GRTH or PRTH. We feel that this clinical distinction will remain useful as a guide to the most appropriate therapy.

Recent analyses of a large number of RTH cases indicate other abnormalities associated with this disorder. A history of attention deficit–hyperactivity disorder (ADHD) in childhood was elicited more frequently in RTH patients (73%) compared to their unaffected siblings (27%) [11]. This may be associated with subsequent learning difficulties in adolescence. Hearing loss (21%), a propensity to upper respiratory tract infections (56%) and cardiac abnormalities (18%; increased contractility, mitral valve prolapse) are also present more frequently than anticipated in RTH [12].

MOLECULAR GENETICS

Following the cloning of thyroid hormone receptors, familial GRTH was shown to be tightly linked to the TRβ gene locus. Since then we and others have reported that affected individuals are heterozygous for mutations in the TRβ gene, consonant with the dominant mode of inheritance of this disorder [13,14]. All RTH mutations identified to date cluster within three areas of the receptor hormone-binding domain (Fig. 2a). In keeping with their location, hormone binding to mutant receptor proteins is moderately or markedly reduced and their ability to modulate target gene expression is impaired, whereas their ability to bind to DNA and form heterodimers with RXR is preserved [15,16]. In addition, the mutant receptors are capable of inhibiting the action of their wild-type counterparts, when coexpressed [17]. Clinical and genetic data from two unusual RTH families provide evidence in favour of such dominant negative inhibition of wild-type receptor action *in vivo*. Affected individuals from the very first kindred with recessively inherited RTH were shown to be homozygous for a complete deletion of both alleles of the TRβ gene, but significantly obligate heterozygotes in this family, harbouring a deletion of one TRβ allele, were completely normal [18]. Conversely, in another kindred, an individual who was homozygous for two mutant TRβ alleles exhibited

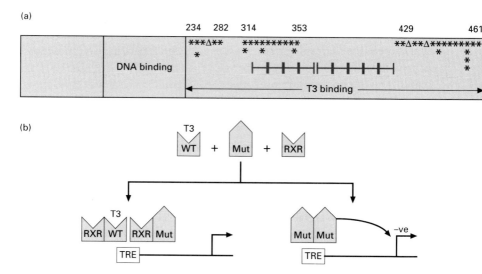

Fig. 2 (a) Schematic representation of the functional domains of hTRβ, illustrating the clustering of resistance mutations within three regions of the hormone-binding domain. Asterisks (*) and triangles (△) denote point mutations and in-frame codon deletions described in resistance to thyroid hormone (RTH). A series of heptad repeats of hydrophobic residues which may constitute a dimerization interface are shown (black bars). One cluster of mutations (αα 314–353) overlaps with the first and second heptad repeats, indicating that they are probably not critical for dimerization. (b) Mechanism of dominant negative inhibition by mutant receptors. One model (left) suggests that transcriptionally impaired mutant thyroid response-retinoid X receptor (TR-RXR) heterodimers compete with their wild-type counterparts at thyroid response elements (TREs). Another model (right) involves the formation of mutant TR homodimers on some TREs. Unlike wild-type receptor, this complex fails to dissociate following hormone binding, allowing continued repression of basal gene transcription.

severe resistance, presumably reflecting the markedly inhibitory effects of a 'double dose' of dominant negative mutant receptor [19]. We and others have also shown that the introduction of artificial mutations which abolish heterodimerization with RXR abrogates the dominant negative activity of natural receptor mutants [15,16]. It has also been suggested that the dominant negative potency of mutant receptors correlates with their ability to form homodimers that fail to dissociate following hormone binding and repress basal gene transcription [20,21] (Fig. 2b). Both models underscore the importance of dimerization for dominant negative activity, which correlates with the clustered distribution of natural mutations outside regions in the carboxy-terminal domain which are involved in dimerization (Fig. 2a) [22].

The observation that hTRβ$_2$ was selectively expressed in the pituitary and hypothalamus had led to the hypothesis that PRTH might represent a distinct genetic entity, possibly associated with mutations in the unique amino-terminal domain of TRβ$_2$. However, recent analyses of a number of PRTH cases [14,23] indicate that these individuals are also hetero-zygous for mutations in the hormone-binding domain of TRβ. Mutations identified in PRTH cases have also been documented in unrelated indivi-duals with GRTH. Even within a single family, the same mutation can be associated with generalized resistance in some individuals and thyrotoxic features suggestive of PRTH in others. These observations indicate that GRTH and PRTH represent different clinical manifestations of a single genetic disorder.

PATHOGENESIS OF RESISTANCE

We suggest that the ability of mutant receptors to exert a dominant negative effect within the pituitary–thyroid axis generates the abnormal thyroid function tests characteristic of RTH. On this background, a variable clinical phenotype is seen in different patients. Variable tissue resistance may also be observed within a single individual, such that normal serum SHBG levels may coexist with tachycardia in the same subject. This latter observa-tion may be partly explicable on the basis of the differing tissue distributions

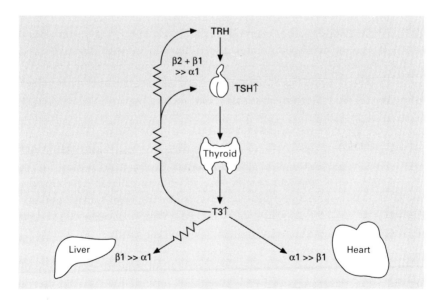

Fig. 3 The influence of tissue distribution of thyroid hormone receptor isoforms on the clinical phenotype. The preponderance of thyroid receptor TRβ$_2$ and TRβ$_1$ isoforms in the pituitary and hypothalamus generates resistance within the feedback axis, leading to elevated serum thyroid hormones and non-suppressed thyroid-stimulating hormone levels. Peripheral tissue responses to raised thyroid hormones are dependent in part on their receptor status. Predominance of TRβ$_1$ in liver is associated with resistance, whereas the relative abundance of TRα$_1$ in myocardium is associated with retention of sensitivity to thyroid hormones and thyrotoxic manifestations.

of receptor isoforms. The liver and pituitary express predominantly $TR\beta_1$ and $TR\beta_2$ receptors respectively, whereas $TR\alpha_1$ is the major species detected in myocardium [24]. Therefore mutations in the $TR\beta$ gene are likely to be associated with pituitary and liver resistance, as exemplified by normal SHBG and non-suppressed TSH levels, whilst the tachycardia or heart failure seen in RTH may represent retention of cardiac sensitivity to thyroid hormones acting via a normal α-receptor (Fig. 3). Another factor which may account for variable resistance is the relative proportion of wild-type to mutant receptor expressed in a given tissue. Marked differences in the relative levels of wild-type and mutant messenger RNA have been documented in skin fibroblasts from two RTH cases and a temporal variation in expression of the mutant allele correlated with the degree of bone resistance [25]. Lastly, the dominant negative potency of mutant receptors, which differs depending on the nature of target gene TREs [16,26], is a third variable which may regulate resistance to hormone action.

MANAGEMENT

One of the most important reasons for recognizing RTH is that its management differs from that of other common forms of thyroid dysfunction. In addition, the distinction between GRTH and PRTH remains useful, since the management of the two states also differs. In most individuals with GRTH, the receptor defect is compensated by high circulating thyroid hormone levels, leading to a euthyroid state not associated with abnormalities other than a goitre. Certain circumstances, such as hypercholesterolaemia in adults or growth retardation in young children, which are indicative of severe resistance and hypothyroid indices in these tissues, may warrant the administration of supraphysiological doses of thyroxine. Although successful in some patients [13], such therapy needs careful monitoring of other indices of thyroid hormone action, to avoid the adverse cardiac effects or excess catabolism associated with overtreatment. Misdiagnosis of RTH, followed by inappropriate thyroid ablation, invariably renders the resistant patient hypothyroid and is another context in which T_4 replacement in supraphysiological dosage is indicated.

In contrast, a general reduction in thyroid hormone levels may be of benefit in the management of PRTH patients with thyrotoxic symptoms. However, the administration of conventional antithyroid drugs usually causes a further rise in serum TSH levels with consequent thyroid enlargement, and may also be associated with a theoretical risk of inducing autonomous TSH-secreting pituitary neoplasia. Accordingly, agents which inhibit pituitary TSH secretion, yet are devoid of peripheral thyromimetic effects, are used to reduce thyroid hormone levels. In a number of cases, the thyroid hormone analogue 3,3,5-triiodothyroacetic acid (TRIAC) has been shown to be beneficial [27]. Dextro-thyroxine $(D-T_4)$ is another useful agent which has been effective in some individuals [28]. If these agents fail, the dopaminergic agent bromocriptine [29] or the somatostatin analogue octreotide [30] may be administered. However, past experience indicates that inhibition of TSH secretion escapes from the effects of bromocriptine [27,28] as well as octreotide [30].

In view of the spontaneous temporal variation of symptoms in PRTH [10], we also advocate periodic cessation of all therapy and re-evaluation of the clinical status of the patient. The treatment of PRTH in childhood again requires careful monitoring to ensure that any reduction in thyroid hormone levels is not associated with growth retardation or adverse neurological sequelae. Indeed, control of cardiac and sympathomimetic manifestations with β-blockade may be the safest course in these circumstances and a cardioselective agent may be preferable to propranolol as the latter may induce hypothyroidism in some tissues by inhibiting the conversion of T_4 to T_3. Thyroid ablation is best used as a last resort in cases with life-threatening dysrhythmias or cardiac failure, as it is irreversible and may worsen the compensated hypothyroidism in some tissues. Finally, the future development of thyroid hormone analogues with selective TRβ agonist activity or TRα1-specific antagonists may represent a more rational basis for the treatment of these disorders.

FUTURE DIRECTIONS

The elucidation of a genetic defect associated with RTH allows the disorder to be diagnosed definitively. Prospective studies of such genetically defined cases will enable the clinical features and their relationship to the associated receptor mutation to be delineated more precisely. The introduction of mutations into the mouse TRβ gene by homologous recombination will generate an animal model for the disorder which will facilitate biochemical and molecular biological analyses to determine the pathogenesis of the variable phenotype.

ACKNOWLEDGEMENTS

Our work is supported by grants from the Wellcome Trust and the Medical Research Council. We are also greatly indebted to many physicians for referrals, without which our studies would not have been possible.

REFERENCES

1 Chatterjee VKK, Tata JR. Thyroid hormone receptors and their role in development. *Cancer Surv* 1992;**14**:147–167.
2 Chin WW. Nuclear thyroid hormone receptors. In: Parker MG ed. *Nuclear Hormone Receptors*, edited by Parker MG. Academic Press, London, 1991;79–102.

3 Horlein A, Naar AM, Heinzel T *et al.* Ligand-independent repression by the thyroid hormone receptor mediated by a nuclear receptor co-repressor. *Nature* 1995;**377**:397–404.

4 Lee JW, Ryan F, Swaffield JC, Johnston SA, Moore DD. Interaction of thyroid hormone receptor with a conserved transcriptional mediator. *Nature* 1995;**374**:91–94.

5 Lazar MA. Thyroid hormone receptors: multiple forms, multiple possibilities. *Endocr Rev* 1993;**14**:184–193.

6 Chatterjee VKK, Beck-Peccoz P. Thyroid hormone resistance. In: *Hormones, Enzymes and Receptors*, vol. 8, edited by Sheppard MC, Stewart PM. Bàllières Clinical Endocrinology and Metabolism London, 1994:267–283.

7 Refetoff S, De Wind LT, De Groot LJ. Familial syndrome combining deaf-mutism, stipple epiphyses, goiter and abnormally high PBI: possible target organ refractoriness to thyroid hormone. *J Clin Endocrinol Metab* 1967;**27**:279–294.

8 Persani L, Asteria C, Tonacchera M, Vitti P, Chatterjee VKK, Beck-Peccoz P. Evidence for the secretion of thyrotropin with enhanced bioactivity in syndromes of thyroid hormone resistance. *J Clin Endocrinol Metab* 1994;**78**:1034–1039.

9 Gershengorn MC, Weintraub BD. Thyrotropin-induced hyperthyroidism caused by selective pituitary resistance to thyroid hormone. A new syndrome of inappropriate secretion of TSH. *J Clin Invest* 1975;**56**:633–642.

10 Beck-Peccoz P, Chatterjee VKK. The variable clinical phenotype in thyroid hormone resistance syndrome. *Thyroid* 1994;**4**:225–232.

11 Hauser P, Zametkin AJ, Martinez P *et al.* Attention deficit–hyperactivity disorder in people with generalized resistance to thyroid hormone. *N Engl J Med* 1993;**328**:997–1001.

12 Brucker-Davis F, Skarulis MC, Grace MB *et al.* Genetic and clinical features of 42 kindreds with resistance to thyroid hormone. *Ann Intern Med* 1995;**123**:572–583.

13 Refetoff S, Weiss RE, Usala SJ. The syndromes of resistance to thyroid hormone. *Endocr Rev* 1993;**14**:348–399.

14 Adams M, Matthews C, Collingwood TN, Tone Y, Beck-Peccoz P, Chatterjee VKK. Genetic analysis of 29 kindreds with generalized and pituitary resistance to thyroid hormone. *J Clin Invest* 1994;**94**:506–515.

15 Nagaya T, Jameson IL. Thyroid hormone receptor dimerization is required for dominant negative inhibition by mutations that cause thyroid hormone resistance. *J Biol Chem* 1993;**268**:15766–15771.

16 Collingwood TN, Adams M, Tone Y, Chatterjee VKK. Spectrum of transcriptional, dimerization and dominant negative properties of 20 different mutant thyroid hormone β receptors in thyroid hormone resistance syndrome. *Mol Endocrinol* 1994;**8**:1262–1277.

17 Chatterjee VKK, Nagaya T, Madison LD, Datta S, Rentoumis A, Jameson JL. Thyroid hormone resistance syndrome. Inhibition of normal receptor function by mutant thyroid hormone receptors. *J Clin Invest* 1991;**87**:1977–1984.

18 Takeda K, Sakurai A, DeGroot LJ, Refetoff S. Recessive inheritance of thyroid hormone resistance caused by a complete deletion of the protein-coding region of the thyroid hormone receptor-β gene. *J Clin Endocrinol Metab* 1992;**74**:49–55.

19 Ono S, Schwartz ID, Mueller OT *et al.* Homozygosity for a dominant negative thyroid hormone receptor gene responsible for generalized thyroid hormone resistance. *J Clin Endocrinol Metab* 1991;**73**:990–994.

20 Yen PM, Sugawara A, Refetoff S, Chin WW. New insights on the mechanism(s) of the dominant negative effect of mutant thyroid hormone receptor in generalized resistance to thyroid hormone. *J Clin Invest* 1992;**90**:1825–1831.

21 Piedrafita FJ, Ortiz MA, Pfahl M. Thyroid hormone receptor β mutants with generalized resistance to thyroid hormone show defects in their ligand-sensitive repression function. *Mol Endocrinol* 1995;**9**:1533–1548.

22 Forman BM, Samuels HH. Interactions among a subfamily of nuclear receptors: the regulatory zipper model. *Mol Endocrinol* 1990;**4**:1293–1301.

23 Mixson AJ, Renault JC, Ramson S, Bodenner DL, Weintraub BD. Identification of a novel mutation in the gene encoding the β-triiodothyronine receptor in a patient with

apparent selective pituitary resistance to thyroid hormone. *Clin Endocrinol* 1993;**38**:227–234.

24 Falcone M, Miyamoto T, Fierro-Renoy F, Macchia E, DeGroot LJ. Antipeptide polyclonal antibodies specifically recognize each human thyroid hormone receptor isoform. *Endocrinology* 1992;**131**:2419–2429.

25 Mixson AJ, Hauser P, Tennyson G *et al.* Differential expression of mutant and normal beta T3 receptor alleles in kindreds with generalized resistance to thyroid hormone. *J Clin Invest* 1993;**91**:2296–2300.

26 Zavacki AM, Harney JW, Brent GA, Larsen PR. Dominant negative inhibition by mutant thyroid hormone receptors is thyroid response element and receptor isoform specific. *Mol Endocrinol* 1993;**7**:1319–1330.

27 Beck-Peccoz P, Piscitelli G, Cattaneo MG, Faglia G. Successful treatment of hyperthyroidism due to nonneoplastic pituitary TSH hypersecretion with 3,5,3'-triiodothyroacetic acid (TRIAC). *J Endocrinol Invest* 1983;**6**:217–223.

28 Dorey F, Strauch G, Gayno JP. Thyrotoxicosis due to pituitary resistance to thyroid hormones. Successful control with D-thyroxine; a study in three patients. *Clin Endocrinol* 1990;**32**:221–227.

29 Dulgeroff AJ, Geffner ME, Koyal SN, Wong M, Hershman JM. Bromocriptine and Triac therapy for hyperthyroidism due to pituitary resistance to thyroid hormone. *J Clin Endocrinol Metab* 1992;**75**:1071–1075.

30 Beck-Peccoz P, Mariotti S, Guillausseau PJ *et al.* Treatment of hyperthyroidism due to inappropriate secretion of thyrotropin with the somatostatin analog SMS 201-995. *J Clin Endocrinol Metab* 1989;**68**:208–214.

MULTIPLE CHOICE QUESTIONS

1 The thyroid hormone receptor

a is a transmembrane G-protein-coupled protein

b binds to DNA as homo- and heterodimers

c is encoded by a single gene in humans

d is organized in distinct functional domains

e enhances gene transcription in a hormone-dependent manner

2 Causes of raised serum thyroxine (T_4) and non-suppressed thyroid-stimulating hormone (TSH) levels are

a amiodarone therapy

b circulating anti-TSH receptor antibodies

c familial dysalbuminaemia

d T_4 replacement

e non-thyroidal illness

3 Commonly recognized features of resistance to thyroid hormone include

a abnormal thyroid function in first-degree relatives

b raised serum TSH levels

c thyrotoxic signs and symptoms

d normal or exaggerated TSH response to thyrotrophic-releasing hormone

e elevated serum sex hormone-binding globulin

4 Resistance to thyroid hormone is characterized by

a resistance within the pituitary–thyroid axis
b mutations in the TRβ gene in both generalized and pituitary resistance
c constitutively active mutant thyroid hormone receptors
d variable resistance in peripheral target tissues
e inhibition of wild-type receptor action by mutant receptor

5 In the management of resistance to thyroid hormone (RTH)

a the development of receptor isoform-specific analogues will be helpful
b thyroid ablation is the treatment of choice
c triiodothyroacetic acid has been shown to be effective
d T_4 therapy is contraindicated
e somatostatin analogues inhibit TSH secretion

Answers

1			2			3		
	a	False		a	True		a	True
	b	True		b	False		b	False
	c	False		c	True		c	True
	d	True		d	True		d	True
	e	True		e	True		e	False

4			5		
	a	True		a	True
	b	True		b	False
	c	False		c	True
	d	True		d	False
	e	True		e	True

Androgen resistance

There cannot be a more dramatic illustration of the clinical consequences of resistance to the action of a hormone than the original description of the testicular feminization syndrome by Morris [1]: a genetic male with normal testicular testosterone production develops phenotypically as a normal female externally. More recent terminology has defined the condition as complete androgen insensitivity syndrome (CAIS) and incomplete resistance to the action of androgens manifesting under the general heading of partial androgen insensitivity syndrome (PAIS). The principal defect resulting in androgen resistance is confined to target cells of androgen action.

PRODUCTION AND BIOLOGICAL ACTIONS OF ANDROGENS

Androgens are C19 steroids produced by the testes, ovaries and adrenals following a series of five enzymatic steps (Fig. 1). Testosterone is the major circulating androgen in the male, with a testicular production rate approximating 6 mg/day. The androgenic effect is amplified by conversion of testosterone to the more potent androgen, dihydrotestosterone (DHT) by way of the enzyme 5α-reductase. Androgens, including testosterone, also act as substrates for the formation of oestrogens through the action of the P450 aromatase complex. The androgen DHT cannot be aromatized because of reduction at carbon atom position 5 in the A ring of the steroid nucleus (Fig. 2).

The biopotency of different androgens is a function of additions to the C19 parent steroid structure, their planar configuration and the affinity with which the androgen binds to androgen receptors within target cells. The structures of some commonly used synthetic androgens are shown in Fig. 3 for comparison with testosterone (Fig. 2). The biological actions of androgens are diverse and some examples are listed in Table 1. Sex dimorphism in muscle development is evident at puberty, with muscle growth being mainly testosterone-dependent. The abuse of anabolic steroids is an unfortunate example of this biological effect of androgens.

479

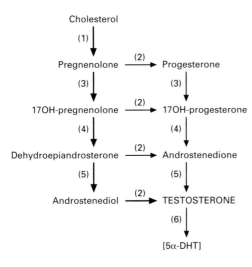

Fig. 1 Pathway of testosterone biosynthesis in the testis, emphasized by the bold arrows. The numbers indicate the enzymes involved: (1) P450scc (cholesterol desmolase); (2) 3β-hydroxysteroid dehydrogenase; (3) 17α-hydroxylase; (4) 17,20-lyase; (5) 17β-hydroxysteroid dehydrogenase; (6) 5α-reductase. Formation of 5α-dihydrotestosterone (DHT) is mainly extraglandular.

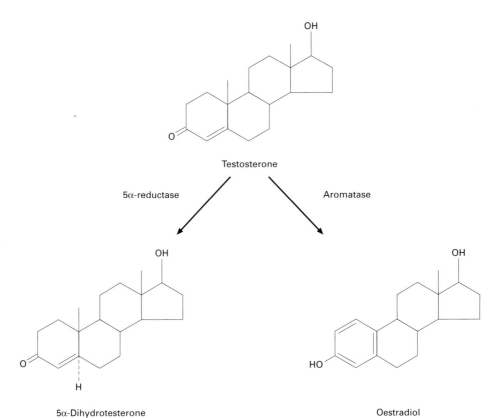

Fig. 2 Testosterone as a substrate for androgen amplification (5α-dihydrotestosterone; DHT) and oestrogen formation.

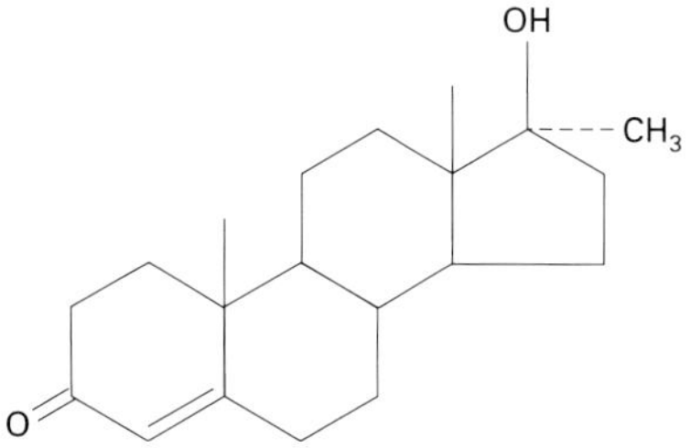

Methyltestosterone

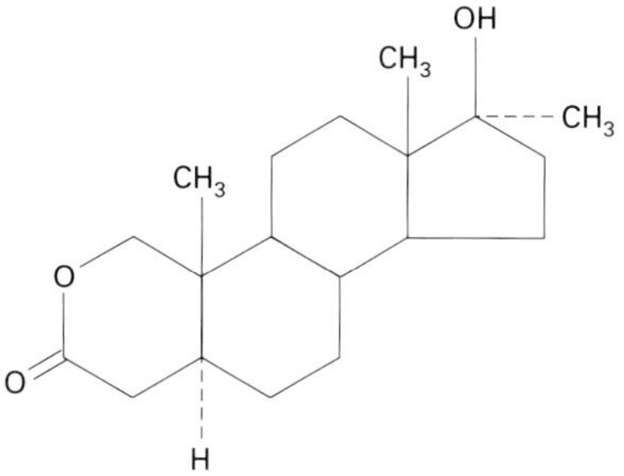

Oxandrolone

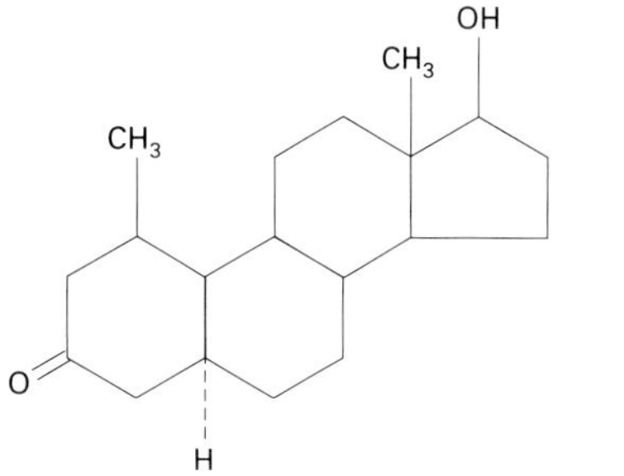

Mesterolone

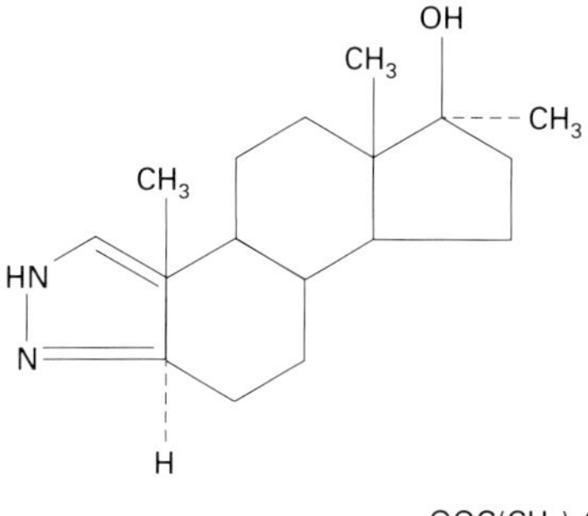

Stanozolol

Other esters:

Testosterone undecanoate (Restandol)

Testosterone proprionate
Testosterone phenylpropionate } (Sustanon)
Testosterone isocaproate

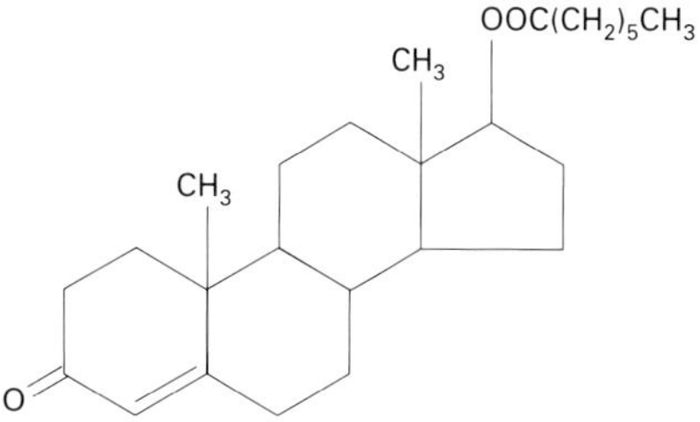

Testosterone enanthate (Primoteston)

Fig. 3 Chemical structure of some commonly used synthetic androgen and anabolic steroids.

Table 1 Some biological actions of androgens.

Muscle growth
Skeletal maturation
Reproductive tissues
External genitalia
Prostate
Seminiferous tubules
Seminal vesicles
Erythropoiesis
Voice maturation
Skin appendages
Hair follicles
Sebaceous glands
Apocrine glands
Behaviour

The growth spurt at puberty is the result of the synergistic effect of increased growth hormone, growth factors and gonadal steroids acting on the growth plate and enhancing skeletal maturation. Recently described isolated cases of aromatase deficiency and an oestrogen-receptor gene mutation in an adult male with unfused epiphyses suggest that androgens merely serve as a local substrate for oestrogenic-mediated closure of the growth plate at the completion of statural growth [2–4].

Androgens have a profound effect on erythropoiesis by enhancing the production of erythropoietin. Maturation of the voice (breaking), as exemplified by a change in fundamental voice frequency, is a relatively late event in male puberty occurring between stages 3 and 4 of the Tanner pubertal classification. Skin appendages are profoundly influenced by androgens. These include sebum production, activity of the apocrine glands and hair growth. Male-pattern baldness is both androgen-dependent and influenced by genetic factors; it does not occur in castrated males or in patients with 5α-reductase deficiency [5,6]. The influence of androgens on behaviour is complex but there is clear evidence from animal studies that a single androgenic stimulus given to females in the early postnatal period can permanently masculinize behaviour.

Androgens play a critical role in male sex differentiation, development and maintenance of normal sexual function in adult life (Fig. 4). Nowhere is this more dramatically illustrated than in the syndrome originally described in detail by Morris [1] where the external phenotypic development is female despite the production of an abundance of testosterone. The intracellular action of androgens in target tissues depends on the presence of a functional receptor which acts as a nuclear transcription factor once bound to ligand [7]. The androgen receptor is part of a large family of transcription factors which includes receptors to all the classes of steroid and thyroid hormones, retinoids, steroidogenic factor-1 (SF-1) as well as

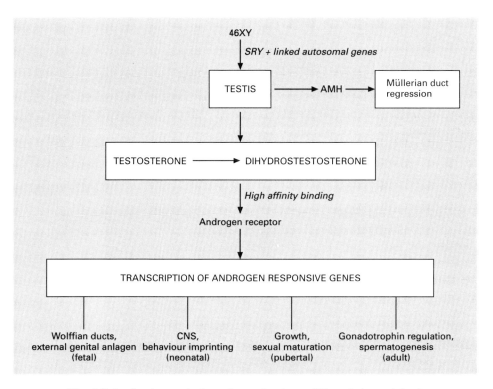

Fig. 4 Role of androgens in the pathway of male sex differentiation and development. SRY, Sex-determining region Y; AMH, anti-Müllerian hormone.

several orphan receptors amongst its members. In common with all the members of this superfamily, the 919-amino-acid androgen receptor is subdivided into three functional domains. The gene encoding for the androgen receptor (AR) is located near the centromeric region on the long arm of the X chromosome and comprises eight exons. Two exons encode a central domain which is highly conserved and is characterized by two zinc finger motifs which are involved in the binding of the ligand-bound receptor complex to chromosomal DNA target sites. A further five exons encode a C-terminal hormone-binding domain which also contains subdomains involved in receptor dimerization as well as probably some element of transcriptional activation. The first exon is the largest and encodes an N-terminal domain which is primarily involved in transcriptional regulation.

Androgen resistance is thus defined in an individual who, despite producing normal or increased testicular concentrations of testosterone which can be metabolized to DHT, shows clinical evidence of complete or partial insensitivity to androgens.

CLINICAL PRESENTATION OF
ANDROGEN INSENSITIVITY SYNDROME (AIS)

The complete form (CAIS) typically presents in an adolescent female who seeks advice for primary amenorrhoea. Breast development is normal, whereas pubic and axillary hair growth is absent or scanty. The external genitalia are female but the vagina is usually shorter than normal and blind-ending. There are no female internal genitalia because of the fetal testicular production and action of anti-Müllerian hormone. The testes are usually intra-abdominal but may present as swellings within inguinal herniae. The karyotype is 46,XY and adult patients are taller than normal females.

The differential diagnosis in the XY female is limited to pure gonadal dysgenesis, 17α-hydroxylase deficiency and Leydig-cell hypoplasia. The last disorder has recently been attributed to a mutation of the luteinizing hormone (LH) receptor gene which affects the transmembrane domain of this member of the G-protein-coupled receptor family [8]. The endocrinology of CAIS is straightforward: elevated LH and testosterone concentrations, while follicle-stimulating hormone (FSH) levels are usually normal. Occasionally, a human chorionic gonadotrophin (HCG) stimulation test may be required to exclude Leydig-cell hypoplasia. CAIS is generally only recognized before puberty if the testes herniate as inguinal swellings, usually in early infancy. Bilateral inguinal herniae are unusual in girls so the karyotype should always be checked in such cases. Because of the X-linked inheritance, a history of surgery for bilateral herniae in an older sister hitherto unrecognized as having CAIS is relatively common.

The partial form of AIS (PAIS) usually presents as ambiguous genitalia of the newborn. In this situation, it is necessary to exclude congenital adrenal hyperplasia due to 21-hydroxylase as the commonest cause of this problem. A 46,XX karyotype and a markedly increased plasma concentration of 17OH-progesterone clinches that diagnosis [9]. The appearance of the external genitalia in PAIS typically shows perineoscrotal hypospadias,

Table 2 Disorders which may produce a phenotype similar to partial androgen insensitivity syndrome (PAIS).

True hermaphroditism
Dysplastic (dysfunctional testes)
Androgen biosynthetic defects
　3β-HSD
　17β-HSD
　5α-reductase
Idiopathic PAIS phenotype (normal AR binding)
Syndromes, e.g. Denys–Drash, Smith–Lemli–Opitz

HSD, Hydroxysteroid dehydrogenase; AR, androgen receptor.

a bifid scrotum, micropenis with chordee and testes which may be cryptorchid. Such a phenotype may also be identical in a 46,XY infant with any one of the disorders listed in Table 2. It is a diagnostic challenge to define a precise cause, but measuring the plasma testosterone and DHT, and urinary androgen metabolite response to hCG stimulation will usually exclude a defect in androgen biosynthesis or metabolism. Dysgenetic testes is a histological diagnosis, although it is suggestive if Müllerian duct remnants are visible on ultrasound examination. The spectrum of genital abnormalities in PAIS can be wide, ranging from almost a CAIS phenotype with just isolated clitoromegaly to an otherwise normal male with an isolated hypospadias [10].

MEASUREMENT OF ANDROGEN BINDING *IN VITRO*

The AR is expressed in many tissues, including skin fibroblasts. Early studies had indicated that androgens bound to a high-affinity, low-capacity

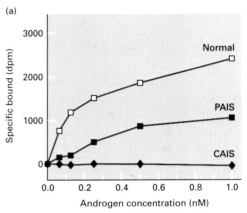

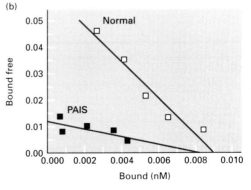

Fig. 5 Androgen-binding assay using cultured genital skin fibroblasts. (a) Saturation curve showing specific androgen binding to the androgen receptor (AR) in normal, partial androgen insensitivity syndrome (PAIS; reduced) and complete androgen insensitivity syndrome (CAIS; absent) fibroblasts. (b) Scatchard plot of the normal and PAIS-binding data. The intercept of the regression line with the ordinate indicates the B_{max} or receptor concentration, while the K_d (binding affinity) is calculated from the negative of the reciprocal of the gradient. In this example, the binding affinity of the AR is about five times lower in PAIS than normal.

protein, typical characteristics for a steroid receptor [11]. Furthermore, the AR was quantitatively greater in fibroblasts grown from genital as compared with non-genital skin [12]. Figure 5 shows the saturation analysis of AR binding when radiolabelled androgen in increasing concentrations was incubated with a normal fibroblast cell line derived from a foreskin sample obtained at the time of circumcision. The Scatchard plot provides a measure of binding affinity (K_d, based on the slope of the regression line) and the receptor concentration (B_{max}, derived from the intercept of the regression line with the ordinate).

Androgen binding to genital skin fibroblasts is usually undetectable or extremely low in CAIS [13]. Even when some binding is detected, the quantity is invariably too low to undertake a Scatchard analysis to derive values for K_d and B_{max}. In the case of PAIS, there is usually androgen binding detectable but the binding affinity (K_d) is abnormal. This is indicated by an alteration in the slope of the regression line, as shown for the Scatchard plot in Fig. 5. Occasionally, androgen binding is normal in fibroblasts from a CAIS patient, and quite often in a patient with PAIS. The results of androgen-binding assays in genital skin fibroblasts provide

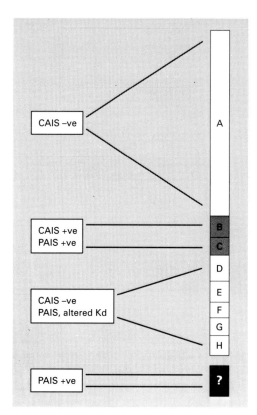

Fig. 6 Relationship between androgen-binding characteristics and likely location of androgen receptor (AR) gene mutations. Exons A, B and C, D–H encode the N-terminal transcriptional, central DNA binding and carboxy-terminal hormone-binding domains, respectively. For example, an altered K_d in partial androgen insensitivity syndrome (PAIS; see Fig. 5) is likely to be associated with a mutation in one of D–H exons.

a useful pointer as to which functional domain of the AR is likely to be affected by a mutation (Fig. 6).

MUTATIONAL ANALYSIS OF THE AR GENE

Absent androgen binding or altered binding affinity are associated with mutations which affect the C-terminal hormone-binding domain of the AR [7,14]. Most are point mutations resulting in amino-acid substitutions. A number of mutations in the first exon which encodes the N-terminal domain have been described which produce frameshift and premature stop codons, resulting in the synthesis of a truncated receptor. Such mutations are usually characterized by decreased or absent androgen binding in patients with the CAIS phenotype. While there is no clearly defined 'hot spot', there is a cluster of point mutations in exon 5 and exon 7 of the hormone-binding domain corresponding to amino acid regions 732–774 and 831–866, respectively. The first of these two clusters corresponds closely to a cluster of mutations identified in the thyroid receptor ß gene of patients with thyroid hormone resistance [15].

A number of interesting mutations have been described involving either exons 2 and 3, which encode the zinc finger-binding motifs of the DNA-binding domain. Since the hormone-binding domain is unaffected, androgen binding in genital skin fibroblasts is normal. Two sisters with phenotypes indistinguishable from typical for CAIS and a 46,XY karyotype had supra-normal levels of androgen receptors based on binding studies in fibroblasts [16]. Subsequent molecular studies showed an in-frame deletion of exon 3, highlighting the role of the second zinc finger in DNA binding [17]. Other mutations affecting the DNA-binding domain include single amino acid substitutions and deletions. This is also the regulatory domain which, in the vitamin D receptor, appears to be more frequently altered in cases of vitamin D hormone resistance [18].

The functional consequences of point mutations in particular are important to study for two reasons. First, as a means of confirming that the amino acid substitution is indeed the cause of the change in phenotype. Second, the recreation of the mutation by site-directed mutagenesis provides an opportunity *in vitro* to study the androgen-binding characteristics of the mutated receptor and the functional ability of the AR complex to bind to DNA and initiate gene transcription. This latter function can be assessed, for example, by use of a transactivation assay which depends on the introduction of an AR expression construct along with a reporter construct into the same cells. The latter construct comprises a gene such as that encoding for chloramphenicol acetyl transferase; this enzyme activity can be induced in the presence of an androgen response element and an androgen ligand [7]. Transactivation assays have provided a useful system to determine which subdomains of the AR appear critical for

androgen-induced gene expression. Of more practical benefit, the hormone induction of reporter gene activity can be quantitated in relation to
the dose and type of androgen. These studies are of particular relevance
in the management of patients with PAIS in whom the sex of rearing is
male and information is needed to predict virilization at puberty. However,
the transactivation assay is complex, time-consuming and impractical
as a simple test to predict androgen responsiveness in newborns with
PAIS. Some promise has been shown with the use of sex hormone-binding
globulin (SHBG) measurements [19]. Exogenous androgens induce a
fall in SHBG concentrations in normal males; no change is observed in
patients with CAIS. However, the response to androgens is variable in
patients with PAIS, which is the subgroup in whom a clear-cut difference
from normals could be of practical benefit.

The androgen-insensitivity syndrome is an X-linked recessive disorder.
Knowledge of the AR gene mutation in an index case may be used for
subsequent prenatal diagnosis and carrier detection [20]. It is important
to realize that phenotypic variability in the expression of a particular mutation in PAIS, both intra- and interfamilial, can pose difficulties in predicting
outcome [21]. The N-terminal portion of the AR contains a polymorphic
stretch of glutamine and glycine amino acid residues whose analysis provides a means of identifying the inheritance pattern of the maternal X
chromosomes. Furthermore, it should be noted that approximately 30%
of mutations arise *de novo*.

The polymorphic glutamine repeat is considerably expanded in spinal
and bulbar muscular atrophy or Kennedy's disease [22]. This neurological
disorder is associated with gynaecomastia and sometimes infertility as the
sole manifestations of androgen insensitivity. How the expanded repeat
produces neuronal dysfunction is unknown, but site-directed mutagenesis
of the AR to include abnormal expansion of the polyglutamine repeat
when recreated *in vitro* leads to reduced transcriptional regulatory competence of the AR protein [23]. Furthermore, there is abnormal binding
affinity of the AR for androgens when suprapubic skin fibroblasts from
patients with Kennedy's disease are studied [24]. Other examples of
diseases associated with expanded trinucleotide repeats include the fragile
X syndrome [25], myotonic dystrophy [26], Huntington's disease [27]
and spinocerebellar ataxia type I [28].

MANAGEMENT OF AIS

The diagnosis in the majority of patients with CAIS is established when
an adolescent female is investigated for primary amenorrhoea. Bilateral
gonadectomy is performed in view of the 2–5% risk of gonadal tumour
formation in later life [29]. Inguinal testes are removed at the time of inguinal
hernia repair; intra-abdominal testes can now be removed laparoscopically.

Oestrogen replacement, administered either orally or transdermally, is required to maintain breast development and prevent the earlier onset of osteoporosis. Additional progesterone treatment is not normally needed because of the absence of a uterus. Vaginoplasty is indicated only in a minority of patients when dilator treatment is not successful. Numerous surgical techniques have been described in an attempt to fashion an adequate vagina.

When the diagnosis of CAIS is made in infancy, there is the option to remove the gonads early or leave *in situ* (assuming there are no troublesome herniae) until after puberty when breast development has occurred. In a recent survey of management practice, the majority of paediatricians were now advocating early gonadectomy, whereas adult physicians and gynae-cologists were more inclined to recommend late gonadectomy (Hughes, personal observation).

The principal management issue in patients with PAIS is the decision about the sex of rearing. This must be undertaken in full consultation with the surgeon, paediatrician and the family. When isolated clitoromegaly is the only sign of virilization, the infant is reared as female and plans made for early clitoroplasty, gonadectomy and perhaps vaginoplasty. The infant with a greater degree of virilization manifest as micropenis, perineoscrotal hypospadias and bifid scrotum requires sophisticated corrective genital surgery if the sex of rearing is male. There is still the later problem of knowing whether adequate virilization will occur at puberty. Testes should be relocated into the scrotum and observed regularly in view of the risk of tumour formation. It is recommended that a testicular biopsy be performed after puberty. High-dose androgen treatment may be necessary if the response to endogenous androgens is inadequate. There is currently little information on the outcome in adult life for patients with PAIS reared as males.

There are other management issues to resolve in AIS. For example, there is no consensus amongst paediatricians, endocrinologists and gynae-cologists about what to tell patients with AIS about the cause of their problems. Should the nature of the karyotype and gonads be disclosed? There is no one answer to this question, but patients with AIS are entitled to more information about their condition than is currently generally the case. An AIS Support Group⋆ has recently been established to work in collaboration with the medical profession to improve the outlook for patients with AIS.

ACKNOWLEDGEMENTS

The secretarial assistance of Mrs Nina Hardman is gratefully acknowledged.

⋆ Androgen Insensitivity Syndrome (AIS) Support Group, c/o Mrs Jacki Burrows, 2 Shirburn Avenue, Mansfield, Notts NG18 2BY.

The author is grateful for helpful discussions with colleagues, especially Dr Alex Tait, Dr Mark Patterson, Ms Helen Davies and Ms Charlotte Bevan.

REFERENCES

1 Morris J. The syndrome of testicular feminisation in male pseudohermaphrodites. *Am J Obstet Gynecol* 1953;**65**:1192–1211.
2 Shozu M, Akasofu K, Harada T, Kubota Y. A new case of female pseudohermaphroditism: placental aromatase deficiency. *J Clin Endocrinol Metab* 1991;**72**:560–566.
3 Conte FA, Grumbach MM, Ito Y, Fisher CR, Simpson ER. A syndrome of female pseudohermaphroditism, hypergonadotrophic hypogonadism, and multi-cystic ovaries associated with missense mutations in the gene encoding aromatase (P450 arom). *J Clin Endocrinol Metab* 1994;**78**:1287–1292.
4 Smith EP, Boyd J, Frank GR *et al.* Estrogen resistance caused by a mutation in the estrogen-receptor gene in a man. *N Engl J Med* 1994;**331**:1056–1061.
5 Hamilton JB. Male hormone stimulation is a prerequisite and an incitant in common baldness. *Am J Anat* 1942;**71**:451–480.
6 Imperato-McGinley J, Miller M, Wilson JD *et al.* A cluster of male pseudohermaphrodites with 5α-reductase deficiency in Papua New Guinea. *Clin Endocrinol* 1991;**34**:293–298.
7 Patterson MN, McPhaul MJ, Hughes IA. Androgen insensitivity syndrome. In: Sheppard MC, Stewart PM eds. Hormones, Enzymes and Receptors, *Clin Endocrinol Metab* 1994;**8**:379–404.
8 Kremer H, Kraaij R, Sergio PA *et al.* Male pseudohermaphroditism due to a homozygous missense mutation of the luteinizing hormone receptor gene. *Nature Genet* 1995;**9**:160–164.
9 Hughes IA, Riad Fahmy D, Griffiths K. Plasma 17OH-progesterone concentrations in newborn infants. *Arch Dis Child* 1979;**54**:347–349.
10 Williams DM, Patterson MN, Hughes IA. Androgen insensitivity syndrome. *Arch Dis Child* 1993;**65**:343–344.
11 Keenan BS, Meyer WJ III, Hadjan AJ, Jones HW, Migeon CJ. Syndrome of androgen insensitivity in man: absence of 5α-dihydrotestosterone binding protein in skin fibroblasts. *J Clin Endocrinol Metab* 1974;**38**:1143–1146.
12 Evans BAJ, Jones TR, Hughes IA. Studies of the androgen receptor in dispersed fibroblasts: investigation of patients with androgen insensitivity. *Clin Endocrinol* 1984;**20**:93–105.
13 Batch JA, Patterson MN, Hughes IA. Androgen insensitivity syndrome. *Reprod Med Rev* 1992;**1**:131–150.
14 Quigley CA, De Bellis A, Marschke KB, El-Awady MK, Wilson EM, French FS. Androgen receptor defects: historical, clinical and molecular perspectives. *Endocr Rev* 1995;**16**:271–321.
15 Chatterjee VKK, Beck-Peccoz P. Thyroid hormone resistance. In: Sheppard MC, Stewart PM eds. Hormones, enzymes and receptors. *Clin Endocrinol Metab* 1994;**8**:267–283.
16 Hughes IA, Evans BAJ, Ismail R, Matthews J. Complete androgen insensitivity syndrome characterized by increased concentration of a normal androgen receptor in genital skin fibroblasts. *J Clin Endocrinol Metab* 1986;**63**:309–315.
17 Quigley CA, Evans BAJ, Simental JA *et al.* Complete androgen insensitivity due to deletion of exon C of the androgen receptor gene highlights the functional importance of the second zinc finger of the androgen receptor *in vivo. Mol Endocrinol* 1992;**6**:1103–1112.
18 Rut AR, Hewison M, Kristjansson K, Luisi B, Hughes MR, O'Riordan JLH. Two mutations causing vitamin D resistant rickets: modelling on the basis of steroid hormone receptor DNA-binding domain crystal structures. *Clin Endocrinol* 1994;**41**:581–590.
19 Sinnecker G, Köhler S. Sex hormone binding globulin response to the anabolic steroid

stanozolol: evidence for its suitability as a biological androgen sensitivity test. *J Clin Endocrinol Metab* 1989;**68**:1195–1200.

20 Davies HR, Hughes IA, Patterson MN. Genetic counselling in complete androgen insensitivity syndrome: trinucleotide repeat polymorphisms, single strand conformation polymorphism and direct detection of two novel mutations in the androgen receptor gene. *Clin Endocrinol* 1995;**43**:69–77.

21 Batch JA, Davies HR, Evans BAJ, Hughes IA, Patterson MN. Phenotypic variation and detection of carrier status in the partial androgen insensitivity syndrome. *Arch Dis Child* 1993;**68**:453–457.

22 La Spada AR, Wilson EM, Lubahn DB, Harding AE, Fischbeck KH. Androgen receptor gene mutations in X-linked spinal and bulbar muscular atrophy. *Nature* 1991;**352**:77–79.

23 Mhatre AN, Trifiro MA, Kaufman M *et al.* Reduced transcriptional regulatory competence of the androgen receptor in X-linked spinal and bulbar muscular atrophy. *Nature Genet* 1993;**5**:184–188.

24 MacLean HE, Choi W-T, Rekaris G, Warne GL, Zajac JD. Abnormal androgen receptor binding affinity in subjects with Kennedy's disease (spinal and bulbar muscular atrophy). *J Clin Endocrinol Metab* 1995;**80**:508–516.

25 Verkerk AJMH, Pieretti M, Sutcliffe JS *et al.* Identification of a gene (FMR-1) containing a CGG repeat coincident with a breakpoint cluster region exhibiting length variation in fragile X syndrome. *Cell* 1992;**65**:905–914.

26 Brook JD, McCurrach ME, Harley HG *et al.* Molecular basis of myotonic dystrophy: expansion of a trinucleotide (CTG) repeat at the 3′ end of a transcript encoding a protein kinase family member. *Cell* 1992;**68**:799–808.

27 The Huntington's Disease Collaborative Research Group. A novel gene containing a trinucleotide repeat that is expanded and unstable on Huntington's disease chromosomes. *Cell* 1993;**72**:921–983.

28 Orr HT, Ming-yi C, Banfi S *et al.* Expansion of an unstable trinucleotide CAG repeat in spinocerebellar ataxia type 1. *Nature Genet* 1993;**4**:221–226.

29 Verp M, Simpson JL. Abnormal sexual differentiation and neoplasia. *Cancer Genet* 1987;**25**:191–218.

The pathogenesis of pituitary tumours

ANDREW LEVY

The pituitary gland is a composite structure derived predominantly from epithelial tissue. It occupies a central place both anatomically and physiologically in the chain of neuroendocrine command from the hypothalamus and higher brain centres to the peripheral endocrine organs. For reasons that are not understood, the pituitary has a propensity to occult adenoma formation. Overt pituitary adenoma formation, presenting with symptoms and signs of space occupation, hypopituitarism, with or without one of the classical syndromes of hormone excess, is fortunately much less common than autopsy evidence of pituitary adenoma formation would lead us to expect. The incidence of acromegaly, Cushing's disease and endocrinologically inactive pituitary adenomas requiring surgery in the UK is around 3.2, 1.8 and 6 per 10^6 respectively, compared to an overall prevalence of pituitary adenomas, from random autopsy examinations, of 20%.

Pituitary adenomas, in addition to being very common, have a number of so-far unexplained characteristics: the first is that distant metastatic spread from pituitary adenomas is very unusual, even though they may be present for several decades before diagnosis and treatment. Second, with the exception of the rare malignant pituitary adenomas, neither classical proto-oncogene activation or antioncogene inactivation — the mechanisms responsible for tumour formation in most other tissues — seems to be implicated in pituitary tumour formation. For the most part, therefore, although the pathogenesis of these lesions remains unknown, it seems likely that a number of quite different mechanisms acting singly or, more probably, in concert, are responsible for pituitary tumour formation.

Before describing some potential specific mechanism of pituitary tumour formation, it is worth bearing in mind that all biological macromolecules are inherently unstable. Even in the absence of γ-rays, cosmic rays, X-rays, ultraviolet radiation and chemical mutagens, deoxynucleotides undergo slow, spontaneous oxidation, hydrolysis and methylation. Fortunately for us, the integrity of double-stranded DNA, and the fidelity with which it is reproduced prior to cell division, is extraordinarily high. The half-life of hydrolytic deamination of a cytosine nucleotide under physiological conditions, for example, is no less than 30 000 years. As the human genome is encoded on roughly 3×10^9 base pairs, however, 2–10 000 purine bases are hydrolysed and repaired in each human cell every day. Whether failure of complete repair is the basis of evolution, ageing or carcinogenesis is not known, but it seems reasonable to predict that a random hit on the coding region for any protein that induces cellular growth or division, inappropriately protects cells from programmed death, impairs the function of nucleotide excision repair genes [1] or disrupts DNA replication, leading to allelic deletion of antioncogene-containing chromosomal tracts, which might, if not repaired, lead to tumour formation. As yet we do not know whether the pattern of 'hits' on the genome is random and if so, whether some parts of the genome are more difficult to repair than others. But from the time of conception and throughout life, the 'balance of power' in the battle to protect the genome from corruption is clearly close-run, and in the final analysis, frequently lost.

To approach the pathogenesis of pituitary adenomas from a less vacuous standpoint, we should ask the question, what are the strategic cellular proteins whose function might, if subverted, lead to tumour formation? Clearly, the genes coding for cell-cycle proteins and the proteins that normally destroy or sequester them when they are no longer needed are prime targets, as are trophic hormones, growth factors and growth factor receptors. Second-messenger transduction systems and the kinases and phosphatases that normally regulate the activity of other proteins are also targets. The human homologues of gene coding for the proteins that control cell death are likely to be determined within the next few years, and may well provide fertile ground for research into new mutations leading to tumour formation. Finally, gene rearrangements and the introduction of exogenous sequences on viral vectors are also potential mutagenic mechanisms.

TROPHIC HORMONE PRODUCTION BY THE PITUITARY GLAND

The isolation of a series of growth factors from pituitary tissue [2,3] and the relative success of hypophysectomy for metastatic breast tumours [4,5] attests to the fact that the pituitary produces growth factors, at least in some cases, at physiologically active concentrations (Table 1). There is also evidence that pituitary adenomas of all types contain clusters of cells that transcribe hypothalamic- releasing factors at levels comparable on a cell-to-cell basis to the releasing hormone-producing cells of the hypothalamus. This is particularly true of somatotroph adenomas, 35% of which transcribe corticotrophin-releasing hormone (CRH), 76% transcribe growth hormone-releasing hormone (GHRH) and 21% transcribe thyrotrophin-releasing hormone (TRH).

Table 1 Growth factors known to be produced by the pituitary gland.

Fibroblast growth factor
Insulin-like growth factor-1 (0.6 ng/100 μg)
Epidermal growth factor (11 ng/pituitary)
Transforming growth factor-β (3–4 ng/pituitary)
Pituitary-derived mammary growth factors
Interleukin-2 and interleukin-6
Growth hormone-releasing hormone
Corticotrophin-releasing hormone
Thyrotrophin-releasing hormone

As a primary mechanism of pituitary adenoma pathogenesis, however, most opinion is swayed against inappropriate exogenous release of growth factors, as the relative incidence of hyperplastic changes in target cells adjacent to adenomas (21% of corticotroph adenomas and 40% of somatotrophinomas) is little more than that found in the normal pituitary glands (13%) [6]. These observations, and the increasing body of evidence to suggest that pituitary tumours are predominantly monoclonal in origin, do not, however, exclude induction of monoclonal cellular expansions by extrapituitary factors.

RECEPTOR ABNORMALITIES

Inappropriate expression

The response of normal and abnormal pituitary cells to microenvironmental factors depends on the complement of cell surface and nuclear receptors that they exhibit. Current dogma maintains that, under normal circumstances, gonadotrophs are the only cells bearing gonadotrophin-releasing hormone (GnRH) receptors [7], and that TRH receptors, for example, are confined to mammotroph and lactotroph cells. It is worth pointing out, however, that whilst the diagnosis of corticotroph adenomas is based to a major extent on demonstrating qualitatively normal CRH receptor responses and corticotroph feedback control, the diagnosis of somatotroph adenomas is confirmed biochemically not by identifying an excessive response to GHRH, but by observing qualitatively abnormal GH secretory responses to a glucose load, and to boluses of TRH and sometimes GnRH. As a paradoxical GH secretory response to TRH, however, can also occur in diabetes mellitus, renal failure, endogenous depression, hypothyroidism and during normal puberty, and as there is evidence that a number of GnRH-responsive cell types other than those secreting gonadotrophins are present in the pituitary [8], there is still doubt about the exact spectrum of receptors expressed by different cell types in the normal pituitary.

Because of this, it is difficult to do more than speculate that the presence of functionally normal receptors expressed in abnormal amounts, or by an apparently inappropriate cell type, might be responsible for tumour formation. The potential trophic implications of these observations are rarely addressed, even though in essence it would not be difficult to do so experimentally.

Receptor structure/coupling abnormalities

At the time of writing, there is no published evidence of specific releasing hormone or growth factor receptor mutations in pituitary adenomas. It is recognized, however, that GnRH receptors in gonadotroph adenomas and endocrinologically inactive adenomas derived from the gonadotroph line are abnormally resistant to down-regulation in response to GnRH superagonists. It has also been observed that adenomatous somatotrophs in acromegaly are sometimes resistant to desensitization in response to continuous exposure to GHRH and that in others dopamine can reduce intracellular calcium ion concentrations but leave adenylyl cyclase levels unchanged.

Abnormal receptor coupling to G-proteins or an abnormal G-protein response following receptor activation are further possible mechanisms of pituitary adenoma formation. Bearing in mind the high frequency of pituitary abnormalities observed at autopsy and the equally high incidence of antibodies to latent cytopathic viruses such as cytomegalovirus in the population at large, it is not too unreasonable to speculate that the presence of coding regions in the cytomegalovirus genome with homology to G-protein-coupled receptors, if constitutively active, might subvert signalling pathways [9]. A less fanciful mechanism by which virus infection might be implicated in pituitary adenoma formation is the recently described ability of cytomegalovirus (CMV) proteins to sequester the cell-cycle regulatory protein P53 [10] (see below).

It has been quite widely observed that a small proportion of somatotroph adenomas (perhaps 5–10%) respond paradoxically to somatostatin analogues *in vivo* and *in vitro* [11]. Under normal circumstances, somatostatin (SRIH) would be expected to reduce basal intracellular calcium ion levels in both normal and adenomatous somatotroph cells to low levels, and block the increase in intracellular calcium ion levels caused by GHRH. In one somatotroph adenoma that we have investigated at length *in vitro*, the addition of SRIH produces a rapid *increase* in intracellular calcium ion levels in all of the cells observed over 3 days of successive experiments (Fig. 1). This paradoxical response — which was not present in dispersed cells from 13 other somatotroph adenomas — does not appear on direct sequencing to be associated with a somatostatin (SSTR2) receptor mutation. Whether this dramatic, qualitatively abnormal response to SRIH disrupts

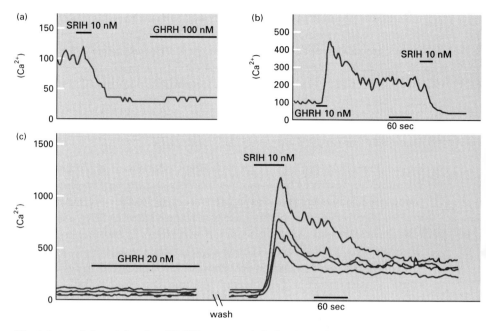

Fig. 1 Intracellular calcium ion ($[Ca^{2+}]_i$) responses in isolated cells from a human somatotroph adenoma. Under normal circumstances, somatostatin (SRIH) reduces baseline $[Ca^{2+}]_i$ (note the different scales on the ordinates) and blocks the $[Ca^{2+}]_i$ increase that would normally be expected in response to growth hormone-releasing hormone (GHRH; a). As expected, the increase in $[Ca^{2+}]_i$ in response to GHRH is also rapidly abolished by the subsequent addition of SRIH (b). In dispersed cells from another somatotroph adenoma, GHRH had no effect, but SRIH caused a dramatic paradoxical increase in $[Ca^{2+}]_i$ in all of the cells examined (c).

hypothalamic control and feedback regulation of somatotroph function sufficiently to predispose to clonal expansion, or indeed, whether it is even responsible for the paradoxical calcium ion response to somatostatin, is presently unknown.

G-protein malfunction

G-proteins play a central role in signal transduction across the cell membrane. The α-subunit, which dissociates from the tightly bound β- and γ-subunits of heterotrimeric Gs when guanosine triphosphate (GTP) displaces its bound guanosine diphosphate (GDP), stimulates adenylyl cyclase to produce cyclic adenosine monophosphate (AMP) from adenosine triphosphate (ATP; Fig. 2). Cyclic AMP activates cyclic AMP-dependent protein kinases and increases intracellular calcium ion concentrations. This is the signal that under certain circumstances tells somatotroph cells to secrete GH, and to grow and divide. The signal is terminated by hydrolysis

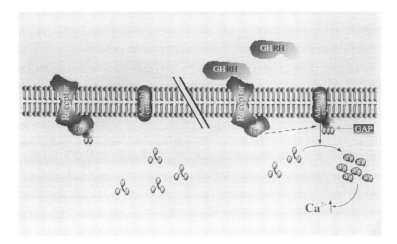

Fig. 2 Schematic diagram of guanosine triphosphatase (GTPase) activity showing a segment of somatotroph cell membrane with an unoccupied growth hormone-releasing hormone (GHRH) receptor (Receptor) in the left-hand panel and an occupied receptor in the right-hand panel. The α-subunit heterotrimeric GTPase Gs is guanosine diphosphate (GDP)-bound in the former and remains associated with the β- and γ-subunits in the inactive state. When the receptor is bound to its ligand the α-subunit binds guanosine tryphosphate (GTP) and dissociates from the β- and γ-subunits. The α-subunit associates with and activates adenylyl cyclase, which converts adenosine triphosphate (ATP) to cyclic adenosine monophosphate (AMP; AP), leading to an increase in intracellular calcium levels with all of the associated epiphenomena. The process is terminated by the intrinsic-GTPase activity of the α-subunit (hence the name of the heterotrimer) and the recently described GTPase activity of adenylyl cyclase itself, enhanced by the activity of the GTPase-activating peptides (GAP). The *gsp* mutation modifies the GTPase α-subunit, making it more resistant to hydrolysis. This results in a constitutive increase in intracellular cyclic AMP level — an effect that is believed to predispose to somatotroph adenoma formation.

of the bound GTP, which leads to dissociation of Gsα from adenylyl cyclase.

GTP hydrolysis is brought about by a number of mechanisms. First, Gsα has weak intrinsic GTPase activity that is potentiated by the GTPase activity of adenylyl cyclase itself [12]. Second, there are a number of GTPase-activating peptides (GAP) [13], the actions of which are self-explanatory, and lastly, a collection of guanine nucleotide-releasing or -exchange proteins [14] that shuffle intracellular GDP molecules with GTP. As the latter is present at higher concentrations, the action of these peptides would tend to antagonize the action of GTPase.

Changes in the intrinsic activity of any of these components [15] may theoretically predispose to adenoma formation. A specific example of this in human pituitary adenomas is the *gsp* oncogene. Activation of the proto-oncogene is brought about by one of two single-point mutations in the Gsα subunit of GTPase, which result in the arginine residue at position

201 being changed to cysteine or histidine, and the glutamine residue at position 227 being replaced by an arginine or leucine. Both of these mutations make the GTP bound by Gsα more resistant to hydrolysis. The result is a longer 'on' time following GTP binding. Although it has not been proved experimentally beyond doubt, this mechanism is thought to be responsible for the induction of approximately 40% of somatotroph adenomas [16]. It also remains unclear why the DNA motifs coding for these two target residues should be predisposed to mutation or perhaps, more to the point, 'beyond repair', once mutated. The obvious but simplistic assumption (entirely unsupported by experimental data) would be that certain critical DNA repair functions are also in some way dependent on the same pathway, and that both are simultaneously disrupted.

Abnormal kinases

Although abnormalities of genes coding for kinases and protein phosphatases would seem to be fertile ground for proto-oncogenes, there are no published reports to suggest that such a mechanism is important in human pituitary adenoma formation. Overexpression of protein kinase C, or in one case, an asparagine to glycine substitution at residue 294 of protein kinase C, has, however, been described in a small series of invasive pituitary adenomas [17].

In addition to cyclic AMP-dependent and inositol phospholipid-dependent protein kinases, many receptors, such as the GH, insulin-like growth factor (IGF-1) and epidermal growth factor (EGF) receptors are either directly associated with, or have intrinsic serine, threonine and/or tyrosine kinase activity. Inappropriate activity of protein kinases or the phosphatases that terminate their effect (some of which are themselves receptor-associated [18]) could disturb the duration of trophic signals and potentially lead to adenoma formation [19].

CLASSICAL ONCOGENE ACTIVATION

The *ras* proto-oncogenes are structurally related to the G-protein family, and although the typical tumour-associated *ras* mutations have not been identified in pituitary adenomas, a change in the H-*ras* gene (Gly to Val) at codon 12 in a highly invasive prolactinoma has been described [20].

Anomalous vascular supply

There has been some speculation that the development of a systemic vascular supply could deprive areas of the anterior pituitary of hypothalamohypophyseal portal blood and prevent dopamine and SRIH from reaching their target cells — a mechanism thought to be in part responsible for the predisposition of certain breeds of rats to mammotroph hyperplasia and prolactinoma formation in response to oestrogen treatment. The same may also be true of releasing factors reaching the anterior pituitary from the neurohypophysis via the short portal system, although there is no direct evidence for this mechanism.

Proteins involved in cell death

Until the importance of programmed cell death during development and as a regulator of turnover and remodelling of mature tissue was recognized, the possibility that tumour formation might result from 'the abnormal absence of cell death' was largely ignored. It is now known that inactivation of genes directly involved in the death pathway, such as p53, can lead to tumour formation by failing to induce apoptosis if genomic integrity cannot be restored after induction of replication arrest. Overactivity of genes which act as 'antidotes to death', such as BCL-2, might theoretically have a similar effect. As human homologues of the genes that control apoptosis in certain lower animals are beginning to be cloned, it seems likely that in the fairly near future, research in this area may well contribute substantially to our knowledge of pituitary adenoma pathogenesis. The importance of dominant antioncogenes is also suggested by the 8–16% incidence of allelic deletion in pituitary adenomas, particularly of parts of the pericentromeric region of the long arm of chromosome 11 [21].

CONCLUSION

Overall it seems likely that a number of mechanisms probably need to act together to induce pituitary tumour formation [22]. Qualitative and quantitative changes in receptor function and signal transduction, sequestration of antioncogenes (perhaps by viral antigens), or allelic deletion of regions coding for the same, may be implicated in the future. Failure of apoptosis, disruption of normal feedback mechanisms by vascular anomalies or local production of growth factors may also play a part, as might disruption of the collection of genes involved in running DNA repair.

Which of these mechanisms accounts for the majority of pituitary adenomas remains an interesting conundrum.

ACKNOWLEDGEMENTS

Data for Fig. 1 kindly provided by Dr Zhen-Ping Chen, Bristol University.

REFERENCES

1 Marx J. DNA repair comes into its own. *Science* 1994;**266**:728–780.

2 Webster J, ten Horn CD, Bevan JS, Ham J, Scanlon MF. Preliminary characterisation of growth factors secreted by human pituitary tumours. *Endocrinol Invest* 1991;207.

3 Halper J, Parnell PG, Carter BJ, Ren P, Scheithauer BW. Presence of growth factors in human pituitary. *Lab Invest* 1992;**66**:639–645.

4 Fernig DG, Smith JA, Rudland PS. Relationship of growth factors and differentiation in normal and neoplastic development of the mammary gland. *Cancer Treat Res* 1991;**53**:47–78.

5 Chomczynski P, Kuryl T, Brar A. Mitogenic effect of a factor from rat somatomam-motrophs on mammary epithelial cells. *Endocrinology* 1992;**131**:228–234.

6 Saeger W, Lüdecke DK. Pituitary hyperplasia. Definition, light and electron micro-scopical structures and significance in surgical specimens. *Virchows Arch A* 1983;**399**:277–287.

7 Clayton RN. Gonadotrophin-releasing hormone: its actions and receptors. *J Endocrinol* 1988;**120**:11–19.

8 Levy A, Lightman SL, Hoyland J, Rawlings S, Mason WT. A gonadotrophin-releasing hormone (GnRH) antagonist distinguishes three populations of GnRH analogue-responsive cells in human and rat pituitary *in vitro* and produces an acute increase in intracellular Ca^{2+} concentration without inducing gonadotropin secretion. *Mol Endocrinol* 1990;**4**:678–684.

9 Ross EM. Viral hijack of receptors. *Nature* 1990;**344**:707–708.

10 Speir E, Modali R, Huang E-S *et al.* Potential role of human cytomegalovirus and p53 interaction in coronary restenosis. *Science* 1994;**265**:391–394.

11 Plöckinger U, Fett U, Bäder M *et al.* Preoperative octreotide therapy of GH-secreting and endocrine inactive pituitary adenomas. Proceedings of the American Endocrine Society's 75th annual meeting, Las Vegas: Endocrine Society, 1993:69 Abst 75.

12 Bourne HR, Stryer L. The target sets the tempo. *Nature* 1992;**358**:541–543.

13 Li Y, Bollag G, Clark R *et al.* Somatic mutations in the neurofibromatosis 1 gene in human tumors. *Cell* 1992;**69**:275–281.

14 Shou C, Farnsworth CL, Neel BG, Feig LA. Molecular cloning of cDNAs encoding a guanine-nucleotide-releasing factor for *Ras* p21. *Nature* 1992;**358**:351–354.

15 Corven EJv, Groenink A, Jalink K, Eichholtz T, Moolenaar WH. Lysophosphatidate-induced cell proliferation: identification and dissection of signaling pathways mediated by G proteins. *Cell* 1989;**59**:45–54.

16 Vallar L, Spada A, Giannattasio G. Altered Gs and adenylate cyclase activity in human growth hormone-secreting pituitary adenomas. *Nature* 1987;**330**:566–568.

17 Alvaro V, Lévy L, Dubray C *et al.* Invasive human pituitary tumors express a point-mutated α-protein kinase-C. *J Clin Endocrinol Metab* 1993;**77**:1125–1129.

18 Streuli M, Krueger NX, Tsai AYM, Saito H. A family of receptor-linked protein tyrosine phosphatases in humans and *Drosophila*. *Proc Natl Acad Sci USA* 1989;**86**:8698–8702.

19 Banks P. Tyrosine phosphatases: cellular superstars in the offing. *J NIH Res* 1990;**2**:62–66.

20 Karga HJ, Alexander JM, Hedley-Whyte ET, Klibanski A, Jameson JL. *Ras* mutations in human pituitary tumors. *J Clin Endocrinol Metab* 1992;**74**:914–919.

21 Boggild MD, Jenkinson S, Pistorello M *et al.* Molecular genetic studies of sporadic pituitary adenomas. *J Clin Endocrinol Metab* 1994;**78**:387–392.

22 Levy A, Lightman SL. The pathogenesis of pituitary adenomas. *Clin Endocrinol* 1993;**38**:559–570.

MULTIPLE CHOICE QUESTIONS

1 Pituitary adenomas

a if left untreated for many years, eventually spread metastatically

b are usually polyclonal in origin

c have been shown to be caused by cytopathic viruses in some cases d of the somatotroph subtype have an incidence of 3/million per year

e of the corticotroph subtype are the most common

2 The formation of pituitary tumours is significantly associated with

a h-*ras* oncogene activation

b v-*myc* oncogene activation

c *gsp* oncogene activation

d p53 mutations

e retinoblastoma gene mutations

3 Somatostatin

a increases cytoplasmic calcium ion levels in somatotroph cells

b antagonizes the metabolic effects of GHRH on somatotroph cells

c analogues are useful in the treatment of thyrotroph adenomas

d has a plasma half-life of 60 minutes

e analogues reduce the size of the majority of somatotroph adenomas

4 The G protein Gs

a is a cellular pump for maintaining cytoplasmic guanosine diphosphate concentrations

b is closely associated with L-type calcium channels

c is in the active form only when its α-, β- and γ-subunits are associated

d γ-subunit is often mutated in somatotroph adenomas

e signalling capacity is inactivated by guanosine triphosphatase-activating peptides

5 Pituitary adenomas

a in most cases respond paradoxically to somatostatin

b of the somatotroph subtype usually exhibit active thyrotrophin-releasing hormone receptors

c of the somatotroph subtype frequently contain GHRH transcripts

d of the corticotroph subtype are usually familiar

e according to autopsy data, are almost always occult

Answers

1 a False	2 a False	3 a False
b False	b False	b True
c False	c True	c True
d True	d False	d False
e False	e False	e False

4 **a** False   5 **a** False
  b False   **b** True
  c False   **c** True
  d False   **d** False
  e True   **e** True

PART 10
BIOCHEMICAL MEDICINE

The role of regulatory peptides in physiology and disease

KEITH D. BUCHANAN

THE PHYSIOLOGY

Until relatively few years ago only a small number of regulatory peptides were known, largely due to the slow and tedious methods of purification and characterization. For example, 10 000 hog guts were required to produce 1 mg of secretin [1]. Immunological techniques such as radioimmunoassay accelerated the process, and latterly molecular biology and rapid methods of purification and peptide sequencing have produced a plethora of peptides presenting the physiologist with a mountainous task of seeking roles for each.

Peptides are encoded in the genes as large precursor molecules and then proteolytically cleaved to produce the biologically active peptides. The secretory products can be complex, consisting of precursor molecules, inactive proteolytically cleaved products and the biologically active products [2].

The sequence of events in the glucagon story is typical. Glucagon was isolated from the pancreas as a side-product of insulin, because of its hyperglycaemic properties [3]. Following the establishment of a radioimmunoassay for glucagon, glucagon, or, more precisely, glucagon-like immunoreactivity (GLI) was also discovered in the gut (enteroglucagon) [4]. But it was not until the era of molecular biology that the whole story unravelled, gene sequences were discovered and differential processing of proglucagon in the pancreas and gut was described. From such came the discovery of glucagon-like peptide-1 (GLP-1), a significant gut insulinotropic peptide [5]. However, the story is not yet ended as the physiological roles of GLP-1 are still being described and the nature of tissue and circulating products of the glucagon gene is still being elucidated.

Although many regulatory peptides were initially discovered in endocrine cells of the pancreas and gastrointestinal tract, their distribution is now known to be widespread and peptides are present in almost every organ system in the body, for example, in heart and central and peripheral nervous systems. The peptides exist not only within endocrine cells but also in neurons where they act as neurotransmitters/neuromodulators. Within the gastrointestinal tract the peptides regulate many exocrine secretory functions, including gastric, pancreatic and intestinal. They are also major factors in intestinal motility, and have significant metabolic roles in carbohydrate, protein and fat metabolism. It is beyond the scope of this review to detail every regulatory peptide's function.

A major distinction of this endocrine system as compared with that of the classical system is the diffuseness of the organization, and this can be referred to as the diffuse endocrine system. Unlike classical endocrine glands, where cells are clustered together, regulatory peptides exist in diffusely scattered cells, frequently adjacent to exocrine cells. This organization may predispose to paracrine actions between the endocrine and exocrine cells. An exception is the islets of Langerhans, where several endocrine cell types are clustered together. The cells are characterized by neurosecretory granules at the electron microscopy level. Such granules can be immunostained not only by antisera to the specific peptide products but also to general neuroendocrine markers such as chromogranin A, neuron-specific enolase and protein gene product (PGP) 9.5. Hence the cell type is usually described as neuroendocrine.

DISEASE

There are many clinical applications of regulatory peptides, both real and potential, but this paper will concentrate only on the neuroendocrine tumours (NETs) mainly of the gastrointestinal tract. Insulinomas will be excluded as they have been extensively covered in the literature over many years, and the paper will concentrate on more recent and uncommon syndromes where significant advances have been made.

Nomenclature

As described in the section on physiology, NETs arise from cells with both neuronal and endocrine characteristics, hence the all-embracing term of 'neuroendocrine tumours' is acceptable. Also acceptable are terminologies relating to site, e.g. islet cell, mid-gut, etc., and relating to hormone production, e.g. insulinoma, glucagonoma. Other terms, like APUDoma cause confusion — APUD is the acronym for amine precursor uptake and decarboxylation, a terminology not likely to be easily remembered and based on rarely used histochemical criteria. The term 'carcinoid' tends to be used ubiquitously by histopathologists to describe the typical histological appearances of NETs at the light microscopy level. If used at all, the term 'carcinoid' should preferably be limited to mid-gut NETs with characteristic amine and peptide profiles.

Diagnostic criteria

The diagnostic criteria include:
1 A typical clinical syndrome, although this may be absent in undetermined or non-secretory types.
2 Elevated levels of peptides or amines in the urine or circulation in the basal or stimulated state.
3 Evidence of target organ overactivity.
4 Characteristic peptide/amine profiles in tumour tissue of NETs. These will include general neuroendocrine markers, e.g. chromogranin, neuron-specific enolase, PGP 9.5 and specific markers, e.g. gastrin, insulin, glucagon, etc. Such markers can be identified by immunocytochemical techniques, by extraction and assay of hormonal contents and by *in situ* hybridization. A comprehensive assessment of the tumour status can only be made if appropriate fixation techniques are employed, and tissues are fresh-frozen at −20°C and −80°C. Such careful foresight in the storage and preservation of tissues allows future studies, which may be of considerable clinical relevance, to be performed.

Characteristics of NETs

1 Some are familial as part of the multiple endocrine neoplasia (MEN) syndromes.
2 The tumours tend to be slow-growing and, although a large proportion metastasize, mainly to the liver, the patients can still survive many years, even with a large burden of metastatic tumour.
3 In most instances the tumours produce peptides/amines that result in characteristic clinical syndromes. Such syndromes may be classified into those produced by hormones where even a small increase can give rise to a syndrome, e.g. insulin or gastrin, and those where relatively massive levels are required before a syndrome emerges, e.g. glucagon. A minority of tumours, although having NET characteristics, do not produce an active hormone and have no syndrome. These are variously described as 'undetermined', 'non-secretory' or 'unknown type' of NETs.

Sporadic or inherited

The majority of NETs are sporadic. However, between 20 and 30%, particularly of islet cell tumours, are part of the MEN syndrome which is Mendelian dominant. The MEN I syndrome is commonly characterized by islet cell and parathyroid tumours, and less commonly by adrenal, pituitary and gonadal tumours. The MEN II syndrome presents with medullary cancer of the thyroid and phaeochromocytoma, often bilateral. Carcinoids of the lung or gut are rarely part of the MEN I syndrome.

Incidence

NETs of the gastrointestinal tract and lung are uncommon. The commonest tumour is the carcinoid, but many are incidentally found in the appendix at appendicectomy and are innocuous. We reported in Northern Ireland an annual incidence of all NETs of about 16 per million of the population per year [6]. Therefore, in Northern Ireland with a population of 1.6 million we should encounter about 25 new patients per year. If the appendiceal carcinoids are removed from this figure, then we would expect to encounter 13 new patients per year.

The diagnosis of such patients has improved, not due to improved diagnostic acumen, but largely due to improved imaging technology where tumours are detected, most frequently as metastases to the liver. Improved methods of biopsy lead to a histopathological diagnosis, although seldom has the real diagnosis been suspected. Where major diagnostic difficulty arises is in the tiny tumours which cannot be visualized. Under such circumstances diagnostic assays are mandatory and should be used freely.

Gastrinoma (Zollinger–Ellison syndrome)

Peptic ulcer disease which is unresponsive to conventional therapy should raise a suspicion of the diagnosis. If this is combined with metastatic liver disease, the diagnosis is probable. The textbook picture of horrific ulceration in unusual sites with severe complications is seldom met now, because patients are almost always receiving potent antacid therapy, even though the dosage may be inadequate for complete symptom relief [7]. The diagnosis is clinched by finding massive hypersecretion of gastric acid, combined with elevated plasma gastrin. Imaging the tumour may be difficult, as some are tiny. The medical management has been revolutionized by H_2-receptor antagonists and proton pump antagonists. The patients may require 10–12 times the usual dosage. Surgical removal of the tumour, if possible, is curative.

Glucagonoma syndrome

The glucagonoma syndrome was thoroughly described by Mallinson *et al.* [8]. The syndrome consists of a characteristic rash (necrolytic migratory erythema), diabetes mellitus and cachexia. Giant intestinal villi may also be present [9]. The tumours are usually metastatic at presentation. Glucagon levels are considerably elevated. It is noteworthy that not all of the features of the syndrome may be present.

Medullary cancer of the thyroid

Although this tumour arises within the thyroid gland, it is not a tumour of the thyroid cells but of the C cells which secrete calcitonin as their main product. A number arise as part of the MEN II syndrome. The patients often present with lymph node metastases to the cervical glands and not as a thyroid swelling. The tumour can metastasize to liver, lungs and bone. Watery diarrhoea is a feature of metastatic medullary cancers of the thyroid. Secretory products include calcitonin, calcitonin gene-related peptide and gastrin-releasing peptide. If surgical cure is not possible, these patients generally have a poorer prognosis than other NETs and are poorly responsive to therapies which are usually successful in NETs.

VIPoma syndrome

This syndrome is alternatively described as the Verner–Morrison syndrome [10] or the WDHA syndrome, the acronym standing for watery diarrhoea, hypokalaemia and achlorhydria. The tumours arise in the islet cells, and will metastasize to liver. Uncommonly, the syndrome may arise from a tumour of neuronal origin, e.g. neuroblastoma or neuroganglioma. The patients suffer from voluminous watery diarrhoea which is characteristically described as 'milky tea' and is odourless. The diarrhoea is rich in potassium and the patients become severely hypokalaemic and may present in a collapsed condition with loss of muscle power. Patients therefore present dehydrated, collapsed and often with radiological evidence of a pancreatic tumour with liver metastases. It is at this point that there is a likelihood of misdiagnosis as metastatic pancreatic cancer with a dreadful prognosis. The mediator of the syndrome is vasoactive intestinal polypeptide (VIP) and elevated circulating levels of VIP in association with the above clinical picture are strongly suggestive of the syndrome. The diagnosis is clinched by biopsy. Peptide histidine methionine (PHM) has also been implicated as a mediator of the syndrome and is nearly always elevated in the circulation in such patients. Pancreatic polypeptide (PP) is frequently elevated in the circulation of such patients but does not appear to be a mediator of the syndrome. The management of the syndrome has been revolutionized by the somatostatin analogues (see below).

Carcinoid tumours and syndromes

The term 'carcinoid' is misleading, especially when used loosely, particularly in histopathological diagnosis. This may lead to confusion by the clinician. The bland term 'neuroendocrine' tumour is much preferred. The term 'carcinoid' should preferably be reserved for NETs of the foregut (lung) and NETs of the mid-gut (ileum) which, when they metastasize, produce a characteristic, although not completely identical, syndrome. Such tumours invariably secrete serotonin. NETs of the hind-gut (colon and rectum) and of the stomach arise from different cell types, secrete different products and should preferably not be described as carcinoids.

NETs of the hind-gut usually do not secrete serotonin, but may secrete somatostatin, glucagon or PP, although not infrequently are undetermined types. They can be malignant. NETs of the stomach secrete chromogranins but no other secretory products have been identified. They are usually benign and arise in atrophic stomachs.

More emphasis will be placed on the NETs of lung and mid-gut which are more highly characterized. Appendiceal NETs, which are quite commonly found at appendicectomy, will not be further described as they are cured by appendicectomy, very rarely metastasize and therefore will rarely produce an endocrine syndrome. Goblet cell 'carcinoids' of the appendix, which are an uncommon type, can be malignant but do not produce an endocrine syndrome [11].

Carcinoids of the mid-gut, usually ileum, are the most frequently met carcinoids which produce an endocrine syndrome (Table 1). The syndrome is nearly always associated with metastatic liver disease, which occurs in about 70%, even when the primary tumour has apparently been completely resected. Sometimes flushing is completely absent, as is diarrhoea. The cardiac lesions are commonly tricuspid incompetence and, less commonly, pulmonary stenosis. The circulating and urinary markers of the syndrome are shown in Table 2. These markers only become elevated when the tumour is metastatic to liver.

The patients may present as an emergency with small-bowel obstruction, unsuspected liver metastases and, less commonly, with the syndrome. The mediators of the syndrome remain uncertain, particularly the flush, although serotonin is strongly implicated as a mediator of the diarrhoea.

Table 1 Carcinoid syndrome from mid-gut carcinoids.

Flushing (in most)
Watery diarrhoea (in most)
Cardiac lesions (in one-third)
Dependent oedema (uncommon)
Wheezing (rare)

Table 2 Circulating and urinary markers of the mid-gut carcinoid syndrome.

Circulation
Tachykinins
  Neurokinin A
  Substance P
Chromogranin and derived peptides, e.g. pancreastatin

Urinary
5-Hydroxyindoleacetic acid
5-Hydroxytryptamine

Table 3 Atypical carcinoid syndrome from lung carcinoids with liver metastases.

Flushing (all)
Diarrhoea (all)

But:
  No cardiac lesions
  No dependent oedema

And:
  Lacrimation (most)
  Salivation (most)
  Facial oedema (most)
  Wheeze (about half)
  Salivary gland enlargement (about half)
  Carcinoid crises (frequent)

Table 4 Atypical (lung) carcinoid syndrome — circulating and urinary markers.

Circulation
Chromogranin and derived peptides, e.g. pancreastatin
Gastrin-releasing peptide
Calcitonin gene-related peptide
Pancreatic polypeptide

Urinary
5-Hydroxyindoleacetic acid
5-Hydroxytryptamine

Metastatic lung carcinoids produce some aspects of the mid-gut carcinoid syndrome, but have additional features. Thus, lung carcinoid syndrome is sometimes referred to as the atypical carcinoid syndrome (Table 3).

The secretory products (Table 4) have some overlap with mid-gut carcinoids but are also distinct, no doubt accounting for the overlapping but also distinct syndromes.

Somatostatinomas

These are uncommon and may arise in pancreas, duodenum (ampulla of Vater) and rectum. They can metastasize. The clinical features are nondescript, including gallstones, steatorrhoea, mild diabetes mellitus but occasionally hypoglycaemia; there may be sensitivity to oral hypoglycaemic agents [12].

Mixed tumour types

Some NETs, both sporadic and MEN, can produce several hormones and multiple syndromes. Most of these tumours are islet cell and not mid-gut or lung carcinoid. In addition to insulinoma, gastrinoma, VIPoma and glucagonoma, adrenocorticotrophic hormone (ACTH) production may be encountered, giving rise to Cushing's syndrome.

Undetermined types

Some NETs, mainly islet cell in origin, produce no active hormone, but have the classical histological pattern of NETs, and can be further characterized by positive immunocytochemistry for non-specific markers such as chromogranin, neuron-specific enolase and PGP 9.5. However, no active secretory product is identified and there is no endocrine syndrome. Such tumours arise more commonly in younger patients, they may be highly malignant and they tend to respond poorly to measures that may be effective in other NETs.

Imaging and localization of NETs

As many NETs present with metastatic disease, imaging is not a problem and ultrasound, computed tomography (CT) and magnetic resonance imaging (MRI) scans are all effective at imaging the tumours. Where problems are encountered in when the tumour is small (< 1 cm in diameter) but may be very active, e.g. gastrinoma and insulinoma. The octreoscan has sometimes been effective at locating some of these lung tumours. Octreoscan is radioactively labelled octreotide (a somatostatin analogue). Most NETs have receptors for octreotide and can be imaged by this technique by nuclear scans. The technique should optimally be used in combination with a more precise anatomical imaging technique such as CT or MRI. Positive octreoscans not only localize tumours but also give information as to the functional nature of the tumour, i.e. that the tumour may be an NET. However, other tumours and pathologies may image with octreoscan [13]. Medullary cancers of thyroid do not image with octreoscan.

Management of NETs

Surgery

Should the tumour be resectable, then surgery offers the only hope of cure. Surgery may also play a role in the debulking of metastatic disease and in symptomatic relief, by removal of tumour obstructing a hollow viscus, e.g. bowel. Surgery may also clear extrahepatic tumour before liver transplantation. When the tumour is metastatic and disabling, other measures must be resorted to, although because of the reasonable life expectancy of some of these patients, a very conservative approach — observation without intervention — may be justifiable.

Chemotherapy and radiotherapy

Streptozotocin is the drug of choice. Many islet-cell tumours respond with remissions up to 1–2 years. Undetermined types and carcinoids of lung and mid-gut respond poorly, if at all. The drug may be given by the peripheral venous route or by the intrahepatic route. Nausea, vomiting and occasional renal failure are the major side-effects.

Conventional multidrug regimes for solid cancers are poorly effective and best avoided. Radiotherapy only has a role in the relief of localized symptoms produced by encroaching tumour; it is ineffective in other situations [14].

Somatostatin analogues

The somatostatin analogues have revolutionized the management of NETs with metastases and disabling endocrine syndromes. The most commonly used drug, octreotide, is effective at controlling the syndromes from carcinoid, VIPomas and glucagonomas. Its effectiveness in insulinomas is variable. It is effective in gastrinomas but the syndrome from these tumours can be alternatively controlled by H_2-receptor antagonists and proton pump antagonists. Less certain is whether these drugs have antitumour properties [15].

Embolization

Embolization of liver tumours is effective, giving remissions of 3 months to 1 year, and it can be repeated.

Liver transplantation

Liver transplantation should be considered for patients with NETs with massive hepatic metastases. Extensive extrahepatic and irresectable disease may be considered a contraindication. The literature on this aspect of transplantation is scanty at present. However, consideration should be given to patients in a deteriorating situation and who are not responding to other therapies.

REFERENCES

1 Jorpes JE. The isolation and chemistry of secretin and cholecystokinin. *Gastroenterology* 1968;55:157–164.
2 Dockray GJ. Regulatory peptides of the intestine. *Curr Opin Gastroenterol* 1990;6:246–250.
3 Collens WS, Murlin JR. Hyperglycaemia following the portal injection of insulin. *Proc Soc Exp Biol Med* 1929;26:485–490.

4 Conlon JM. The glucagon-like polypeptides — order out of chaos? *Diabetologia* 1980;**18**:85–88.
5 Holst JJ. Glucagon like peptide 1: a newly discovered gastrointestinal hormone. *Gastroenterology* 1994;**107**:1848–1855.
6 Watson RGP, Johnston CF, O'Hare MMT *et al*. The frequency of gastrointestinal endocrine tumours in a well-defined population — Northern Ireland 1970–1985. *Q J Med* 1989;**72**:647–657.
7 Collins JSA, Buchanan KD, Kennedy TL *et al*. Changing patterns in presentation and management of the Zollinger–Ellison syndrome in Northern Ireland, 1970–1988. *Q J Med* 1991;**78**:215–225.
8 Mallinson CN, Bloom SR, Warin AP, Salmon PR, Cox B. A glucagonoma syndrome. *Lancet* 1974;**i**:1–5.
9 Stevens FM, Flanagan RW, O'Gorman D, Buchanan KD. A glucagonoma syndrome demonstrating giant duodenal villi. *Gut* 1984;**25**:784–791.
10 Verner JV, Morrison AB. Islet cell tumour and a syndrome of refractory water diarrhea and hypokalemia. *Am J Med* 1958;**35**:374–379.
11 Anderson NH, Somerville JE, Johnston CF, Hayes DM, Buchanan KD, Sloan JM. Appendiceal goblet cell carcinoids: a clinicopathological and immunohistochemical study. *Histopathology* 1991;**18**:61–65.
12 Larsson L-I, Hirsch MA, Holst JJ *et al*. Pancreatic somatostatinoma: clinical features and physiological implications. *Lancet* 1977;**1**:666–669.
13 Nauck C, Ivanevi V, Emrich D, Creutzfeldt W. In-pentetreotide (somatostatin analogue) scintigraphy as an imaging procedure for endocrine gastro-entero-pancreatic tumors. *Z Gastroenterol* 1994;**32**:323–327.
14 Kvols LK. Hormonal and chemotherapy of metastatic carcinoid and islet cell tumours. In, Gastrointestinal APUDomas, edited by Buchanan KD. International Congress and Symposium series no 138, Royal Society of Medicine Services, London and New York.
15 Buchanan KD. Effects of sandostatin on neuroendocrine tumours of the gastrointestinal system. In: *Recent Results in Cancer Research: Peptides in Oncology II*, edited by Hoffken K. Springer-Verlag, Berlin, 1993:45–55.

Amyloid — can we cure it?

MARK B. PEPYS

Amyloidosis is a disorder of protein metabolism characterized by the extracellular deposition of abnormal insoluble protein fibrils [1]. These may be either organ-localized or distributed throughout the body (Table 1), and they can cause tissue damage and serious morbidity. Major visceral involvement, especially of the kidneys and heart, is usually fatal.

The fibrils which form the bulk of amyloid deposits are derived from different precursor proteins in different forms of the disease but are always intimately associated with sulphated glycosaminoglycans. In addition, the normal circulating glycoprotein, serum amyloid P component (SAP), specifically binds to the fibrils and is a universal constituent of amyloid deposits. Although SAP is only a trace constituent of plasma, 20–40 mg/l, it is remarkably concentrated in amyloid. Traces of other, much more abundant serum proteins, including apolipoprotein E, some serine proteinase inhibitors and complement components, may also be present.

Amyloid is defined by its staining with the dye Congo red, giving pathognomonic apple-green birefringence when viewed in polarized light, and by the characteristic ultrastructural morphology of the rigid, non-branching approximately 10-nm diameter fibrils. Amyloidosis is now class--ified on the basis of the chemical identity of the amyloid fibril protein in each case, rather than according to clinicopathological features, as in the past (Table 1).

Asymptomatic amyloid deposition in a variety of tissues is a universal accompaniment of ageing and clinical amyloidosis is not rare. Intracerebral and cerebrovascular β-protein amyloid deposits are a hallmark of the pathology of both sporadic and familial Alzheimer's disease, amyloid derived from β_2-microglobulin (β_2M) is a common complication of long-term haemodialysis, and islet amyloid polypeptide is the fibril protein in the universal islet amyloidosis of type II diabetes mellitus.

The development of radiolabelled SAP scintigraphy [2,3] has allowed amyloid to be diagnosed non-invasively *in vivo* for the first time, has provided unique insight into the distribution and size of amyloid deposits, and yielded novel information on the natural history and the effects of treatment. Amyloid deposits are in a state of dynamic turnover and can

Table 1 Classification of the most common types of amyloid and amyloidosis.

Type	Fibril protein precursor	Clinical syndrome
AA	Serum amyloid A protein	Reactive systemic amyloidosis associated with acquired or hereditary chronic inflammatory diseases. Formerly known as secondary amyloidosis
AL	Monoclonal immunoglobulin light chains	Systemic amyloidosis associated with myeloma, monoclonal gammopathy, occult B-cell dyscrasia. Formerly known as primary amyloidosis
ATTR	Normal plasma transthyretin	Senile systemic amyloidosis with prominent cardiac involvement
	Genetically variant transthyretin	Familial amyloid polyneuropathy, usually with systemic amyloidosis. Sometimes prominent amyloid cardiomyopathy or nephropathy
$A\beta_2M$	β_2-Microglobulin	Periarticular and, occasionally, systemic amyloidosis associated with renal failure and long-term dialysis
$A\beta$	β-Protein precursor (and rare genetic variants)	Cerebrovascular and intracerebral plaque amyloid in Alzheimer's disease Occasional familial cases
AIAPP	Islet amyloid polypeptide	Amyloid in islets of Langerhans in type II diabetes mellitus and insulinoma

regress if new fibril formation is halted. Recent work on SAP, including the findings that it is structurally invariant, that it is totally unaltered in tissue amyloid deposits, and that it can protect amyloid fibrils from proteolytic degradation, strongly suggest that it may play a key role in the pathogenesis of amyloidosis [4,5]. Elucidation of the three-dimensional structure of human SAP, which we lately reported [6], may enable design of specific therapeutic agents. Other groups are exploring alternative pharmacological avenues for disrupting amyloid fibril formation: polysulphates and polysulphonates [7] and iododeoxydoxirubicin [8].

IN VIVO SCINTIGRAPHY WITH ^{123}I-LABELLED HUMAN SERUM AMYLOID P COMPONENT

When SAP labelled with [123]I (a pure medium-energy γ-emitter) is injected into the circulation in patients with amyloidosis, it rapidly and specifically localizes to the deposits in proportion to the quantity of amyloid present, allowing the deposits to be visualized and quantified by scintigraphy [2,3,9,10] (Fig. 1). This has enabled important observations regarding amyloid to be made for the first time *in vivo*, including the different pattern of distribution of amyloid in different forms of the disease, the demonstration of amyloid in sites not normally available for biopsy and

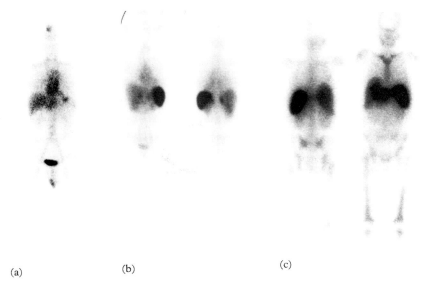

(a)   (b)   (c)

Fig. 1 Whole-body scintigraphs 24 hours after intravenous injection of ^{123}I-labelled human serum amyloid P (SAP). (a) Anterior view of normal control subject showing distribution of residual tracer in the blood pool and radioactive breakdown products in urine in the bladder; note the absence of localization or retention of tracer anywhere in the body. (b) Anterior (left) and posterior (right) views of patient with juvenile chronic arthritis complicated by AA amyloidosis. There is uptake of tracer in the spleen, kidneys and adrenal glands — a typical distribution of AA amyloid in which the spleen is involved in 100% of cases, kidneys in 75% and adrenals in 40%. (c) Posterior (left) and anterior (right) views of patient with monoclonal gammopathy complicated by extensive AL amyloidosis. There is uptake and retention of tracer in the liver, spleen, kidneys, bone marrow and soft tissues around the shoulder. Note the complete absence of blood pool or bladder signal compared to (a) indicating a heavy whole-body amyloid load. This pattern of amyloid distribution revealed by scintigraphy is pathognomonic for AL amyloidosis; bone marrow uptake has never been seen in any other type.

the demonstration of a poor correlation between the quantity of amyloid present in a given organ and the level of organ dysfunction.

This last finding is of interest with regard to the mechanism by which amyloid deposits cause tissue damage, since there is usually no inflammation associated with amyloid and little evidence of necrosis. It has generally been considered that the deposits exert their effects simply by structural disruption of the tissues leading to impaired function, but recent work *in vitro* suggests that several types of amyloid fibrils can cause cell death by inducing apoptosis [11,12]. If it also occurred *in vivo* this process would be 'invisible' histologically since the affected cells are promptly cleared and do not elicit inflammation. Different fibril types apparently have different capacities for inducing apoptosis in different target cells *in vitro* [11], and this may explain our observations of poor correlation between amyloid load and organ dysfunction *in vivo*.

Histological demonstration of amyloid, identified by the pathognomonic green birefringence after Congo red staining, remains a gold standard for diagnosis of amyloidosis and is very useful in the case of cardiac amyloid, where for technical reasons SAP scintigraphy has poor sensitivity. However, in most respects biopsy methods are severely limited by comparison with SAP scintigraphy. They are significantly more invasive but yield only tiny samples of single organs or tissues and they can never be quantitative with respect to either organ or whole-body amyloid load. Also, in non-expert hands there is a significant incidence of both false-positive and false-negative histology reports.

REGRESSION OF AMYLOIDOSIS

Scintigraphy with labelled SAP allows the natural history of the disease and the effects of treatment on amyloid itself to be studied, rather than just organ dysfunction. In untreated patients most types of amyloid usually persist and accumulate relentlessly. However, amyloid deposits can regress once supply of the precursor proteins is reduced. Evidence for this was previously available only from histological studies in isolated case reports [13]. However, there are now prospective data from serial studies with ^{123}I-SAP scans demonstrating regression of amyloid deposits following treatment to reduce precursor protein levels in patients with reactive systemic (AA) [10], monoclonal immunoglobulin light chain (AL) [9,14,15], haemodialysis-associated ($A\beta_2M$) [16], and hereditary trans-thyretin (ATTR) amyloidosis [17] (Table 2).

In AA amyloid, treatment is aimed at suppression of the acute-phase production of the fibril precursor, serum amyloid A protein (SAA), either

Table 2 Reducing the supply of fibril precursors in systemic amyloid.

Disease	Aim of treatment	Example of treatment
AA amyloid	Suppress acute-phase response	Immunosuppression in rheumatoid arthritis, Still's disease (chlorambucil). Colchicine for familial Mediterranean fever, even if clinical episodes are not fully suppressed. Surgery for osteomyelitis and rare cytokine-producing tumours
AL amyloid	Suppress production of monoclonal immunoglobulin light chains	Chemotherapy for myeloma and monoclonal gammopathy
Hereditary ATTR amyloidosis	Eliminate source of genetically variant protein	Orthotopic liver transplantation for variant transthyretin-associated familial amyloid polyneuropathy
Dialysis amyloidosis	Reduce plasma concentration of β_2-microglobulin	Renal transplantation

by removal of the stimulus, as in surgical resection of tumour or chronic infective focus, by disease-specific therapy, as with colchicine in familial Mediterranean fever, or by aggressive use of anti-inflammatory therapy in chronic rheumatic diseases. In AL amyloid the aim of treatment is to reduce or obliterate the B-cell or plasma cell clone that is producing the monoclonal light-chain precursors of the amyloid fibrils. The only treatment that adequately reduces $\beta_2 M$ levels in chronic haemodialysis patients is renal transplantation. In patients with amyloidogenic transthyretin mutations the only effective treatment is liver transplantation which removes the source of the circulating pathogenic variant transthyretin and replaces it with a source of normal wild-type protein [17].

Amyloid deposits are thus not immutable but are, as might be expected, in a state of dynamic turnover, at least for some of the time in some patients. The appearance of indefinite persistence and often remorseless progression is a reflection of the persistent and usually incurable nature of the diseases responsible for production of the amyloid fibril precursor proteins.

AMYLOID AND ALZHEIMER'S DISEASE

Alzheimer's disease, a progressive dementia in the elderly leading to complete mental and physical incapacity and death, is the fourth most common cause of death in the western world after myocardial infarction, stroke and cancer. Its cause is unknown but the characteristic neuropathology consists of neuronal loss associated with intracerebral and cerebrovascular amyloidosis, and neurofibrillary tangles (paired helical filaments) [18]. The latter are composed of an abnormally phosphorylated form of the neurofilament protein τ and, although they stain with Congo red and give green birefringence, their ultrastructural morphology is completely different from all other types of amyloid fibril.

The actual cerebral amyloid fibrils themselves are composed of the so-called amyloid β-protein (Aβ), a 39–43 residue cleavage fragment of the much larger β-amyloid precursor protein (APP) [18]. There are also more diffuse, apparently non-amyloid accumulations of Aβ within the brain. The gene for APP is on chromosome 21 and all patients with trisomy 21 (Down's syndrome) develop Alzheimer's disease and do so much earlier than individuals with a normal karyotype. In some kindreds hereditary Alzheimer's disease is caused by mutations in the APP gene and these are associated with overproduction of Aβ. Very recently a transgenic mouse has been constructed in which there is massive overexpression of human APP in the brain and which develops Aβ deposits, amyloid plaques and neuronal damage closely similar to that seen in human Alzheimer's disease [19]. Finally, Aβ readily forms amyloid fibrils *in vitro*, and these fibrils are cytotoxic for neuronal cells *in vitro* and possibly also *in vivo* [18]. There is thus compelling evidence that Aβ amyloid deposition and/or APP itself are intimately related to the pathogenesis of Alzheimer's disease. However, just as with systemic forms of amyloid, there is some evidence that the cerebral deposits in Alzheimer's disease are in a dynamic state with both formation and resolution in progress [20,21].

All the amyloid, amyloid-like and Aβ lesions in the brain of Alzheimer's-disease patients, including cerebral amyloid plaques, cerebrovascular amyloid deposits, diffuse Aβ plaques and neurofibrillary tangles, contain SAP [22,23].

SERUM AMYLOID P COMPONENT BINDS TO AMYLOID FIBRILS AND PROTECTS THEM FROM PROTEOLYSIS

SAP undergoes specific calcium-dependent binding to all known types of amyloid fibrils, including, as we have lately demonstrated, fibrils formed *in vitro* from pure synthetic Aβ [5,24]. This binding is responsible for the universal presence of SAP in amyloid deposits *in vivo* and we proposed some years ago that SAP might contribute to the pathogenesis of amyloidosis by protecting amyloid fibrils from degradation [25]. Amyloid fibrils are abnormal structures and, although they are relatively resistant, they can be digested by proteinases *in vitro*. The body is generally extremely efficient at remodelling tissues and abnormal extracellular accumulations of protein during normal development and during healing after trauma or inflammation. We therefore hypothesized that coating with normal, unaltered SAP molecules, identical to the circulating precursor, might mask the abnormal amyloid fibrils and prevent their recognition as targets for clearance by macrophages or other cells.

Subsequently it has become evident that SAP itself is remarkably resistant to proteolysis [26] and this is compatible with its three-dimensional structure, consisting of a flattened β-jelly roll with compact loops joining the strands and tightly bonded to the body of the molecule [6]. We have therefore lately investigated whether the binding of SAP to amyloid fibrils protects the fibrils from digestion by proteolytic enzymes, and found that indeed SAP is very potent in this respect [5]. Thus it can greatly reduce cleavage of various types of amyloid fibrils *in vitro* by such powerful digestive and bacterial enzymes as trypsin, chymotrypsin and pronase, as well as protecting against more physiological enzymes, such as cathepsin G, and whole living macrophages and neutrophils in culture. SAP is not itself an enzyme inhibitor and it has no effect on digestion of fibrils unless it is actually bound to them. It seems to act simply as a proteinase-resistant coating, and clearly if this effect is operative *in vivo* it could make a significant contribution to the damaging persistence of amyloid deposits.

A STRATEGY FOR TREATMENT OF AMYLOIDOSIS

Our work with radiolabelled SAP as a specific quantitative *in vivo* diagnostic probe for systemic amyloidosis has demonstrated that in most patients the deposits can regress if the supply of amyloid fibril precursor molecules is sufficiently reduced. In addition, the most active possible supportive management is indicated, including, if required, renal, hepatic and/or cardiac transplantation, in order to keep patients alive long enough to benefit from disease-specific treatment aimed at reducing fibril precursor production [27].

Our recent discovery that SAP protects fibrils from degradation when it is bound to them suggests a potential new avenue for amyloid therapy. Pharmaceutically acceptable molecules which inhibit and reverse binding of SAP to amyloid fibrils could enable the body's own mechanisms to remove such fibrils from the tissues, and even a small increase in the rate of clearance might have a very significant clinical impact when the rate of fibril deposition was also being restricted. We have already identified and synthesized low-molecular-weight carbohydrate ligands that inhibit and reverse the SAP-fibril interaction *in vitro* [25,28] and have solved the three-dimensional structure of ligand–SAP complexes [6]. Although the present compounds are not themselves suitable for use as drugs *in vivo*, our state of knowledge constitutes an exciting starting point for drug discovery. Any agents that were effective in systemic amyloid would be interesting candidates for investigation in Alzheimer's disease, and would provide a further test of the hypothesis that amyloid is responsible for its pathogenesis. Positive results would open the possibility of prophylactic use to prevent amyloid deposition and thereby Alzheimer's disease.

Can we cure amyloid? No, not yet, but the prospects are brighter than they have ever been!

ACKNOWLEDGEMENT

The work of the Immunological Medicine Unit, Royal Postgraduate Medical School, is supported by Medical Research Council Programme Grant G7900510.

REFERENCES

1 Pepys MB. Amyloidosis. In: *Samter's Immunologic Diseases*, 5th edn, edited by Frank MM, Austen KF, Claman HN, Unanue ER. Little, Brown, Boston, 1994:637–655.
2 Hawkins PN, Myers MJ, Lavender JP, Pepys MB. Diagnostic radionuclide imaging of amyloid: biological targeting by circulating human serum amyloid P component. *Lancet* 1988;**i**:1413–1418.

3 Hawkins PN, Lavender JP, Pepys MB. Evaluation of systemic amyloidosis by scintigraphy with ^{123}I-labeled serum amyloid P component. *N Engl J Med* 1990;**323**:508–513.

4 Pepys MB, Rademacher TW, Amatayakul-Chantler S *et al.* Human serum amyloid P component is an invariant constituent of amyloid deposits and has a uniquely homogeneous glycostructure. *Proc Natl Acad Sci USA* 1994;**91**:5602–5606.

5 Tennent GA, Lovat LB, Pepys MB. Serum amyloid P component prevents proteolysis of the amyloid fibrils of Alzheimer's disease and systemic amyloidosis. *Proc Natl Acad Sci USA* 1995;**92**:4299–4307.

6 Emsley J, White HE, O'Hara BP *et al.* Structure of pentameric human serum amyloid P component. *Nature* 1994;**367**:338–345.

7 Kisilevsky R, Lemieux LJ, Fraser PE, Xianqi K, Hultin PG, Szarek WA. Arresting amyloidosis *in vivo* using small molecule anionic sulphonates or sulphates: implications for Alzheimer's disease. *Nature Med* 1995;**1**:143–148.

8 Merlini G, Ascari E, Amboldi N *et al.* Interaction of the new anthracycline 4′-iodo-4′-deoxydoxorubicin with amyloid fibrils: inhibition of amyloidogenesis. *Proc Natl Acad Sci USA* 1995; (in press).

9 Hawkins PN, Richardson S, MacSweeney JE *et al.* Scintigraphic quantification and serial monitoring of human visceral amyloid deposits provide evidence for turnover and regression. *Q J Med* 1993;**86**:365–374.

10 Hawkins PN, Richardson S, Vigushin DM *et al.* Serum amyloid P component scintigraphy and turnover studies for diagnosis and quantitative monitoring of AA amyloidosis in juvenile rheumatoid arthritis. *Arthritis Rheum* 1993;**36**:842–851.

11 Lorenzo A, Razzaboni B, Weir GC, Yankner BA. Pancreatic islet cell toxicity of amylin associated with type-2 diabetes mellitus. *Nature* 1994;**368**:756–760.

12 Lorenzo A, Yankner BA. β-Amyloid neurotoxicity requires fibril formation and is inhibited by Congo red. *Proc Natl Acad Sci USA* 1994;**91**:12243–12247.

13 Gertz MA, Kyle RA. Response of primary hepatic amyloidosis to melphalan and prednisone: a case report and review of the literature. *Mayo Clin Proc* 1986;**61**:218–223.

14 Hawkins PN, Hall M, Hall R *et al.* Regression of AL amyloidosis and prolonged survival following cardiac transplantation and chemotherapy. In: *Amyloid and Amyloidosis 1993*, edited by Kisilevsky R, Benson MD, Frangione B, Gauldie J, Muckle TJ, Young ID. Parthenon Publishing, Pearl River, New York; 1994:657–659.

15 Hawkins PN, Vigushin DM, Richardson S, Seymour A, Pepys MB. Evaluation of 100 cases of systemic AL amyloidosis by serum amyloid P component (SAP) scintigraphy. In: *Amyloid and Amyloidosis 1993*, edited by Kisilevsky R, Benson MD, Frangione B, Gauldie J, Muckle TJ, Young ID. Parthenon Publishing, Pearl River, New York, 1994:209–211.

16 Nelson SR, Hawkins PN, Richardson S *et al.* Imaging of haemodialysis-associated amyloidosis with ^{123}I-serum amyloid P component. *Lancet* 1991;**338**:335–339.

17 Holmgren G, Ericzon B-G, Groth C-G *et al.* Clinical benefit and regression of amyloidosis following liver transplantation in patients with familial amyloid polyneuropathy due to transthyretin variant Met-30. *Lancet* 1993;**341**:1113–1116.

18 Selkoe DJ. Amyloid β-protein precursor: new clues to the genesis of Alzheimer's disease. *Curr Opin Neurobiol* 1994;**4**:708–716.

19 Games D, Adams D, Alessandri R *et al.* Alzheimer-type neuropathology in transgenic mice overexpressing V717F β-amyloid precursor protein. *Nature (Lond)* 1995;**373**:523–527.

20 Maggio JE, Stimson ER, Ghilardi JR *et al.* Reversible *in vitro* growth of Alzheimer disease β-amyloid plaques by deposition of labeled amyloid peptide. *Proc Natl Acad Sci USA* 1992;**89**:5462–5466.

21 Hyman BT, Marzloff K, Arriagada PV. The lack of accumulation of senile plaques or amyloid burden in Alzheimer's disease suggests a dynamic balance between amyloid deposition and resolution. *J Neuropathol Exp Neurol* 1993;**52**:594–600.

22 Coria F, Castano E, Prelli F *et al.* Isolation and characterization of amyloid P component from Alzheimer's disease and other types of cerebral amyloidosis. *Lab Invest* 1988;**58**:454–458.

23 Duong T, Pommier EC, Scheibel AB. Immunodetection of the amyloid P component in Alzheimer's disease. *Acta Neuropathol* 1989;**78**:429–437.

24 Pepys MB, Dyck RF, de Beer FC, Skinner M, Cohen AS. Binding of serum amyloid P component (SAP) by amyloid fibrils. *Clin Exp Immunol* 1979;**38**:284–293.

25 Hind CRK, Collins PM, Caspi D, Baltz ML, Pepys MB. Specific chemical dissociation of fibrillar and non-fibrillar components of amyloid deposits. *Lancet* 1984;**ii**:376–378.

26 Kinoshita CM, Gewurz AT, Siegel JN *et al.* A protease-sensitive site in the proposed Ca^{2+}-binding region of human serum amyloid P component and other pentraxins. *Protein Sci* 1992;**1**:700–709.

27 Tan S-Y, Pepys MB, Hawkins PN. Treatment of amyloidosis. *Am J Kidney Dis* 1995;**26**:267–285.

28 Hind CRK, Collins PM, Renn D *et al.* Binding specificity of serum amyloid P component for the pyruvate acetal of galactose. *J Exp Med* 1984;**159**:1058–1069.

Naturally occurring mutations that down-regulate expression of the human α-globin genes and cause α-thalassaemia

DOUGLAS R.HIGGS, DAVID J. PICKETTS & RICHARD J. GIBBONS

Over the past 20 years the application of molecular biology to medicine has provided a new dimension to our understanding of the pathology of both inherited and acquired disorders. Many new and important principles have been established by studying the molecular genetics of haemoglobin and its naturally occurring variants of structure and synthesis. This review summarizes our current knowledge of the human α-globin gene family and some of the mutations that give rise to underproduction of the α-globin chains of haemoglobin — a group of disorders referred to as the α-thalassaemias. The clinically severe forms of α-thalassaemia (HbH disease and the Hb Bart's hydrops fetalis syndrome) are particularly common in South-East Asia where it has been estimated that up to 17 000 severely affected individuals are born each year [1]. These syndromes also occur less frequently in and around the Mediterranean basin. Analysis of the determinants of α-thalassaemia is directed towards providing a rational basis for genetic counselling and prenatal diagnosis of these disorders. In addition, these naturally occurring molecular defects often provide important insights into the mechanism by which genes are normally regulated.

THE STRUCTURE OF HAEMOGLOBIN

Haemoglobin is a tetrameric molecule made up of two identical α-like (α or ζ) and β-like (ε, γ, δ, β) globin chains encoded by genetically distinct loci on chromosomes 16 and 11 respectively (reviewed in [2,3]). Throughout development there is a series of coordinated switches controlling the activity of these loci so that different types of haemoglobin are made during embryonic ($\alpha_2\varepsilon_2$, $\zeta_2\varepsilon_2$ and $\zeta_2\gamma_2$), fetal ($\alpha_2\gamma_2$) and adult ($\alpha_2\delta_2$ and α_2, β_2) life (reviewed in [4]). In fetal life the predominant haemoglobin comprises α and γ chains ($\alpha_2\gamma_2$ (HbF)) and in adult life α and β chains ($\alpha_2\beta_2$ (HbA)).

THE PATHOPHYSIOLOGY OF α-THALASSAEMIA

The α-thalassaemias are common genetic disorders of synthesis of the

524

α-globin chains which are present in fetal and adult haemoglobins (see above). Reduced α-chain synthesis in fetal and adult life results in an excess of γ or β chains which produce Hb Bart's (γ_4) and HbH (β_4) respectively (Fig. 1). The clinical and haematological features of α-thalassaemia are due to the abnormal properties of these haemoglobins, together with an inability to produce sufficient fetal (HbF) or adult haemoglobin (HbA; reviewed in [2,5]).

In the 1960s and early 1970s, classical genetic analysis of families with α-thalassaemia indicated that normal individuals have four functional α-globin genes. Furthermore, it appeared that carriers of α-thalassaemia, with a very mild hypochromic microcytic anaemia, have either three or two functional α genes. Clearly, in regions where such individuals are common, some of their offspring may have only one functional gene (Fig. 2). These subjects have a moderately severe hypochromic microcytic anaemia and produce a large excess of β chains, which from HbH (β_4). HbH eventually precipitates in the red blood cells, causing membrane damage and premature destruction of the cells. Patients with HbH disease have the signs of chronic haemolytic anaemia (pallor, jaundice and hepatosplenomegaly) and have 1–40% HbH in their peripheral blood. Most patients with HbH disease lead a relatively normal life and only occasionally require blood transfusion (see [4] for review).

Less commonly, some offspring inherit no functional α genes (Fig. 2) and this condition is almost always incompatible with life. An affected

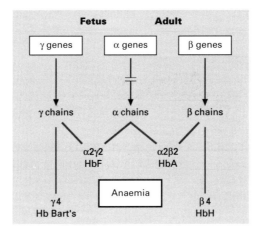

Fig. 1 Abnormal pattern of globin synthesis is α-thalassaemia. Reduced synthesis of α-globin chains in fetal life results in underproduction of fetal haemoglobin (HbF; $\alpha_2\gamma_2$) and excess γ chains from Hb Bart's (γ_4). Reduced synthesis of α chains in adult life results in underproduction of adult haemoglobin (HbA; $\alpha_2\beta_2$) and excess β chains form HbH (β_4).

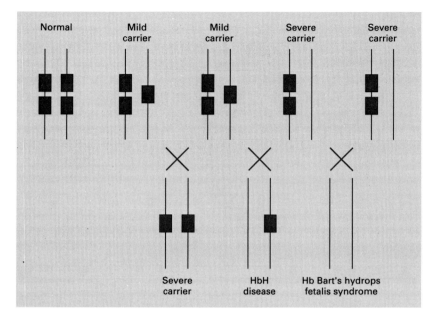

Fig. 2 The pattern of inheritance of the deletional forms of α-thalassaemia.

fetus produces large amounts of Hb Bart's (γ_4), which is functionally useless. The affected infant is born with signs of chronic intrauterine hypoxia and usually dies at or soon after birth. The condition is known as the Hb Bart's hydrops fetalis syndrome (see [4–6] for review).

THE NORMAL STRUCTURE AND REGULATION OF THE α-GLOBIN CLUSTER

The α-globin cluster lies near the tip of chromosome 16 within band p13.3 (Fig. 3). It includes the duplicated α genes (α_2 and α_1), an embryonic α-like gene (ζ) and a gene of undetermined function (θ_1) arranged in the order $5'-\zeta-\alpha_2-\alpha_1-\theta_1-3'$ [2].

Both α and ζ genes are expressed in the primitive erythroblasts in the yolk sac (up to 6–7 weeks of gestation), although ζ globin synthesis predominates during this period; definitive line erythroblasts almost exclusively synthesize α-globin (from 6 weeks onwards) [7]. The expression of the α_2 gene predominates over the α_1 gene by approximately 3 : 1 throughout development [8]. Using more sensitive assays, low levels of ζ-globin expression can be detected throughout fetal life [9] and in up to 80% of cord bloods [10]. Similarly, low levels of θ messenger RNA can be detected at all stages of development [11]. None of these genes is expressed in non-erythroid tissues.

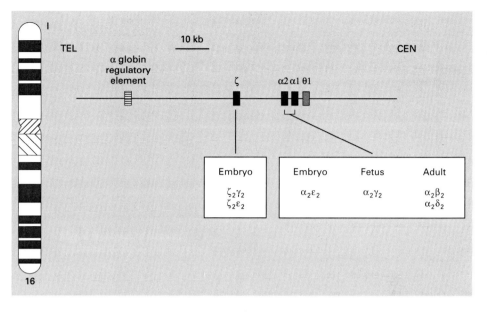

Fig. 3 The organization of the α complex at the tip of chromosome 16, within band p13.3, as described in the text. Filled boxes indicate the position of the structural genes. A stippled box denotes the position of the θ₁ gene. A striped box shows the position of the α-globin-regulatory element 40 kb upstream of the ζ gene. Below is shown the haemoglobins synthesized at different stages of development. TEL and CEN denote the orientation of the α cluster with respect to the telomere and centromere.

From the analysis of naturally occurring mutations (see below) and expression studies in transgenic mice we have shown that expression of the ζ, α and θ genes is dependent on a remote regulatory element located 40 kb upstream of the ζ-globin messenger RNA cap site [12]. In the absence of this regulatory element, ζ- and α-globin synthesis is virtually undetectable in erythroid cells (reviewed in [13,14]). The role of this regulatory element and its putative mechanism of action are discussed in more detail below.

α-THALASSAEMIA MOST FREQUENTLY RESULTS FROM DELETIONS INVOLVING THE α-GLOBIN GENES

Characterization of the α complex in large numbers of non-thalassaemic individuals has confirmed previous genetic studies which suggest that normal individuals have four α-globin genes, two on each chromosome 16 (denoted αα/αα). It has now been shown that α-thalassaemia most commonly results from deletions of various segments of DNA from the α-globin cluster. Deletions removing one of the duplicated α genes (denoted −α) are common throughout all tropical and subtropical regions. Deletions involving both α genes (denoted −−) are most commonly seen in South-east Asia and the Mediterranean basin. This explains why patients with HbH disease, who have the genotype $--/-\alpha$ or the Hb Bart's hydrops fetalis syndrome (genotype $--/--$) are most frequently observed in these regions of the world. Extensive mapping of DNA from patients with α-thalassaemia has shown that at least seven different deletions may give rise to the $-\alpha$ haplotype and 16 different deletions may account for the $--$ haplotype; these are summarized in [5].

Less commonly, α-thalassaemia is the result of single-base or oligo-nucleotide mutations affecting either the α_2 (denoted $\alpha^T\alpha$) or α_1 (denoted $\alpha\alpha^T$)-globin gene, so called non-deletional α-thalassaemia. Mutations of the dominant α_2 gene produce a more severe phenotype than those affecting the α_1 gene (reviewed in [5]). Some cases of HbH disease result from the interaction of non-deletional and deletional types of α-thalassaemia (usually $--/\alpha^T\alpha$). Some homozygotes for non-deletional forms of α-thalassaemia also have HbH disease ($\alpha^T\alpha/\alpha^T\alpha$). The currently described types of non-deletional α-thalassaemia are summarized in [5].

It is of interest that all of these determinants of α-thalassaemia are predominantly found in tropical or subtropical regions where they are thought to confer an increased fitness in the presence of endemic falciparum malaria [15].

Taken together, these deletional and non-deletional mutations probably represent a significant proportion of all the common determinants of α-thalassaemia to be found throughout the world. Thus it is becoming possible to use this information to provide a useful genetic counselling and prenatal testing service for those at risk of producing offspring with the most severe forms of α-thalassaemia.

α-THALASSAEMIA OCCASIONALLY RESULTS FROM DELETIONS OF THE α-GLOBIN REGULATORY ELEMENT

Over the past 10 years we have seen occasional patients with α-thalassaemia who have no deletions or point mutations affecting the structural α genes. In these cases, although the cluster appears to be intact, the α genes are expressed at very low levels (> 1%), if at all. We have now shown that such patients have deletions involving the α-globin-regulatory element. Altogether we have observed 6 patients of this type and in each case the α-globin-regulatory element has been deleted from the chromosome along with a variable amount of the flanking DNA (see [5,14] for review).

HOW DOES THE REGULATORY ELEMENT CONTROL α-GLOBIN GENE EXPRESSION?

At present the mechanism by which the α-globin-regulatory element controls α gene expression is unknown and so this process has become an important focus of our research. One way into this problem is to determine which proteins can bind to the α-globin-regulatory element and its putative targets, the α-globin promoters. We now know that the regulatory element binds at least two erythroid-restricted transcription factors (called GATA-1 and NF-E2) together with poorly defined, ubiquitously expressed proteins. By contrast, the α-globin promoter is thought to bind only ubiquitously expressed proteins (reviewed in [16]).

In an erythroid environment it is proposed that an erythroid-specific protein–DNA complex at the α-regulatory element interacts with a protein–DNA complex at the α promoter and by an as yet undefined mechanism increases the efficiency with which the α gene is transcribed (Fig. 4). At some point in the activation process it seems likely that the chromatin structure at the α promoter and regulatory element are derepressed, although again the underlying mechanism for this is unknown.

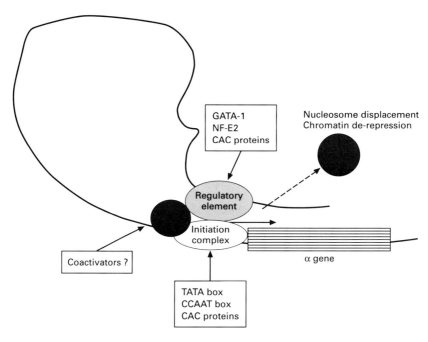

Fig. 4 Hypothetical model describing an interaction between the α-globin-regulatory element and the α-globin promoter. The α-globin-regulatory element binds erythroid (GATA-1, NF-E2) and ubiquitous (CAC box) factors. The initiation complex at the α promoter includes the TATA-box and CCAAT-box binding factors and may also include upstream activator proteins such as Sp1. The interaction may require coactivators and would be preceded by nucleosome displacement or some other form of chromatin derepression. The model shows a loop forming between the regulatory element and the promoter; this is only one of several models that could explain the interaction. The *XH2* protein (see text) could be involved in facilitating one or more of the steps involved in this interaction.

MUTATIONS IN A *TRANS*-ACTING FACTOR THAT DOWN-REGULATE α-GLOBIN EXPRESSION

Nearly all cases of α-thalassaemia occur in patients from tropical and subtropical regions of the world, and are due to inherited *cis*-acting mutations (usually deletions) involving the α-globin genes. However, during the past 15 years we have identified 40 individuals (26 families), nearly all of Northern European origins, with an unusual mild type of HbH disease, severe mental retardation and urogenital abnormalities [17]. Careful family studies have shown that none of the parents has the typical haematological features of α-thalassaemia.

Initially, our studies concentrated on the α-globin cluster but we did not detect any abnormality in structure, sequence or pattern of methylation of the α-genes. Similarly, the α-globin-regulatory element appeared normal. Subsequently, linkage studies demonstrated that the mutation causing α-thalassaemia in these families was not encoded on chromosome 16. As additional families came to our attention it became clear that only boys are affected by this condition and the pattern of inheritance suggested it is encoded on the X chromosome (so-called ATR-X syndrome; X-encoded α-thalassaemia with mental retardation).

Linkage studies have now localized the ATR-X syndrome to the proximal region of the X chromosome Xq13.1–q21.1, close to the X-inactivation

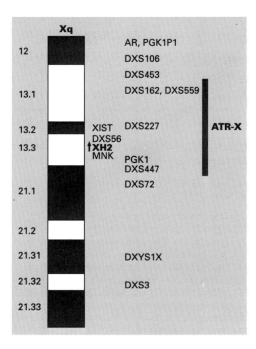

Fig. 5 The order and cytogenetic positions of loci in and around the X-encoded α-thalassaemia with mental retardation (ATR-X) candidate region (black bar). The position of the affected gene (*XH2*) between the X inactivation centre (XIST) and the previously described locus for Menke's disease (MNK) is shown.

centre (Fig. 5). This region (estimated to be 15 Mb) contains many genes and initial studies using cytogenetic, Southern blot, pulsed-field gel electrophoresis and polymerase chain reaction (PCR) analysis revealed no abnormality in boys with the ATR-X syndrome [18]. Recently, however, several complementary DNAs from this area of the X chromosome have been isolated and we have examined these genes as candidates for the ATR-X syndrome.

Using a small (84 bp) complementary DNA fragment from one of these genes (called *XH2*) we discovered a ~2 kb deletion in 1 out of 26 patients studied: this deletion severely down-regulates messenger RNA expression of *XH2* in this patient and a similarly affected cousin, suggesting that it is a good candidate for the ATR-X syndrome. We have further characterized the *XH2* complementary DNA, which encodes a gene of the putative helicase family. Analysis of *XH2* in ATR-X patients identified two premature in-phase stop mutations and seven missense mutations in addition to the gene deletion (see above) that severely down-regulates expression of this gene, proving beyond reasonable doubt that mutations in this gene are responsible for the ATR-X syndrome [18].

CONCLUSION

α-thalassaemia most frequently results from deletions of the α-globin genes or the α-globin-regulatory element. The proteins that bind these critical *cis*-acting sequences have been identified and a model for their interaction has been proposed. The identification of diverse mutations in an X-encoded protein (*XH2*) that down-regulate expression of the α genes suggests that this protein may normally be involved in regulation of the α genes. The precise mechanism by which this might occur is currently unknown. However, other members of the putative helicase family, to which *XH2* belongs, are involved in a wide range of nuclear functions including DNA recombination/repair (RAD16, RAD54, ERCC6) and regulation of transcription (SW12/SNF2, MOT1, brahma). The complex ATR-X phenotype suggests that *XH2*, when mutated, down-regulates expression of several genes, including the α genes, indicating that it could be a transcriptional regulator. The identification of mutations in a *trans*-acting factor provides an entirely novel, albeit rare, mechanism that causes the thalassaemia.

REFERENCES

1 Report of the Vth Annual Meeting of the WHO Working Group on the Feasibility Study on Hereditary Disease Community Control Programmes. (Hereditary Anaemias: Alpha Thalassaemia). 1987.
2 Higgs DR, Vickers MA, Wilkie AOM, Pretorius I-M, Jarman AP, Weatherall DJ. A review of the molecular genetics of the human α-globin gene cluster. *Blood* 1989;73:1081–1104.

3 Stamatoyannopoulos G, Nienhuis AW, Majerus PW, Varmus H. (eds) *The Molecular Basis of Blood Diseases.* W.B. Saunders, Philadelphia, 1994.
4 Weatherall DJ, Clegg JB. (eds) *The Thalassaemia Syndromes.* Blackwell Scientific Publications Oxford, 1981.
5 Higgs DR. α-Thalassaemia. In: *Baillière's Clinical Haematology. International Practice and Research:The Haemoglobinopathies,* edited by Higgs DR,Weatherall DJ. Baillière Tindall, London, 1993:117–150.
6 Liang ST,WongVCW, SoWWK, Ma HK, ChanV,Todd D. Homozygous α-thalassemia: clinical presentation, diagnosis and management. A review of 46 cases. *Br J Obstet Gynaecol* 1985;**92**:680–684.
7 Peschle C, Mavilio F, Care A *et al.* Haemoglobin switching in human embryos: asynchrony of ζ-α and ε-γ-globin switches in primitive and definite erythropoietic lineage. *Nature* 1985;**313**:235–238.
8 Liebhaber SA, Cash FE, Ballas SK. Human α-globin gene expression. The dominant role of the α$_2$-locus in mRNA and protein synthesis. *J Biol Chem* 1986;**261**:15327–15333.
9 Hill AVS, Nicholls RD, Thein SL, Higgs DR. Recombination within the human embryonic ζ-globin locus: a common ζ-ζ chromosome produced by gene conversion of the ψζ gene. *Cell* 1985;**42**:809–819.
10 Chui DHK, MentzerWC, Patterson M *et al.* Human embryonic ζ-globin chains in fetal and newborn blood. *Blood* 1989;**74**:1409–1414.
11 Albitar M, Peschle C, Liebhaber SA. Theta, zeta and epsilon globin messenger RNAs are expressed in adults. *Blood* 1989;**74**:629–637.
12 Higgs DR, Wood WG, Jarman AP *et al.* A major positive regulatory region located far upstream of the human α-globin gene locus. *Genes Dev* 1990;**4**:1588–1601.
13 Sharpe JA,Wells DJ,Whitelaw E,Vyas P, Higgs DR,Wood WG. Analysis of the human α-globin gene cluster in transgenic mice. *Proc NatlAcad Sci USA* 1993;**90**:11262–11266.
14 Flint J, Craddock CF,Villegas A *et al.* Healing of broken human chromosomes by the addition of telomeric repeats. *Am J Hum Genet* 1994;**55**:505–512.
15 Flint J, Hill AVS, Bowden DK *et al.* High frequencies of α thalassaemia are the result of natural selection by malaria. *Nature* 1986;**321**:744–749.
16 Higgs DR, Wood WG. Understanding erythroid differentiation. *Curr Biol* 1993;**3**:548–550.
17 Gibbons RJ,Wilkie AOM,Weatherall DJ, Higgs DR. A newly defined X linked mental retardation syndrome associated with α thalassaemia. *J Med Genet* 1991;**28**:729–733.
18 Gibbons RJ, Picketts DJ,Villard L, Higgs DR. X-linked mental retardation associated with α thalassaemia (ATR-X syndrome) results from mutations in a putative global transcriptional regulator. *Cell* 1995;**80**:837–845.

MULTIPLE CHOICE QUESTIONS

1 Patients with HbH disease
  a die at or around the time of birth
  b are often of North European extraction
  c have a moderately severe hypochromic/microcytic anaemia
  d have the equivalent of only one functional α gene
  e usually require blood transfusion

2 Carriers of α-thalassaemia
  a are common in all tropical and subtropical areas of the world
  b are almost exclusively seen in individuals of South-East Asian origin
  c may have an increased fitness for survival in the presence of endemic falciparum malaria

d always have detectable changes in their red cell indices
e may be identified at birth by haemoglobin electrophoresis

3 The Hb Bart's hydrops fetalis syndrome
a can be detected by prenatal DNA analysis
b is only lethal in 50% of cases
c occurs most commonly in patients of Mediterranean origin
d affected individuals inherit no functional α-globin genes
e affected individuals die from intrauterine hypoxia

4 X-encoded α-thalassaemia/mental retardation syndrome (ATR-X)
a is associated with mild mental retardation
b may cause severe mental retardation in female carriers
c is usually due to cytogenetically visible rearrangements affecting the X chromosome
d often has the haematological phenotype of HbH disease
e is usually associated with urogenital abnormalities

Answers

1		2		3	
a	False	a	True	a	True
b	False	b	False	b	False
c	True	c	True	c	False
d	True	d	True	d	True
e	False	e	True	e	True

4 a False
b False
c False
d True
e True

The biochemistry of human disease through magnetic resonance

GEORGE K.RADDA

Wouldn't it be wonderful if we could look inside a living cell and study directly with a non-invasive method the various chemicals that are responsible for maintaining and controlling physiological events? The network of chemicals is very complex and there are at least 500 separate compounds that are interconvertible, the rates being catalysed by a variety of enzymes. What hope is there of looking at this network and getting valuable information? Fortunately, nature has helped us in that we can focus down on to a central pathway, the one involved in the production and utilization of chemical energy. In all living cells the central currency of life is adenosine triphosphate (ATP). Because of the importance of ATP in providing the energy for muscle contraction, for beating of the heart, for pumping ions in the brain and synthesizing proteins in the liver, there are a number of processes that make sure that we never run out of ATP. These are the oxidative metabolism of sugars, fats, amino acids (oxidative phosphorylation), the rapid conversion of phosphocreatine to ATP catalysed by the enzyme creatine kinase and the utilization of stored sugars in the form of glycogen, particularly under conditions of extreme stress or oxygen deprivation. The key molecules in these series of reactions, namely ATP, phosphocreatine, sugar phosphates, inorganic phosphate, can be observed by magnetic resonance spectroscopy (MRS) when the instrument is tuned on to the phosphorus nucleus (^{31}P MRS). So we can study individual concentrations, fluxes through the different pathways and how the three reactions of ATP production are coordinated and controlled.

Hydrogen ions (H$^+$) play an important role in several stages in these reactions, particularly at the equilibrium catalysed by creatine kinase and when lactic acid is produced under anaerobic conditions. The linkage of intracellular pH or hydrogen ion concentration to other ionic events such as the maintenance of the membrane potential through the sodium potassium ATPase or the role of calcium in the cell is an important component of the overall ionic homeostasis in cells. The various ionic processes are closely interlinked and interact with the energetics of the tissue. These processes, too, can be studied by magnetic resonance.

There are different ways one might imagine that the biochemical information derived from MRS can be used in medicine. In some circumstances it might provide diagnostic information while in other situations it may help in the management of patients and decisions taken about the form of treatment necessary. Most importantly, however, biochemical observations in normal and pathological states in humans provide us with a new approach to understanding the mechanisms of disease processes.

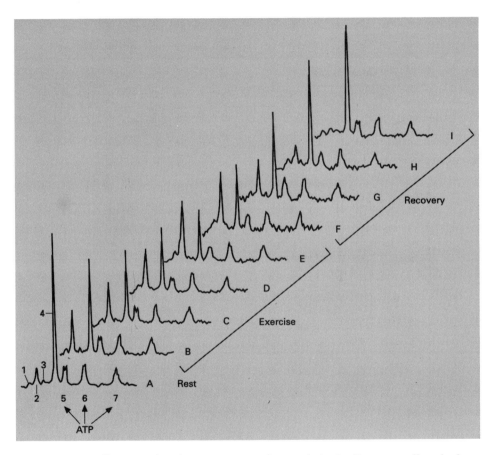

Fig. 1 ^{31}P spectra from human gastrocnemius muscle *in vivo*. Data were collected using a 6-cm diameter surface coil with an 80 second pulse length and a 2 second interpulse delay. The 1.9 T magnet (Oxford Magnet Technology) was interfaced to a Bruker spectrometer. On the x axis is the chemical shift in parts per million, and on the y axis the signal intensity. Peak assignments: (1) phosphomonoesters (PME); (2) P_i; (3) phosphodiesters (PDE); (4) phosphocreatine (PCr); (5) γ phosphate of adenosine triphosphate (ATP); (6) α-ATP + NADH and NAD^+; (7) β-ATP. The spectra show muscle (A) at rest, (B–E) during aerobic, dynamic exercise and (F–I) in recovery from exercise. The number of accumulations for each spectrum was (A) 64, (B–E,I) 32, (F,G) 8, (h) 16. The pH_i at rest (A) was 7.03, decreasing to 6.74 at the end of exercise (E).

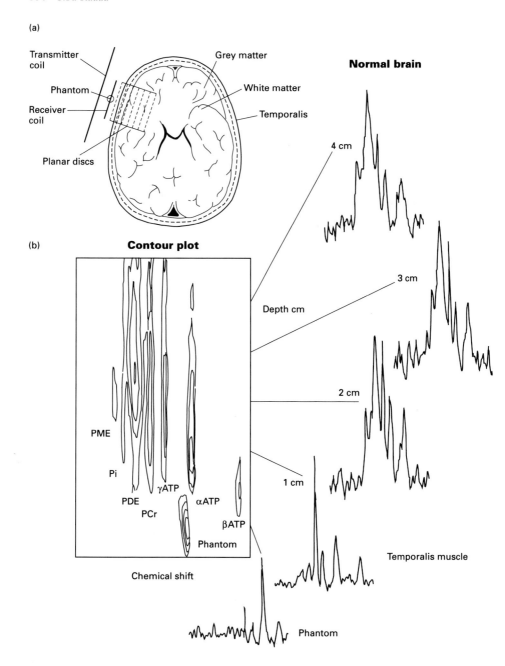

536   *G.K. Radda*

(a)

Transmitter coil

Phantom

Receiver coil

Planar discs

Grey matter

White matter

Temporalis

Normal brain

4 cm

3 cm

Depth cm

2 cm

1 cm

(b)   **Contour plot**

PME

Pi

PDE

γATP

PCr

αATP

βATP

Phantom

Chemical shift

Temporalis muscle

Phantom

Fig. 2 The diagram (a) shows the anatomical regions from which the phosphorus signal is received from the normal subjects. The magnetic resonance spectroscopy contour plot (b) combines chemical shift on the x axis with depth into the brain on the y axis. Note that the ridge caused by the P_i peak remains parallel with the phosphocreatine peak, with increasing depth into the brain. This demonstrates that pH_i does not change with depth into normal brain. Spectra are selected at increasing depth into normal brain.

We can enhance the value of the MRS measurement by observing the response to a perturbation, that is, use the method as a dynamic tool to follow fluxes and reaction rates. For example, if one observes the phosphorus MR spectrum in human muscle at rest, during exercise and in recovery (Fig. 1) [1], we can follow the rates of oxidative phosphorylation during recovery, [2] we can derive quantitative information about the relative contributions of oxidative and glycogenolytic rates to ATP maintenance during exercise [3] and we can also obtain the quantitative measure of the rates of proton removal and production both in exercise and in recovery [4]. The other way of enhancing the information content of the measurement, which of course is very important in many situations, is to resolve the spectra in space. We can effectively get one- and two-dimensional metabolic images of the brain or of the human heart using several techniques that have been developed over the past decade. A one-dimensional spatially resolved set of spectra from the human head is shown in Fig. 2 [5]. I shall illustrate some of the uses of ^{31}P MRS in the study of human diseases according to the groupings shown in Table 1.

First we may consider a group of diseases where oxygen or substrate delivery is impaired. Some of the common disorders associated with impaired oxygen delivery include blocked arteries such as in stroke and ischaemic heart disease, vasospasm, anaemia where the haemoglobin content of the blood or the nature of haemoglobin is altered, anatomically based heart disease, lung diseases and a number of genetic disorders where oxygen delivery is affected. Then there are conditions where there is abnormal control, such as altered hormonal status, rapid cellular growth

Table 1 Groups of diseases studied by ^{31}P nuclear magnetic resonance.

Impaired oxygen and substrate delivery
Peripheral vascular disease
Ischaemic heart disease
Stroke
Birth asphyxia in children
Cerebral vasospasm
Anaemia
Abnormal haemoglobin

Abnormal control
Hormonal: diabetes (muscle, liver)
Hypothyroidism (muscle)
Growth control: tumours (brain, liver, muscle)

Genetic diseases
Enzyme defects (muscle, liver)
Mitochondrial (muscle, brain)
Dystrophy (muscle, brain)

Foreign substrates
Viral infection (brain, liver)
Toxic substances (e.g. paracetamol, alcohol, liver)

(cancer) and so on. Genetic diseases provide a separate group. Finally we may study the effect of external agents like viruses and toxic substances.

Reduced oxygen delivery

There is a well-known problem in patients suffering from subarachnoid haemorrhage. The condition leads to instability in the level of consciousness over a period of days or up to a week and, it is thought, for reasons as yet unknown, that transient ischaemic episodes are produced as a result of vasospasm. We have now studied well over 20 patients with this condition and have been able to show that a few days after the initial event different parts of the brain become transiently acidotic [6]. In Fig. 3 I show a pH map as derived from a one-dimensional ^{31}P MRS imaging experiment in a control subject and in a patient at a time when the consciousness level is low. While in the control brain pH is steady as we scan from the front to the back of the brain (i.e. from the cortex white matter), in the patient 8 days after the haemorrhage we see a clear acidification and can detect phosphate resonances in two different pH environments, both corresponding to a lower pH at about 6.9 and 6.5. These phenomena are reversible and the time course of the clinical condition of the patients can be related to the appearance of high acidity. These observations indicate that oxygen delivery is impaired (possibly as a result of microvessel vasospasm) and that glycogen breakdown leads to the production of lactic acid that causes the acidic regions. These measurements may provide a new way of following interventions and of testing new forms of therapy to prevent the vascular spasm.

Mitochondrial diseases

Abnormal mitochondria are increasingly recognized as the basis of a variety of disorders affecting muscle, brain and heart. By looking at the energetics of the muscle we have been able to characterize the effects of mitochondrial dysfunction on skeletal muscle metabolism. In our studies of over 29 cases we have shown that in a number of situations phosphocreatine recovery following exercise is slow and is associated with a decrease in the maximal mitochondrial capacity (Q_{max}) [7]. At the same time, and contrary to expectations, we observed that the pH recovery after exercise is more rapid than in control subjects. This has two consequences: one, that, in spite of the need for increased lactate production, the intracellular accumulation of hydrogen ions and presumably lactate is less. This observation is consistent with the observed high blood lactate levels in patients suffering from mitochondrial disease. The second consequence of a rapid proton removal is that, as a result of the creatine kinase equilibrium, the concentration of adenosine diphosphate (ADP), which is affected by

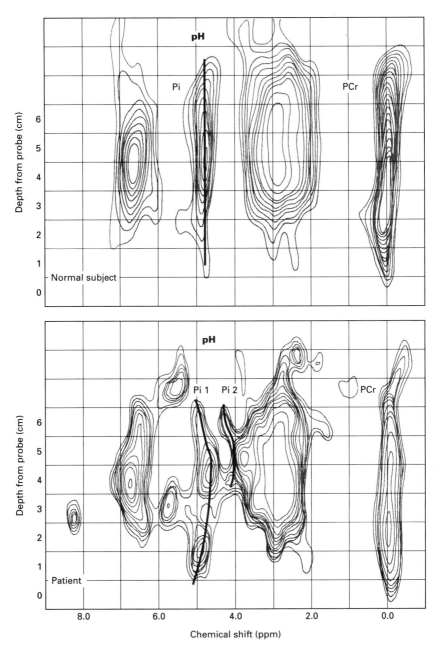

Fig. 3 Measurement of acidosis in subarachnoid haemorrhage. (Lower) Contour plot of patient 1 on day 8. The contour plot was generated by connecting points of equal intensity in the image analogue to altitude on a map. The horizontal axis represents chemical shift (p.p.m., parts per million), and the vertical axis represents depth (cm) from the probe. The level of the lowest intensity in the contour plot was set to be above the noise level in the data. The intensity of signal decreases with depth due to the inherent decrease in sensitivity of the surface coil. The plot shows the distribution of metabolites in a cylinder of tissue 6 cm in diameter and 6 cm in depth. The phosphocreatine (PCr) peak is seen to follow a straight line through the matrix. The P_i peak, however, bends towards the PCr peak, implying a decrease in pH_i. Deeper into the brain, two P_i peaks (P_i1 and P_i2) at different pH_i are seen. (Upper) Normal contour plot. The separation between the PCr and P_i peak remains the same with depth. There is virtually no spatial variation in pH_i in the brain. Adapted from [6].

the concentration of H^+, is increased if the cellular proton concentration is kept high. Since ADP has been shown to be a major factor in controlling the rate of oxidative phosphorylation it makes biological sense to increase the ADP levels when the mitochondria are damaged so as to maintain the ATP synthesis rates close to maximal activities. So an increase in the rate of sodium hydrogen antiport not only protects the muscle cell from acidotic damage but also leads to a compensatory effect for the low mitochondrial capacity, i.e. we have a favourable adaptation in terms of proton efflux to provide an energetic advantage to the diseased muscle. We have summarized elsewhere the results of our studies on the skeletal muscle in 29 patients with mitochondrial myopathy [7]. In 86% of the patients abnormalities were detected in resting muscle. In most cases there was a low phosphocreatine (PCr) to ATP ratio, a high calculated free ADP and a low phosphorylation potential, the last one being the best discriminator of the abnormality. These observations are in contrast to some other conditions where intracellular phosphate levels are also elevated, for example in patients suffering from renal failure where both extracellular and intracellular phosphate (P_i) concentrations are increased in the muscle. There is a linear relationship between P_i outside and the cellular P_i but the change in P_i is considerably attenuated. In spite of that, in these patients the phosphorylation potential is maintained at a constant value [8].

Studies on the heart

Several methods are now available to observe ^{31}P MR spectra from the human heart. We used two of these with very similar conclusions. In our study of patients with cardiac hypertrophy resulting from valve disease we have been able to show that the PCr to ATP ratio is a good parameter of the energy state of the heart (as it is in the muscle) and that in the failing heart this ratio is considerably reduced from the normal value of around 1.5–1.8 to around 1. [9] We have concluded from literature data as well as from animal heart experiments that this reduced ratio is a result of the reduction in the total creatine content of the hypertrophied failing heart. We have, therefore, considered the possibility that the restoration of the creatine levels by feeding creatine might be clinically beneficial. In thinking of how one might achieve this it became clear that relatively little is known about the regulation of the cellular content of total creatine (PCr + creatine) which is a fundamental bioenergetic parameter. We investigated creatine transport and accumulation in cultured G8 myoblast cells [8]. Creatine uptake is rapid, saturable and sodium-dependent. Total cellular concentration is relatively independent of extracellular creatine levels and this is consistent with a high-affinity active uptake balanced by a slow passive afflux. We showed that several agents stimulated creatine uptake and these included isoproterenol noradrenaline and a cyclic adenosine monophosphate (AMP) analogue, but not the α_1-adrenergic receptor agonist methoxamine. Net creatine uptake was also increased by 3, 3', 5 triiodothyronine and by amylin. Both of these are known to stimulate the sodium potassium ATPase. Indeed, the relationship between the sodium-potassium ATPase activity and net creatine influx has been shown to be particularly important. It would be of interest to see how these different processes are altered in the failing heart and whether by particular pharmacological manipulations the creatine concentrations can be increased.

Genetic diseases

The spectacular advances in the mapping of human disease genes has changed our approach to modern medicine. It is, however, not sufficient to have the gene mapped — we need to characterize the abnormal gene product and in the end we need to be able to understand the biochemical functional consequences of that abnormal gene product so as to relate genetics to function. MRS is an ideal way of looking at function *in vivo* and we have now studied a variety of genetic conditions where functional abnormalities can be detected. For example, in patients with Duchenne muscular dystrophy at the very early stages or in the mild forms of Becker dystrophy and even in some carriers of the disease the most easily detected abnormality is that of a change (an alkalinization) of the muscle-cell pH [10]. The same is observed in the mouse model for the human disease, the mdx mouse, where not only were we able to observe an abnormal pH at rest but managed to show that this is associated with a slow clearance of protons, probably as a result of an altered sodium hydrogen antiport [11]. This is linked to a high cellular sodium concentration, which is probably the reason for the slow hydrogen ion clearance and also results in an increase in cellular calcium. That is, an easily detectable metabolic abnormality in these patients is the perturbation of the ionic homeostasis.

We can now use these measurements as a way of finding out whether correction of the genetic defect, for example by gene therapy, will also correct the functional consequences of the disease. In addition to the ionic abnormalities in the diseased Duchenne muscle there is a clear elevation of the P_i concentration and a decrease in the PCr levels.

Since about 30% of the boys suffering from Duchenne muscular dystrophy also show mental retardation, we have embarked on a study to see if similar biochemical abnormalities can be observed in the brain of such patients. We indeed found elevated phosphate in our studies of over 22 cases of Duchenne muscular dystrophy (DMD) [12]. By carrying out detailed neuropsychological testing we have also been able to show that there was a relationship between the biochemical abnormality and the full-scale IQ of such boys. Our MRS protocol was designed to address the difficulties of obtaining reliable data quickly and without discomfort from young DMD patients. We have, therefore, used a measurement where we detected signal from the cerebral cortex extending from the frontal lobes to the parietal region and did not attempt any further localization. Using proton spectroscopy ^{1}H MRS, the signal-to-noise ratio is better and we were therefore able to obtain spatially resolved information in patients with DMD. We found, by localizing the spectroscopic measurement on the basis of a proton image, that the signals observed from creatine, choline and N-acetyl aspartate (NAA) were at the same ratio in DMD boys and in controls when taken from the cortex, but there was a significant difference in the intensity of the choline signal relative to that of creatine and NAA when the measurement was localized on to a region of the cerebellum with a volume of $3 \times 3 \times 3$ cm. The observations suggested an increase in the choline concentration in the cerebellum of these patients. Both the energetic abnormalities and the change in the amount of choline in the brain of DMD boys presumably reflect the lack of expression of dystrophin in the brain as it is in the muscle. It is important that we observed similar changes in studies of the brain in the mdx mouse, both with ^{31}P and ^{1}H spectroscopy. It is possible that the ionic imbalance and some alterations in cholinergic receptors both result from the absence of dystrophin that may provide an anchor between the cell membrane and the cytoplasmic environment in the cell.

CONCLUSIONS

MRS is at a stage where it can be used to study a variety of human conditions and diseases non-invasively and with relative ease. In a number of cases we, and others, have been able to characterize energetic and ionic abnormalities that have resulted in a better understanding of the mechanisms underlying the disease. One may then be in a position to design and test new forms of treatment. This has been done in several situations. The study of genetic diseases by MRS is likely to be an important aspect of future work, because of the rapid advances in mapping human disease genes and the potential of MRS to observe the biochemical consequences of the genetic defect.

REFERENCES

1 Radda GK, Taylor DJ. The study of bioenergetics *in vivo* using nuclear magnetic resonance. In: *Molecular Mechanisms in Bioenergetics*, edited by Ernster L. Elsevier, Amsterdam, 1992:463–481.
2 Kemp GJ, Taylor DJ, Thompson CH *et al.* Quantitative analysis by ^{31}P magnetic resonance spectroscopy of abnormal mitochondrial oxidation in skeletal muscle during recovery from exercise. *NMR Biomed* 1993;**6**:302–310.
3 Kemp GJ, Thompson CH, Barnes PRJ, Radda GK, Comparisons of ATP turnover in

human muscle during ischaemic and aerobic exercise using ^{31}P magnetic resonance spectroscopy. *Magn Reson Med* 1994;**31**:248–258.

4 Kemp GJ, Radda GK. Quantitative interpretation of bioenergetic data from ^{31}P and ^{1}H magnetic resonance spectroscopic studies of skeletal muscle: an analytical review. *Magn Res Q* 1994;**10**:43–63.

5 Cadoux-Hudson TAD, Wade K, Taylor DJ. Persistent metabolic sequelae of severe head injury in humans *in vivo*. *Acta Neurochir* 1990;**104**:1–7.

6 Brooke NSR, Ouwerkerk R, Adams CBT, Radda GK, Ledingham JGG, Rajagopalan B. [31]Phosphorus magnetic resonance spectra reveal prolonged intracellular acidosis in the brain following subarachnoid haemorrhage. *Proc Natl Acad Sci* 1994;**91**:1902–1907.

7 Taylor DJ, Kemp GJ, Radda GK. Bioenergetics of skeletal muscle in mitochondrial myopathy. *J Neurol Sci* 1994;**127**:198–206.

8 Radda GK, Odoom J, Kemp GJ, Taylor DJ, Thompson CH. Assessment of mitochondrial function and control in normal and diseased states. *Biochim Biophys Acta* 1995;**1271**:15–19.

9 Conway MA, Allis J, Ouwerkerk R, Tiioka T, Rajagopalan B, Radda GK. Detection of low phosphocreatine to ATP ratio in failing hypertrophied human myocardium by ^{31}P magnetic resonance spectroscopy. *Lancet* 1991;**338**:973–976.

10 Kemp GJ, Taylor DJ, Dunn JF, Frostick SP, Radda GK. Cellular energetics of dystrophic muscle. *J Neurol Sci* 1993;**116**:201–206.

11 Dunn JF, Tracey I, Radda GK. A ^{31}P NMR study of muscle exercise metabolism in mdx mice: evidence for abnormal pH regulation. *J Neurol Sci* 1992;**113**:108–113.

12 Tracey I, Scott RB, Thompson CH *et al*. Brain abnormalities in Duchenne muscular dystrophy: a ^{31}P magnetic resonance spectroscopy and neuropsychological study. *Lancet* 1995;**345**:1260–1264.

Venoms and antivenoms

DAVID A.WARRELL

EVOLUTIONARY DIVERSITY OF VENOMS

Toxins have evolved in many groups of animals — notably, mammals, birds, reptiles, amphibians, fish, arthropods, molluscs, echinoderms, annelids and coelenterates — to immobilize and digest prey and to repel enemies. The diversity of their chemical structure, targets and biological functions is quite astonishing. There are also examples of evolutionary convergence in structure and function in disparate groups. The toxin recently found in the skin and feathers of members of a genus of passerine birds (Pitohui, Pachycephalidae) in Papua New Guinea is homobatrachotoxin, structurally identical to a skin toxin of the Latin American 'poison dart' frogs (Phyllobates, Dendrobatidae) [1,2]. Anticoagulant factors in the saliva of vampire bats (Desmodontinae) and the hypostomal secretions of leeches (Hirudinea), which promote the flow of blood during feeding, have attracted interest as potential therapeutic agents. The evolution of toxins which are antagonists or agonists of a very wide range of receptors/acceptors and ion channels has provided the medical scientist with an array of tools with which to investigate normal structure and function, to study deranged function in diseased patients and, in a few cases, the means for therapeutic intervention (Table 1).

VENOMS IN SCIENCE AND MEDICINE

Snake venom toxins in the haemostasis laboratory [3] (Table 2)

Procoagulant enzymes from Russell's viper venom contributed to the elucidation of the blood-clotting cascade [4]. Many of these enzymes, and other venom components which affect other clotting factors, fibrinolysis and platelet function, are currently used in experimental and clinical haemostasis laboratories. Batroxobin (Reptilase) from the venom of Brazilian lance-headed vipers (fer de lance, *Bothrops atrox*, *B. moojeni*) is a fibrinogen-clotting enzyme used to monitor the fibrinogen–fibrin reaction in patients being treated with heparin and other protease inhibitors

Table 1 Lessons from animal toxins.

Mechanism of:

Blood clotting (e.g. procoagulant enzymes — Russell's viper venom)

Neuromuscular transmission (e.g. bungarotoxins — krait venoms)

Central nervous system functions (e.g. fasciculins and dendrotoxins — mamba venoms)

Blood pressure control (e.g. angiotensin-converting enzyme inhibitors — jararaca snake venom)

Endothelin receptor subtypes (sarafotoxins — Israeli burrowing asp venom)

Complement activation (e.g. cobra venom factor — elapid venoms)

Protein/enzyme chemistry (e.g. phospholipases, endopeptidases, L-amino acid oxidases — snake venoms)

Table 2 Snake venoms used in haemostasis laboratories.

Venom component	Snake	Assay
Batroxobin (Reptilase)	*Bothrops atrox*, *B. moojeni*	Fibrinogen–fibrin reaction
Bistatin	*Bitis arietans*	Plasminogen activator inhibitor type 1
Botrocetin	*Bothrops* spp.	von Willebrand's variants
Ecarin	*Echis* spp.	Abnormal prothrombin
Echistatin	*Echis* spp.	Platelet aggregation
Protein C activator (Protac C)	*Agkistrodon c contortrix*	Protein C
Russell's viper venom (Stypven)	*Daboia russelii*	X, lupus anticoagulant
Taipan venom	*Oxyuranus scutellatus*	Prothrombin, lupus anticoagulant
Textilin	*Pseudonaja textilis*	Lupus anticoagulant

(hirudin, ε-aminocaproic acid and aprotinin). Russell's viper venom (Stypven, RVV) contains a factor X activator which is employed in the Stypven time to distinguish factor VII and factor X deficiencies and for characterizing factor X dysproteinaemias. It is also used in factor X assays and as a test for platelet phospholipid availability (platelet procoagulant activity). The dilute Russell's viper venom time detects lupus anticoagulant and antiphospholipid coagulation inhibitor. Other snake venoms such as those of the Eastern brown snake (*Pseudonaja textilis*) [5] and taipan (*Oxyuranus scutellatus*) have also been used for the detection of lupus anticoagulant. A specific protein C activator (Protac C) from the venom of the southern copperhead (*Agkistrodon contortrix*) is useful for assaying protein C, a measurement of particular interest in patients who may have an inherited thrombotic tendency associated with deficiency of this endogenous inhibitor of coagulation [6].

Platelet-aggregating and inhibiting factors [7,8]

Many snake venoms have been found to contain components which either induce platelet aggregation (for example, crotalocytin from the venom of the timber rattlesnake, *Crotalus horridus*) or inhibition (such as bitistatin from the venom of the puff adder, *Bitis arietans*. In the haemostasis laboratory, botrocetin (from *Bothrops* venoms), is used, together with ristocetin, to distinguish the molecular variants of von Willebrand's disease. Fibrinogen receptor antagonists such as echistatin from the venom of the saw-scaled viper (*Echis* species), trigramin from the venom of the Taiwanese bamboo viper (*Trimeresurus stejnegeri*) and kistrin from the venom of the Malayan pit viper [9] (*Calloselasma rhodostoma*) are of particular interest because of their potential therapeutic use. These possess an Arg-Gly-Asp (RGD) adhesion site recognition sequence through which they bind to glycoprotein (GP)IIb–IIIa, blocking the interaction of platelets with adhesive proteins such as fibrinogen and inhibiting platelet aggregation.

Snake venom procoagulant enzymes in therapy (Table 3)

Ancrod and batroxobin are fibrinogen-clotting enzymes which cause therapeutic defibrinogenation which prevents thrombus formation or the extension of pre-existing thrombi, promotes fibrinolysis and, by reducing blood viscosity, improves blood flow through diseased and narrowed vessels. These snake venom enzymes caused fewer haemorrhagic, thromboembolic and allergic effects than heparin or streptokinase and their effects can be rapidly reversed by the use of specific antivenoms [10–12]. However, they are more expensive than heparin or streptokinase, are less effective than streptokinase and no more effective than heparin. Antibody formation can be expected to cause resistance to treatment during prolonged therapy. Ancrod or batroxobin are indicated in patients in whom heparin is contraindicated, such as those with heparin-induced thrombocytopenia with thrombosis and heparin antibodies and in those with protamine

Table 3 Snake venom procoagulant enzymes in therapeutic use.

Venom component	Snake	Use
Ancrod (Arvin, Arwin, Venacil)	*Calloselasma rhodostoma*	Antithrombotic
Batroxobin (Reptilase, Defibrase)	*Bothrops atrox, B. moojeni*	Antithrombotic
Bothropase	*B. jararaca*	Antithrombotic
Stypven	*Daboia russelii*	Topical haemostasis

hypersensitivity in whom anticoagulation cannot be rapidly reversed using this drug. Ancrod or batroxobin may also be useful in acute or progressive ischaemic cerebral infarction [12] in thrombotic lupus glomerulonephritis, thromboangiitis obliterans, central retinal vein thrombosis, priapism and hyperviscosity syndrome [11].

Snake venoms and the discovery of angiotensin-converting enzyme inhibitors

While studying the physiological action of the venom of the jararaca snake (*Bothrops jararaca*; Fig. 1) in dogs, Rocha e Silva and his colleagues discovered bradykinin [13]. This nonapeptide was released from its α_2-globulin precursor (bradykininogen) in the dog's blood by the venom, causing a fall in blood pressure and delayed (hence brady-) contraction of isolated guinea-pig ileum. Jararaca venom also contains a number of peptides (bradykinin-potentiating factors, BPFs) which inhibit both kininase II, responsible for inactivating bradykinin, and angiotensin-converting

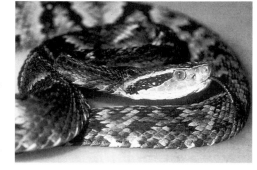

Fig. 1 Jararaca (*Bothrops jararaca*) from Brazil: a snake whose venom led to the discovery of bradykinin, bradykinin-potentiating factors and angiotensin-converting enzyme inhibitors. (Copyright DA Warrell.)

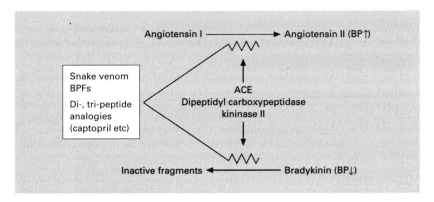

Fig. 2 Action of snake venom (*Bothrops jararaca*) bradykinin-potentiating factors (BPFs) in inhibiting angiotensin-converting enzyme (ACE) and kininase II.

enzyme (ACE [14,15]; Fig. 2). These discoveries led to the synthesis of competitive inhibitors of ACE, such as captopril and enalapril, an important new class of hypotensive agents [15].

> The discovery of potent inhibitors of converting enzyme provides one of many illustrations of the utility of seemingly esoteric pharmacological enquiry on the properties of poisons of plant or animal origin [15].

Snake venom sarafotoxins and endothelins

Atractaspididae is an interesting family of burrowing snakes which includes the genus *Atractaspis* (burrowing asps, burrowing or mole vipers/adders). Bites by several species of *Atractaspis* in Africa and the Middle East have proved rapidly fatal and in some envenomed patients there was evidence of cardiovascular disturbances, including atrioventricular conduction defects and profound hypotension. In the past few years, the venom of the Israeli burrowing asp (*A. engaddensis*) has been found to contain four 21-amino-acid isotoxins, known as sarafotoxins (SRTXa–d) which are so similar in structure and function to the endothelins (potent vasoconstrictor peptides from vascular endothelium) as to suggest a common evolutionary origin. These compounds have a variety of different effects — coronary artery vasoconstriction, atrioventricular block and a positive inotropic action. They bind to different receptors in brain, atrium and smooth muscle, causing hydrolysis of phosphoinositides and the mobilization of intracellular Ca^{2+}. Competitive binding studies with labelled endothelins and sarafotoxins have allowed identification of receptor subtypes [16].

Venom neurotoxins: tools in experimental neurophysiology and neuropharmacology

The evolution of neurotoxins, whose function is to immobilize prey species, has resulted in a wide diversity of compounds which are agonists or antagonists of almost every known class of receptor/ion channel in the excitable tissues of animals.

Snake venoms contain toxins which act at different sites in the nervous system. The postsynaptic toxins (α-neurotoxins) bind to and block nicotinic acetylcholine receptors of vertebrate neuromuscular junctions. They are polypeptides — 60–62 (short) and 70–74 (long) amino acid residues in length. A well-known example is α-bungarotoxin from the venom of the Chinese krait (*Bungarus multicinctus*) which has been used to study the structure and function of the neuromuscular junction [17]. κ-bungarotoxin binds to neuronal nicotinic acid receptors. The venoms of the African mambas (genus *Dendroaspis*) contain some unusual presynaptic neurotoxins — dendrotoxins, which facilitate acetylcholine release by

Table 4 Geography cone shell (*Conus geographus*).

Toxin	Size (number of amino acids)	Target (tissue acceptor)
ω-Conotoxin CVIA	27	Voltage-sensitive Ca^{2+} channel
α-Conotoxin GI	13	Acetylcholine receptor
μ-Conotoxin GIII	22	Voltage-sensitive Na^+ channel
Conopressin-G	9	Vasopressin receptor
Conantokin-G	17	N-methyl-D-aspartate receptor

Venoms of other *Conus* species contain excitotoxins, α-adrenergic and cholinomimetic toxins.

blocking voltage-dependent potassium channels fasciculins which inhibit cholinesterases and muscarinic toxins [18,19].

Phospholipase A_2 toxins act at the presynaptic site of neuromuscular junctions, somehow inhibiting the release of acetylcholine transmitter before they damage the nerve and muscle. Examples are β-bungarotoxin (from the venom of *B. multicinctus*), toxins from Australasian elapid snakes (e.g. taipoxin, textilitoxin) and from viper venoms (e.g. crotoxin from the venom of the tropical rattlesnake, *Crotalus durissus terrificus*).

Many other groups of animals possess neurotoxic venoms. A particularly remarkable example is the *coneshells* (genus *Conus*). These are carnivorous marine snails which can immobilize their prey (e.g. relatively large fish and other molluscs) by harpooning them with a venom-filled dart. The numerous conotoxins are peptides, 10–30 amino acids in length, which have a wide range of targets [20] (Table 4).

Venoms: other constituents of scientific interest

For biochemists, snake venoms are a rich source of enzymes (Table 1). Cobra venom factor, a C3b-like protein found in elapid venoms, activates the alternative complement pathway by binding to factor B and has been used to explore the complement system and to depress complement activity in patients [21]. After the submaxillary glands of male mice, some snake venoms are the richest source of nerve growth factors [22].

ANTIVENOMS AND THE TREATMENT OF ENVENOMING

Following closely the introduction of equine diphtheria antitoxin by Roux in 1894, Albert Calmette, working in the Institut Pasteur in Saigon, developed an equine cobra antivenom, which was first tried in human victims of snake bite 100 years ago [23]. It was soon realized — but not initially by Calmette — that antivenoms would neutralize only those venoms used in their production. Until recently, unrefined hyperimmune horse serum/plasma was still used to treat human patients in some countries, but most manufacturers concentrated the immunoglobulin G (IgG) fraction by ammonium sulphate precipitation and removed the complement-activating Fc fragment by pepsin digestion (Fig. 3). Antivenoms are now available against the venoms of species of snakes, fish, box jellyfish, spiders, scorpions and ticks.

No randomized, comparative clinical trials of therapeutic antivenoms were carried out before 1973, but there is now good evidence that antivenoms can reverse antihaemostatic, cardiovascular, postsynaptic and rhabdomyolytic effects of snake venoms. Efficacy against local tissue necrosis, presynaptic toxicity and nephrotoxicity remains unproven [24]. Equine antivenoms carry a considerable risk of inducing early anaphylactic, pyrogenic and late serum sickness-type reactions which are potentially fatal. In 1957, a 13-year-old boy bitten by an adder near Poole died of an anaphylactic reaction to Pasteur antivenom [25]. This led the *British National Formulary* to publish, up until September 1981, the statement that 'the adder bite itself may be less dangerous than the so-called specific snake bite antiserum which is therefore not recommended'. However, modern antivenoms, such as Immunolski Zavod-Zagreb Vipera polyspecific (currently supplied to British hospitals) and the new Therapeutic Antibodies Inc Beritab are effective and safe.

In the hope of improving the efficacy and safety of antivenoms, a new generation of antivenoms is now being raised in sheep — animals which produce higher and more persistent antibody titres than horses. Instead of conventional pepsin digestion of concentrated IgG to produce $F(ab)_2$ fragments, papain digestion is used to produce Fab fragments (Fig. 3). Specific Fab can be isolated by passing the total Fab down columns coated with the specific venom antigens against which neutralization is required [26]. An ovine Fab antitoxin against digoxin (Digibind) has proved effective in the treatment of poisoning by this drug. Theoretical advantages of Fab, compared to $F(ab)_2$ antivenoms, are more rapid tissue penetration, allowing neutralization of the venom depot at the site of the bite or sting; a larger apparent volume of distribution and reduced risk of anaphylactic reactions resulting from complement activation. Other innovations in antivenom design and production are immunization with venom fractions or even purified toxins (subunit antivenoms) and monoclonal antibodies raised against important toxin epitopes. However, these refinements are unlikely to be commercially viable. Most antivenom producers have now recognized that they must be far more critical in selecting venoms for immunization, bearing in mind the variations in venom composition and antigenicity with the age and geographical origin of snakes, even with a single species.

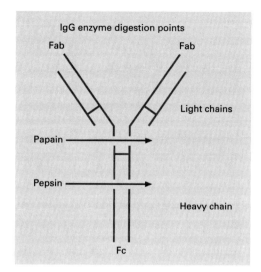

Fig. 3 Sites of enzyme cleavage in the ovine immunoglobulin G (IgG) molecule resulting in F(ab)$_2$ (conventional) and Fab (new-generation) antivenoms and antitoxins.

VENOMOUS BITES AND STINGS IN THE UK

There is a dearth of venomous animals in the UK, but weeverfish stings, adder bites and bee and wasp sting anaphylaxis are sufficiently frequent and occasionally severe enough to be of medical importance. More than 100 weeverfish stings occur around the British coast each year, especially in Cornwall and usually in August or September. Paddlers are stung when they tread on the fish. Usually stings are not dangerous but they can be very painful. Immersion of the stung part in uncomfortably hot but not scalding water ($< 45°C$) can bring dramatic relief.

Adder bites

The adder (*Vipera berus*) is the only indigenous venomous snake in the British Isles and is the only snake found in Scotland. It is absent from Ireland, the Orkneys and Shetlands, Outer Hebrides, the Isle of Man and the Channel Islands. More than 100 bites occur each year in the UK, the peak months being June to August. The commonest symptoms (Table 5) are local pain, swelling and bruising, which are usually apparent within 30 minutes of the bite and may advance to involve the whole limb and extend on to the trunk within 24 hours. Gastrointestinal and anaphylactic systemic symptoms may appear within 5 minutes of the bite. Shock, causing syncope, is the most dramatic. It may be transient or persistent, recurrent, progressive and potentially fatal. Severe manifestations of envenoming (Table 6), although unusual, have been seen in infants, children and adults

Table 5 Adder bites: common symptoms and signs.

Local	Systemic
Pain	Vomiting
Swelling	Colic
Bruising	Diarrhoea
Blistering	Shock
Lymphangitis	Angio aedema
Lymphadenopathy	Urticaria
Bronchospasm	Fever

Table 6 Adder bites: unusual severe features.

Persistent hypotension
Bleeding, coagulopathy
Coma, seizures, cerebral oedema
Acute renal failure
Adult respiratory distress syndrome
Cardiac arrhythmias, atrioventricular block, ECG ST segment/T-wave abnormalities
Gastric dilatation, paralytic ileus

ECG, Electrocardiogram.

in the UK over the last 20 years, and it is surprising that there have been no more than 12 deaths from adder bites in this country this century, the last being in 1975 [25]. Common laboratory abnormalities in adder-bite victims are a peripheral neutrophil leukocytosis, elevated serum creatine kinase concentration, thrombocytopenia, mild coagulopathy and metabolic acidosis.

Treatment of adder bites

There is persuasive evidence that modern specific antivenoms can prevent morbidity and reduce the length of convalescence in patients with moderately

Table 7 Adder bites: indications for antivenom.

Systemic envenoming
Hypotension
Vomiting
Haemostatic abnormalities
Leukocytosis > $15 \times 10^9/l$

Local envenoming
Swelling & more than half limb within 48 hours of the bite
(Adults) beyond wrist/ankle within 4 hours of the bite

severe envenoming and can save the lives of severely envenomed patients [25,27,28]. Slow intravenous injection of 10–20 ml of Zagreb antivenom or 100–200 mg of Beritab is recommended for patients in whom antivenom is indicated (Table 7). Adrenaline should always be available to treat early antivenom reactions.

Bee or wasp sting anaphylaxis

In the UK, 4–8 people are reported to die of bee or wasp sting anaphylaxis each year — more than 50 times the mortality from adder bites. Some surveys have suggested that between 0.4 and 4% of the population would develop systemic symptoms if stung by a bee or a wasp. Bee-keepers and their families have an increased risk. The development of hypersensitivity is suggested by a progressive increase in the extent and duration of the local reaction to the sting (swelling and inflammation) with successive stings. Systemic signs include urticaria, angioedema, bronchospasm, shock and gastrointestinal symptoms. Adults who develop such symptoms have a more than 50% chance of suffering at least as severe a systemic reaction if they are stung again by the same species. There is a also a risk that the next reaction may be more rapidly evolving and more severe.

Severe and potentially fatal reactions can be prevented by prompt subcutaneous self-injection of adrenaline (0.5–1.0 ml of 0.1% for adults) by the victim. People at high risk should carry an adrenaline kit (for example EpiPen, Min-i-Jet or Anakit. Patients should be shown how to use this equipment. A Medic Alert tag is also useful to identify the patient's risk of anaphylaxis in case he or she is found unconscious. Adults who have had a systemic reaction to a sting and have evidence of type I IgE-mediated hypersensitivity to bee or wasp venom, revealed by skin testing or radioallergosorbent test, can be desensitized. The value of desensitization has been proved by controlled clinical trials [29,30]. Children and young adults can lose this hypersensitivity spontaneously and, in these cases, desensitization may not be justified.

CONCLUSIONS

In the UK, venom diseases range in importance from bee or wasp sting anaphylaxis, which is responsible for much morbidity and occasional mortality, to adder bites, in which appropriate use of antivenom can reduce morbidity and virtually eliminate mortality, and to the painful but otherwise innocuous sting of the weeverfish. Animal venoms have proved extremely useful as tools to examine physiological mechanisms, as laboratory agents and in a few cases as therapeutic agents. The study of animal venoms and their antidotes — antivenoms — will continue to be relevant and revealing in medical science.

REFERENCES

1 Dumbacher JP, Beehler BM, Spande TF, Garraffo HM, Daly JW. Homobatracho-toxin in the genus *Pitohui*: chemical defense in birds? *Science* 1992;**258**:799–801.
2 Myers CW, Daly JW, Malkin B. A dangerously toxic new frog (*Phyllobates*) used by Embera Indians of western Colombia, with discussion of blowgun fabrication and dart poisoning. *Bull Am Mus Nat Hist* 1978;**161**:307–366.
3 Hutton RA, Warrell DA. Action of snake venom components on the haemostatic system. *Blood Rev* 1993;**7**:176–189.
4 Macfarlane RG. Russell's viper venom, 1934–64. *Br J Haematol* 1967;**13**:437–451.
5 Triplett DA, Stocker KF, Unger GA, Barna LK. The Textarin/Ecarin ratio: a confirmatory test for lupus anticoagulant. *Thromb Haemost* 1993;**70**:925–931.
6 Schafer AI. Hypercoagulable states: molecular genetics to clinical practice. *Lancet* 1994;**344**:1739–1742.
7 Teng CM, Huang TF. Snake venom constituents that affect platelet function. *Platelets* 1991;**2**:77–87.
8 Teng CM, Huang TF. Inventory of exogenous inhibitors of platelet aggregation. *Thromb Haemost* 1991;**65**:624–626.
9 Adler M, Lazarus RA, Dennis MS, Wagner G. Solution structure of Kistrin, a potent platelet aggregation inhibitor and GPIIb-IIIa antagonist. *Science* 1991;**253**:445–448.
10 Latallo ZS. Retrospective study on complications and adverse effects of treatment with thrombin-like enzymes: a multicentre trial. *Thromb Haemost* 1983;**50**:604–609.
11 Southar RL, Ginsberg JS. Anticoagulant therapy with ancrod. *Crit Rev Oncol Hematol* 1993;**15**:23–33.
12 The Ancrod Stroke Study Investigators. Ancrod for the treatment of acute ischemic brain infarction. *Stroke* 1994;**25**:1755–1759.
13 Rocha e Silva M, Beraldo WT, Rosenfeld G. Bradykinin, a hypotensive and smooth muscle stimulating factor released from plasma globulin by snake venoms and by trypsin. *Am J Physiol* 1949;**156**:261–273.
14 Ferreira SH, Bartelt DC, Greene LJ. Isolation of bradykinin-potentiating peptides from *Bothrops jararaca* venom. *Biochemistry* 1970;**9**:2583–2593.
15 Douglas WW. Polypeptides — angiotensin, plasma kinins and others. In: *Goodman and Gilman's the Pharmacological Basis of Therapeutics*, edited by Goodman AG, Gilman LS, Rall TW, Murad F, 7th edn. Macmillan, New York, 1985:639–659.
16 Sokolovksy M. Minireview. Endothelins and sarafotoxins: receptor heterogeneity. *Int J Biochem* 1994;**26**:335–340.
17 Albuquerque EX, Barnard EA, Porter CW, Arnick JE. The diversity of acetylcholine receptors and their sensitivity in the post-synaptic membrane of muscle end plates. *Proc Natl Acad Sci* 1974;**71**:2818–2822.
18 Harvey AL. (ed.) Snake toxins. In *International Encylopedia of Pharmacology and Therapeutics*, section 134. Pergamon, New York, 1991.
19 Harvey AL. (ed.) *Natural and Synthetic Neurotoxins*. Academic Press, London, 1993.
20 Olivera BM, Rivier J, Scott JK, Hillyard DR, Cruz LJ. Minireview: conotoxins. *J Biol Chem* 1991;**266**:22067–22070.
21 Vogt W. Snake venom constituents affecting the complement system. In: *Medical Use of Snake Venom Proteins*, edited by Stocker KE. CRC Press, Boca Raton, 1990:79–96.
22 Hogue-Angeletti RA, Bradshaw RA. Nerve growth factors in snake venoms. In: *Snake Venoms Handbook of Experimental Pharmacology*, edited by Lee CY, vol. 52. Springer-Verlag, Berlin, 1979:276–294.
23 Calmette A. The treatment of animals poisoned with snake venom by the injection of antivenomous serum. *Lancet* 1896;**ii**:449–450.
24 Warrell DA. The global problem of snake bite: its prevention and treatment. In: *Recent Advances in Toxicology Research*, edited by Gopalakrishnakone P, Tan CK. vol. 1. National University of Singapore. Venom and Toxin Research Group, Singapore, 1992:121–153.
25 Reid HA. Adder bites in Britain. *Br Med J* 1976;**2**:153–156.
26 Sullivan JB. Past, present and future immunotherapy of snake venom poisoning. *Ann Emerg Med* 1987;**16**:938–944.

27 Persson H, Irestedt B. A study of 136 cases of adder bite treated in Swedish hospitals during one year. *Acta Med Scand* 1981;**210**:433–439.
28 Karlson-Stiber C, Persson H. Antivenom treatment in *Vipera berus* envenoming — report of 30 cases. *J Intern Med* 1994;**235**:57–61.
29 Hunt KJ, Valentine MD, Sobotka AK *et al*. A controlled trial of immunotherapy in insect hypersensitivity. *N Engl J Med* 1978;**299**:157–161.
30 Mueller UR. *Insect Sting Allergy. Clinical Picture, Diagnosis and Treatment*. Gustav Fischer, Stuttgart, 1990.

MULTIPLE CHOICE QUESTIONS

1 In haemostasis laboratories, snake venom components are used for the following
  a detection of lupus anticoagulant
  b diagnosis of Diamond–Blackfan syndrome
  c assay of protein C
  d as antifibrinolytic agents
  e diagnosis of von Willebrand's disease

2 Snake venom components have been used therapeutically for the following purposes in human patients
  a topical haemostasis
  b neuromuscular blockade (anaesthesia)
  c treatment of migraine
  d reduction of blood viscosity
  e treatment of lupus glomerulonephritis

3 Snake venom components have proved useful tools in the laboratory investigation of the following
  a effect of antidiuretic hormone on the renal tubule
  b mechanism of neuromuscular transmission
  c function of N-methyl-D-aspartate receptors
  d alternative pathway of complement activation
  e types of endothelin receptors

4 Common symptoms of adder bite are
  a nausea, vomiting and diarrhoea
  b swelling of the lips, gums or tongue
  c bleeding from the gingival sulci
  d early, recurrent or persistent hypotension
  e ptosis and external ophthalmoplegia

5 Laboratory investigations may reveal the following abnormalities in victims of adder bites
  a neutrophil leukocytosis exceeding $20 \times 10^9/l$
  b raised creatine kinase

c reduced serum albumin concentration
d metabolic acidosis
e eosinophilia

6 The following are indications for antivenom treatment of adder bite victims
a reliable history of an adder bite
b swelling of more than half of the bitten limb
c local bruising at the site of the bite
d fever
e hypotension

Answers

1 a True	2 a True	3 a False
b False	b False	b True
c True	c False	c False
d False	d True	d True
e True	e True	e True
4 a True	5 a True	6 a False
b True	b True	b True
c False	c False	c False
d True	d True	d False
e False	e False	e True

Index

interaction with insulin 285
growth hormone binding protein in
   IDDM 287
growth hormone-releasing hormone
   production by pituitary
   tumours 493
guanylate cyclase 207

H₂-receptor antagonists 508
H-ras gene 498
haemangioma in childhood 33
haemochromatosis, HLA association *334,*
   339
haemodialysis
   amyloid deposition 515
   in the elderly 324, 325–6
haemoglobin
   glycosylated, in diabetes control 434–5
   reaction with nitric oxide 206–7
   structure 524
haemophilia, and ischaemic heart
   disease 93
haemostasis, and snake venom
   toxins 544–6
Hb Bart's hydrops fetalis syndrome 524
   α-globin gene deletions 528
   pathophysiology 526
HbH disease 524
   α-globin gene deletions 528
   pathophysiology 525
HDL *see* high-density lipoproteins
headache
   cluster 175
   nitrate-induced 175
   tension 175
Health Promotion Strategy 104
hearing loss and resistance to thyroid
   hormone 471
heart
   ³¹P magnetic resonance
      spectroscopy 540–1
   abnormalities and resistance to thyroid
      hormone 471
   compensatory mechanisms 134, 135–6
   failure 7
   see also chronic heart failure
Helicobacter pylori 96
Henry's law 204
heparin 231, 546
hepatitis B 382
   carrier status 394
hepatocyte growth factor in epithelial
   tubulogenesis 44–7, *48*
herpes simplex virus type 1 *see* HSV-1
15-HETE 237
HG-A gene 310
HG-B gene 310
HG-C gene 310
hepatocyte growth factor in epithelial
   tubulogenesis 44–7, *48*

5-hydroxytryptamine in migraine 172
high-density lipoproteins
   in polycystic ovary syndrome 462
   protective effects 4
   and risk factors 104
high-output heart failure 138
hirsutism in polycystic ovary
   syndrome 461
hirudin 545
histamine 154
HIV infection 382, 389, 391, 392
HLA system 333
   association with rheumatoid
      arthritis 53–4, *334,* 340, 347–8
   disease association mechanisms 339–40
   functions of molecules 335–7
   genetics 337–8
   linkage disequilibrium 338–9
   structure of molecules 333–5
Hodgkin's lymphoma, HLA
   association 333
Hoe 140 130
homobatrachotoxin 544
homocysteine 106
hormone replacement therapy 464, 489
house dust mite allergens 355–6
HPV *see* hypoxic pulmonary
   vasoconstriction
HRPT deficiency *see* hypoxanthine
   phosphoribosyltransferase
   deficiency
HSV-1
   as gene therapy vector 406, 407–9
      in brain injury repair 410
      in brain tumours 410–11
      ethical issues 412
      examples 412–13
      ideal properties 411–12
      in inherited metabolic brain
         diseases 409
      in neurodegenerative disorders 409–
         10
      in neurological disease 409–11
      potential problems 411–12
   latency 408
5-HT *see* serotonin
human chorionic gonadotrophin
   stimulation test 484
human immunodeficiency virus
   infection 382, 389, 391, 392
human leukocyte antigen system *see* HLA
   system
Huntington's disease 14, 69, 488
   anticipation in 17, 19
   classical genetic studies *15*
   clinical features *15*
   gene therapy 409–10
   genetic instability in 19–20, *21, 22*
   juvenile 14, 15–16, 20–2, 24
   mutational mechanism 19, 26–30
   origin of mutation 25